COMMON MEDICAL EMERGENCIES

COMMON MEDICAL EMERGENCIES

Shivaprakash S. Shirale

MBBS, PGDHM

Assistant Medical Officer
(Nodal officer of JSSK Scheme, Nodal officer of Disaster Management Committee, Assistant Warden)
Hinduhridaysamrat Balasaheb Thackeray Medical College And
Dr. Rustum Narsi Cooper Municipal General Hospital
Juhu, Mumbai, Maharashtra

Former
Assistant Medical Officer
GTB Hospital
Sewri, Mumbai, Maharashtra

Former
House Officer
Department of Pediatrics
Government Medical College
Nanded, Maharashtra

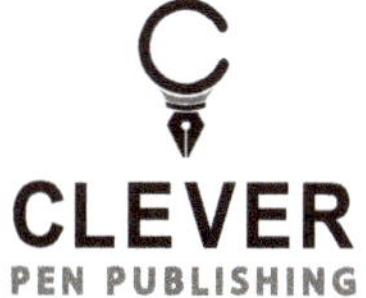

First Edition: 2022

Published by:

Clever Pen Publishing
D-2 Neelkanth Business Park Co-op. Premises Society Ltd.
Nathani Road
Vidyavihar (West)
Mumbai 400086
Mob.: 09867214519

Email: cleverpen9@gmail.com

ISBN 978-93-92215-05-6

Printed & Bound in India

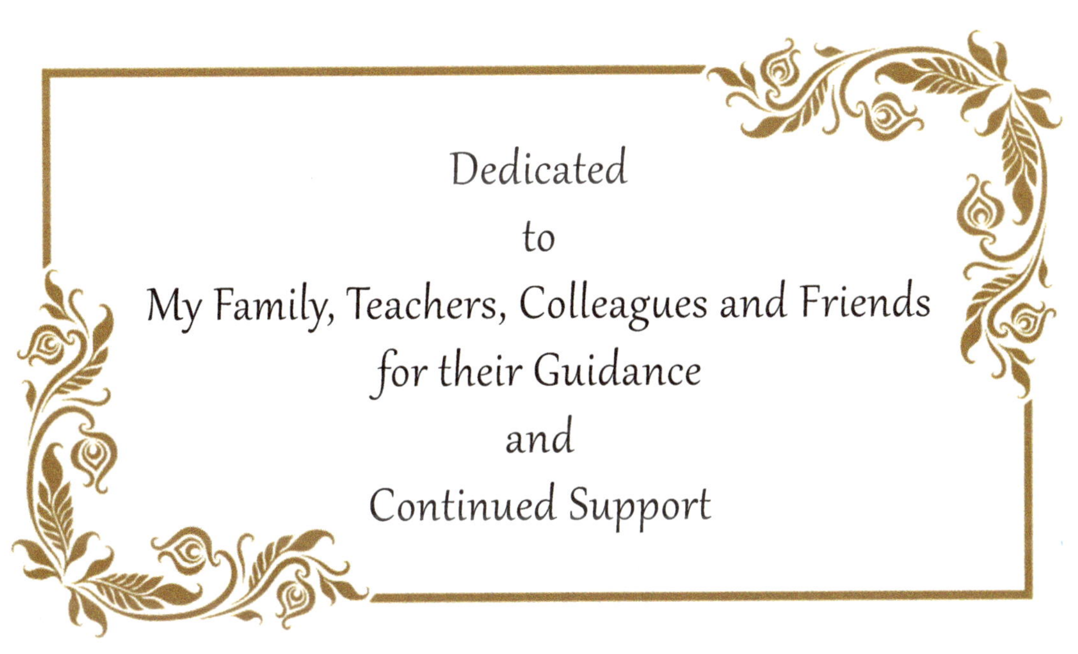

Dedicated

to

My Family, Teachers, Colleagues and Friends

for their Guidance

and

Continued Support

PREFACE

Each and every doctor has to face different kinds of emergencies in their regular practice and has to deal with them in a very effective manner to save the lives of patients or reduce morbidity.

A general Practitioner should be able to understand which patient is an emergency based on the patient's clinical presentation, should be able to stabilize & treat the patient and if needed refer the patient to the concerned speciality for further management.

So every doctor needs a book which includes different kinds of common medical emergencies and their management in day to day practice.

In medical internship programs students need orientation of emergencies in each speciality.

So I have decided to write a book which includes common medical emergencies under the guidance of specialists.

The main purpose of this book is to assist the Medical interns, casualty medical officers, General practitioners in understanding and in decision making while dealing with emergencies, which will be of great help to them.

Shivaprakash S. Shirale

FOREWORD

Medical emergencies not only requires medical management of patient but also emotional and social management of relatives. A thorough knowledge of treatment protocols can help to save numerous lives. Doctors handling emergencies is the first line of contact and at most of the places a Medical Officer is responsible and is incharge of the casualty unit. Triage, patient examination and necessary lifesaving treatment needs to be done with lightning speed in the Emergency Department. Doctors should be well aware of various emergencies and exact management protocols.

Dr Shivaprakash Shirale is a very hard working and a sincere doctor. He has been working in the Casualty Department as Medical Officer for the last 5 years at HBT medical college and Dr. R.N. Cooper hospital, Mumbai . His expertise in the management of Trivial to Life threatening emergencies makes a tremendous difference in the casualty. He believes in transferring knowledge and teaching to upcoming generations. This passion of his has converted into a well descriptive and highly informative book on Medical Emergencies.

He has concisely compiled all the sub-specialty emergencies and explained protocol based management of each in very lucid language. This is an extremely useful reference book and a guide in and during the casualty to learn and understand management of trivial to grievous injuries. I am sure that this is a must read book for all Medical Students, Medical Interns, Medical Officers, General Practitioners. It will definitely help them to make the right decision while dealing with emergencies.

I congratulate Dr Shivaprakash Shirale on his achievement and wish him best for all his future endeavors.

Dr Tatyarao P. Lahane
M.S. (Ophthalmology)
Padma-Shri Awardee
Ex Dean of Grant Medical College and J.J. Hospital, Mumbai
Ex Director of Medical Education and Research, Maharashtra Mumbai

FOREWORD

In the emergency department, well trained and clinically efficient doctors are required to manage all common medical emergencies and their complications in the right way. A good knowledge of triaging of patients and its management will definitely save numerous lives. So, every doctor needs a book which will cover various emergencies and their management.

Dr. Shivaprakash Shirale, is known to me as a very hard working, sincere and creative minded Assistant Medical Officer. He has been working in the Casualty and Administrative Department of our hospital for the last 5 years.

He has written a book which includes all common medical emergencies and which is written in very lucid language with good illustrations. This is a very useful book to understand the necessary management while dealing with emergencies.

I am sure that this book is a must read book for medical students, medical interns, medical officers, general practitioners and will definitely help them to make the right decisions while dealing with emergencies.

I wish him all the best for his future endeavors.

Dr. Shailesh C. Mohite
MD,DFM, DNB, PGDHA, MBA (HCS), LLB
Dean
H.B.T Medical College &
Dr R.N. Cooper Hospital
Mumbai

FOREWORD

Dr. Shivaprakash Shirale is known to me as a very enthusiastic,sincere and hard working Assistant Medical officer. He has been working in the Casualty Department and Hospital Administration of our hospital since last 5 years. He has authored this book covering important topics of Common Medical Emergencies. This book has covered all important emergencies commonly seen in day to day clinical practices. It is written in simple and understandable language with good illustrations .Very few books have been authored with so much attention in detail as demonstrated in this book.

I am sure that this book is a must read book for Medical Students, Medical Interns,Medical Officers, General Practitioners and will definitely help them to make the right decisions while dealing with emergencies.

I wish all the best to Dr Shivaprakash Shirale.

Dr Prasad Pandit
MBBS, MD
Head of Department of Pharmacology and
Medical Superintendent at HBT Medical College &
Dr R.N. Cooper Hospital, Mumbai

FOREWORD

Dr Shivaprakash Shirale is known to me ever since he joined as Assistant Medical Officer at Dr Rustom Narsi Cooper hospital. He has always shown his sincerity, enthusiasm, creative mind and new concepts of visualization and innovative ideas in the capacity as a Casualty Medical Officer and is playing an active role in administrative management.

He has authored this book covering important topics of Common Emergencies in clinical practice. Very few books have been written on this topic. This book has covered all important emergencies commonly seen in day to day clinical practice and in emergency Medical Service Department of major hospitals and in all broad specialties. Well written, Comprehensive, Methodical with good illustrations are evident in this book.

I am sure that this book will be very useful for all Medical Students, Medical Interns and Medical Officers in public healthcare system who are attending the patients requiring emergency lifesaving management and procedures in the golden hours, where quick decision making is essential so as to provide quality emergency medical care at the right time, at right place and at a right way.

This book is surely the need of the hour, especially when the National Medical Commission has brought the Emergency Medical Service Department in Medical Colleges all across the country for Undergraduate and Postgraduate Medical Students.

This book is boon for all Medical Professionals and guides them in taking right decisions while dealing with all types of Medical Emergencies in their day to day clinical practice.

I wish Dr Shivaprakash Shirale all the best.

Dr Jiten M. Bhavsar
M.B.B.S, D.H.A.
HBT Medical College and
Dr. R.N. Cooper Hospital, Mumbai 400056

FOREWORD

I have known Dr Shivaprakash Shirale for many years as a very enthusiastic and hard-working Medical Officer at Dr. R.N. Cooper hospital.

I congratulate Dr Shirale for authoring an extremely well written book on an important topic: Common Medical Emergencies in Practice .Very few books have been authored with so much attention to detail as demonstrated in this book. The simple yet methodical approach has impressed me the most.

I am sure that this book will be a must read book for all Medical Professionals and will help them make the right decision while dealing with emergencies.

I wish Dr Shirale all the best.

Dr Samir Bhargava
D.L.O. (London), M.S. (E.N.T), D.O.R.L.,
Diplomat of national Board
National president: Association of ENT
Surgeons of India (2020)

ACKNOWLEDGMENTS

I am thankful to my co-author and all my editors who have provided valuable guidance, clinical pictures and made necessary corrections which have helped me a lot in completing the book with accuracy.

I would like to thank my seniors, colleagues, friends and medical interns for their support and valuable suggestions: Dr Jiten Bhavsar, Dr Ajit Israni, Dr Sulbha Sadaphule, Dr Devidas Walke, Dr Pratibha Badole, Dr Bhumika Keny, Dr Nehal Mehta, Dr Arefa Khan, Dr Lalit Hulhule, Dr Abhijeet Kondar, Dr Tulsidas Karpe, Dr Niranjan Ksirsagar, Dr Mihir Vaidya, Dr Shrikrishna Parab, Dr Himanshu Prasad, Dr Mohammad Parkar, Dr Priyanka Bhagtani, Dr Balaji Mane, Dr Lata Naik, Dr Harish Kumar, Dr Shaziya Ansari, Dr Jagruti Munje, Dr Harsh Trivedi, Dr Shreenivas, Dr Shivkumar Shete, Dr Vivek Mane, Dr Nishid Trivedi, Dr Divya Kotkar, Dr Shravan, Sheetal Shete, Dr Vilaksh Jain, Dr Tanvi Garg, Dr Sobriety Awasthi, Dr Aakanksha Pandey, Dr Soham Tokale.

I also thank our editorial team **Mr. Rajesh Bhalani & Mr. Rushabh Bhalani and Mrs. Harsha Shah** from **Clever Pen Publishing** along with the DTP typesetter who were excellent and supportive from the start and helped me in realizing what sort of textbook will be appropriate and best suited for the reader.

Finally, my deep and sincere gratitude to my family members Mr. Sambhaji Shirale, Mrs. Sangeeta Shirale, Mrs. Jijabai Shirale, Mr. Kishanrao Shirale, Mrs. Kusum Anerao, Mr. Chandrashekhar Anerao, Mr. Ratnakar Anerao, Mrs. Shilpa Shete, Mr. Avinash Shirale, Mr. Hanumant Shirale, Dr Sushma Shirale for their continuous love, help and support.

Shivaprakash S. Shirale

CO-AUTHORS AND EDITORS

Subject	Co-authors and editors
Surgery	**Dr Vipul Nandu** (Editor) (MBBS, MS general surgery) Assistant Department of Surgery Hinduhridaysamrat Balasaheb Thackeray Medical College & Dr RN Cooper Medical College, Mumbai **Dr Uttareshwar Honrao** (MBBS,MS general surgery, MCh neurosurgery) SMC Department of Neurosurgery Hinduhridaysamrat Balasaheb Thackeray Medical College & Dr RN Cooper Medical College, Mumbai
Ear, nose and throat	**Dr Vinod Gite** (Editor) (MBBS, MS ENT) Associate Professor in the department of ENT at Hinduhridaysamrat Balasaheb Thackeray Medical College & Dr RN Cooper Medical College, Mumbai **Dr Neeraj R. Shetty** (Editor) (MBBS, DNB ENT fellow Head, Neck Oncosurgery) Assistant professor Department of ENT Hinduhridaysamrat Balasaheb Thackeray Medical College & Dr RN Cooper Medical College, Mumbai
Ophthalmology	**Dr Amrita Ajani** (Co-author) (MBBS, MS Ophthalmology, DNB, FCPS, DOMS, Fellowship in Cornea and Refractive surgery Associate Professor Hinduhridaysamrat Balasaheb Thackeray Medical College & Dr RN Cooper Medical College, Mumbai Former Assistant Professor Department of Ophthalmology KEM Hospital, Parel, Mumbai **Dr Rameshwar Chamle** (Editor) (MBBS, DOMS)

Subject	Co-authors and editors
Orthopedic	**Dr Ganesh R Yeotiwad** (Editor) (MBBS, MS Orthopedic) Fellowship in trauma (South Korea) Fellowship in joint replacement (Mumbai) Fellowship in Sports Medicine (France) Associate Professor Department of Orthopedic Hinduhridaysamrat Balasaheb Thackeray Medical College & Dr RN Cooper Medical College, Mumbai **Dr Mohit R. Upadhyaya** (Co-editor) (MBBS, MS Orthopedics, DNB Orthopedics) Assistant Professor Department of Orthopedics Hinduhridaysamrat Balasaheb Thackeray Medical College & Dr RN Cooper Medical College, Mumbai
Obstetric and gynecology	**Dr Arvind B Mulay** (Editor) (MBBS, DGO, DNB OB GYN) SMO/SR Department of (OB GYN) Hinduhridaysamrat Balasaheb Thackeray Medical College & Dr RN Cooper Medical College, Mumbai
Medicine	
Cardiovascular system	**Dr Shrikant Mandge** (Editor) (MBBS, MD General Medicine)
Respiratory system	**Dr Anuj Tiwari** (Editor) (MBBS, DNB Medicine) Assistant Professor Department of Medicine Hinduhridaysamrat Balasaheb Thackeray Medical College & Dr RN Cooper Medical College, Mumbai
Gastrointestinal, hepatobiliary system and Endocrinology and Metabolism	**Dr Sweta Jadav** (Editor) (MBBS, MD General Medicine) Assistant Professor Hinduhridaysamrat Balasaheb Thackeray Medical College & Dr RN Cooper Medical College, Mumbai
Nervous system	**Dr Sharad Awachar** (Editor) (MBBS, MD General Medicine)
Acute febrile illness, Hematology and Dog bite, Snake bite and Poisoning	**Dr Faisal Memon** (Editor) (MBBS, MD General Medicine) Assistant Professor Hinduhridaysamrat Balasaheb Thackeray Medical College & Dr RN Cooper Medical College, Mumbai

Subject	**Co-authors and editors**
Skin	**Dr Radha Mundhra** (Editor) (MBBS, MD, DNB Dermatology, MRCP SCE Dermatology) Assistant Professor Department of dermatology at Hinduhridaysamrat Balasaheb Thackeray Medical College & Dr RN Cooper Medical College, Mumbai **Dr Sachin chamle** (Editor) (MBBS, MD)
Psychiatric	**Dr Angeline Thangiah** (MBBS, DNB Psychiatry)
Pediatric	**Dr Baraturam Bhaisara** (Editor) (MBBS, MD Pediatrics) Associate Professor Department of Pediatrics Hinduhridaysamrat Balasaheb Thackeray Medical College & Dr RN Cooper Medical College, Mumbai

CONTENTS

SECTION 1 - SURGICAL EMERGENCIES

SECTION 2 - EAR, NOSE AND THROAT EMERGENCIES

SECTION 3 - OPHTHALMOLOGY EMERGENCIES

SECTION 4 - ORTHOPEDIC EMERGENCIES

SECTION 5 - OBSTETRIC AND GYNECOLOGY EMERGENCIES

SECTION 6 - MEDICINE EMERGENCIES

SECTION 7 - SKIN EMERGENCIES

SECTION 8 - PSYCHIATRIC EMERGENCIES

SECTION 9 - PEDIATRIC EMERGENCIES

SECTION 10 - NORMAL LABORATORY VALUES

Section 1

Surgical Emergencies

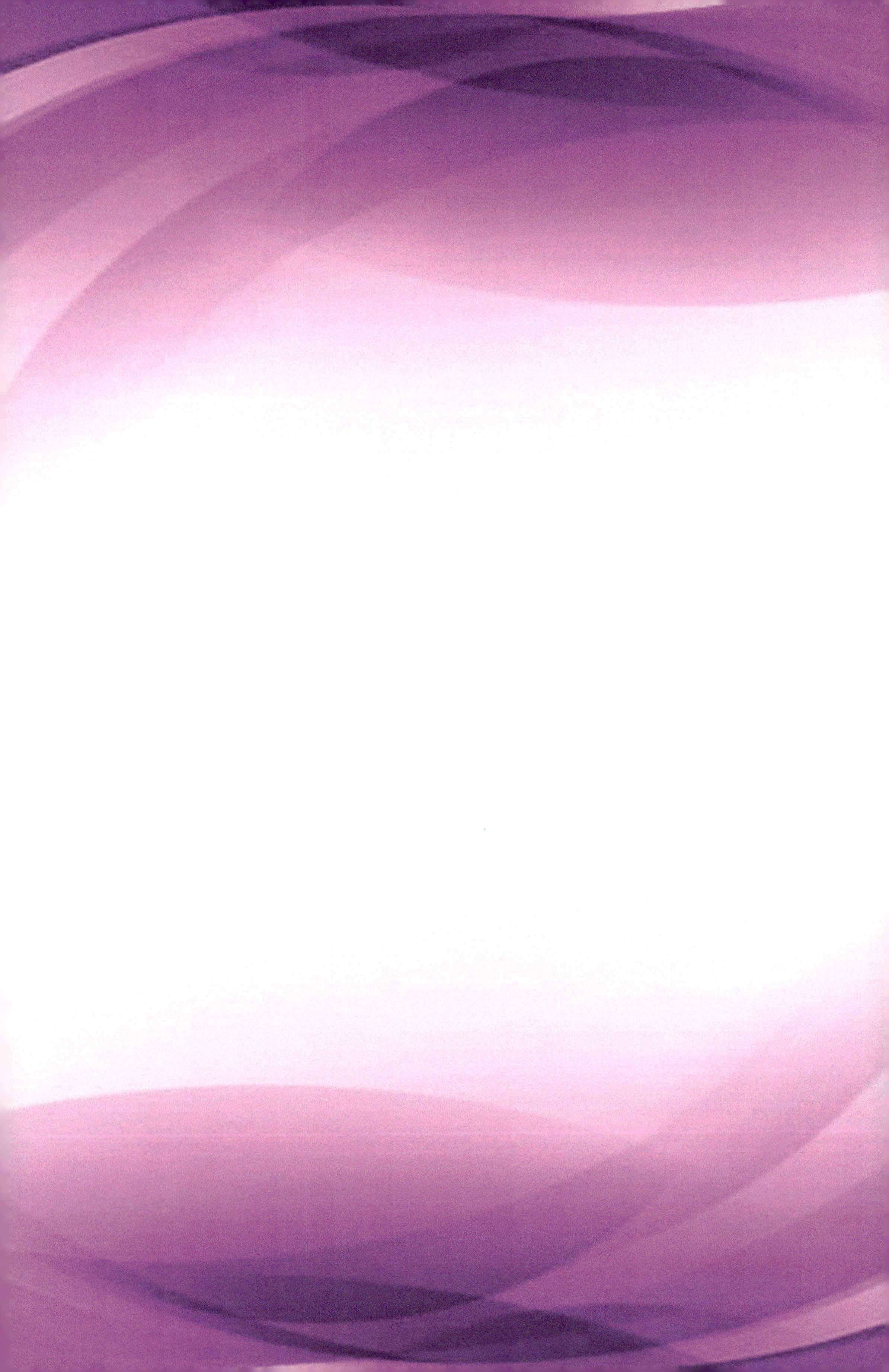

CHAPTER

1 Surgical Emergencies

ACUTE WOUND MANAGEMENT

1. When evaluating a patient that comes to you with an acute wound, the first step is to control active blood loss and evaluate the need for other emergency procedures.
2. Examine the wound for the site, type (Tidy or Untidy) and possible structures damaged (tendon, nerve, muscles, vessels).
3. In bleeding wounds the limb should be elevated and a pressure pack and immobilisation applied.
4. The site injured, the structures involved in the injury and the mechanism of injury all affect healing and recovery of function

5. Timing of injury is important for management of acute wounds.
6. If less than 6 hours between injury and evaluation, the wound can usually be closed with suture after cleaning.
7. If more than 6 hours have passed, the wound should not be closed due to high infection risk.
8. In facial wounds as face has an excellent blood supply, face wound may be closed even 24 hours after injury, if it is a clean wound.
9. In wound management, in order to facilitate examination and repair, adequate analgesia and/ or anesthesia (local, regional or general) are required.
10. General anesthesia is often needed for acute wound management in children.
11. It is essential to assess movement and sensation of affected limb for understanding distal neurological deficit.
12. Classification of wound into tidy and untidy

Tidy wound	Untidy wound
Incised	Crushed or avulsed
Clean	Contaminated
Healthy tissues	Dead tissues
Not often tissue loss	Often tissue loss

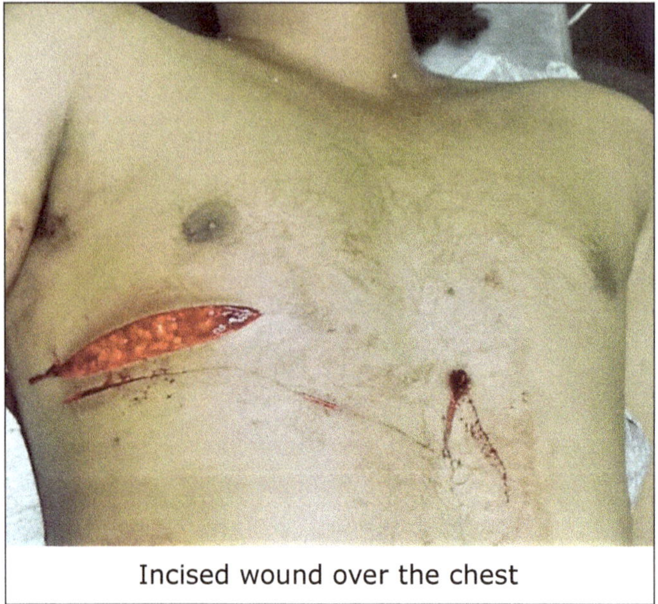
Incised wound over the chest

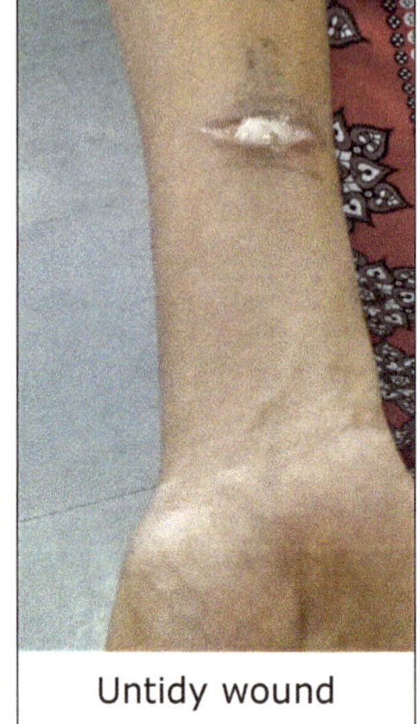
Untidy wound

13. The aim is to convert untidy wound to a tidy wound by removing all contaminated and devitalised tissue

14. Order of management of wound:

1. Cleaning of wound
2. Exploration and Diagnosis
3. Debridement of wound
4. In certain wounds repair of structures e.g. muscles, nerves, vessels
5. Replacement of lost tissues wherever indicated
6. Skin cover if required
7. Skin closure without tension

15. After assessment, a thorough wash given and debridement done.

16. Primary repair of all structures (e.g. bone, tendon, vessel and nerve) may be possible in a tidy wound.

17. In untidy wound, vessels can be repaired first but bone, tendon and nerve should be kept as it is after marking for repair at later date.

18. A contaminated wound with dead tissue requires debridement one or several times before definitive repair can be carried out.

19. The use of copious saline irrigation which is less destructive is preferred than knife or scissors while debriding the wound.

20. In debridement unviable tissue must be excised until bleeding healthy tissue is seen.

21. Nerves, vessels and tendons may survive with adequate revascularisation subsequently or after being covered with viable tissue such as skin or muscle flaps.

22. Muscle viability is judged by the color, bleeding pattern and contractility.

23. In a tidy wound, repair of all damaged structures may be attempted.

24. Classification of wound healing:

a. **Primary intention:**

1. Healing of a clean wound without tissue loss
2. This process is faster than healing by secondary intention
3. Less scarring associated with primary intention, as there are no large tissue losses to be filled with granulation tissue
4. In primary intention, wound edges are adjacent to each other and re-approximation with sutures is possible and should be attempted.

b. **Secondary intention:**

1. This procedure is implemented when primary intention is not possible

2. A significant loss in tissue or tissue damage
3. This healing process is slower.
4. Granulation results in a broader scar.
5. Wound care must be performed daily to encourage wound debris removal to allow for granulation tissue formation

c. **Tertiary intention (also called delayed primary intention)**

1. The wound is initially cleaned, debrided and observed, typically 4 or 5 days before closure.
2. The wound is purposely left open.

26. The technique of suturing depends on site, tissue involved.

27. The correct choice of suture technique and suture material is also important.

28. For any wound to heal well, there must be a good blood supply, no tension on the edges for closure and no infection.

29. Types of sutures:

a. **Natural**

1. **Absorbable material**
   a. **Catgut suture (Plain or chromic)**
2. **Non absorbable material**
   a. **Silk**
   b. **Linen**

b. **Synthetic**

1. **Absorbable material**
   a. **Dexon (Polyglycolic acid)**
   b. **Vicryl (Polyglactin)**
   c. **Maxon (Polyglyconate)**
   d. **Polydiaxone (PDS)**
2. **Non absorbable material**
   a. **Nylon (Polyamide)**
   b. **Dacron (Polyester)**
   c. **Prolene (Polypropylene)**
   d. **Stainless steel wire/suture**

30. Types of suture technique:

Four frequently used suture techniques are as follows:

1. Interrupted sutures
2. Continuous sutures
3. Mattress sutures
4. Subcuticular suture

31. Dressing: A dressing is a sterile pad or compress applied to a wound to promote healing and protect the wound from further harm.

A dressing is designed to be in direct contact with the wound, as distinguished from a bandage which is most often used to hold a dressing in place.

32. Types of dressing:

1. Dry or impregnated gauze
2. Plastic films
3. Gels & foams
4. Hydrocolloid
5. Alginates
6. Hydrogel
7. Polysaccharide pastes
8. Granules and beads

Uses of dressing:

1. Aim of a dressing is to promote healing of the wound by providing a sterile, breathable and moist environment that facilitates granulation and epithelialization.
2. Protect the wound against infection and mechanical damage due to trauma.
3. Soak up blood, plasma, and other fluids exuded from the wound and prevent maceration of wound and skin.
4. Helps to seal the wound to expedite the clotting process
5. Prevents pain due to further trauma
6. Helps the wound to heal more quickly, and reduce scarring.

HEAD INJURY

1. Head injury is any trauma to the scalp, skull or brain.
2. Head injury causes damage to the head's content (i.e. Brain and cranial nerves) or its coverings (Dura, skull and scalp)

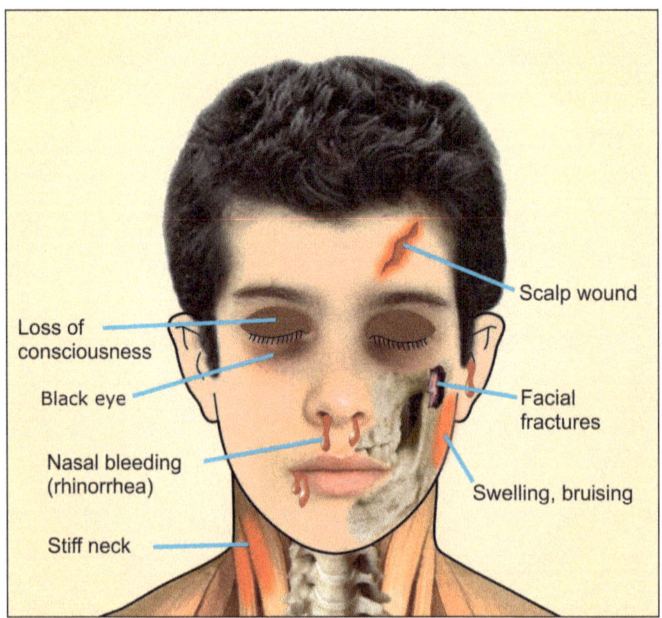

3. Damage to brain can occur at the time of impact (Primary damage) or during subsequent minutes, hours or days (Delayed damage)
4. Most of the patients admitted to hospital after head injury do not need operative management, but most of them need good non operative care directed to brain function to promote recovery from brain injury.
5. Intracranial pressure and other parameters are important to reduce secondary injury.
6. **Causes:** Common causes of head injuries are road traffic accidents, fall, assault, sports related injuries, firearm related injuries.
7. **Head injury classification using the Glasgow Coma Scale (GCS) score:**
   a. Minor head injury [GCS 15 with no loss of consciousness (LOC)]
   b. Mild head injury (GCS 14 or 15 with LOC)
   c. Moderate head injury (GCS 9–13)
   d. Severe head injury (GCS 3–8)

8. **Types of head injuries (Simply we can divide the head injuries as follows:**
   a. **Scalp injury**
   b. **Skull bones fracture**
   c. **Intracranial hemorrhage**
   d. **Traumatic Brain injury**
9. **Scalp injuries:** Abrasion, Contusion, laceration, subgaleal hematoma.

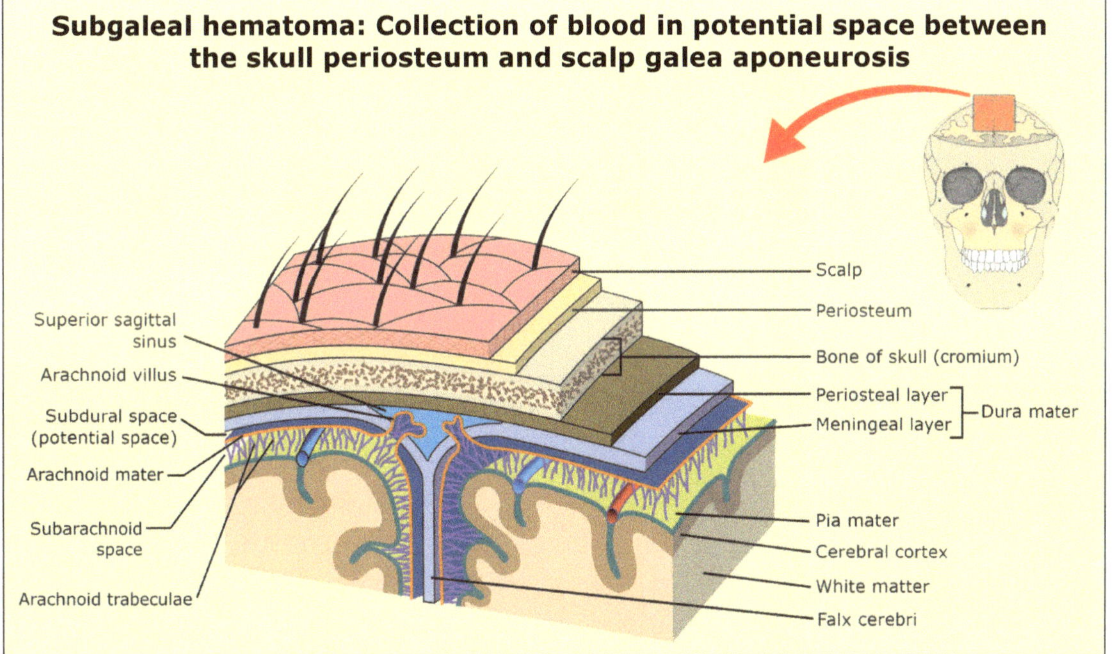

Figure showing different layers of head

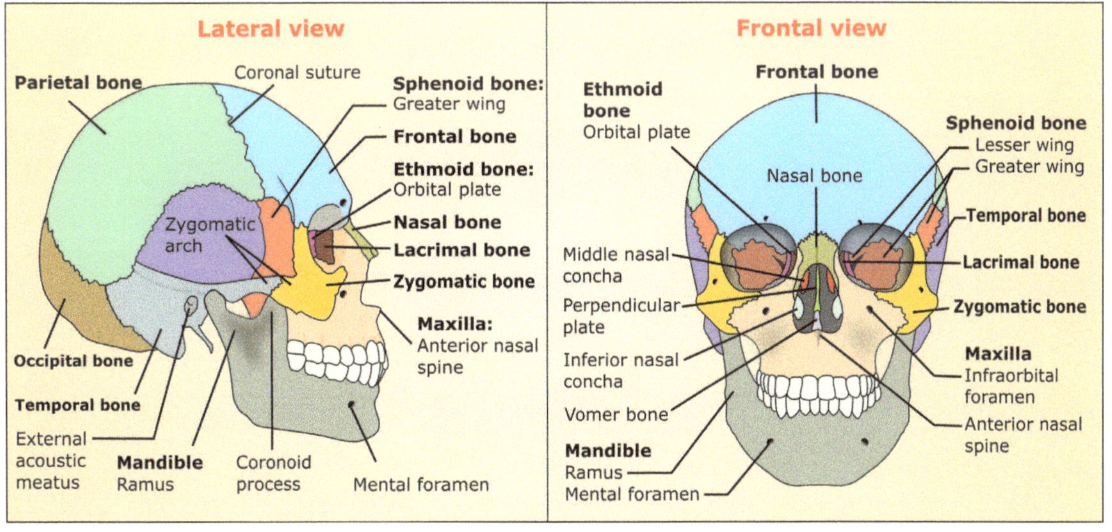

10. A skull fracture is a break in the continuity of skull bone. There are four major types of skull fractures, including the following:

a. **Linear skull fractures:**

1. This is the most common type of skull fracture.
2. In a undisplaced linear fracture, there is a break in the bone, but it does not move the bone.
3. Usually, no interventions are necessary.

b. **Depressed skull fractures**:

1. This type of fracture may be seen with or without a cut in the scalp.
2. In this fracture, part of the skull is actually sunken inside due to blunt force trauma
3. This type of skull fracture may require surgical intervention, depending on the severity of fracture to lift the bone off the brain, if it is pressing on it.
4. Strict neurological monitoring

c. **Diastatic skull fractures:**

1. These are fractures that occur along the suture lines in the skull.
2. In this type of fracture, the normal one or more suture lines are widened.
3. These fractures are more often seen in newborns and young children.

d. **Basilar skull fracture:**

1. This is the most serious type of skull fracture, and involves a fracture at the base of the skull & may be complicated by neurological deficits, meningitis.
2. Patients with this type of fracture mostly have bruises around their eyes (Raccoon or Panda eyes) and a bruise behind their ear (Battle sign).

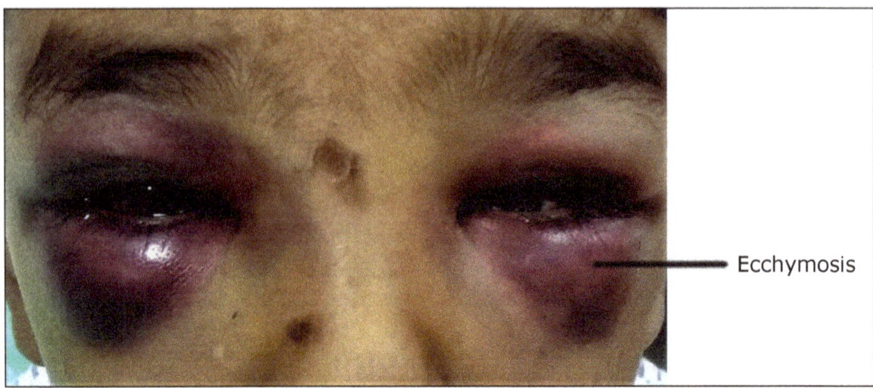

Figure showing Raccoon eye's

3. Clear CSF fluid draining from their nose (Rhinorrhea) or ear (Otorrhea) is highly suggestive of a fracture skull base.
4. Patients require close observation & CSF leak may resolve spontaneously or require repair.

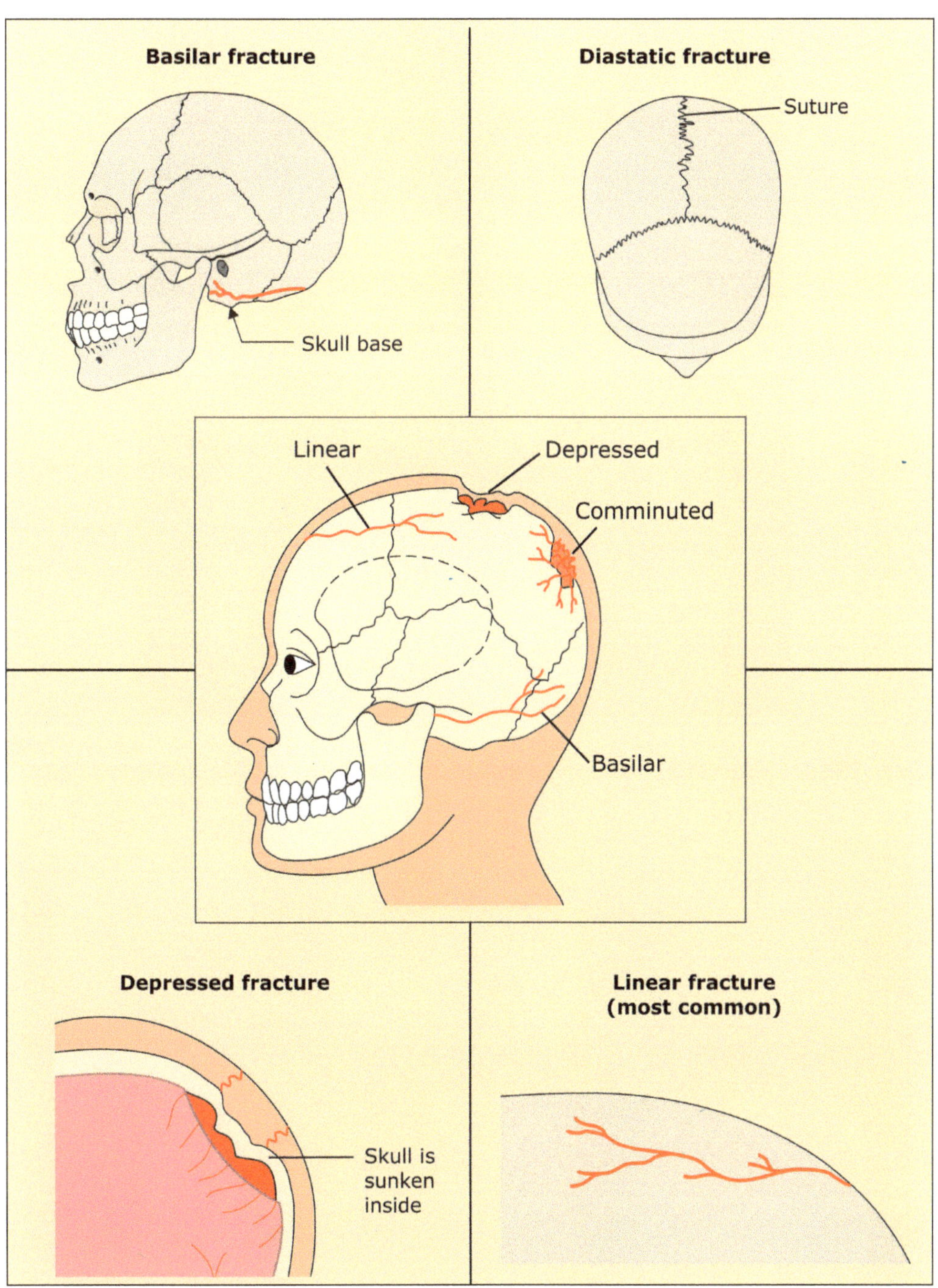

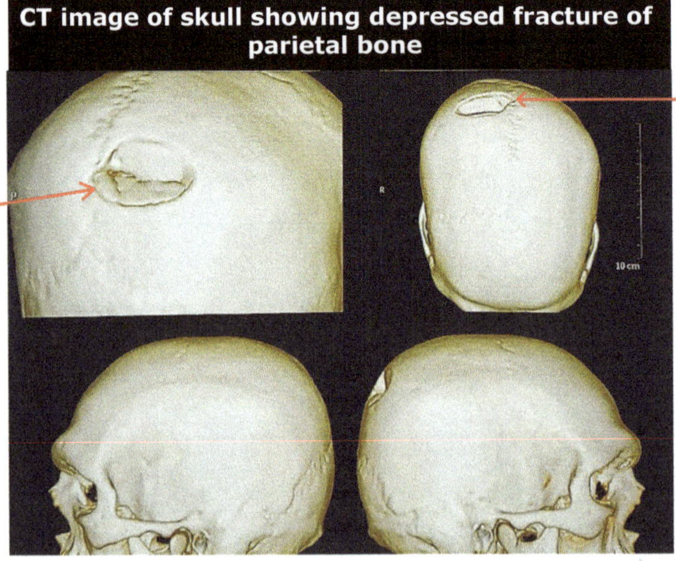
CT image of skull showing depressed fracture of parietal bone
Parietal bone
Depressed skull
10 cm

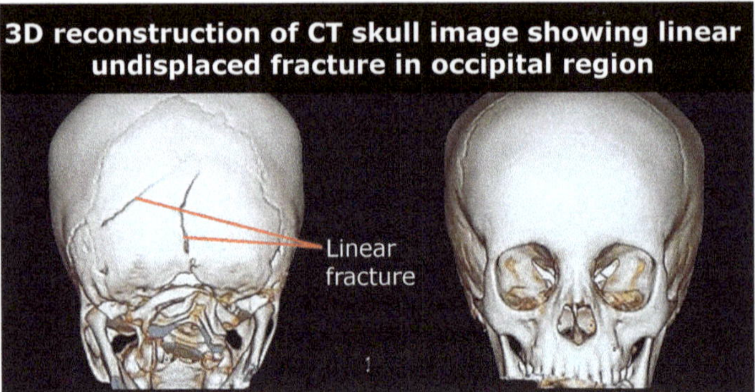
3D reconstruction of CT skull image showing linear undisplaced fracture in occipital region
Linear fracture

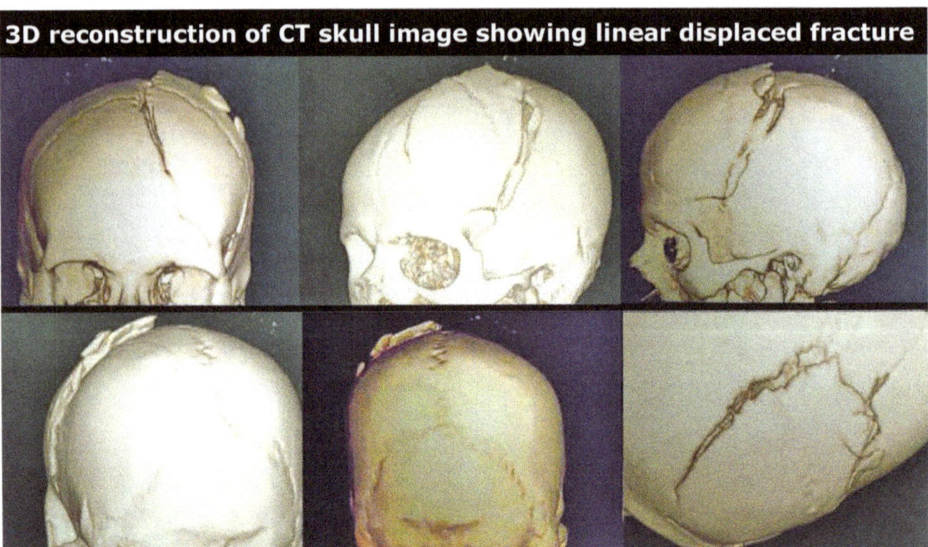
3D reconstruction of CT skull image showing linear displaced fracture

11. Location of fracture and associated symptoms and signs:

Temporal bone	Parietal bone	Orbital	Basilar skull
Bruise behind the ear in mastoid region called as Battle sign CSF Otorrhea Bleeding from ear	Deafness, Scalp hematoma, Neurological deficit due to trauma to nerves	Periorbital ecchymosis damage to eye ball	Bruising around the eye, Battle sign, facial paralysis, CSF otorrhea, rhinorrhea, meningeal irritation sign like vertigo, neck rigidity, bleeding from ear and nose.

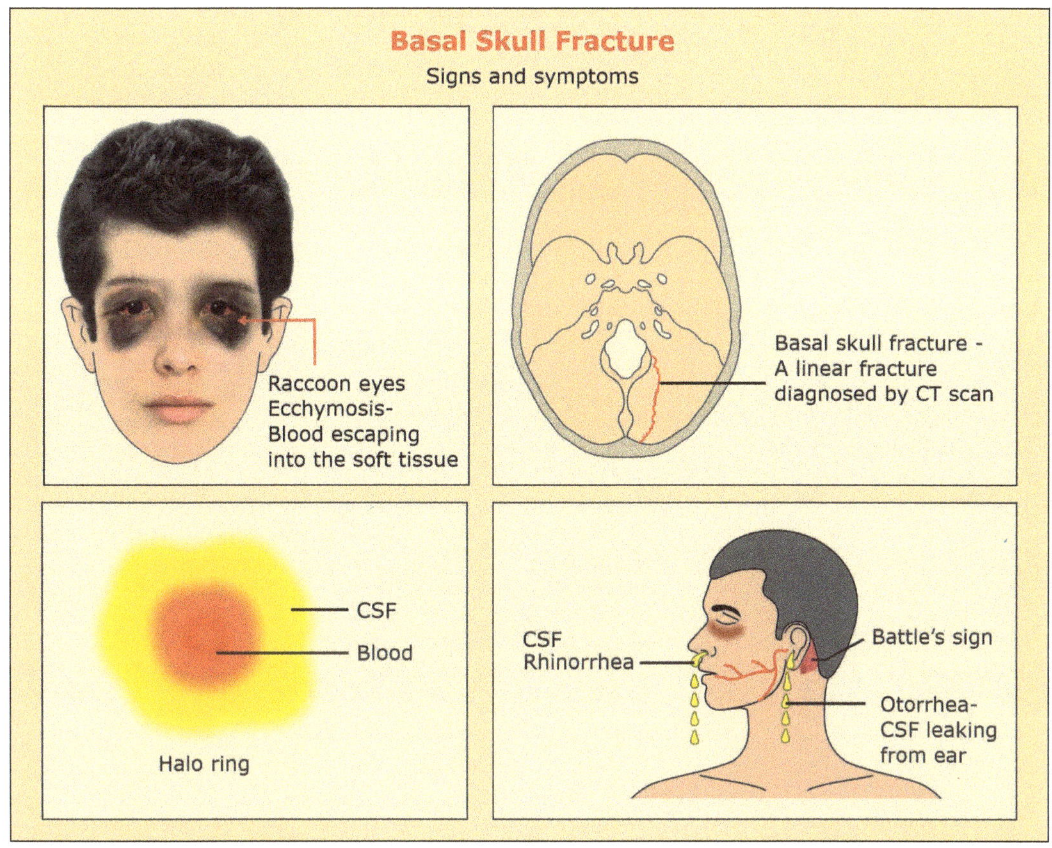

12. Intracranial hemorrhage

a. Extra axial hemorrhage

1. Epidural hematoma
2. Subdural hematoma - acute and chronic
3. Subarachnoid hemorrhage

	EDH	SDH	SAH	Chronic subdural hematoma
Mechanism of injury	Blow to head	High energy trauma to head	Trauma to head Or spontaneous due to rupture of an aneurysm or arteriovenous malformation	Even trivial trauma to head can cause
Location	Bleeding in between inner surface of skull and dura Usually does not crosses a sutures	Bleeding in between the dura and arachnoid Develop slowly It can crosses sutures	Bleeding in between arachnoid and Pia mater	Bleeding in between the dura and arachnoid types It can crosses sutures
Clinical manifestation	Brief LOC with lucid intervals associated with headache, nausea and vomiting.	Severe headache, vomiting, loss of consciousness progress from the drowsy state then to confused state finally complete loss of consciousness	Severe headache, nausea, vomiting, LOC, signs of meningeal irritation may present	Occurs in elderly patient especially on anticoagulant therapy Headache, Drowsiness, Seizure or Neurological deficit
Involvement of vessels and venous sinus	Middle meningeal artery	Venous bleeding due to tearing of bridging veins running from cerebral cortex to dural sinus	Berry Aneurysmal bleed, skull base fracture leading to internal carotid aneurysm.	Cerebral atrophy commonly found in elderly with stretch bridging veins that rupture with trauma.
On CT appearance	Lentiform, biconvex, lens shaped, hyperdense lesion	Concave, hyperdense Lesion	Increased attenuation seen in the CSF spaces over cerebral hemisphere.	Diffuse hypodense lesion
Management	Decisions should be taken by neurosurgeon for evacuation. Immediate evacuation of concealed clot and decompression is required for prevention of herniation and it will improves the outcome.	Decisions should be taken by neurosurgeon for evacuation. Craniotomy/ Craniectomy for evacuation of clot and decompression of brain	Aneurysmal bleeds will need coiling or surgical clipping of aneurysm.	Depends on neurological condition Drainage is performed by **burrhole**

- Strict neurological monitoring is required for patient (Pulse, blood pressure, respiratory pattern, GCS, pupillary size & reaction, neurological response).
- Repeat CT scan or emergency surgery will be needed in case of neuro deterioration.

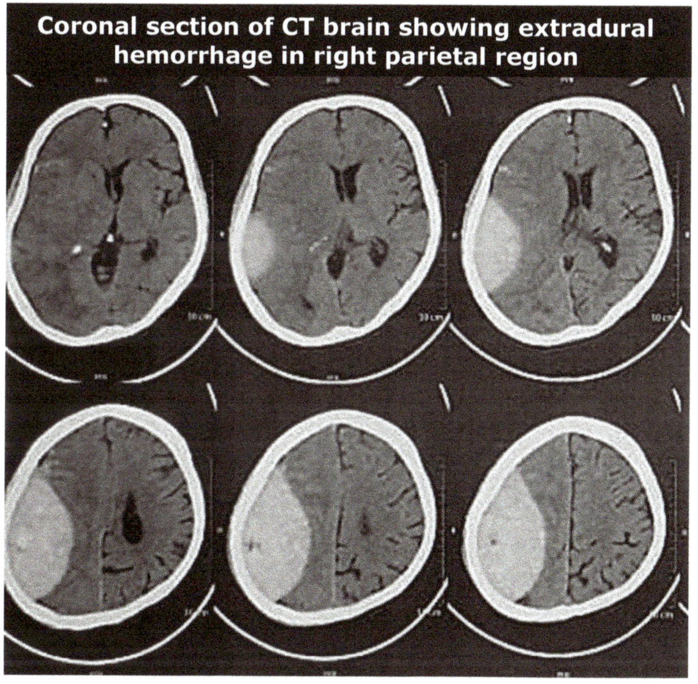

Coronal section of CT brain showing extradural hemorrhage in right parietal region

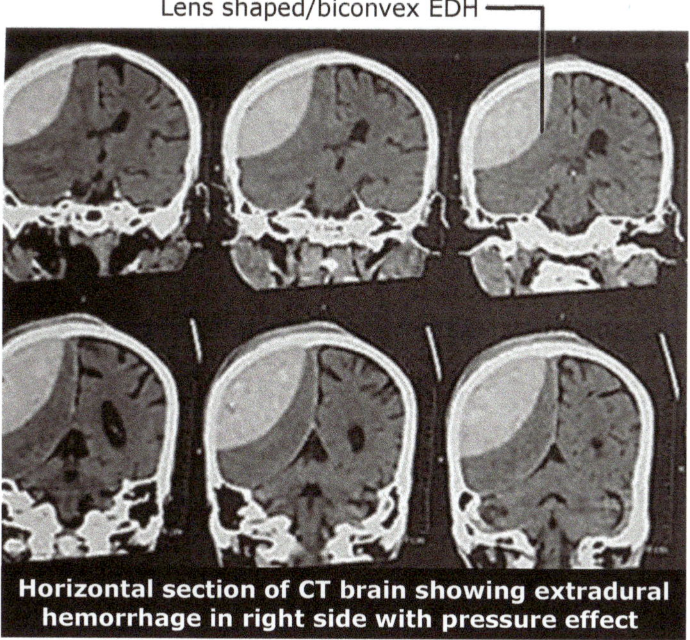

Horizontal section of CT brain showing extradural hemorrhage in right side with pressure effect

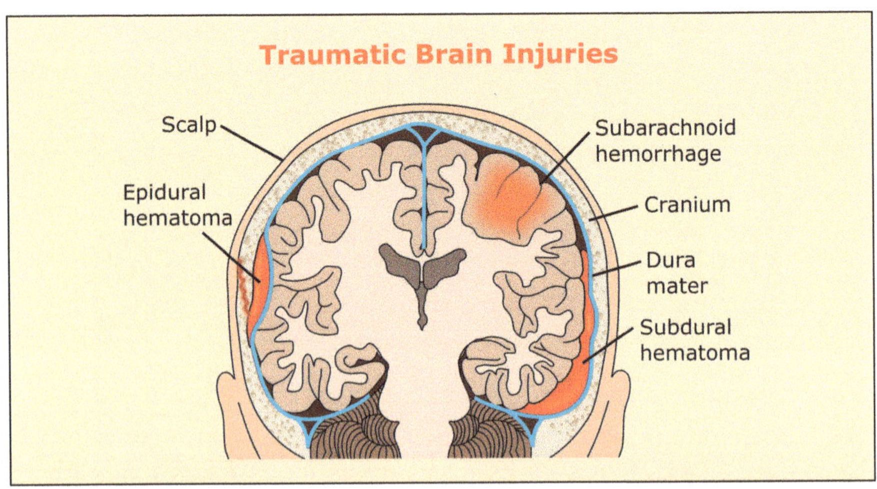
Traumatic Brain Injuries
Scalp
Epidural hematoma
Subarachnoid hemorrhage
Cranium
Dura mater
Subdural hematoma

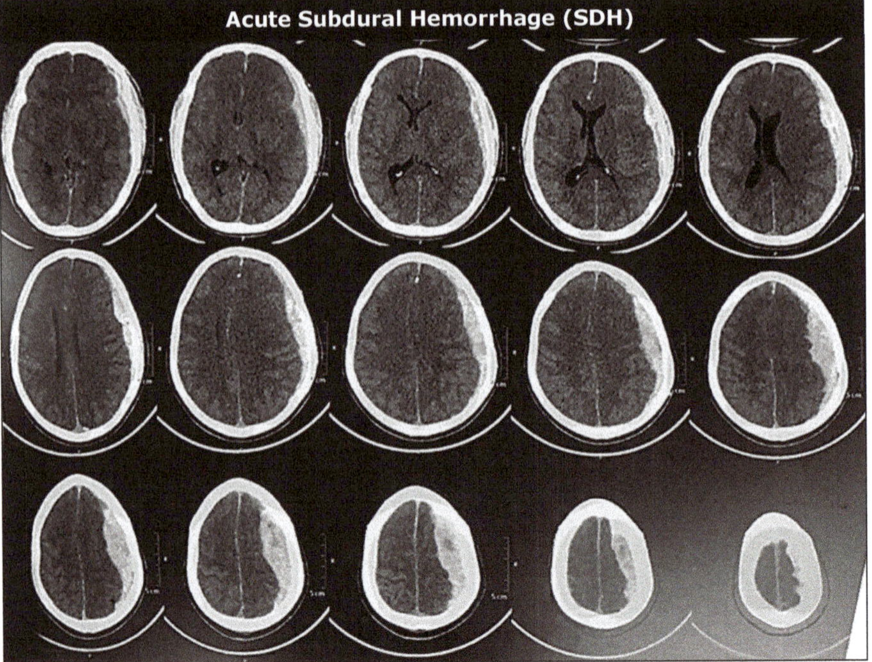
Acute Subdural Hemorrhage (SDH)

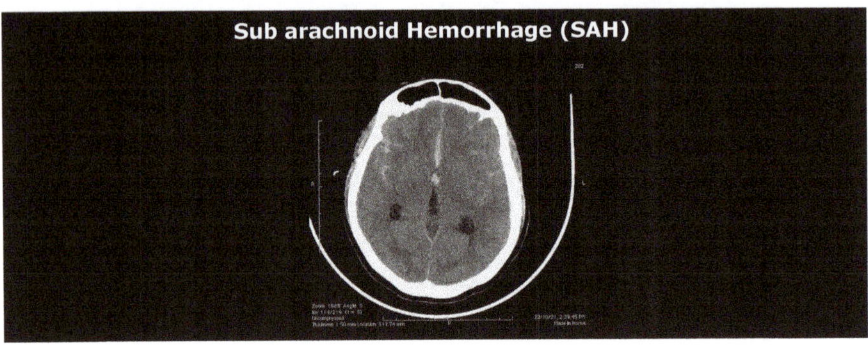
Sub arachnoid Hemorrhage (SAH)

b. **Intra-axial hemorrhage:**

1. **Intraparenchymal bleed:** Hemorrhage within the brain parenchyma and accompanying edema may disrupt or compress adjacent brain tissue which leads to neurological dysfunction.

   Substantial displacement of brain parenchyma may cause elevation of ICP and may cause fatal herniation syndrome.

2. **Intraventricular bleed:** Bleeding into the brain ventricular system, where the cerebrospinal fluid is produced and circulates through the subarachnoid space.

   a. **Primary intraventricular hemorrhage:** It is caused by intraventricular trauma, aneurysm, vascular malformation, or tumors, particularly of the choroid plexus.

   b. **Secondary intraventricular bleeding:** Resulting from an expansion of an existing intraparenchymal or subarachnoid hemorrhage

13. **Injuries to brain:**

a. In brain injuries there is direct transmission of energy due to impact on head leading to trauma and accumulation of blood within the cranium.

b. Energy transmitted to the cranium and underlying brain tissue can cause direct injury at the location of contact **(coup injury)** and on the contralateral part of the brain **(counter-coup injury)**.

c. Injured brain develops edema after injury that can become worse by ongoing bleeding, ischemia and rise in intracranial pressure.

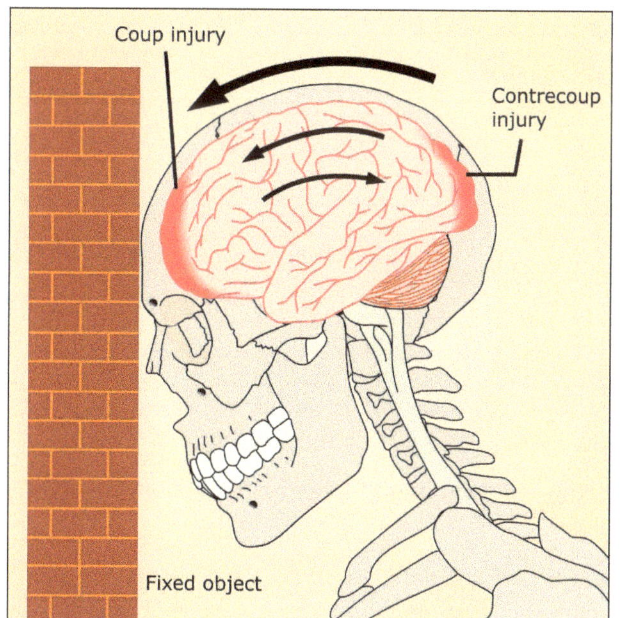

d. Head trauma leads to tearing of blood vessels due to injury resulting in accumulation of blood within the cranium.

e. Increase in intracranial volume results in an exponential increase in ICP once the total volume exceeds the volume of cranial vault.

f. The brain requires continuous perfusion of oxygen and glucose delivery for its survival and proper functioning.

g. This significant elevated ICP worsens cerebral perfusion and oxygenation which results in further edema.

h. Cerebral edema raises ICP which will further compromise cerebral perfusion, resulting in a cycle of secondary brain injury and swelling.

i. **Signs and symptoms of raised ICP:**
   1. Headache
   2. Vomiting without nausea
   3. Altered level of consciousness
   4. Papilledema

j. Cushing triad of signs which develop due to body response to rising intracranial pressure.

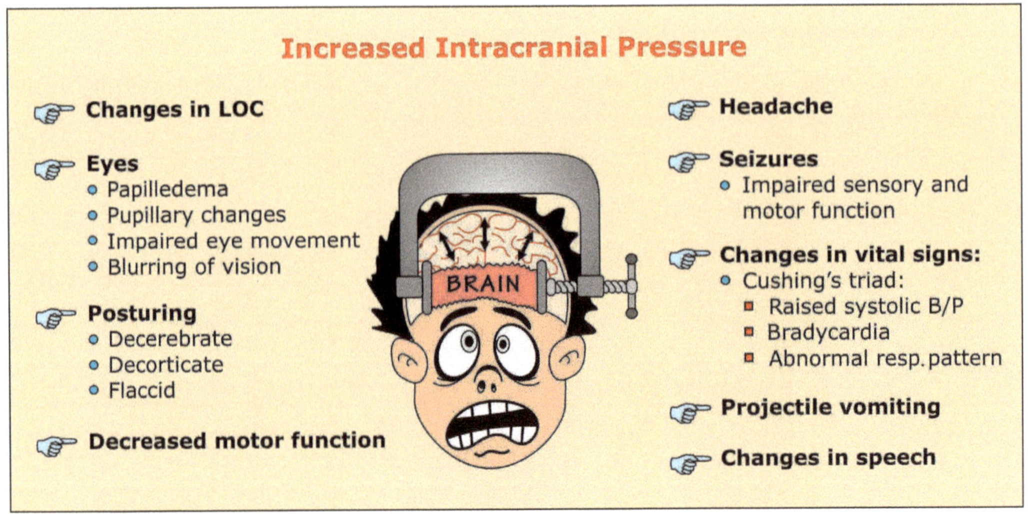

k. **Cushing triad:** It involves an increased systolic blood pressure, a widened pulse pressure, bradycardia and abnormal respiratory pattern.

l. Mass effect present due to traumatic brain injury which results in cerebral herniation.

m. **Cerebral herniation:** Shift of cerebral tissue from its normal position into the adjacent space as a result of mass effect

n. **Additional signs in herniation includes:**

1. Pupillary dilation
2. Abducens palsies

14. **Diffuse brain injury (DAI):** Usually caused by shaking of the brain back and forth, which can happen in car accidents, from falls.

Diffuse injury can be mild, such as with concussion or very severe as in diffuse axonal injury

PRIMARY SURVEY:

Use a systematic approach based on ABCDE to assess and treat an acutely injured patient

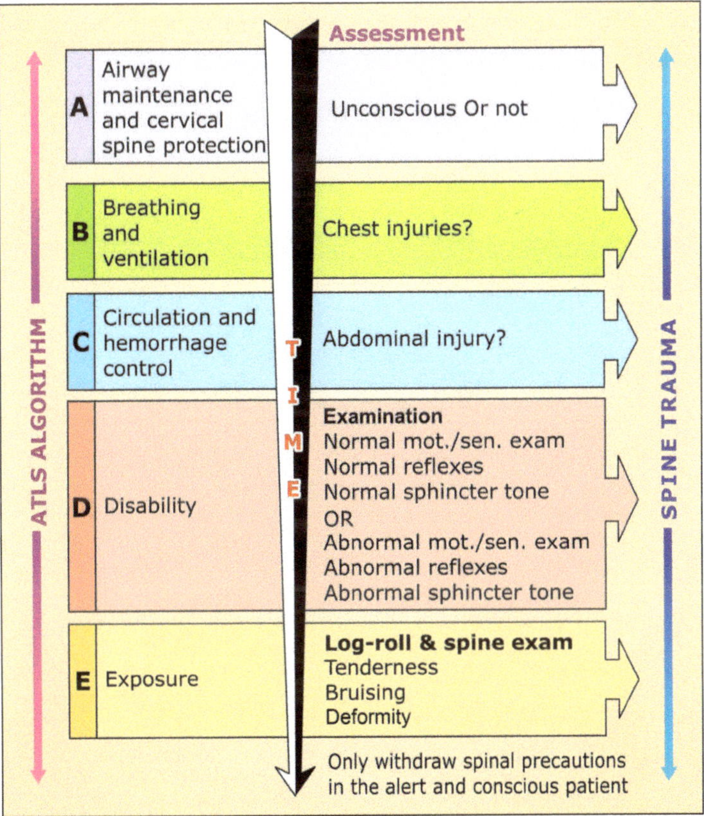

1. The goal is to manage any life threatening condition and identify any emergent concern, especially in a neurotrauma patient who may present with other multi system injuries.
2. **Initial evaluation and management**

   In initial management we should follow ATLS system, that is "ABCDE" of trauma care

Airway with cervical spine protection	1. Clearing the mouth and airway by suction. 2. Removal of foreign body 3. Maneuvres such as jaw thrust or chin lift used 4. Do not rotate hyper extend or hyper flex the head or neck. 5. Stabilisation of cervical spine manually or by loose cervical collar. 6. Check the trachea whether it is in midline or not. 7. In case of severe head injury (GCS 8 or less) then definitive airway may be required i.e. endotracheal intubation and electively to preserve airway and prevent aspiration. 8. Protection of airway is important to prevent risk of aspiration 9. If patient communicates verbally then the airway is patent 10. Pulse oxymeter is attached to measure the oxygen concentration 11. Use mouth gag to avoid tongue fall.

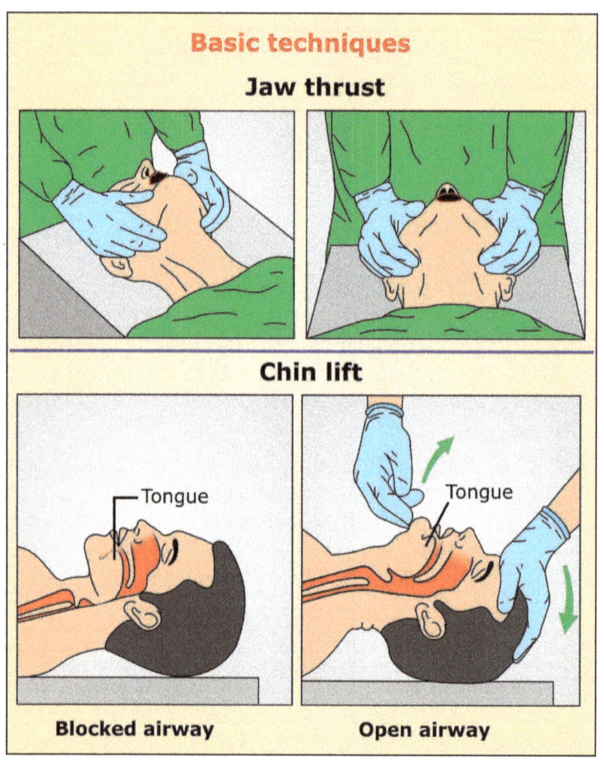

3.

Breathing and ventilation	1. Oxygen should be administered with high concentration O_2 with reservoir in patient with respiratory distress 2. Check for movement of chest wall while breathing 3. Tension pneumothorax, flail chest with contusion, a massive hemothorax and open pneumothorax are the life threatening injuries that must be identified and treated.

4.

Circulation and hemorrhage control	1. Check level of consciousness 2. Can indicate perfusion of brain 3. Pulse: Rapid and thready pulse indicate hypovolemia 4. BP <90 mmHg may lead to the worst outcome as it causes secondary brain injury. 5. If hypovolemic then consider internal or external bleeding. 6. Large bore cannulas should be placed. 7. Administer warm IV crystalloids and control the site of bleeding. 8. Check the potential sites of major blood loss including chest cavity, Abdomen, Pelvis and long bone fracture and achieve hemostasis. 9. Take blood for blood grouping and cross matching. 10. Arterial blood gases: Lactate to measure the degree of shock and administer the blood and blood products if unresponsive to the crystalloid fluid.

5.

Disability	1. Neurological status of the patient should be rapidly assessed by GCS scale. 2. Repeated regularly to access how the treatment is going on 3. Other causes of altered level of consciousness-hypoglycemia, alcohol consumption, drug abuse and hypovolemia should be evaluated and treated.

6.

Exposure	Patient should be fully exposed to examine the front and back by controlled log roll. All the wounds are and its details are noted and concerned system evaluated accordingly.

7. **GCS scale for clinical classification:**

Eye opening	Verbal response	Motor response
Spontaneous 4	Well oriented 5	Obeys command 6
To verbal command 3	Confused 4	Localise to pain 5
To painful stimulus 2	Inappropriate words 3	Withdrawal to pain 4
Do not open 1	Incomprehensible sound 2	Abnormal flexion to pain 3
	No response 1	Abnormal extension to pain 2
	Intubated patient VT	None 1

8. **Associating initial evaluation and management, following investigation should be done**

   a. **Blood test:** Blood sugar, CBC, blood grouping and cross match, serum electrolyte, creatinine, PT/INR

   b. **Urinary catheter and RT tube**

   c. **Radiograph:** Chest, skull and pelvic along with desired long bones as per the injuries.

   d. **ECG**

   e. **Arterial blood gas analysis**

   f. **USG FAST**: To rule out abdominal collection

   g. **CT scan brain:** More specialised form of investigation should be done after stabilization of patient

9. **NICE guidelines for indication of doing CT scan in head injury:**

   NICE [National institute for health and clinical excellence]

1. GCS <13 At any point
2. GCS 13 OR 14 At 2 hours
3. Focal neurological deficit
4. Suspended open, depressed or basal skull fracture
5. Seizures after trauma
6. More than one episode of vomiting after head injury.
7. Any patient with mild head injury over the age of 65 yrs or with coagulopathy on warfarin
8. Dangerous mechanism of injury or integrate amnesia >30 min warrants CT within 8 hours

SECONDARY SURVEY:

1. The secondary survey is rapid but thorough head to toe examination assessment to identify all potential injuries.
2. It should be performed after the primary survey and initial stabilization is complete.
3. It is helpful to determine the priorities for continued evaluation and management.
4. The purpose of the secondary survey is to obtain history about the patient and his or her injuries as well as to evaluate and treat injuries not found during the primary survey.
5. **History:** History taken from bystanders or patients and paramedics.

   a. Mechanism of injury

   b. Loss of consciousness and amnesia (Ask regarding the event).

   c. Episodes of vomiting

d. Evidence of seizure
e. Consumption of alcohol
f. Medical history/conditions like IHD, seizure disorders or pregnancy.
g. Medication history: anticoagulant like warfarin, heparin
h. Allergy to any drugs and tetanus immunisation status

6. **Secondary survey includes:**
   a. Head, neck and face examination:
   b. Examination of chest
   c. Examination of abdomen
   d. Examination of extremities
   e. Pelvic examination neurological examination: reassess
   f. Skin examination
7. **Tertiary survey:** It includes re-evaluation of patient after patient stabilisation, priorities identified, treatment started and all the investigations available.

MANAGEMENT:

a. **Medical management:** Medical management strategies aim to minimise secondary brain injury, through avoidance of hypoxia and hypotension and control of ICP
   1. Head up (avoided in spinal injury)
   2. Cervical collar to stabilise the cervical spine tight enough to prevent movement but should not be so tight so as to compromise venous return.
   3. Airway protection
   4. High concentation O_2 with reservoir
   5. IV fluids warmed crystalloid solution.
   6. Scalp wound closure.
   7. Tetanus toxoids
   8. Foley's catheterization
   9. Seizure control by administration of INJ. phenytoin dose 10-15 mg/kg or any other anticonvulsant drugs.
   10. Injection mannitol administered with dose of 1.5 to 2 mg/kg IV over 30-60 minutes.
   11. Sedation with or without muscle relaxant (If required)
   12. Antibiotics
   13. In case of a base of skull fracture pneumococcal vaccine and 3rd generation

cephalosporins are given.

14. Anticonvulsant in the depressed fracture of the skull is given.
15. In certain cases thiopental coma induced so as to decrease brain metabolic rate and decrease intracranial pressure (dose 100 mg IV or 150-200 mg IM).

b. **Surgical management**

1. **Burr hole:** Opening in the cranium with drill.
2. **Decompressive Craniotomy:** Temporary bone flap is removed to access the brain tissue.
3. **Craniectomy:** Remove the part of skull to relieve pressure.
4. **Cranioplasty:** Surgical repair of deformity of skull.

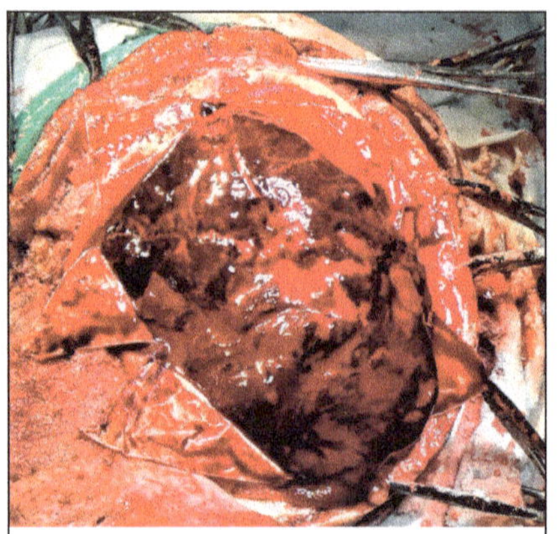

Subdural hematoma - white layer opened is the dura

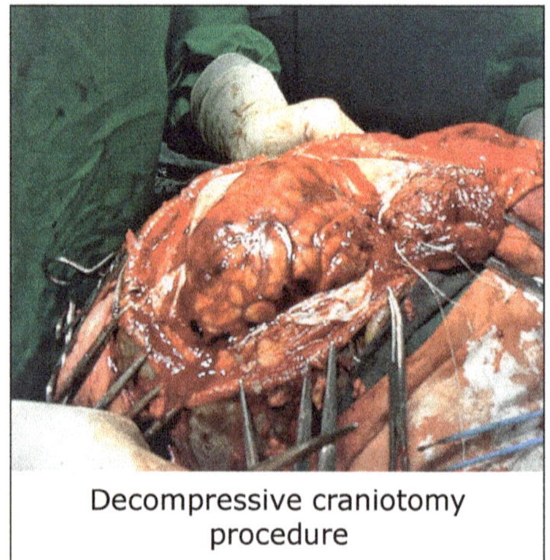

Decompressive craniotomy procedure

Criteria for discharge from the casualty with head injury.

a. GCS 15/15
b. Normal CT
c. Patient not under the influence
d. Patient is with responsible persons
e. No any dangerous signs and symptoms present.

Written and verbal advice is given to patient and relatives regarding the following symptoms and if they develop to take immediate medical treatment.

a. Persistent worsening headache
b. Persistent vomiting
c. Drowsiness
d. Visual disturbance
e. Numbness and weakness in limb

THORACIC INJURY

1. Chest trauma accounts for 25% of all severe cases in the emergency department.
2. Blunt injury to the chest can cause injury to anyone or all components of the chest wall and thoracic cavity.
3. It includes the bony skeleton (ribs, clavicles, scapulae, and sternum), the lungs and pleura, the tracheobronchial tree, the esophagus, the heart, the great vessels of the chest, and the diaphragm.

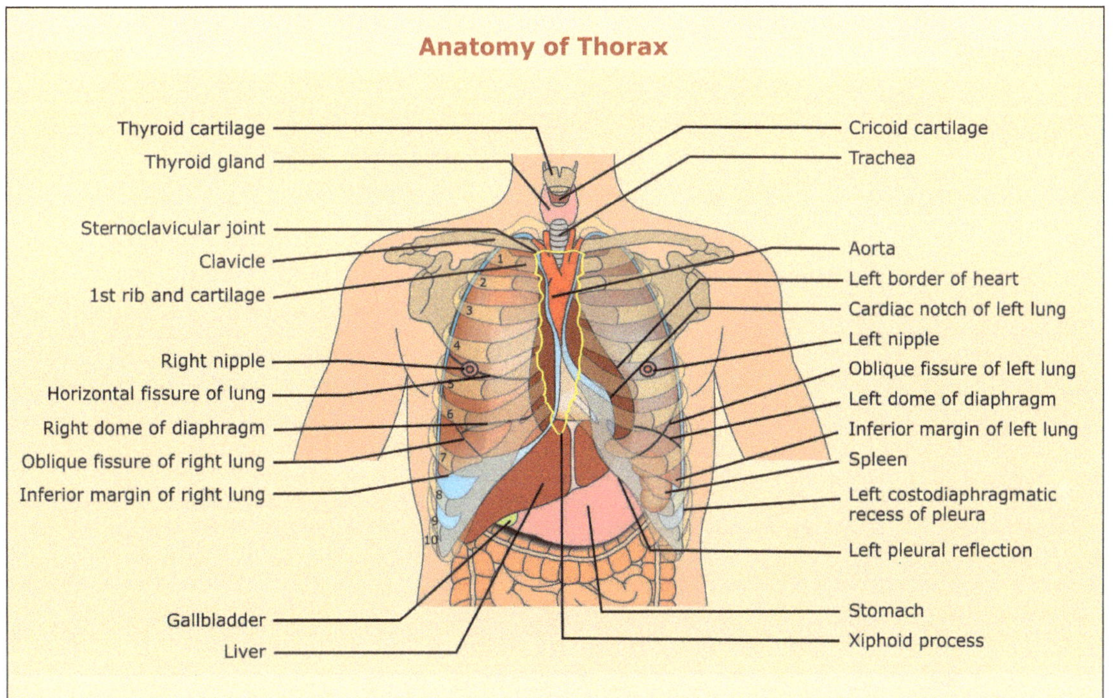

4. In most of the cases of thoracic injuries cause of death is hemorrhage.
5. Thoracic injuries range from simple rib fracture to complex life threatening rupture of organs.
6. **Blunt thoracic injuries may be divided into the following three broad categories:**
   1. Chest-wall bony fractures, dislocations, and barotrauma (including diaphragmatic injuries)
   2. Blunt injuries of the pleurae, lungs, and aerodigestive tracts
   3. Blunt injuries of the heart, great arteries, veins and lymphatic vessels.

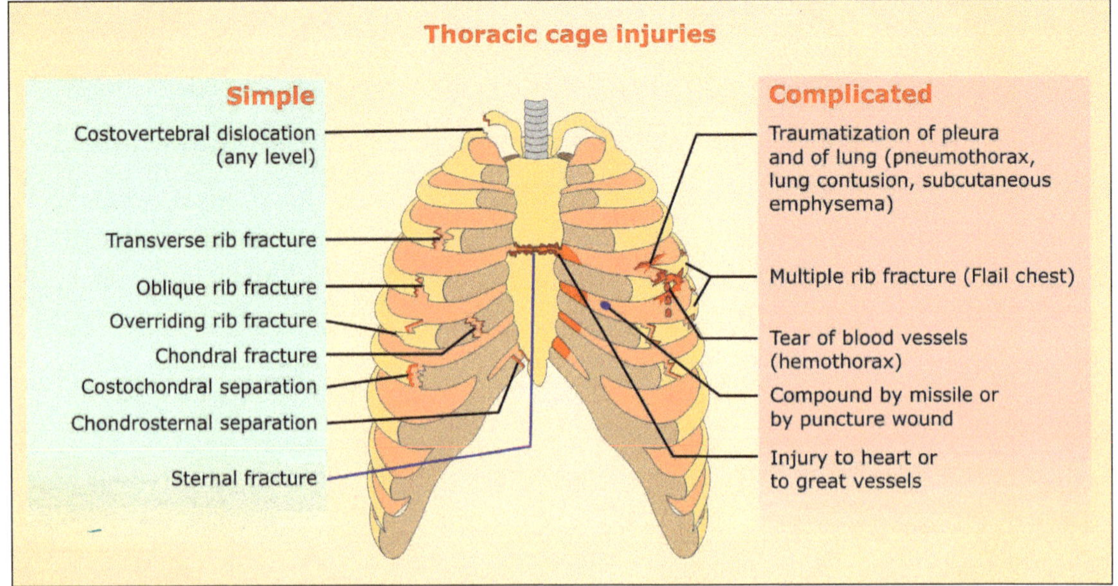

7. **Mechanism of injuries:**
   a. **Blunt trauma**
   b. **Penetrating trauma**
   c. **Iatrogenic**
8. **Pathophysiology**
   a. Chest trauma leads to disturbance in the flow of air, blood supply, or both in combination.
   b. Sepsis occurs due to leakage of alimentary tract contents in thoracic cage, as occurs in esophageal perforations.
   c. Chest-wall injuries like rib fractures, the pain associated with these injuries can make breathing difficult, and this may compromise ventilation.
   d. Direct lung injuries, such as pulmonary contusions may cause impairment in ventilation and ultimately oxygenation.
   e. Space-occupying lesions like pneumothorax, hemothorax & hemopneumothorax interfere with oxygenation and ventilation by compressing lung parenchyma.
   f. In tension pneumothorax, in which pressure continues to build in the affected hemithorax as air leaks from the pulmonary parenchyma into the pleural space. This can compress the mediastinal contents toward the opposite hemithorax.
   g. Blunt trauma that may cause significant cardiac injuries (e.g., chamber rupture)

or severe great-vessel injuries (e.g., thoracic aortic disruption) which causes hypovolemic or cardiogenic shock and death.

h. The key to good outcome is early resuscitations followed by correct diagnosis and management.

9. **History and Physical Examination:**
   a. Information should be obtained directly from the patient whenever possible and from other witnesses (bystanders) to the accident, if available.
   b. The presentation depends on the mechanism of injury & the organ systems injured.
   c. Obtain a detailed clinical history (DM, HTN) and detailed physical examination.
   d. The time of injury, mechanism of injury, motor vehicle speed and deceleration all play important role in estimating damage due to injury.
   e. Evidence of associated injury to other systems like head injury, spinal cord injury, extremity trauma.

10. **Investigations**
    a. Complete blood count
    b. ABG analysis,
    c. Serum electrolyte
    d. Coagulation profile
    e. ECG
    f. Chest X-ray
    g. Thoracic USG
    h. The focused assessment with sonography for trauma (FAST)
    i. CT chest
    j. CT angiography
    k. D-dimer test
    l. Serum troponin I, CK-MB
    m. Serum Lactate
    n. Echocardiography
    o. Transesophageal echocardiography (TEE)
    p. Aortography
    q. Contrast esophagography
    r. Esophagoscopy
    s. Bronchoscopy

11. **Types of injuries (Deadly dozen)**
    a. **Immediately life threatening**
        1. Airway obstruction
        2. Tension pneumothorax
        3. Massive hemothorax
        4. Flail chest
        5. Pericardial tamponade
        6. Open pneumothorax
    b. **Potentially life threatening**
        1. Pulmonary contusion
        2. Thoracic Aortic injuries
        3. Tracheobronchial injuries
        4. Esophageal injuries
        5. Diaphragmatic injury
        6. Myocardial contusion

Immediately life threatening injuries

Type of injury	Clinical features and diagnosis	Management
Airway obstruction	Difficulty in breathing Confusion Agitation High pitched breathing noise **Diagnosis: Clinically**	**Relieve and prevent the obstruction** Early intubation is required, particularly in cases of neck hematoma or possible airway edema
Tension pneumothorax **A** tension pneumothorax develops when air leak from the damaged lung parenchyma like a "one way valve" Air is trapped in the thoracic cavity without any escape which leads to completely collapsing affected lung of the thoracic cavity and mass effect on mediastinum and opposite lung.	Restlessness which is continuously increasing Dyspnea Tachypnea Trachea is deviated away from the side of injury Absent breath sound on the affected side Distended neck vessels Hyperresonant sound on percussion **Diagnosis:** Clinical and should not wait for radiological confirmation as every minute is crucial.	Immediate decompression by rapid insertion of large bore needle into 2nd Intercostal space in the midclavicular line of affected hemithorax. After that ICD is inserted through 5th intercostal space in "safe triangle The commonly recommended site for insertion of a chest drain is the '**safe triangle**', formed anteriorly by the lateral border of the pectoralis major, laterally by the lateral border of the latissimus dorsi, inferiorly by the line of the 5th intercostal space and superiorly by the base of the axilla.

(Continued)

Type of injury	Clinical features and diagnosis	Management
Massive hemothorax Accumulation of blood within the pleural space Bleeding occurs from injured intercostal vessels or occasionally from the internal mammary artery	Feelings of restlessness chest pain, especially when breathing cold, pale, or clammy skin Increased respiratory efforts Tachycardia Low blood pressure Dull note on percussion Decreased air entry on affected side **Diagnosis:** Physical exam X-ray CT scan Sonography	Correction of hypovolemic shock Insertion of intercostal drain In some cases intubation Pain control & pulmonary toilet. Blood in the pleural space should be removed gradually over a time period to prevent hypotension and sudden release, dislodging, decompression of clot. **Urgent thoracotomy:** If initial drain more than 1500 ml of blood and >200 ml/hr ongoing hemorrhage over 3-4 hours. Physiotherapy and active mobilisation should begin as soon as possible.
Flail chest When 2 or more ribs fracture in two or more planes it is called a flail chest. The blunt force typically also produces an underlying pulmonary contusion.	Paradoxical movement of chest wall segment during respiration i.e. chest wall segment moves inside on inspiration or outside on expiration. May be associated with lung contusion There is a high risk of developing a pneumothorax or hemothorax. **Diagnosis:** Clinically CT scan with 3D reconstruction with contrast	Oxygen administration, Adequate analgesia (including opiates), If a chest tube is in situ, topical intrapleural local analgesia introduced via the tube, can also be used. Physiotherapy Ventilator with positive pressure ventilation is required for cases developing respiratory failure despite adequate analgesia and oxygen. Surgery to stabilise the flail segment using internal fixation of the ribs.
Pericardial tamponade Accumulation of small amount of blood into the non distensible pericardial sac which can produce physiological obstruction to the heart. All patients with penetrating injury anywhere near the heart with shock should be considered for pericardial tamponade.	Increased venous return Tachycardia Muffled heart sound Cyanosis Decrease in arterial pressure. **Diagnosis:** Chest X-ray shows enlarged heart shadow **eFAST:** Showing fluid in the pericardial sac	**Needle pericardiocentesis:** To get enough time to shift the patient to operation theatre. **Sternotomy or left thoracotomy**

(Continued)

Type of injury	Clinical features and diagnosis	Management
Open pneumothorax	Signs and symptoms depends on the size of defect	**Initial management**
If there is a > 3 cm defect present then intrathoracic pressure becomes equal to atmospheric Pressure leading to profound hypoventilation of affected side and hypoxia If valvular effect present may develop tension pneumothorax.	Respiratory distress Absent breath sounds Shift of contents of the mediastinum to the opposite side Decreasing the return of blood to the heart, leading to hemodynamic instability.	Application of sterile occlusive dressing on three sides to act like flutter type valve Pain control & pulmonary toilet Chest tube insertion from the site remote from the injury site. **Definitive management** Formal debridement and closure Early referral to higher centre

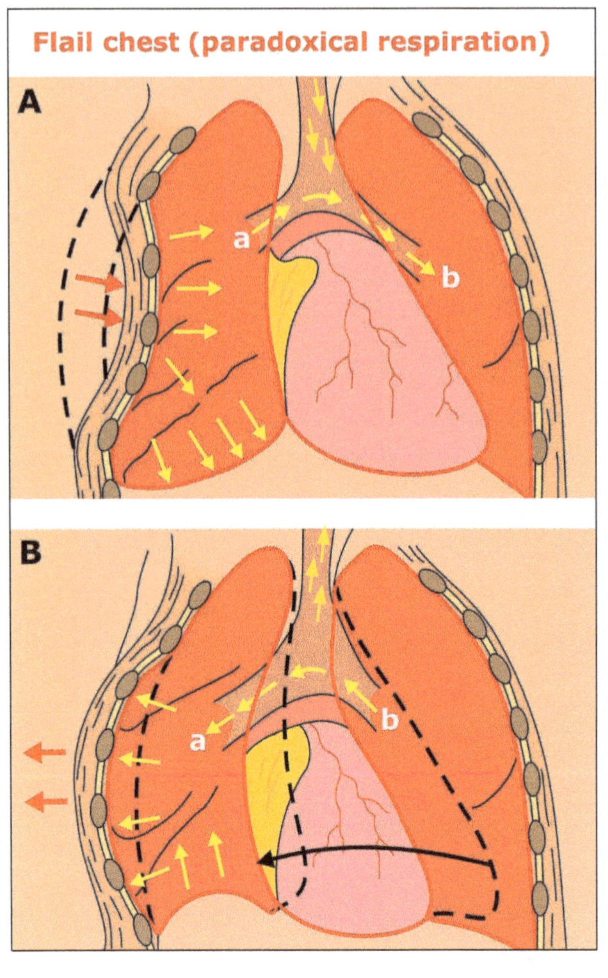

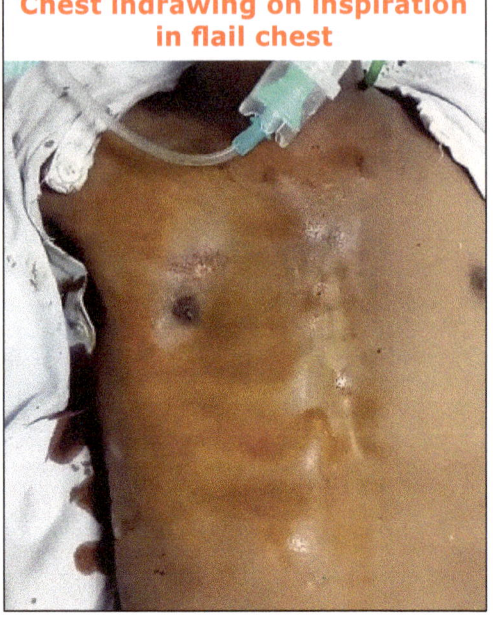

Management

Complications: **Hematoma, intercostal neurovascular injury, thoracic and abdominal visceral injuries, infections.**

Tube malposition (i.e. not in pleural cavity) or slippage

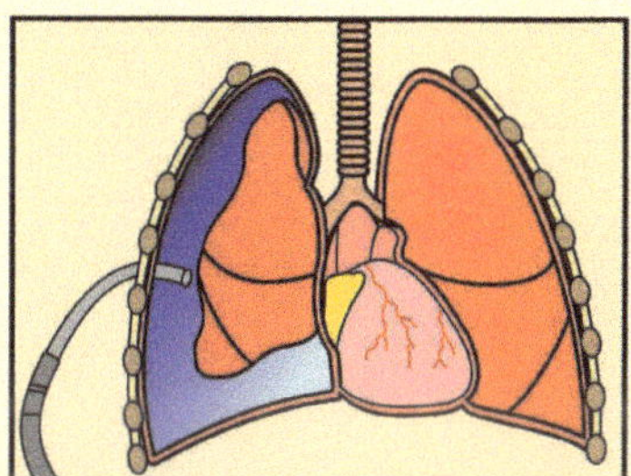

Pneumothorax

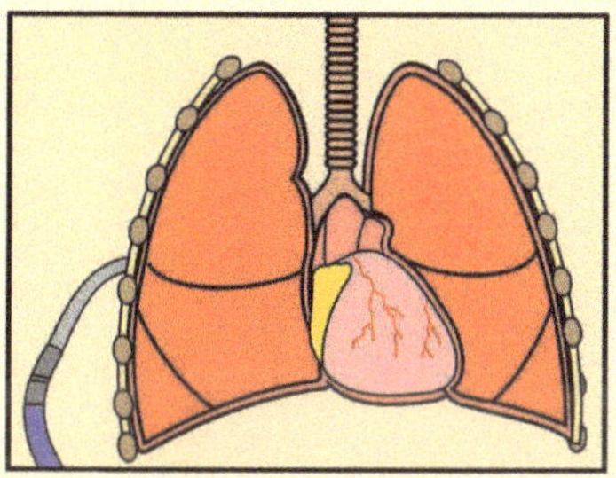

Re-expanded lung
Flail chest
(tube inserted)

3D reconstruction of chest images showing multiple ribs fractures

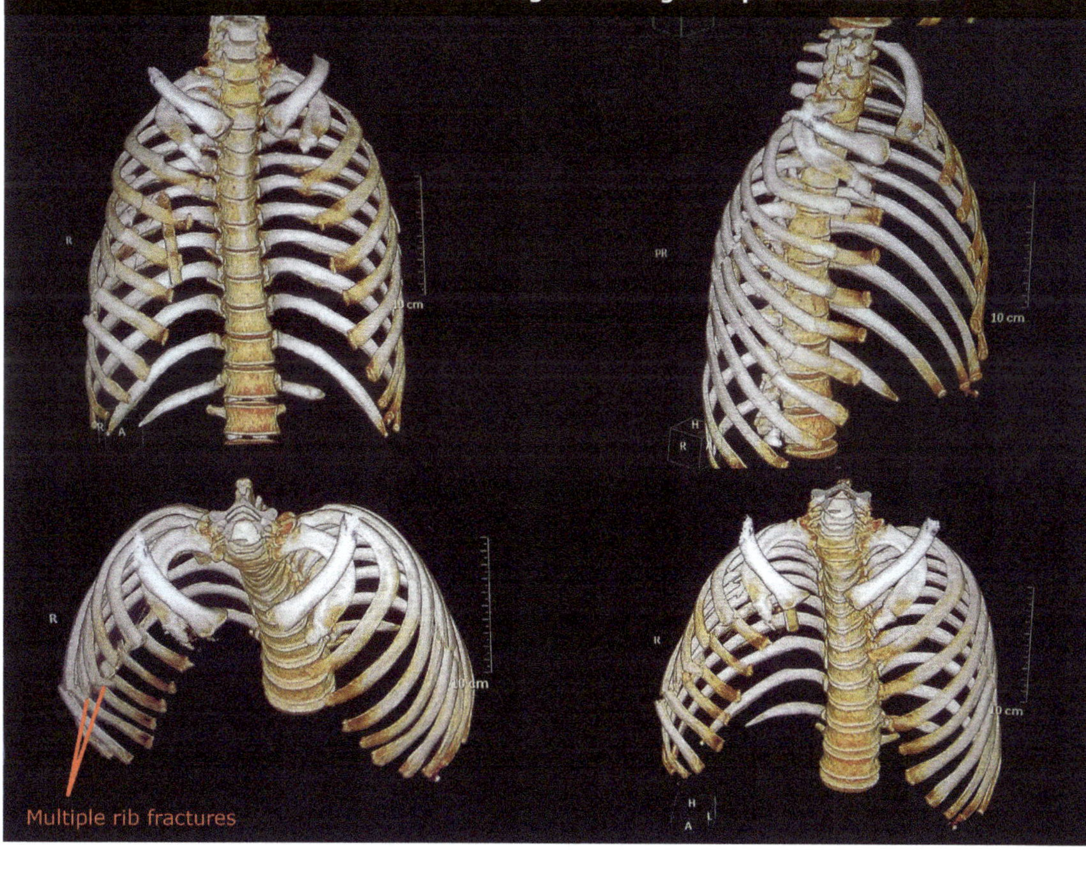

Multiple rib fractures

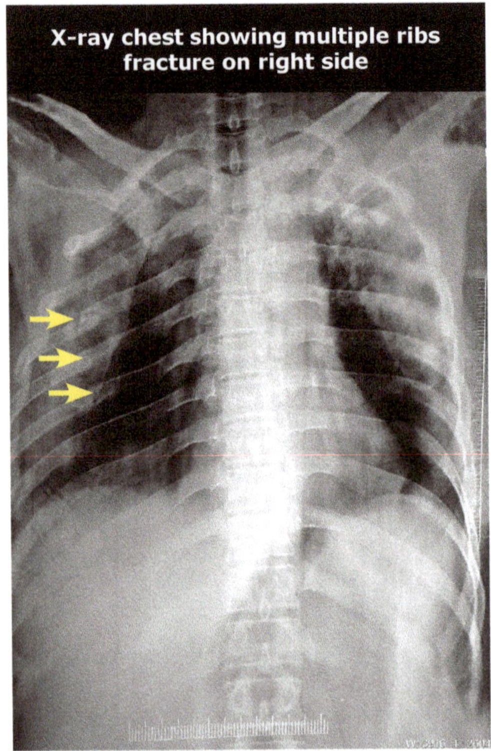
X-ray chest showing multiple ribs fracture on right side

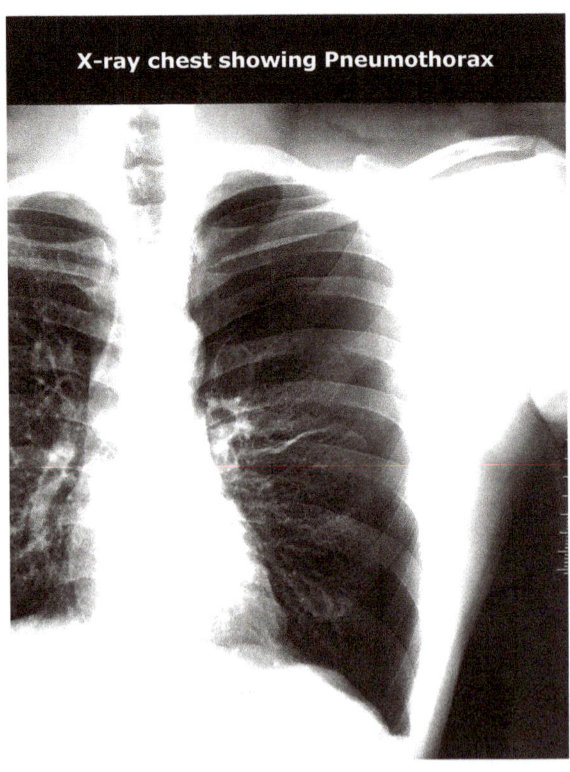
X-ray chest showing Pneumothorax

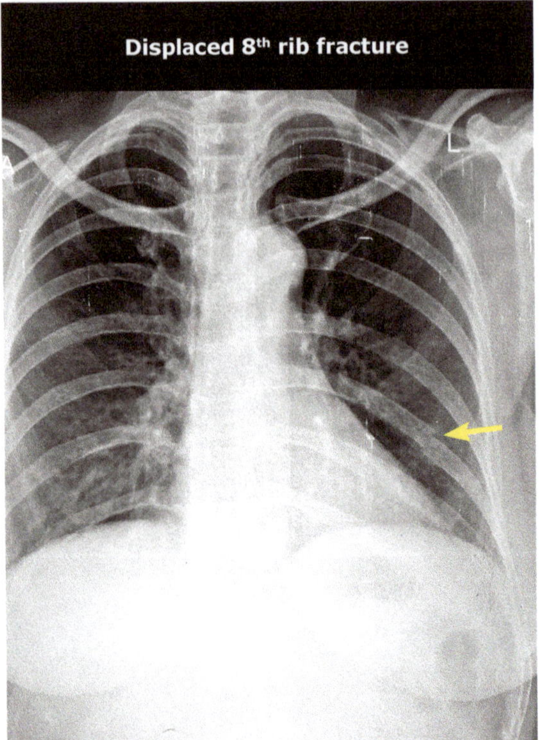
Displaced 8th rib fracture

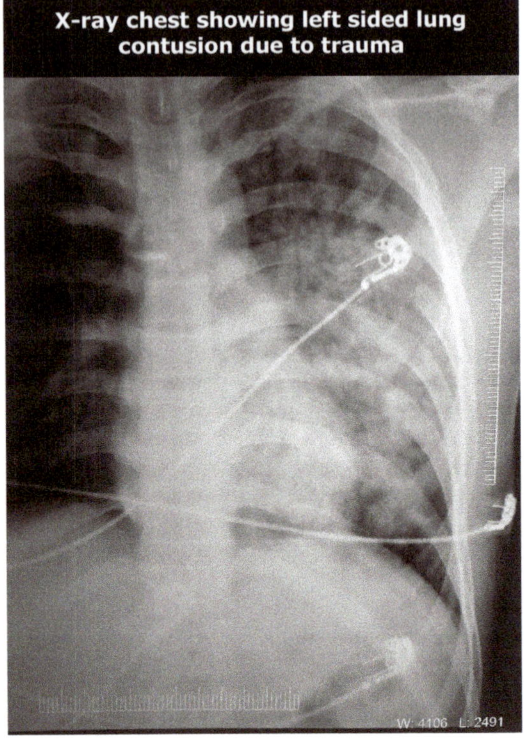

X-ray chest showing left sided lung contusion due to trauma

HRCT chest showing right sided pneumothorax with bilateral contusions

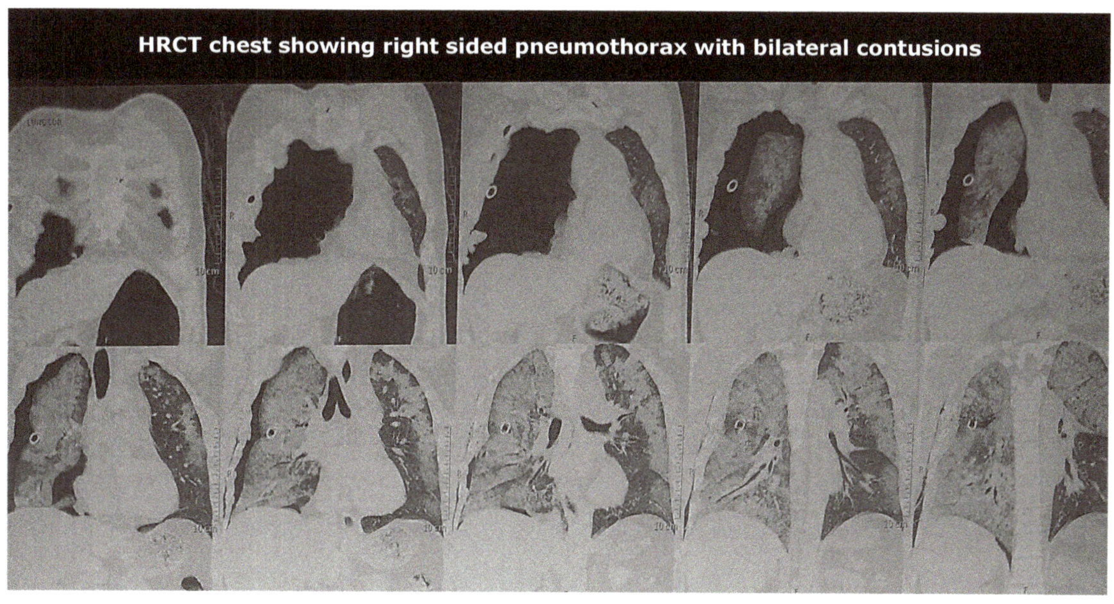

Potentially life threatening injuries

Type of injury	Clinical features and diagnosis	Management
Pulmonary contusion Usually associated with a flail segment or fractured ribs Develops worsening hypoxia for first 24-48 hours after trauma. Further worsening after 48-72 hours due to secondary infection.	Difficulty in breathing Decreased breath sounds Hemoptysis or blood in the endotracheal tube is a sign of pulmonary contusion Major cause of hypoxemia after blunt trauma **Diagnosis** Chest radiographic findings may be typically delayed. CT chest with contrast is used for confirmation	**In mild contusion** Oxygen therapy, pulmonary toilet, drainage and adequate analgesia **In more severe cases** Mechanical ventilation is necessary.
Thoracic aortic disruption It is due to road traffic accident or fall from height Shearing force after collision impact disruption of the intima and media of aorta.	Asymmetry in the upper and lower extremities blood pressure Widened pulse pressure Chest wall contusion **Diagnosis:** **Erect chest X-ray:** Thoracic aortic disruption and widened mediastinum **CT scan of mediastinum:** Confirmatory **Transesophageal echocardiography**	Adequate resuscitation with blood and blood products Operative repair with dacron graft/intra-aortic stent

(Continued)

Type of injury	Clinical features and diagnosis	Management
Tracheobronchial injuries Tracheobronchial trees are well protected, so it normally takes a large amount of force to injure them.	Severe subcutaneous emphysema Difficulty in breathing Dysphonia and abnormal breath sounds **Diagnosis:** Bronchoscopy is diagnostic	Intubation of unaffected bronchus followed by operative repair. Chest drain insertion on the affected side
Esophageal Injury Esophageal injuries are partial tear or complete disruptions of the esophagus that subsequently lead to leakage of intraluminal contents into the surrounding mediastinum. This causes sepsis that results in significant morbidity and mortality Esophageal injury is a rare but challenging clinical finding in the setting of trauma.	Odynophagia (pain on swallowing food or fluids) Unexplained fever Subcutaneous or mediastinal emphysema Pleural effusion Air in paraesophageal space **Diagnosis:** A combination of esophagogram in decubitus position and esophagoscopy to confirm diagnosis. CT scan with oral contrast	The mortality rate rises exponentially if treatment is delayed. Operative repair and drainage.
Diaphragmatic injury Any penetrating injury below the fifth intercostal space should raise suspicions of diaphragmatic penetration Blunt injury to the diaphragm is usually caused by compressive force over the pelvis and abdomen	**Signs and symptoms** **Early complications** Dyspnea Decreased breath sound Paradoxical movement of abdominal wall **Late complications** Abdominal pain Intestine obstruction Audible bowel sounds in chest area **Following investigations are helpful in diagnosis:** Chest radiography after insertion of a nasogastric tube may be diagnostic Contrast studies of upper or lower gastrointestinal tract CT scan abdomen Diagnostic peritoneal lavage Video assisted thoracoscopy (VATS) OR laparoscopy most accurate evaluation.	Operative repair is recommended in all cases **ICD** insertion if pneumo or hemothorax

(Continued)

Type of injury	Clinical features and diagnosis	Management
Blunt myocardial injury **B**lunt myocardial injury may cause cardiac wall rupture, transient arrhythmias	**A**rrhythmias and hypotension **P**ericardial friction rub **A**n S3 gallop rhythm **Crepitations are heard in lung fields** **E**levated central venous pressure **N**on specific chest pain arising from non cardiac chest structures **Diagnosis:** **E**KG, Holter monitoring **I**ncreased level of cardiac enzymes **2**D echo show wall motion abnormalities Transesophageal (TEE) or transthoracic (TTE) echocardiogram.	**P**roper cardiac evaluation Appropriate cardiac monitoring and treatment is to be given as per symptoms. Cardiac wall rupture repair once the patient is stabilised.

ABDOMINAL TRAUMA

1. In the patients with blunt trauma abdomen, solid organs often sustain contusion or laceration, causing bleeding that may require surgical management.
2. Force of blunt trauma can cause rupture of hollow viscera due to rapid compression of segments of intestine containing fluid and air.

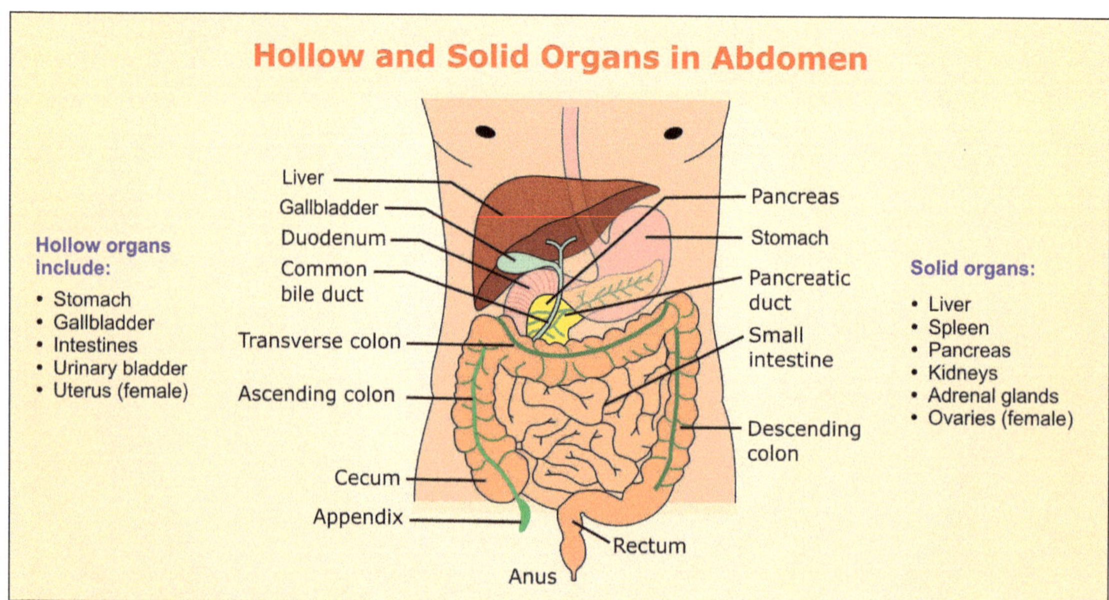

3. In penetrating injury, direct laceration of solid or hollow viscera, results in bleeding and intra-abdominal contamination that often require surgical repair.

4. **Classification of injuries:**
   a. **Blunt trauma**
   b. **Penetrating trauma**
      1. **Stab injury**
      2. **Gunshot injury**
   c. **Iatrogenic trauma**

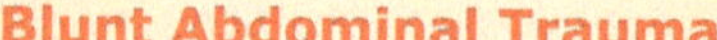

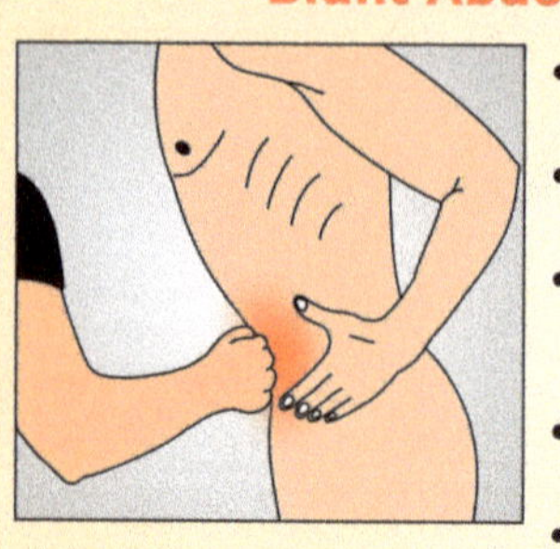

- Direct impact or movement of organs
- Compressive, stretching or shearing forces are involved
- Solid organs often sustains contusion or laceration causing bleeding
- Rupture of hollow organs containing air and fluid
- Retroperitoneal>Often asymptomatic initially

5. **Management**
   a. **Initial resuscitation**:
      1. Proper position of patient
      2. Spine and neck immobilisation
      3. **ATLS principles of resuscitation should be followed:**

      A Airway B Breathing C Circulation D Disability (Neurology) E Environment and Exposure.

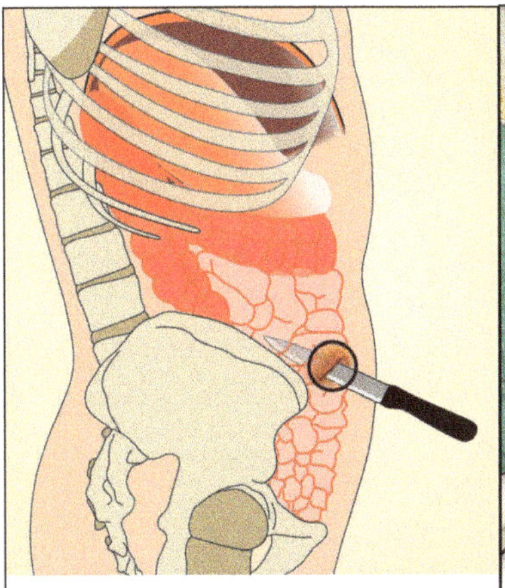
Penetrating injury of the abdomen

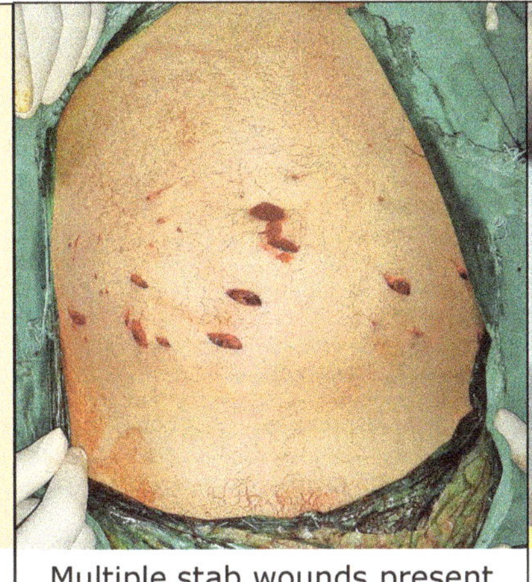
Multiple stab wounds present over abdomen

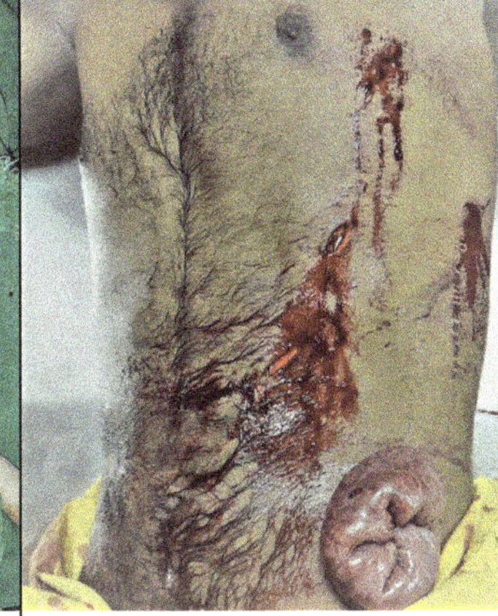
Stab injury over the abdomen with evisceration

4. Rapid assessment for blood loss in abdomen
5. Intravenous fluids (Crystalloid solution) and blood product (If indicated) to support cardiovascular function in shock.
6. **In case of penetrating injury:** Retained foreign bodies transversing the abdominal wall should be maintained throughout the initial evaluation and protected from excessive movement.
7. Pain control by Intravenous analgesics
8. Insert foleys catheter and RT tube
9. Tetanus toxoid prophylaxis
10. Intravenous antibiotics covering aerobic and anaerobic bacteria.
11. Rectal examination for bleeding and for any injury.
12. Prompt transfer to operative room when needed.

b. **Abdominal trauma patients can generally be classified into the following categories depending on their hemodynamic condition:**

Hemodynamically 'normal'	Complete investigation can be done
Hemodynamically 'stable'	Investigation is more limited and aimed to understand whether the patient can be managed non-operatively or whether surgery is required.
Hemodynamically 'unstable'	Investigations need to be suspended as immediate surgery required.

6. **History and Physical examination:**

a. S - Symptoms

b. A - Allergies

c. M - Medication

d. P - Previous history

e. L - Last meal

f. E - Events

7. **Inspection:**

Signs	Refers to	Suggest the diagnosis
Grey turner sign	Bluish discoloration of lower flank, lower back	Retroperitoneal bleeding of pancreas, kidney and pelvic fracture
Cullen sign	Bluish discoloration around umbilicus	Peritoneal bleed Pancreatic hemorrhage
Kehr sign	Shoulder pain while supine caused by diaphragmatic irritation	Splenic injury, free air, intra-abdominal bleeding
Balance sign	Dull percussion in LUQ	Sign of splenic injury Blood accumulation in sub capsular or extracapsular spleen

Kehr Sign

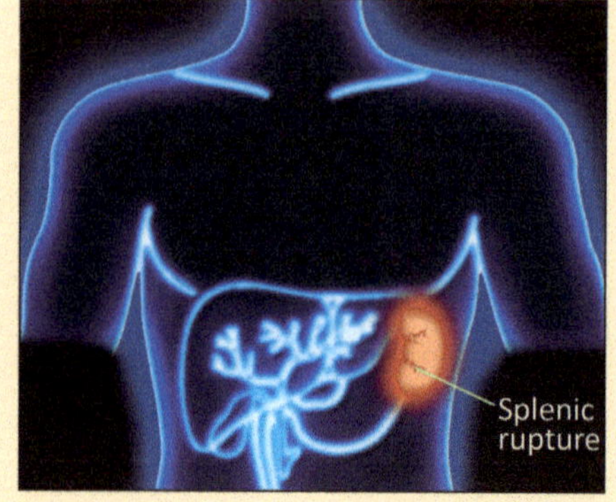

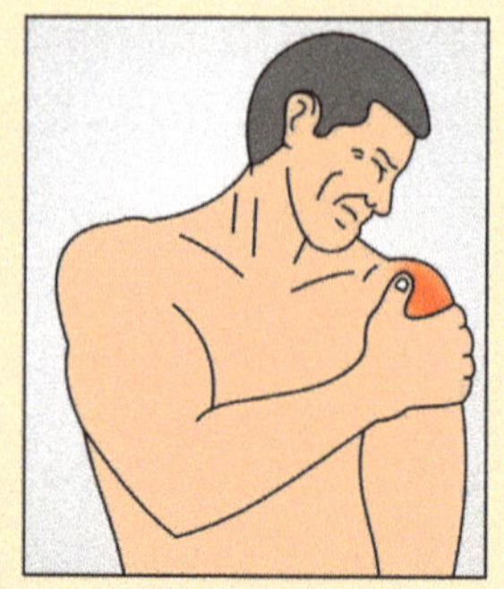

Sign of splenic injury

Referred pain in to left shoulder

- **Kehr sign**- is symptom of pain near tip of left shoulder, due to referred pain from the diaphragmatic irritation
- Because of diaphragmatic irritation due to hemoperitoneum
- P/A- generalised tenderness or LUQ tenderness
- Patient may present with tachycardia, tachypnea, anxiety, hypotension due to hemorrhegic shock

8. **Investigation:**
   a. **Blood investigation:**
      1. Complete blood count, Hb
      2. Blood grouping and cross matching
      3. Random blood sugar
      4. Arterial blood gas
      5. Serum creatinine
   b. **Radiological and ancillary diagnostic investigation**
      1. Local wound exploration if penetrating injury
      2. Chest X-ray and X-rays of extremities for fractures
      3. Focused abdominal sonar for trauma (FAST)
      4. Deep peritoneal lavage (DPL)
      5. CT scan
      6. Urethro-cystography
      7. Intravenous pyelography (IVP)
9. **Investigation and finding**
   a. **X-ray abdomen:**
      1. **Ground glass appearance:** Massive hemoperitoneum
      2. **Obliteration of psoas shadow:** Retroperitoneal bleeding
      3. **Free air under diaphragm:** Perforation
      4. **Lower rib fracture:** Possibility of liver/splenic injury
   b. **Chest X-ray:** Pneumothorax, Hemothorax
   c. **Pelvic X-ray:** For pelvic fracture
   d. **Focused assessment sonar for trauma (FAST)**
      1. Used to assess the presence of free blood in abdominal cavity or in pericardium
      2. Focused in 6 areas: Pericardium, areas around the liver, spleen, left and right paracolic gutter, Peritoneal space in the pelvis (pouch of Douglas)
      3. Detect >100 ml of blood or free fluid
      4. **Advantage**
         - Early diagnosis
         - Non invasive

- Performed rapidly
- Repeatable

e. **CT scan:**

CT scan of abdomen showing splenic laceration with hemoperitoneum

Splenic rupture

Splenic rupture

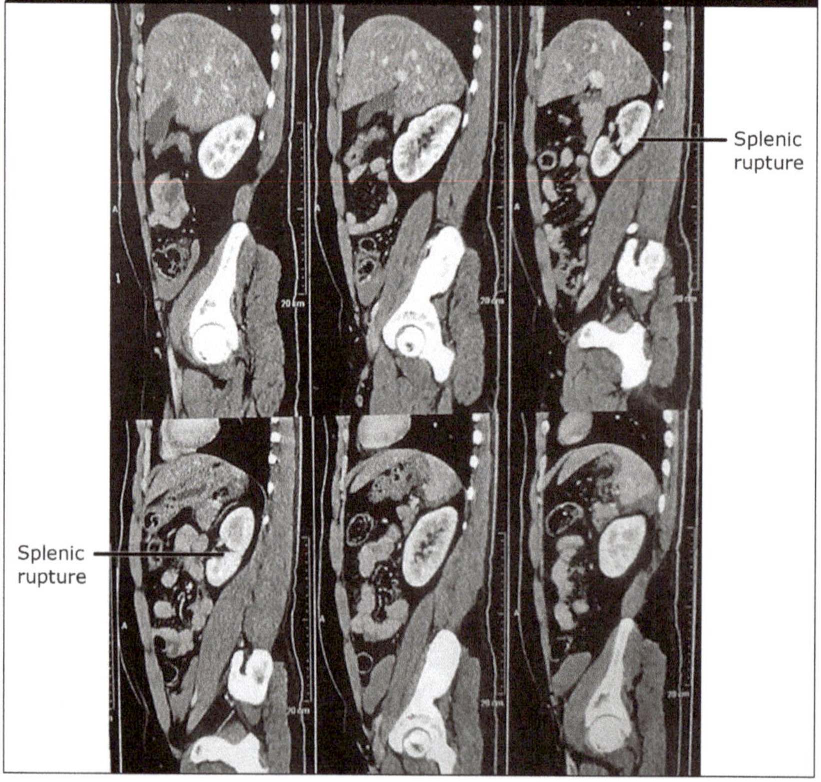

Resected specimen of rupured spleen due to trauma

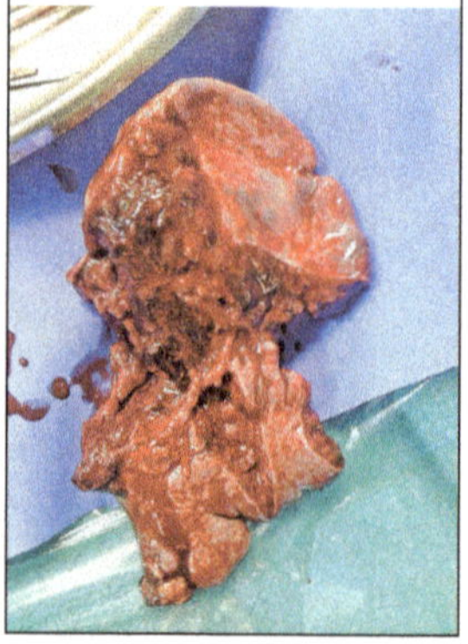

CT scan of abdomen in coronal view showing liver laceration with hemoperitoneum

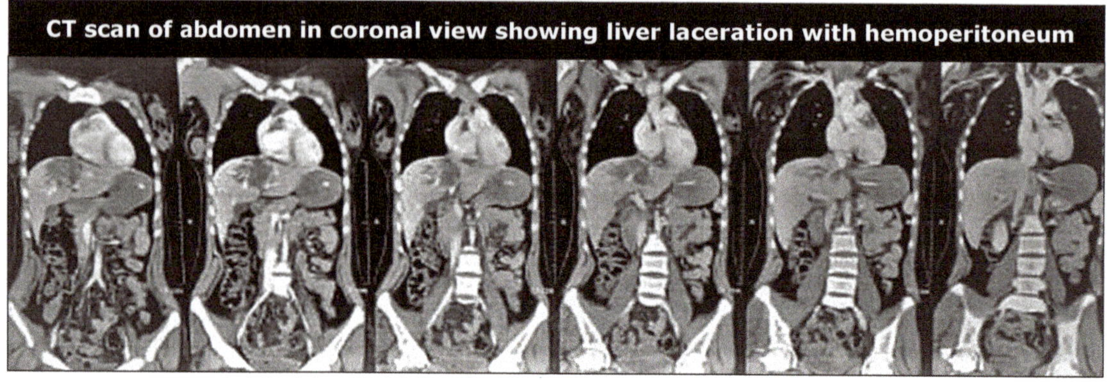

CT scan abdomen in horizontal view showing liver laceration

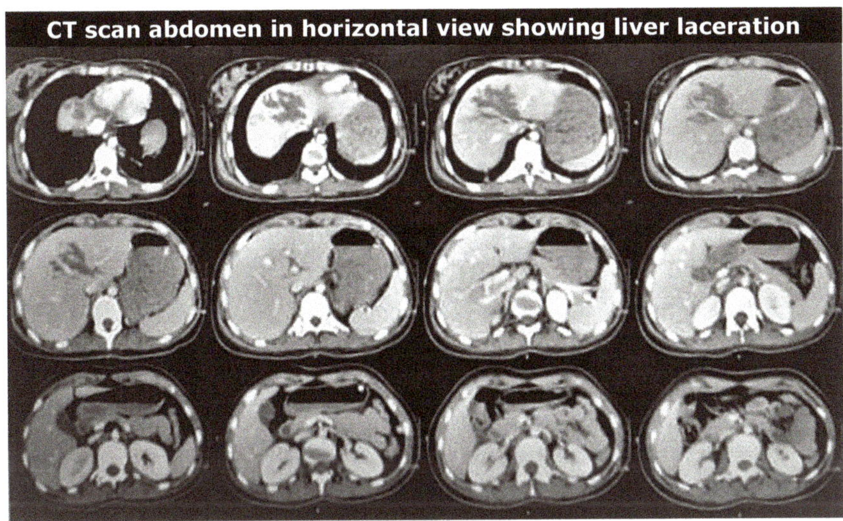

1. Gold standard for the intra-abdominal diagnosis of injury in a stable patient
2. Sensitive for blood, individual organs, retroperitoneal injury.
3. Abdominal CT is mostly performed with IV administration of a contrast agent
4. Abdominal CT provides the necessary visualization of the solid organs to allow the determination of injury severity, including the presence of active bleeding.
5. 3D imaging CT is also useful to visualize the retroperitoneum.
6. **Disadvantages:**
   - Less sensitive to detecting injuries to the hollow viscera.

f. **Diagnostic peritoneal lavage:**

1. **Indication**
   - If FAST is not available.
   - If imaging is equivocal
   - If changes in abdominal examination or vitals with negative initial imaging
   - If cannot be safely transported from the resuscitation bay for investigation
2. **Advantages**
   - Early diagnosis
   - Performed rapidly
   - Detects bowel injury

3. **Disadvantages**
   - Invasive procedure
   - Low specificity

10. **Management:**

a. **Steps to be followed in Blunt abdominal trauma management:**

1. Initial resuscitation as per ATLS guidelines as mentioned above.
2. Investigation depending on the hemodynamic status of the patient whether to suspend or do complete work up.
3. The patient's hemodynamic condition is often more important for the need of laparotomy than the presence of injury alone.
4. Any patient with significant abdominal trauma whether stable or unstable, blood group and cross match should be sent immediately & blood and blood products are kept ready for emergency availability.
5. If a patient is unstable and there is a significant drop in hemoglobin or the patient becomes pale, emergency blood & blood product transfusion is needed.
6. All patients will undergo evaluation, exploratory laparotomy is performed if indicated.
7. Patients who are unstable and have peritoneal fluid identified on USG (FAST) require emergent laparotomy to manage active bleeding.
8. If FAST scan is not available in the hospital, diagnostic peritoneal lavage done if revealing 10 ML or more of gross blood suggests an intra abdominal bleeding with shock requiring emergency operation.
9. The presence of peritonitis is also an indication for immediate patients requiring surgical exploration.
10. Continuous reassessment is done in patients with significant abdominal trauma if initial negative imaging.
11. Serial examinations of the abdomen is important to know worsening tenderness and peritoneal irritation and
12. If changes in the imaging or positive DPL or changes in abdominal findings with change in hemodynamic stability then explorative laparotomy is done.
13. Repair of individual organs during exploration of abdomen
14. Damage control surgery protocol to be followed if the patient is unstable.

b. **Steps to be followed in Penetrating abdominal trauma management:**

1. Any penetrating injury that could have entered the peritoneal cavity or retroperitoneum inflicting causing damage to the abdominal contents.

2. Penetrating abdominal injury can be due to stab injury or gunshot injury
3. **Stab injury:**
   - In anterior abdominal stab injury, determine whether the wound enters the peritoneal cavity by visually exploring the wound.
   - Local exploration done by infiltrating local anesthesia, after which the wound is prepped and draped.

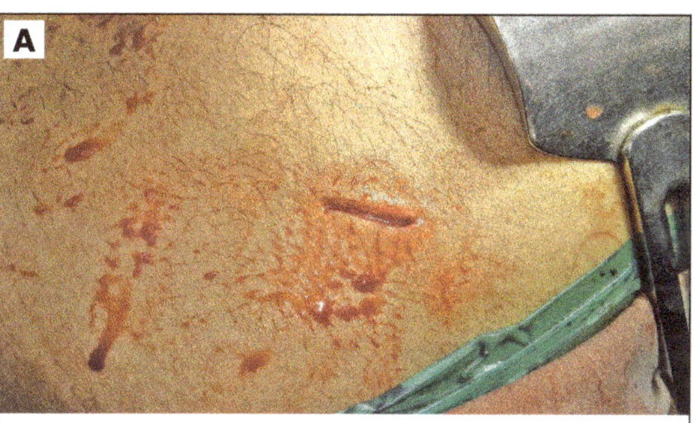

(A) Stab injury to abdomen

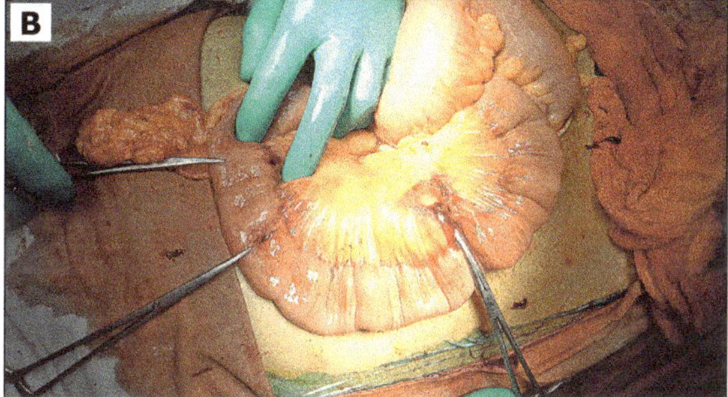

(B) Intraoperative photo showing stab injury causing injuries to bowel and mesentery

   - Detailed wound examination findings should be documented for medicolegal purpose.
   - The wound is extended if necessary to allow a visual inspection of the wound to determine its depth
   - If the wound does not penetrate the anterior fascia, then the wound can be debrided, irrigated and closed and the patient may be discharged, if no other injuries exist.
   - If the local wound exploration reveals any evidence of possible anterior fascial penetration then patients should be monitored with serial abdominal examinations and laboratory investigations for any changes.
   - All patients with anterior fascia penetration who are not taken for the operation should be admitted for observation.
   - Patients with hemodynamic instability, presence of peritonitis, or evisceration require immediate laparotomy
   - Laparotomy is also indicated in patient with gross hematemesis or blood from nasogastric tube
   - The development of peritonitis, hemodynamic instability, significant decrease in the hemoglobin level, or leukocytosis should be promptly evaluated and usually such patient requires laparotomy.
   - Laparoscopy can be used to know the presence of peritoneal penetration, which can be then followed by laparotomy to repair of injury.

4. **Gunshot injury:**
   a. Generally, the entry wounds for an abdominal injury extend from the fifth intercostal space to the perineum.
   b. Gunshot injury involving the upper abdomen may also require evaluation of the chest for mediastinal, pleural or pulmonary injuries.
   c. Injury identified with radio-opaque markers and plain radiographs to determine their location and relation to missile position.
   d. 3D CT scan of abdomen/chest or both is useful to understand injury track, injured organs and vital structures including the vertebral column, spinal cord, pelvis and blood vessels.
   e. All gunshot wounds with path or other evidence of intraperitoneal penetration or retroperitoneal organ injury require immediate operative intervention.
   f. Such patients should be explored under C -arm guidance only.
   g. Forensic opinion is required for medico legal purpose

11. **Exploratory laparotomy:**
   a. **Indication for exploratory laparotomy:**
      1. **Clinical:**
         - Obvious peritoneal signs on physical examination
         - Hypotension with distended abdomen
         - Abdominal gunshot wound with peritoneal penetration
         - Abdominal stab wound with evisceration, hypotension or peritonitis
      2. **Paraclinical**
         - Positive FAST with hemodynamic instability or DPL
         - Finding with any other diagnostic intervention.
   b. A laparotomy is performed to explore the abdomen and to repair the injured abdominal organs and other structures that are identified
   c. It is important that the exploration of the abdomen be performed systematically to avoid missing injuries that may be subtle.
   d. As standard technique, the abdomen is opened from the xiphoid process to the pubic symphysis to provide adequate exposure.
   e. When the injuries are identified they are repaired with admissible techniques.
   f. The development of physiologic compromise lead to the need to shorten the operation and to proceed with damage control surgery.
   g. This decision is to be taken by the surgery and anesthesia team.

h. If the operation can be completed without conversion to damage control, then abdominal fascia is closed.

12. **Damage control surgery:**

    a. Damage control is a staged process.

    b. Stages involved in damage control surgery as follows:

        1. **Patient resuscitation**
        2. **Control of hemorrhage and control of contamination**
        3. **Resuscitation continued in the intensive care unit for physiological stabilisation**
        4. **Definitive surgery**

    c. The initial focus is hemorrhage control, followed by control and limitation of contamination.

    d. Damage control surgery includes simple ligation of bleeding vessels, therapeutic packing, shunting of major arteries and veins, drainage, temporary stapling of bowel and therapeutic packing are used.

    e. Then the abdomen is closed temporarily (If suitable) or left open with a dressing/bogota bag to cover the abdomen.

    f. Suction/Vac dressing can be applied to collect abdominal fluid.

    g. As soon as damage control has been achieved, then the patient is transferred to the intensive care for resuscitation.

    h. The next stage following damage control surgery and physiological stabilisation is definitive surgery.

    i. In definitive surgery team will perform definitive anastomoses, vascular reconstruction and closure of the body cavity is done within 24–72 hours of injury.

APPROACH IN ACUTE ABDOMEN

1. Acute abdomen is most common cause of surgical emergency admission
2. Acute abdomen includes conditions which are varying from trivial to life threatening.
3. In any patient with an acute abdomen the main aim is to identify the patients requiring immediate resuscitation and treatment.
4. Some patients with acute abdomen may present with septic or hypovolemic shock depending on etiology of acute abdomen which need resuscitation and treatment
5. So, proper history, clinical examination and radiological investigation is needed for proper diagnosis and management
6. **Differential causes of acute abdomen**

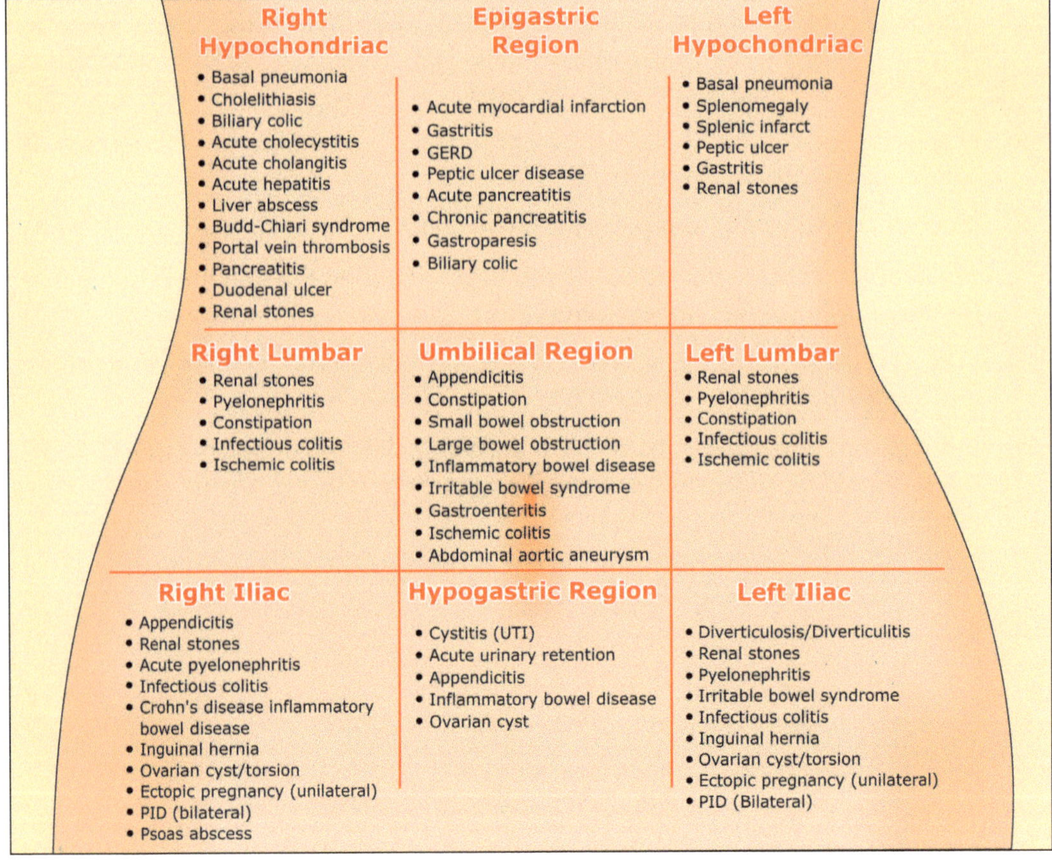

7. **History**
   a. **Abdominal pain:**
      1. **Determine the site**

2. **Mode of onset** (Explosive i.e. within seconds (Perforation, stones, torsion), rapidly progressive i.e. within 1-2 hours, gradual i.e. over several hours)
3. **Character** (Colicky, burning, throbbing, agonising)
4. **Severity** (Pain intensity score)
5. **Frequency** (Continuous, intermittent or occasional)
6. **Radiation and shift:**

Surgical cause	Pain begins at	Pain spread/shift to
acute appendicitis	Umbilicus	Right iliac fossa
In duodenal ulcer perforation	Epigastrium	Entire abdomen
Acute pancreatitis	Epigastrium	Back

7. **Timing**
   a. In duodenal ulcers pain improves after meal but becomes severe in evening or night
   b. In gastric ulcers pain intensifies after meals
8. **Aggravating and relieving factors** (Colicky pain relieved by pressure and inflammatory pain aggravated by pressure).

b. **Vomiting:**

1. **Character of vomiting** (Projectile or regurgitant)
2. **Frequency** (Repetitive and profuse in acute pancreatitis and Intestinal obstruction; periodical and infrequent in duodenal ulcer perforation)
3. **Quantity and Association with pain and nausea**
4. **Nature of vomitus** (Gastric, bilious, intestinal, feculent or blood stained).
5. **Vomiting that follows the onset of abdominal pain tends to imply a surgical cause**
6. **Whereas vomiting preceding pain is often non surgical**

c. **Bowel disturbances: Constipation** (Mechanical bowel obstruction), **bleeding, diarrhea** (IBD, ischemic colitis)

d. **Urinary disturbances:** Hematuria, hesitancy, painful urination

e. **Other symptoms:** Fever, chills and rigors

f. **Past history** (Medical, surgical, gynecological, medications, personal history, travel history)

8. **Physical examination**

a. **General examination:** Appearance, vitals (Pulse, BP, RR, hydration, temperature), pallor, cyanosis, Icterus.

b. **Abdominal examination:**

1. Inspection (Movement with respiration, skin, contour, visible peristalsis, hernial orifices)
2. Palpation (Tenderness, guarding and rigidity)
3. Percussion (To check free fluid)
4. Auscultation (Bowel sounds are increased in early phase of intestinal obstruction)

c. **Digital examination of rectum**

d. **Examination of external genitalia**

e. **Pervaginal examination**

9. **Investigations**

a. **Radiological investigations**

b. **Specific investigations as per the differential diagnosis.**

ACUTE GASTRITIS

1. **Definition:** Gastritis is an inflammation of the lining of the stomach.
2. **Classified according to the underlying etiology:**
   a. **H. Pylori gastritis:** Colonization of the gastric mucosa with Helicobacter pylori results in the development of chronic gastritis
   b. **Erosive gastritis:** This is due to erosion of gastric mucosa commonly caused by NSAIDs, alcohol
   c. **Reflux gastritis:** This is caused by enterogastric reflux (Biliary reflux)
   d. **Stress gastritis:** This is due to reduction of the blood supply to superficial mucosa of the stomach
   e. **Autoimmune gastritis:** It occurs due to destruction of parietal cells of stomach by circulating antibodies
   f. **Other rare forms of gastritis:** Lymphocytic gastritis, Eosinophilic gastritis, Granulomatous gastritis, Acquired immunodeficiency syndrome (AIDS) gastritis, Phlegmonous gastritis
3. **Diagnosis:**
   a. Based on the patient's description of his symptoms
   b. Urea breath test for Presence of H. pylori
   c. Endoscopy, to check for stomach lining inflammation and mucous erosion
4. **Treatment:**
   a. **For mild gastritis antacids are prescribed:** Neutralise acid pepsin formation

      E.g. milk of magnesia, magnesium hydroxide, aluminium hydroxide.
   b. **H2 blocker and proton-pump inhibitors:** When antacids do not provide enough relief then these are prescribed that help reduce the amount of acid production.
   c. **Mucosal barrier:** Formation of protective coat e.g. sucralfate
   d. **H pylori infection eradication.**
5. **Complications of gastritis**
   a. **Bleeding**
   b. **Gastric ulcers**
   c. **Gastric cancer:** Gastric ulcers may become malignant and an ulcerated gastric cancer may mimic a benign ulcer.

PEPTIC ULCERS

1. **Definition:** Erosions in the lining of the stomach or duodenum caused by the digestive action of pepsin and stomach acid.
2. **Types:**
   a. **Gastric ulcer**
   b. **Duodenal ulcers**
3. **Pathophysiology:**
   a. Normally, there is a balance between the aggravating factors and defensive mechanism.
   b. When balance is disturbed, it leads to mucosal injury and thus peptic ulcer.

Defensive factors	Aggravating factors
Bicarbonate secretion	H. pylori infection
Local Prostaglandins	NSAIDs
Epithelial cells renewal	Pepsins
Mucus production	Bile acids
Sub-mucosal blood flow	Smoking and alcohol

4. **Risk factors or etiological factors:**
   a. **Lifestyle**: Smoking, alcoholic, acidic drink, medications like NSAIDs
   b. **H. pylori**: Found in 90% of peptic ulcers
   c. **Age:**
      1. Duodenal ulcer is common in 30-40 age group
      2. Gastric ulcer is common in over 50 years
   d. **Genetic factors**: Positive history in the family
   e. **Stress ulcer**: Develop after major surgery or traumatic injury (**"Cushing ulcer"**), burns (**"Curling ulcer"**), or severe infections
5. **Difference between the gastric ulcer and duodenal ulcers:**

	Gastric ulcer	Duodenal ulcer
Age	Middle age specially 40-50	At Any age but specially 30-40
Sex	More common in female	More common in male
Pain	Epigastric region can be referred to back	Epigastric discomfort
Onset	Immediately after eating	2-3 hours after eating
Aggravated by	After Eating	On fasting
Relieved by	Lying down or vomiting	Eating
Vomiting	Common	Uncommon

6. **Investigation:**
    a. **Complete blood count**
    b. **Stool examination**: For examination of fecal occult blood
    c. **Diagnostic Endoscopy:** EGD (esophagogastroduodenoscopy) to visualise the ulcers and to take biopsy to rule out cancer
    d. **Urea breath test:** To detect H. Pylori infection
    e. **Barium swallow:** To visualise the upper GI
    f. **Alarming signs for endoscopy to rule out cancer**
        1. Dysphagia
        2. Weight loss
        3. Vomiting
        4. Anorexia
        5. Melena and hematemesis
7. **Management:**
    a. **Lifestyle modification:** Discontinue alcohol, smoking cessation, decrease NSAIDs use, reduction of stress
    b. **Hyposecretory drug therapy:**
        1. **H2 receptors antagonists:**

            Decrease the histamine stimulated gastric secretion

            E.g. Ranitidine, Cimetidine, Famotidine
        2. **Proton pump inhibitors:**

            Decreases acid secretion

            E.g. Omeprazole, Rabeprazole, Pantoprazole
        3. **Antacids:**

            Neutralise acid pepsin formation

            E.g. Milk of magnesia, Magnesium hydroxide, Aluminium hydroxide.
        4. **Prostaglandin analog:**

            Decrease acid secretion and mucosal resistance

            E.g. Misoprostol
        5. **Mucosal barrier:**

            Formation of protective coat

            E.g. Sucralfate

c. **H pylori eradication: Triple therapy for 10-14 days**

PPIS + Metronidazole (500 mg) + Clarithromycin (500mg)

PPIS + Clarithromycin (500 mg) + Amoxicillin (1 gm)

d. **Surgery**: Principle is to decrease the acid and pepsin secretion.

1. **Indication:**
    - Failure to medical therapy
    - Development of complications

8. **Complication of peptic ulcers:**

a. Hemorrhage

b. Perforation

c. Narrowing and deformity of stomach

d. Gastric outlet obstruction

LIVER ABSCESS

1. Liver abscess is formation of suppurative cavity in the liver resulting from the invasion and multiplication of the microorganism in the liver parenchyma.
2. **Two main etiology for liver abscess:**
   a. **Amebic**
   b. **Pyogenic**
3. Both these types are important causes of mortality and morbidity in tropical countries.
4. **Classification of liver abscess**
   A. **Pyogenic abscess**
   B. **Amebic abscess**
   C. **Fungal abscess (Less common)**
   D. **Iatrogenic abscess**

A. PYOGENIC ABSCESS

1. Etiology is unexplained in most cases but some frequent conditions which are involved in development of pyogenic abscess are Cholelithiasis, appendicitis and diverticular disease.
2. Incidence is higher in elderly, diabetic and immunocompromised individuals.
3. Mixed growth of organisms is commonly associated in pyogenic abscess.
4. The most commonly involved organisms are Escherichia coli, staphylococcus aureus, enterococcus and klebsiella pneumoniae.
5. The right lobe of the liver is more commonly affected.
6. **Clinical presentation:**
   a. Fever with chills
   b. Anorexia and weight loss
   c. Right quadrant tenderness on palpation
   d. Nausea and vomiting
   e. Jaundice
   f. Involvement of the diaphragm may result in symptoms of cough or dyspnea
   g. Rupture may lead to peritonitis.

7. **Involved Investigation:**

   a. **Laboratory investigation**

      1. **Complete blood count:** Neutrophilic leukocytosis and Anemia.
      2. **Erythrocyte sedimentation rate:** Increased ESR count
      3. **LFT**: Deranged i.e. Increased ALP (Alkaline Phosphatase), Increase in total bilirubin

         Hypoalbuminemia or mild elevations of the PT and INR can be present and reflect a degree of chronicity.
      4. **Culture and sensitivity:** Aspirated fluid for the microbiological diagnosis.

   b. **Specific investigation:** Most essential element to establish the diagnosis of hepatic abscess is radiographic imaging.

      Ultrasound and CT are the mainstays of diagnostic investigations for hepatic abscess.

      1. **Sonography:** Cystic mass is seen on ultrasound.
      2. **CT scan:** The diagnosis is suggested by the finding of a multiloculated cystic mass on CT scan.

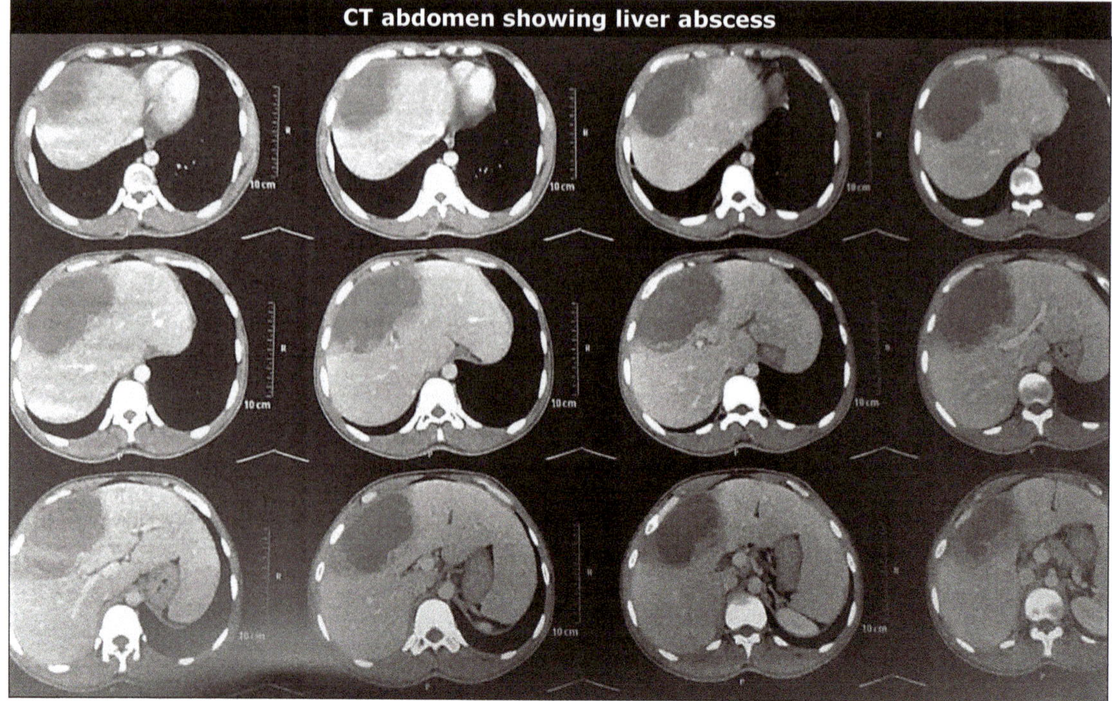
CT abdomen showing liver abscess

8. **Treatment:**
    a. **Medical treatment**
        1. **Analgesic and antipyretics**
        2. **Broad spectrum antibiotics:** 1st line antibiotics used are penicillin, aminoglycoside and metronidazole Or cephalosporins and metronidazole
        3. **Specific antibiotics:** According to culture sensitivity
        4. **Fluid resuscitation:** To prevent hepatorenal syndrome
    b. **Drainage**
        1. **Percutaneous drainage:** USG guided or CT guided drainage done
            a. **Needle aspiration**
            b. **Catheter drainage**
        2. **Surgical drainage:**
            a. **Open**
            b. **Laparoscopic**
            c. **ERCP in case of biliary obstruction**

B. AMEBIC LIVER ABSCESS

1. Amebic liver abscess is an inflammatory space occupying lesion of the liver
2. Causative parasite is Entamoeba histolytica.
3. Ingestion of E. histolytica cysts through a fecal-oral route is the cause of amebiasis.
4. Humans are the principal host, and the main source of infection is human contact with a cyst-passing carrier
5. Contaminated water and vegetables are also the sources of infection
6. Trophozoites reach the liver through the portal venous system.
7. Most common site is para-cecal and liver.
8. **Clinical presentation:**
    a. **Abdominal pain** (Right hypochondrium which may be dull or pleuritic)
    b. **Fever**
    c. **Abdominal tenderness**

d. **Hepatomegaly**

e. **Anorexia**

f. **Weight loss**

g. **Diarrhea**

h. **Jaundice** (Not a common finding but a large abscess can cause compression of bile ducts and produce obstructive jaundice at a later stage)

i. **Thumping sign:** Hepatomegaly with intercostal tenderness is a characteristic finding but may be absent in deep or centrally located lesions.

9. **Investigation:**

a. **Complete blood count:** A mild to moderate leukocytosis without eosinophilia. Anemia is also common in chronic cases.

b. **Liver function test:** Mild abnormalities include fall in albumin, elevated PT INR, elevated ALP, AST and bilirubin levels.

c. **Stool examination:** Trophozoites is usually negative, at least 3 stool specimens should be evaluated after concentration and staining.

d. **Ultrasonography:** Gold standard test for liver abscess

e. **CT scan/ MRI scan:** Abdominal CT scanning is probably more sensitive than ultrasound and is helpful in differentiating amebic from pyogenic.

CT scan also detects signs of colitis.

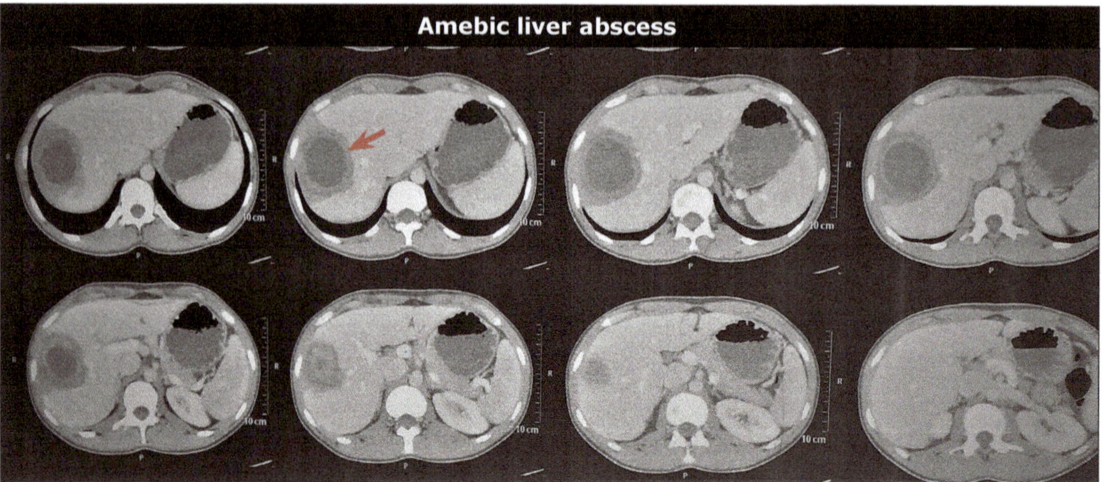
Amebic liver abscess

f. **Amebisis Serological test:** Indirect hemagglutination IHA and ELISA tests for amebiasis are confirmatory tests. A negative IHA should be repeated after one week and if found again negative then it definitely rules out amebic abscess.

g. **Diagnostic aspiration:** When diagnosis is uncertain and there is a high possibility of the pyogenic abscess then aspiration is done for gram staining and culture which will help in diagnosis.

10. **Treatment:**

a. **Medical:**

1. **Relief of pain and fever with analgesics**

2. **Drug therapy (Amebicidal drugs):**

a. Treated empirically by metronidazole 400-800 mg TDS for 7-10 days.

b. Other nitroimidazole used in treatment includes secnidazole, tinidazole or ornidazole.

c. **Second line alternatives:** Emetine hydrochloride and chloroquine 500 mg bid for 2 days and then 500 mg daily for 3 weeks should be reserved for non-responder.

3. Resolution of the abscess can be monitored using ultrasound.

b. **Surgical**

1. **Aspiration of abscess:**

- Routine aspiration is not indicated in the abscess as it does not change the disease course, most of the patients respond well to medical therapy.
- Repeated aspiration should be avoided to avoid the conversion of amebic liver abscess into the pyogenic abscess.
- **It can be done in following situations:**

i. No response to medical line management for 5 days

ii. Impending rupture, the thin rim of size < 1 cm between abscess and liver capsule on USG.

iii. Abscess in the left lobe of the liver carries a higher risk of rupture so it is aspirated to avoid rupture.

iv. Large abscess of size > 10 cm

v. When distinction from the pyogenic abscess and amebic abscess is uncertain.

c. **Catheter drainage:** To treat the abscess with complications like rupture.

11. **Complications & management:**

a. **Pleuropulmonary rupture/abscess:** Drainage and medical therapy.

b. **Hepato-bronchial abscess:** Abscess ruptured in the lungs: Drainage and antiamebic therapy.

c. **Rupture of abscess into peritoneum:** Percutaneous catheter drainage and antiamebic therapy.

d. **Rupture of abscess into pericardium:** Pericardiocentesis and medical therapy

e. **Rupture with generalised peritonitis**

f. **Rupture with localised peritonitis**

ACUTE CHOLANGITIS

1. Acute cholangitis is due to an acute, ascending infection of the biliary tree caused by an obstruction.
2. Cholangitis can be life-threatening and delay in appropriate treatment results in multiorgan failure secondary to septicemia.

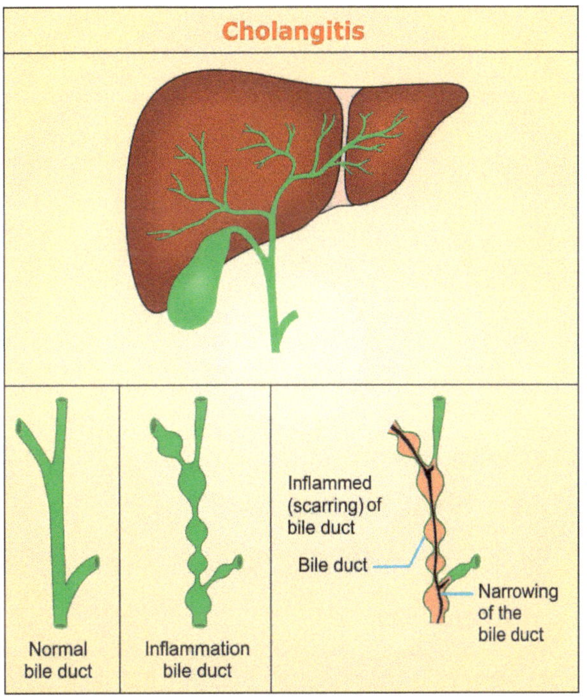

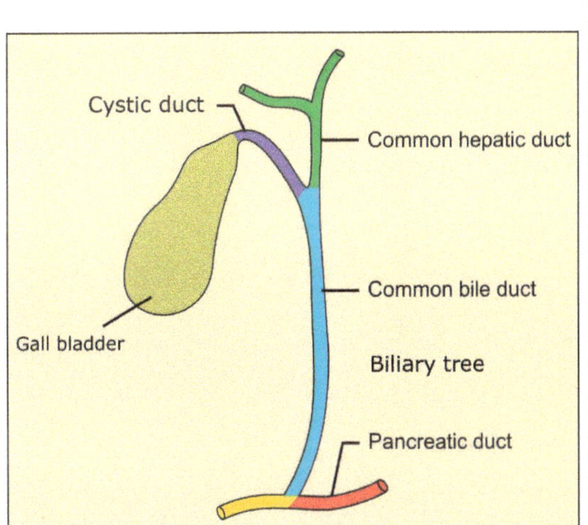

3. **Two absolute requirements for the development of acute cholangitis:**
   a. **Bacteria in biliary tree (**Klebsiella, E. coli, enterobacter, pseudomonas, or citrobacter spp)
   b. **Obstruction of flow with increased intraluminal pressure (Stones, malignant neoplasm).**

Clinical features:

1. Abdominal pain (Particularly in the right upper quadrant of the abdomen), fever, rigors (uncontrollable shaking) and a feeling of uneasiness (Malaise)
2. Classical presentation of cholangitis is that of charcot triad, with **fever, jaundice, and right upper quadrant pain.**
3. When infection begins to manifest with shock, then two additional finding seen
   a. **Septic shock**
   b. **Mental confusion**

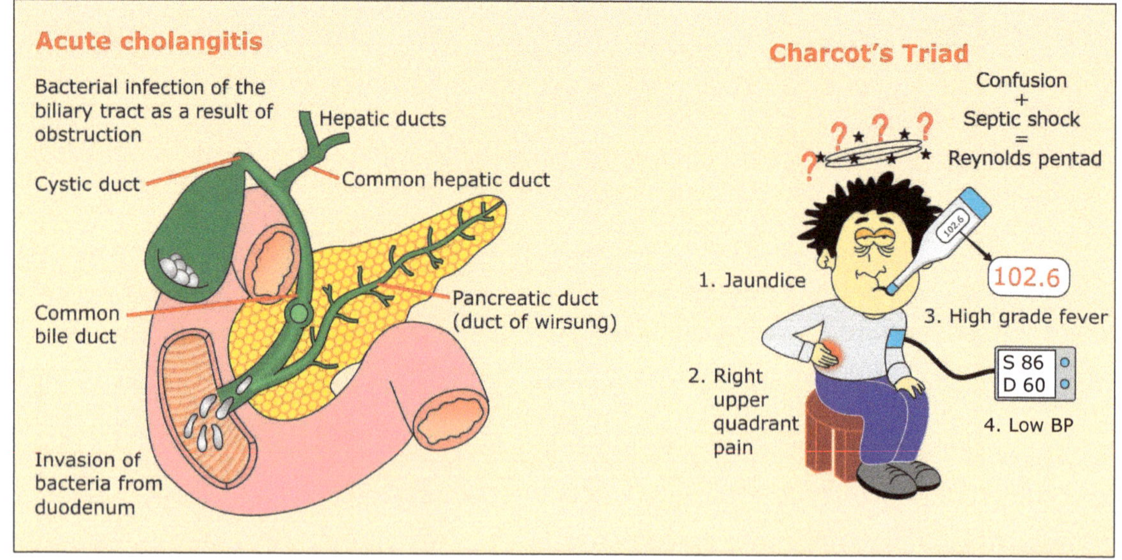

4. **Charcot's triad** associated with above two additional findings is known as **Reynolds pentad**.

5. **Investigation:**

   a. **Blood investigation:**

      1. **Complete blood count:** Leukocytosis (Infection and inflammation)

      2. **CRP:** Elevated level (Inflammation and infection)

      3. **Liver function test:** Elevated serum transaminase and alkaline phosphatase levels. (Hepatocellular damage due to infection and obstruction).

      4. **Blood cultures** are often performed in people with fever and evidence of acute infection.

   b. **Specific investigation:**

      1. **Abdominal sonography:** Commonly show dilation of the biliary tree

      2. **Cholangiography:** This procedure is useful for identification of obstruction site, cause of obstruction and biliary drainage.

      3. **Magnetic resonance cholangiopancreatography (MRCP):** Non invasive procedure having a comparable

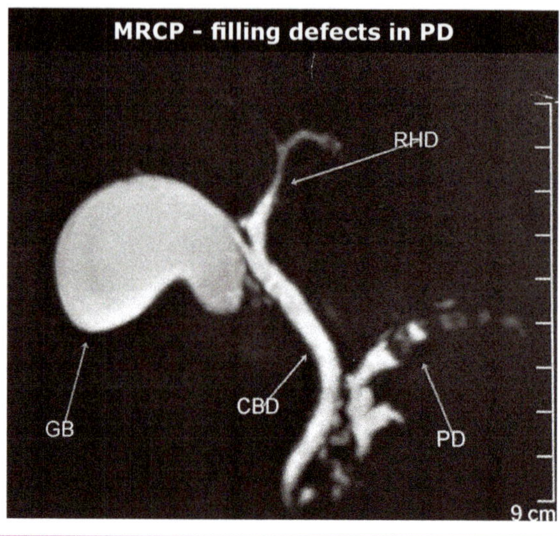

sensitivity to ERCP, but small gallbladder stones can be missed.

4. **CT scan with IV contrast: Useful to diagnose acute cholangitis and type of obstruction.**
5. **HIDA scan (**Hepatic iminodiacetic acid scan):
    1. In atypical cases, a HIDA scan may be used to demonstrate obstruction of the cystic duct.
    2. Scan is performed with Tc-99m DISIDA (Given intravenously)
    3. In acute cholecystitis no visualisation of the gallbladder is due to edema of cystic duct so dye does not enter in gallbladder
    4. In biliary tree, infection reduces the secretion of these agents so used cautiously.
6. **Bile fluid & pus for culture and sensitivity.**

6. **Treatment:**
    a. Patient should be managed actively in intensive care unit as it may progress quickly to septic shock.
    b. Start intravenous fluid resuscitation to maintain adequate hydration
    c. Analgesics to relieve pain
    d. Monitor blood pressure, heart rate and urine output
    e. Start intravenous antibiotics: Blood culture should be taken into consideration before antibiotics are started.
    f. Empirical treatment with broad spectrum antibiotics is usually started until antibiotics sensitivity report.
    g. Any one of the following procedures can be used for biliary tree decompression and to permit normal drainage of bile:
        1. Endoscopic
        2. Percutaneous
        3. Surgical: T-tube placement
    h. Definitive treatment of etiology
7. **Complications:**
    a. Septic shock
    b. Multiorgan failure

ACUTE CHOLECYSTITIS

1. **Definition:** Acute bacterial inflammation of the gallbladder with or without stone.
2. More than 90% of the time acute cholecystitis is from blockage of the cystic duct by a gallstone.
3. Primary pathophysiologic event in a cholecystitis is the obstruction of cystic duct and infection is secondary event that follows stasis and inflammation.
4. Most cases of acute cholecystitis is complicated by superinfection of inflamed gallbladder.
5. **Types of cholecystitis**
   a. **Calculus**
   b. **Acalculus**

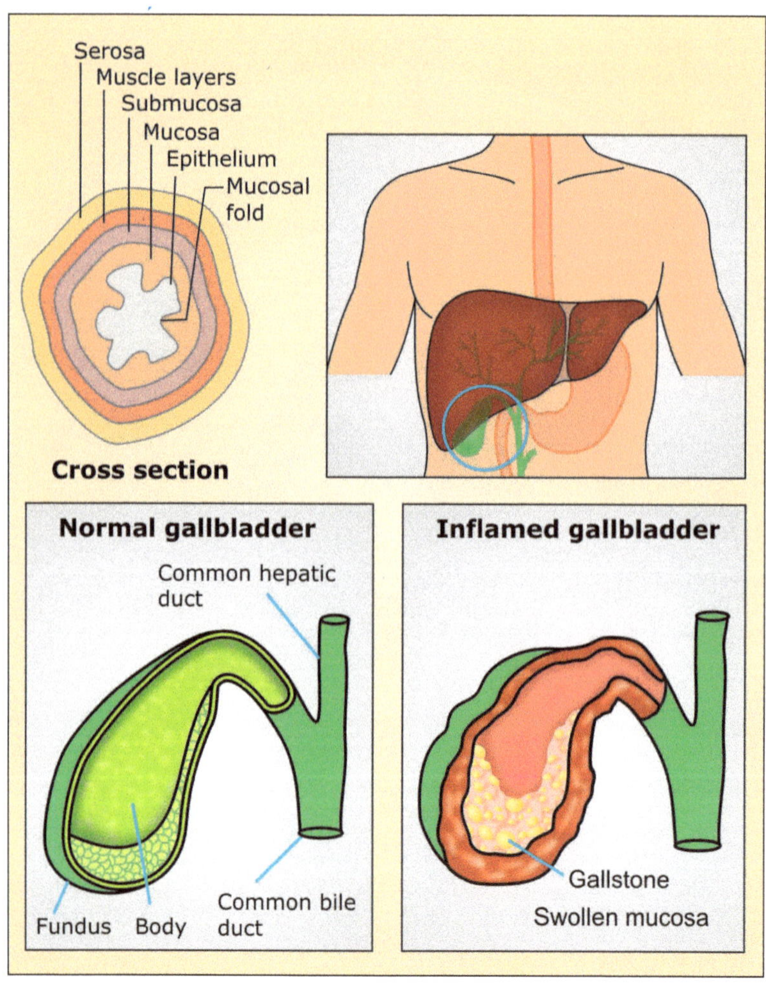

ACUTE CALCULUS CHOLECYSTITIS

1. It is the obstructive cholecystitis due to gallstones
2. Blockage of bile flow due to gallstones causing an enlarged, red & tense gallbladder. Without resolution of obstruction, the gall bladder progresses to ischemia and necrosis.
3. **Modes of infection**
   a. **Hematogenous**
   b. **Through portal vein**
   c. **Through bile**
4. Clinical features
   a. **Symptoms:**
      1. **Pain:**
         - Intense pain occurs in the right upper quadrant of the abdomen, in addition to this referred pain in the right shoulder.
         - In some patients pain may radiate to the back.
         - Pain is colicky but in most cases it is dull and constant.
         - The pain is usually severe and may last for minutes or even several hours. Frequently, the pain starts during the night or after a heavy meal.
      2. Fever
      3. Nausea, vomiting are also common.
      4. Anorexia
      5. Other symptoms include dyspepsia, flatulence, change in bowel habits.
      6. Jaundice may result, if stone obstructs the common bile duct.
      7. Rarely, a gallstone can lead to bowel obstruction (gallstone ileus).

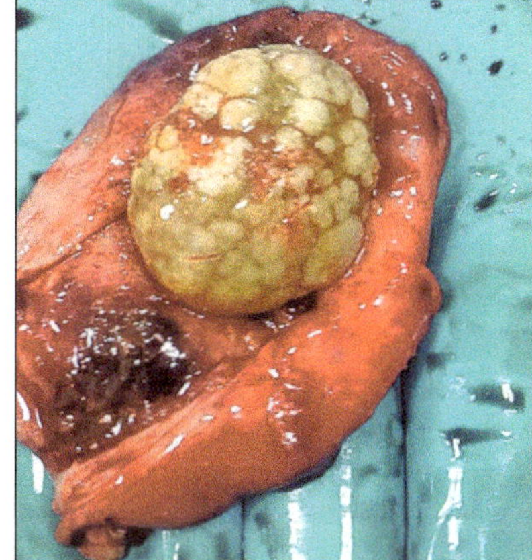

Resected specimen of inflamed gall bladder with gall stone

   b. **Signs:**
      1. **Murphy sign:**
         - Keep the finger on the right hypochondrium and tell a patient to take a deep breath. At the height of inspiration, there is a sudden catch on breathing.
         - It is due to inflamed gallbladder
      2. **Boas sign:** Feeling of hyperesthesia between 9th and 11th ribs posteriorly on right side.
      3. **Palpable tender gallbladder**
      4. **Guarding and Rigidity of upper abdominal wall**

5. **Investigation:**

   a. **Laboratory studies:**

      1. **Complete blood count:** Leukocytosis is present
      2. **Liver function test:** Mild elevation of bilirubin, ALP, SGOT, SGPT

   b. **Transabdominal ultrasonography:**

      1. Identifying gallstones, gall bladder thickening, and can show pericholecystic fluid
      2. Sonographic Murphy's sign
      3. It is the most sensitive, inexpensive and reliable tool for diagnosis of acute cholecystitis

   c. **HIDA scan (**Hepatic iminodiacetic acid scan): In atypical cases, a HIDA scan may be used to demonstrate obstruction of the cystic duct.

      1. Definitely diagnose the acute cholecystitis.
      2. Scan is performed with Tc-99m DISIDA (Given intravenously)
      3. In acute cholecystitis no visualisation of the gallbladder is due to edema of cystic duct so dye does not enter in gallbladder

   d. **CT scan:**

      1. CT is less sensitive than ultrasound for diagnosis of acute cholecystitis.

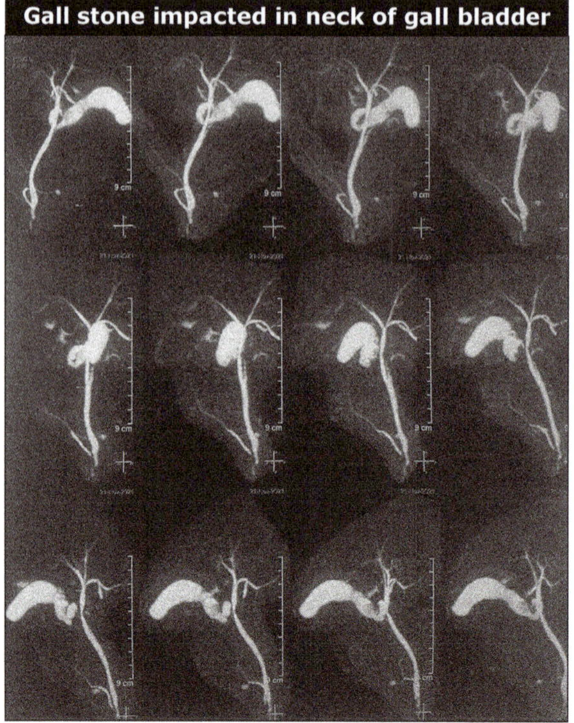

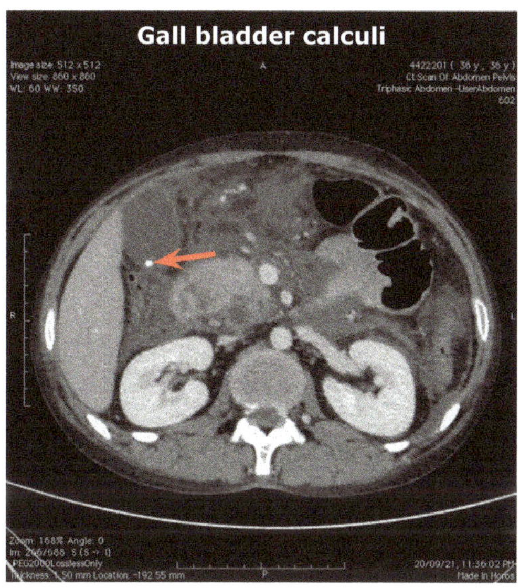

Gall bladder calculi

2. CT may show similar findings to ultrasound with pericholecystic fluid, gallbladder wall thickening and emphysematous gall bladder.

6. **Diagnosis:** It is based on the history, clinical examination and radiological investigations

7. **Management:**

   a. Admission

   b. Nil by mouth

   c. IV fluids

   d. Parenteral broad spectrum antibiotics started

   e. Analgesics (Parenteral narcotics are usually required to control pain)

   f. Antispasmodics

   g. **Finally cholecystectomy:** Open or laparoscopic is the treatment of choice

      1. **Early cholecystectomy:** Early removal of the gallbladder, preferably within the first few days.

      2. **Interval cholecystectomy:** Performed approximately 6 weeks after initial episode.

   h. **Some patients present with acute cholecystitis but have a high operative risk:** In these patients, a percutaneously placed cholecystostomy tube should be considered.

   i. Percutaneous drainage results in improvement in symptoms and hemodynamic stability.

   j. Finally delayed cholecystectomy 3 to 6 months after medical fitness for surgery.

8. Complications of acute cholecystitis:

a. **Perforation**

b. **Peritonitis**

c. **Pericholecystic abscess**

d. **Pancreatitis**

e. **Empyema**

f. **Septicemia**

g. **Cholangitis**

h. **Gangrenous gallbladder**

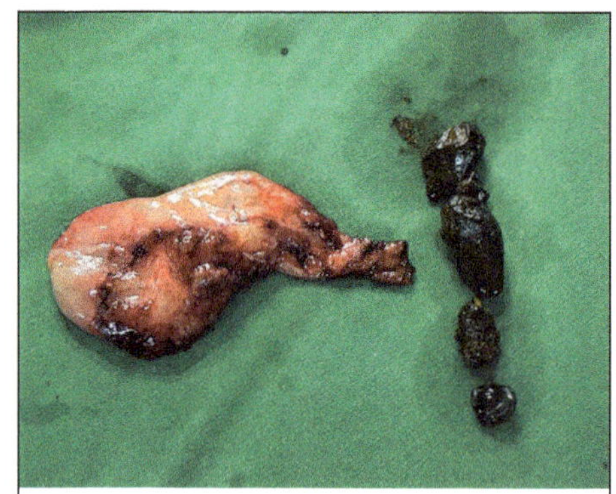

Cholecystectomy specimen - showing gall bladder with stones

ACUTE ACALCULUS CHOLECYSTITIS

1. Inflammation of gallbladder is known as acute cholecystitis.
2. In acalculus cholecystitis, there is no stone in the biliary duct & still there is blockage of gall bladder.
3. Acalculus cholecystitis is typically seen in people who are hospitalized and critically ill
4. It has a more fulminant disease course and may progress to gangrene and perforation of the gallbladder.
5. Development of acalculus cholecystitis is associated with older age, critical illness, burns, trauma, prolonged use of total parenteral nutrition, diabetes and immunosuppression.
6. **Clinical features:**

   a. Most of the patients are critically ill, possibly septic

   b. **Pain:**

      1. Pain in the right upper quadrant, additional to this the right shoulder pain may be present.
      2. It may radiate to the back
      3. It is colicky but more often is dull and constant.
      4. The pain is usually severe and may last for minutes or even several hours. Frequently, the pain starts during the night or after heavy meal.

   c. Fever

   d. Nausea, vomiting are also common.

   e. Anorexia

   f. Other symptoms include dyspepsia, flatulence, food intolerance particularly to fats and some alteration in bowel frequency.

7. **Investigation:**
   a. **USG scan:** The gallbladder will show a significantly thickened wall with pericholecystic fluid
   b. **CT scan:** Shows similar findings like ultrasonography
   c. **HIDA scan:** Definitely diagnose obstruction of cystic duct
8. **Treatment:**
   a. Admission in ICU.
   b. Nil by mouth (NPO)
   c. Intravenous fluids administration
   d. Parenteral broad spectrum antibiotics started.
   e. Analgesics (Parenteral narcotics are usually required to control pain)
   f. Antispasmodics
   g. Cholecystectomy is either laparoscopic or open if repeated attack.
   h. If the patient is unstable for surgery then the percutaneous drainage of the distended and inflamed gallbladder is carried out.
   i. The cholecystostomy tube used to drain the gallbladder can be placed by ultrasound or CT scan guidance, 90% of patients will improve with percutaneous drainage
   j. If in follow up studies no stones are observed then generally, interval cholecystectomy is not needed.

ACUTE PANCREATITIS

1. Pancreatitis is inflammation of the pancreas.
2. For clinical purposes, it is useful to divide the pancreatitis into acute condition which is emergency condition and chronic, which is prolonged and frequently lifelong disorder resulting from development of fibrosis & calcification within the pancreas.
3. Acute on chronic pancreatitis is a phase of chronic pancreatitis.

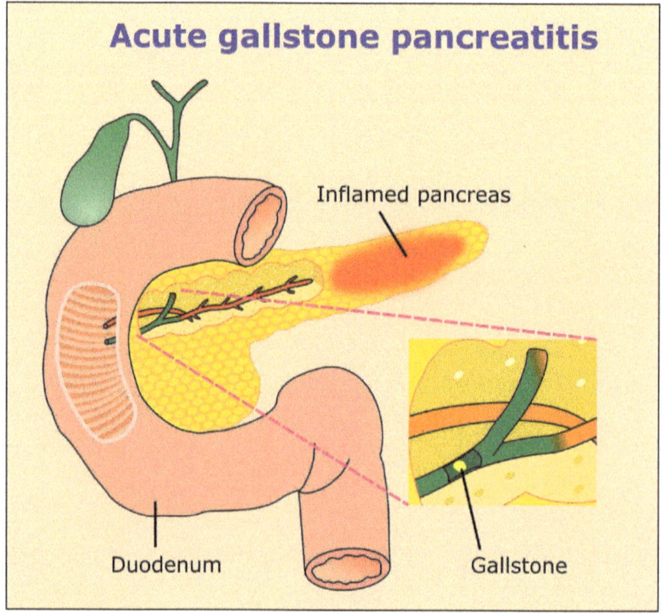

ACUTE PANCREATITIS

1. **Definition:** An acute condition presenting with abdominal pain and is usually associated with raised pancreatic enzyme levels in the blood or urine as a result of pancreatic inflammation
2. The most common cause of death in this patient is multiorgan dysfunction syndrome.
3. **There are two main types:**
   a. **Acute pancreatitis**
   b. **Chronic pancreatitis.**
4. **In ATLANTA classification acute pancreatitis is classified in three groups:**
   a. **Mild acute pancreatitis**
      1. No organ failure

2. No local or systemic complications

b. **Moderately severe acute pancreatitis**

1. Organ failure that resolves within 48 hours (transient organ failure) and/or
2. Local or systemic complications without persistent organ failure.

c. **Severe acute pancreatitis**

1. Persistent organ failure (> 48 hours);
2. Single organ failure,
3. Multiple organ failure.

5. **Etiology:**

The two most common causes of acute pancreatitis are a gallstone blocking the common bile duct and heavy alcohol use.

a. **Gallstones** 50–70%
b. **Alcohol** 25%
c. **Congenital**: Pancreatic divisum
d. **Metabolic**: Hyperlipidemia, hypercalcemia.
e. **Toxic**: Scorpion bite
f. **Viral infection**: Mumps, coxsackie B
g. **Abdominal trauma**
h. **Autoimmune**: Hereditary pancreatitis.
i. **Post ERCP**
j. **Ampullary tumor**
k. **Drugs**: Estrogen, thiazides, corticosteroids, valproate
l. **Idiopathic**

6. **Symptoms:**

a. **Pain:**

1. Pain occurs in upper abdominal region
2. It is sudden in onset and remains for hours or even days.
3. Pain is sharp, severe, continuous, radiates to the back
4. Pain may be felt diffusely throughout the abdomen.
5. Some patient gains benefits by leaning forward or seating

b. **Nausea and repeated non projectile vomiting**

   c. **Retching**
   d. **Hiccups** due to gastric distension or gastric irritation
   e. **Fever and weakness**
   f. **Anorexia**

7. **Signs:**
   a. Patient is distressed, moving continuously, or sitting in leaned forward position
   b. Patient is pale, confused
   c. Tachycardia, hypotension
   d. Tachypnea
   e. Low grade fever
   f. Mild icterus in the gallstone induced pancreatitis
   g. Abdominal distension (ileus or more rarely, ascites with shifting dullness)
   h. Patient with significant abdominal distension, generalized rebound tenderness and abdominal rigidity represent severe pancreatitis.
   i. Patient has rebound tenderness, rigidity and muscle guarding over the upper abdomen.
   j. **Grey turner's sign** (Bluish discoloration of flank), **Cullen's sign** (umbilical blue discoloration) and **Fox sign** (Bluish discoloration of upper outer aspect of thigh region)
   k. Above signs are indicative of retroperitoneal bleeding associated with severe pancreatitis.

8. **Differential diagnosis:**

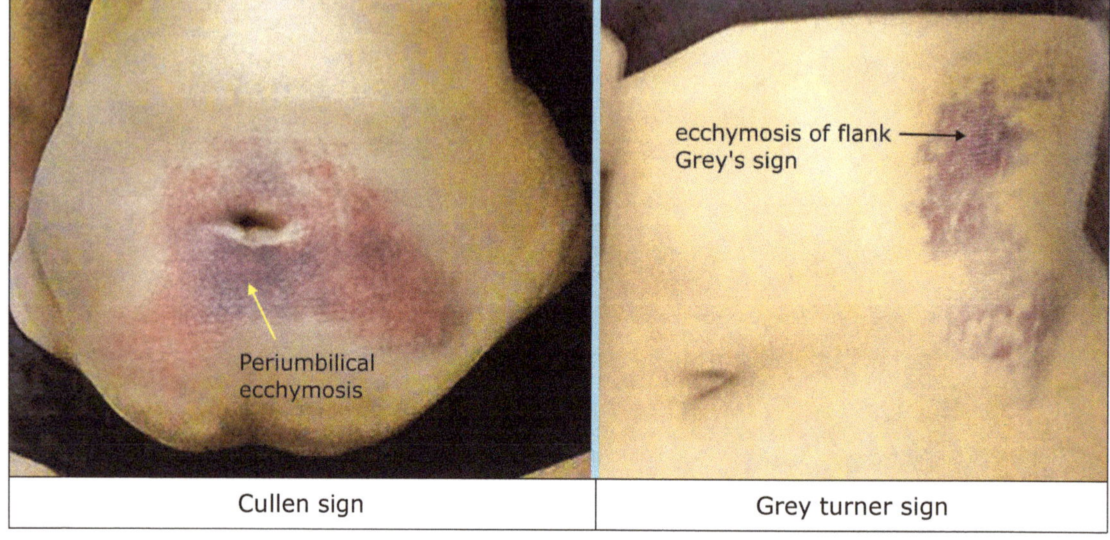

Cullen sign	Grey turner sign

a. Acute cholecystitis, biliary colic
b. Acute intestinal obstruction
c. Renal colic
d. Perforated viscus
e. Mesenteric vascular obstruction
f. Myocardial infarction
g. Basal pneumonia

9. **Investigation:**
   a. **Blood investigation:**
      1. **CBC**: WBC, Hematocrit count
      2. **Serum albumin**
      3. **Serum amylase**
         a. Level more than 3 to 4 fold above normal indicates disease
         b. Normal serum amylase level does not exclude the acute pancreatitis, released within 6-12 hours of the onset & remain elevated for 3-5 days.
         c. To be higher in gallstone pancreatitis
      4. **Serum lipase:**
         a. Slightly more sensitive and specific than the amylase
         b. Useful in patient presenting late to the physician
         c. Higher in the alcohol induced pancreatitis.
      5. **Arterial blood gases**
      6. **Renal function test:** Blood urea nitrogen
      7. **Liver function test: AST/ALT level**
      8. **C reactive protein**
      9. **Clotting profile**
      10. **Blood glucose**
      11. **Lipid profile**
      12. **Serum electrolyte**
      13. **LDH level:**
   b. **Radiological investigation:**

1. **Chest X-ray:** Rule out other D/D like pleural effusion and diffuse infiltrate (ARDS)
2. **Abdominal plain X-ray**: Helpful to diagnose & to exclude other causes like obstruction and perforation.
   - **Mild disease:** Localized ileus of a segment of small intestine **(Sentinel loop) -** Observed in acute pancreatitis.
   - **Severe disease:** Abrupt termination of gas filling within the proximal colon at the level of radiological splenic flexure **(Colon cutoff sign)-** Usually related with acute pancreatitis.
3. **Abdominal ultrasound:** Alone cannot establish acute pancreatitis but, combined with elevations of liver transaminase and pancreatic enzyme levels and the presence of gallstones have high sensitivity and specificity for diagnosing acute biliary pancreatitis.
4. **CT Scan:** Contrast-enhanced computed tomography (CT) is currently the best modality for evaluation of the pancreas.

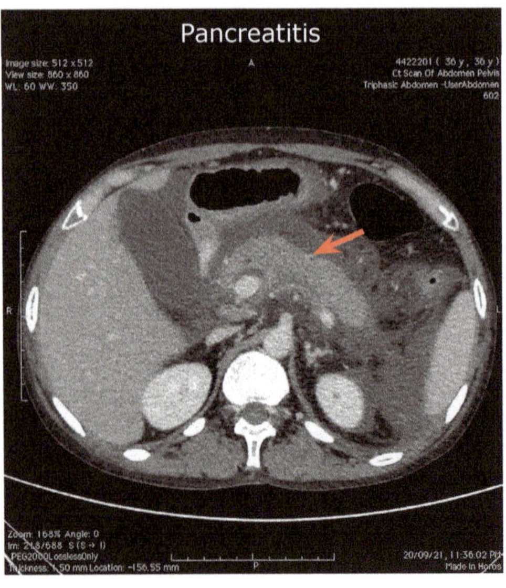

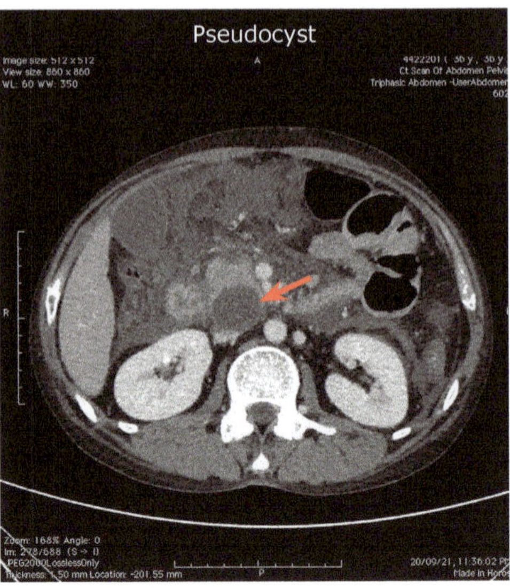

5. **MRCP:** It is used to evaluate the biliary & pancreatic ducts, CBD stone detection and assessment of pancreatic parenchyma.
6. **ERCP:** It is used to identify and remove CBD stone

c. **Investigation should be aimed at answering three questions**

1. For diagnosis of acute pancreatitis
2. How severe is attack of acute pancreatitis
3. What is the etiology of acute pancreatitis

10. Severity of attack:

a. Assessments should be performed in patients at the time of admission, 24 hours, 48 hours and 7 days after admission for severity of attack.

b. The **Ranson and Glasgow** scoring systems are specific for acute pancreatitis, and a score of 3 or more at 48 hours indicates a severe attack

c. **Scoring systems to predict the severity of pancreatitis**

Ranson score
On admission
1. Age >55 years
2. White blood cell count >16000/L
3. Blood glucose >200 mg/dL
4. Lactate dehydrogenase level >350 units/L
5. Aspartate aminotransferase level >250 units/L
Within 48 hours
1. Hematocrit fall of 10% or greater
2. Blood urea nitrogen rise >5 mg/dL(1.8 mmol/L) despite fluids
3. Arterial oxygen saturation (PaO2) <8 kPa (60 mmHg)
4. Serum calcium <2.0 mmol/L
5. Base deficit >4 mmol/L
6. Fluid requirement >6 litres

d.

Glasgow score
Within 48 hours
1. Age >55 years
2. White blood cell count > 15000/L
3. Blood glucose >10 mmol/L (non diabetic case)
4. Lactate dehydrogenase > 600 units/L
5. Serum urea >16 mmol/L (no response to intravenous fluids)
6. Arterial oxygen saturation (PaO2) <8 kPa
7. Serum calcium <2.0 mmol/L
8. Serum albumin <32 g/L

e. **In both systems disease is classified as severe, if three or more factors are present.**

11. **Management: The treatment of pancreatitis is supportive and depends on severity**
    a. **Admission to ICU**
    b. **Analgesia:** Adequate analgesia should be administered
    c. **Antiemetics**
    d. **Prompt intravenous fluid infusion:** Early fluid resuscitation within 24 hours helps to maintain pancreatic perfusion and to avoid secondary organ failure due to hypotension
    e. **Supplemental oxygen:** Patients should receive supplementary oxygen to maintain arterial saturation above 95%
    f. **Monitoring of vitals:** Blood pressure, oxygen saturation, central venous pressure, urine output, blood gases.
    g. **Monitor blood glucose, liver function, renal function, PTINR, serum calcium, arterial blood gases frequently.**
    h. **Central venous catheter insertion:** Often required in patients who do not respond to initial fluid resuscitation or have significant renal, cardiac, or respiratory comorbidities.
    i. **Foleys catheter insertion.**
    j. **Nasogastric tube inserted and nasogastric drainage is done initially.**
    k. **Nutritional support is vital in the treatment of acute pancreatitis.**
    l. Nutritional support is provide with eternal feeding and total parenteral nutrition (TPN).
    m. **Antibiotics:**
        1. If cholangitis suspected; prophylactic antibiotics can be started
        2. Prevents local and other septic complications
        3. Commonly used antibiotics are ceftriaxone/cefuroxime, or ciprofloxacin along with metronidazole or imipenem
        4. Antibiotic therapy is given for 14 days
    n. **Supportive therapy:** In organ failure patients the patients may require inotropic support, ventilatory support, hemofiltration, etc.
    o. CT scan essential if organ failure, clinical deterioration or signs of sepsis develops in patient.
    p. ERCP required within 72 hours for severe gallstone pancreatitis or signs of cholangitis.
    q. In cholangitis and to avoid infective complication, sphincterotomy to be done or biliary stent should be placed to drain the duct.

12. Complications:

a. Systemic complications:

Cardiovascular	Shock, arrhythmias
Pulmonary	Acute respiratory distress syndrome (ARDS)
Renal	Acute renal failure
Metabolic	Hypocalcemia, hypoglycemia, hyperlipidemia
Hematological	DIC
Gastrointestinal	Ileus
Neurological	Visual disturbance, confusion, irritability, encephalopathy
Miscellaneous	Subcutaneous fat necrosis, arthralgia

b. Local complication:

1. Acute peripancreatic fluid collection
2. Sterile pancreatic necrosis
3. Infected pancreatic necrosis
4. Pancreatic abscess
5. Pseudocyst
6. Pancreatic ascites & pancreatico-pleural fistula
7. Pleural effusion
8. Portal or splenic vein thrombosis
9. Pseudoaneurysm of the splenic vein

ACUTE APPENDICITIS

1. **Definition:** Inflammation of an appendix.
2. Acute appendicitis is the most common abdominal emergency.
3. Infections associated with appendicitis should be considered polymicrobial, includes both gram-negative bacteria and anaerobes e.g. Escherichia coli, pseudomonas aeruginosa, anaerobic bacteroides fragilis.

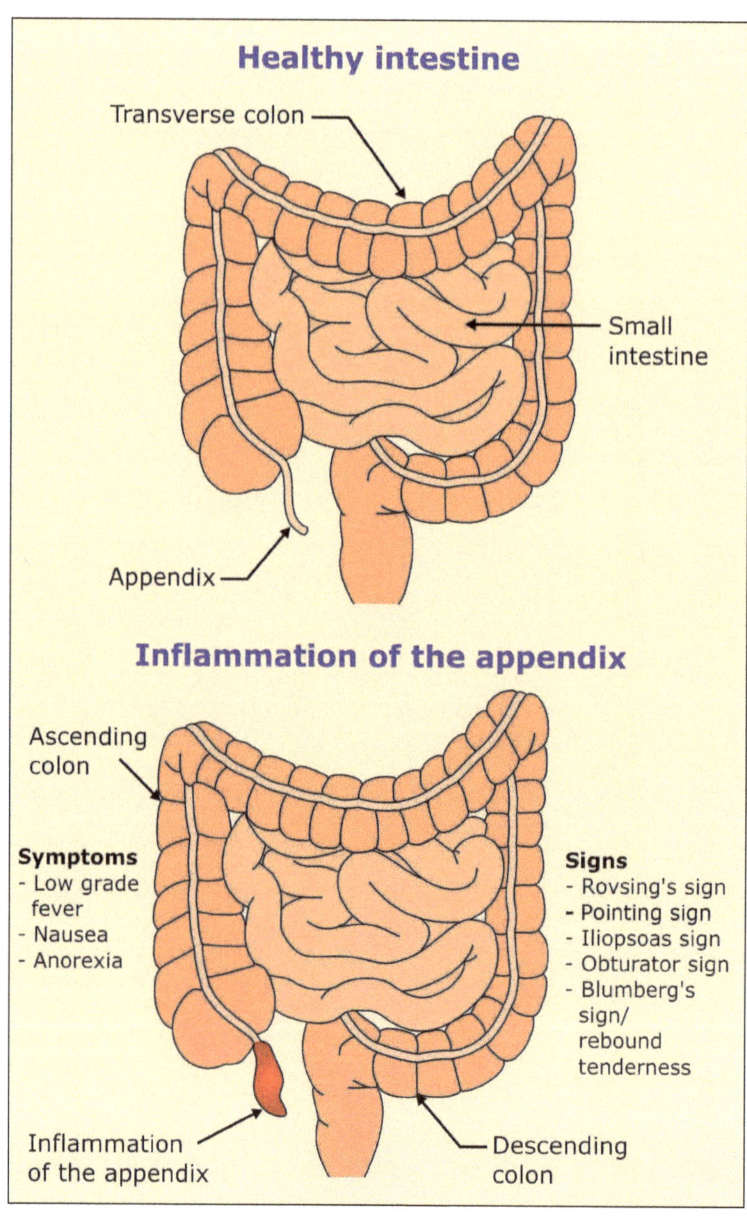

4. **Etiology:**
   a. Appendicitis is caused by luminal obstruction
   b. Decrease in intake of dietary fibre and increased consumption of refined carbohydrate
   c. Luminal obstruction either by the fecolith or stricture
   d. Obstruction of appendicular orifice by tumor, particularly by CA cecum.

5. **Clinical features:**

   As the appendix becomes more swollen and inflamed, it begins to irritate the adjoining abdominal wall which results in symptoms and signs
   a. Initial periumbilical pain migrates to right iliac fossa afterwords
   b. Anorexia
   c. Nausea and vomiting
   d. Sudden pain relief suggestive of rupture of appendix

6. **Clinical signs:**
   a. Pyrexia
   b. Localised tenderness in right iliac fossa at Mc burney's point.
   c. Muscle guarding
   d. Rebound tenderness
   e. Tachycardia: Perforation, gangrene and peritonitis.
   f. Obesity can obscure and diminish all the local signs of acute appendicitis and the clinician may have to remain dependent on imaging to establish the diagnosis.

7. **Signs to elicit the appendicitis:**
   a. Pointing sign: Asked to point to where pain began and where it moved
   b. Rovsing sign: Deep palpation or the left iliac fossa may cause pain in the iliac fossa
   c. Psoas sign: If inflamed appendix lies on the psoas muscle then patient lies with right hip flexed for pain relief.
   d. Obstructor sign: Pain on passive internal rotation of the flexed thigh.
   e. Blumber sign/Rebound tenderness: Patients feels pain after removal of pressure from abdomen.

8. **Differential diagnosis:**

Children	Adult
Gastroenteritis	Regional enteritis
Meckel's Diverticulitis	Pancreatitis
Mesenteric adenitis	Perforated peptic ulcer
Intussusception	Torsion of testis, orchitis
Lobar pneumonia	Ureteric colic
Henoch schonlein purpura	Rectus sheath hematoma

Adult female	Elderly
Pelvic inflammatory disease (PID)	Intestinal obstruction
Pyelonephritis	Diverticulitis (Right sided)
Ectopic pregnancy	Carcinoma of colon
Torsion or rupture of ovarian cyst, tubo-ovarian abscess	Torsion testis, orchitis, renal colic
Endometriosis	Mesenteric infarction

9. **Investigations**

   a. **Preoperative investigation:**

      1. **Routine:**
         - **Full blood count:** Leukocytosis
         - **Urinalysis**
      2. **Selective:**
         - **Pregnancy test:** In reproductive age groups
         - **Urea and electrolyte**
         - **Supine abdominal radiograph**

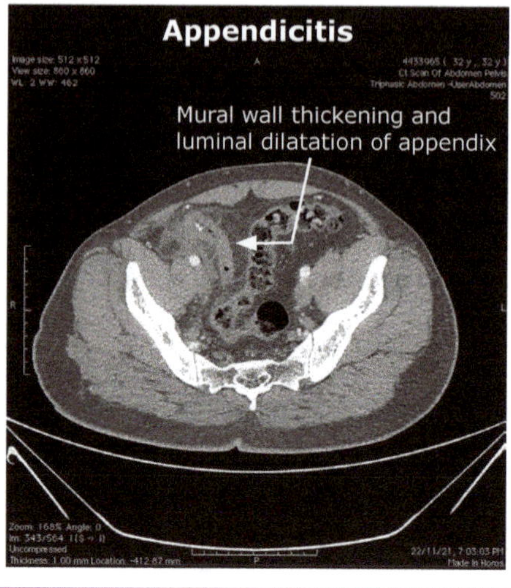

- **Ultrasound of the abdomen:** if clinical diagnosis is equivocal
- **Contrast enhanced CT of abdomen and pelvis:** Especially in equivocal cases

10. **Diagnosis**

a. The diagnosis of acute appendicitis is essentially clinical

b. Number of scoring systems available to assist diagnosis

c. Most widely used scoring system is **Alvarado score & RIPASA Score**.

d. **In patient with equivocal score 5-6:** Patient advised abdominal USG or CT Scan

e. USG scan is more useful in children, thin adults and in some patients if we are suspecting gynecological pathology.

f. CT scan with contrast is useful when there is diagnostic uncertainty particularly in older patients, in whom acute diverticulitis, intestinal obstruction, neoplasm are likely differential diagnosis.

g. **Alvarado score:**

Symptoms	1. Migratory RIF pain	**1**
	2. Anorexia	**1**
	3. Nausea and vomiting	**1**
Sign	4. RIF Tenderness	**2**
	5. Rebound tenderness	**1**
	6. Elevated temperature	**1**
Lab findings	7. Leukocytosis	**2**
	8. Shift to left of Neutrophils	**1**
Total score	To remember (MANTRELS)	**10**

h. **Interpretation:**

<4	Excludes diagnosis
5-6	Equivocal
>7	Strongly suggestive of appendicitis

11. **Treatment of acute appendicitis:**

a. **Rest and NPO**

b. **IV fluid administration**

c. **Analgesics**

d. **Antibiotics:** Usually metronidazole and third generation cephalosporins

e. **Appendectomy:** Types of appendectomy procedures

1. **Conventional/open**
2. **Laparoscopic**

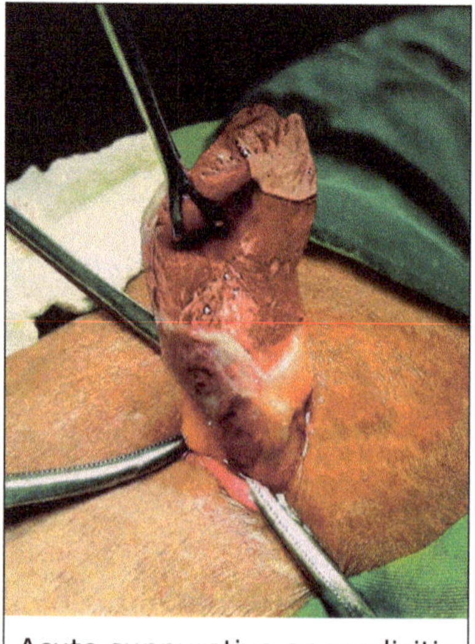

Acute suppurative appendicitis

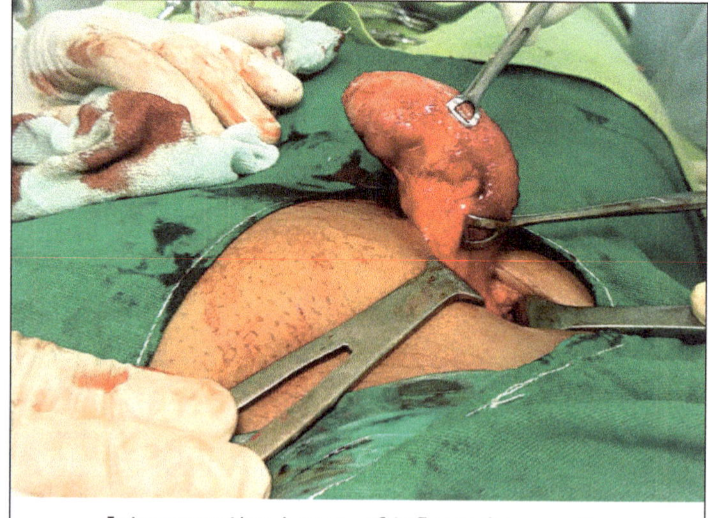

Intraoperative image of inflamed appendix

12. **Indication of appendectomy:**
   a. Acute appendicitis
   b. Recurrent appendicitis
   c. Mucocele of appendix
   d. Carcinoma confined to the mucosa
13. **Appendicectomy can be elective, emergency or interval**

INTESTINAL OBSTRUCTION

1. **Definition**: Intestinal obstruction is a partial or complete blockage of the bowel that prevents the content of the intestine from passing through.
2. A mechanical or functional obstruction of the intestines, prevents the normal movement of the products of digestion.
3. In intestinal obstruction either the small bowel or large bowel may be affected
4. Small bowel obstructions are most often due to adhesions and hernias while large bowel obstructions are most often due to tumors, diverticulosis or volvulus.

Classification:

5. **On the basis of type of obstruction**
   a. **Dynamic obstruction:** In this type peristalsis is working against a mechanical obstruction
   b. **Adynamic obstruction:** In this type there is no mechanical obstruction but peristalsis is absent or inadequate e.g. paralytic ileus or pseudo-obstruction
6. **On the basis of nature:**
   a. **Acute**
   b. **Chronic**
   c. **Acute on chronic**
   d. **Subacute**
7. **On the basis, Whether obstruction is**
   a. **Simple**
   b. **Strangulated**
   c. **Closed loop**
8. **Intestinal obstruction clinically classified into**
   a. **Small bowel obstruction: High or low**
   b. **Large bowel obstruction**
9. **Cause of intestinal obstruction:**

Dynamic obstruction	Causes
1. Intraluminal (In the lumen)	1. Fecal impaction 2. Ingested foreign bodies 3. Bezoars (Trichobezoars & Phytobezoars) 4. Gallstones ileus

(Continued)

Dynamic obstruction	Causes
2. Intramural (In the wall)	1. Stricture 2. Malignancy 3. Intussusception 4. Volvulus
3. Extramural (Outside the wall)	1. Bands/adhesions 2. Hernia 3. Peritoneal metastasis

Adynamic obstruction
1. Paralytic ileus 2. Pseudo-obstruction 3. Spinal injuries 4. Electrolyte imbalance 5. Post operative period

10. Causes of large and small bowel obstruction:

Small bowel obstruction	Large bowel obstruction
1. **Adhesions** (Usually postoperative) 2. **Hernia:** Inguinal, femoral, umbilical, or ventral hernias congenital defects such as paraduodenal, foramen of Winslow, and diaphragmatic hernias or postoperative secondary to mesenteric defects 3. **Neoplastic: Benign or malignant** 4. **Intra-abdominal abscess** 5. **Congenital** a. Malrotation (Volvulus) b. Intestinal duplication c. Cysts d. Atresia or stenosis 6. **Inflammatory** **a. Crohn's disease** **b. Infections:** Tuberculosis, eosinophilic, gastroenteritis Actinomycosis Diverticulitis 7. **Traumatic** Hematoma (Trauma, anticoagulant, blood dyscrasias) Ischemic stricture 8. **Gallstone** 9. **Enterolith** 10. **Bezoar** 11. **Foreign body** 12. **Miscellaneous** a. Intussusception b. Endometriosis c. Radiation enteropathy/stricture	1. Neoplasms/ cancer 2. Diverticulitis/ Diverticulosis 3. Hernias 4. Inflammatory bowel disease 5. Colonic volvulus (sigmoid, cecal, transverse colon) 6. Adhesions 7. Constipation 8. Fecal impaction 9. Fecaloma 10. Colon atresia

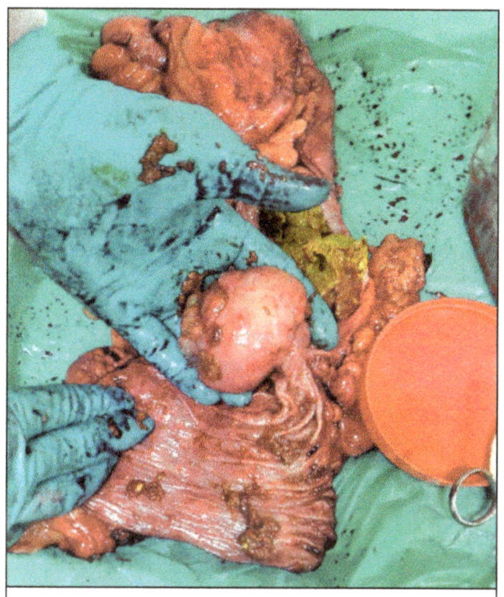
Resected specimen of bowel with polyp causing obstruction

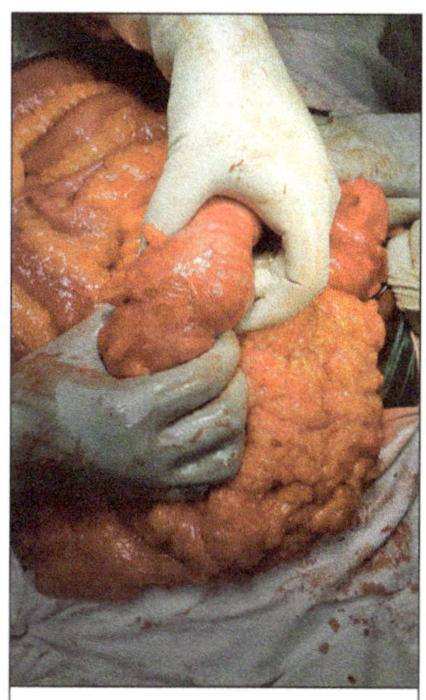
Intraoperative image showing polyp causing obstruction

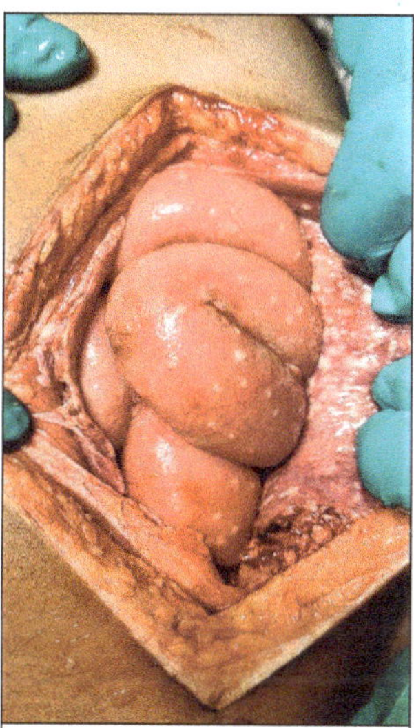
Tubercles on intestine

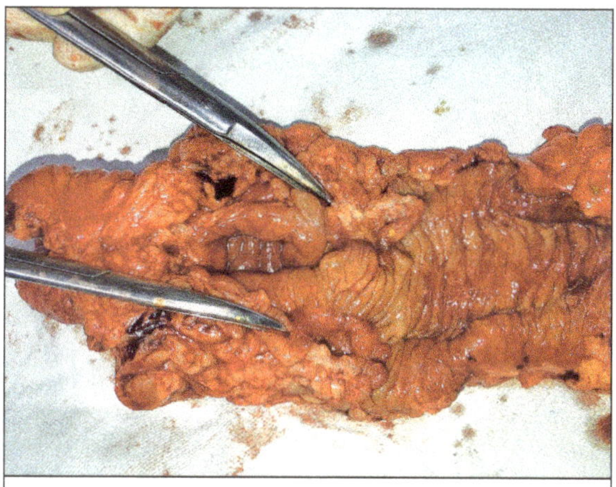
Intestinal stricture

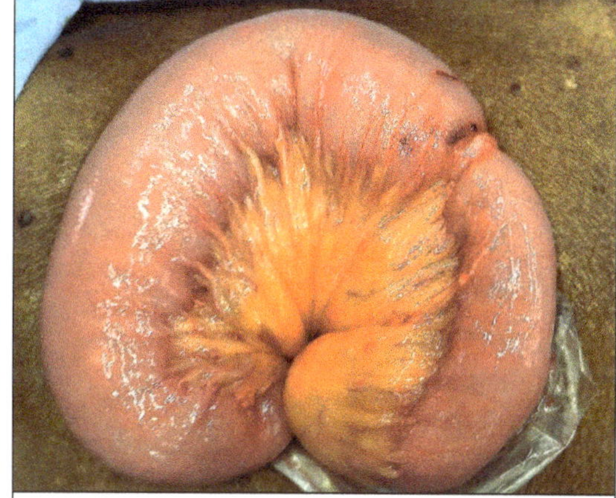
Intraoperative image showing bowel stricture (Courtesy Dr. Prashant Rao from the book Clinics in Surgical Gastroenterology.)

11. **Clinical features:** The Diagnosis of dynamic intestinal obstruction is based on the classic quarter of pain, vomiting, abdominal distension, constipation.

Clinical features of obstruction varies according to:

1. Location of the obstruction
2. Duration of the obstruction
3. Underlying pathology
4. Presence or absence of intestinal ischemia

a. **Pain:**

1. Pain is the first symptom that occurs in obstruction which is sudden in onset and usually severe colicky and centred on the umbilicus (small bowel) and Lower abdomen (large bowel)
2. The pain increases with increased peristalsis activity of intestines
3. As distension of abdomen increases colicky pain is replaced with mild and continuous diffuse abdominal pain.
4. If patient develops severe and continuous abdominal pain then it is mostly due to strangulation.

b. **Vomiting:**

1. The more distal the obstruction, the longer the interval between the onset of symptoms and the appearance of nausea and vomiting.
2. Character of vomiting changes from digested food to feculent material due to progression in obstruction and as a result of overgrowth of the bacteria

c. **Abdominal distension:**

1. In small bowel, the degree of distension is dependent on the site of obstruction
2. Distal the obstruction greater is the distension of abdomen
3. Visible intestinal peristaltic movement may be present.

d. **Constipation**

1. Constipation may be absolute (i.e. neither feces nor flatus is passed) or relative (where only flatus is passed)
2. Failure to pass flatus or feces through the rectum are important symptoms of bowel obstruction.
3. Absolute constipation is cardinal feature of complete intestinal obstruction
4. Administration of enemas should be avoided in case of suspected cases of obstruction.

e.

High small bowel obstruction	Low small bowel obstruction	Large bowel obstruction
Vomiting is early and persistent	Vomiting is delayed	Vomiting is late feature
Dehydration is rapid	Dehydration is later	Dehydration is later
Distension is minimal with little evidence of dilated small bowel loops on radiograph	Central distension with multiple dilated small loops visible on radiograph	Colon proximal to the obstruction is distended on radiograph
Pain is intermittent	Pain is predominant with central distension	Pain is less severe

12. **Physical examination:**

a. **Inspection:**

1. Abdominal distension
2. Movement of the abdominal wall/ visible peristalsis
3. Umbilicus: Everted
4. Visible loop of bowel/visible peristalsis
5. Operative scar
6. Prominent veins
7. Hernial orifices

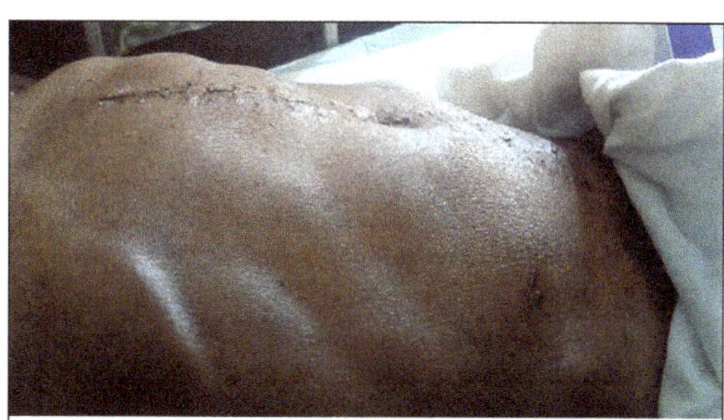

Inspection of abdomen showing Step-ladder pattern of peristalsis in a patient with intestinal obstruction (Courtesy Dr. Prashant Rao from the book Clinics in Surgical Gastroenterology.)

b. **Palpation:**

1. Muscle guarding may present on palpation during colic
2. Tenderness and rigidity at the sight of obstruction usually indicates strangulation
3. All hernial orifices should be palpated to exclude the presence of hernia.

c. **Percussion:**

1. Percussion is useful method in detecting intestinal obstruction
2. Tympanic sounds are heard on percussion due to gas filled bowel loops.
3. A hyperresonant note would be heard in intestinal obstruction..

d. **Auscultation**

1. Bowel sounds are initially loud and frequent
2. As bowel distends the sounds become more resonant and high pitched
3. In strangulation bowel sound is completely absent

e. **Rectal examination:**

1. Presence of mass on rectal examination within or outside the lumen will give clue to diagnosis
2. Presence or absence of feces in the rectum should be noted. Absence means obstruction is higher up.
3. If present it should be studied for presence of occult blood which includes mucosal lesion e.g. cancer, intussusception or infarction.

f. **Tachycardia and hypotension**

g. **Fever:** Suggests the possibility of strangulation.

13. **Investigation:**

a. **Blood investigation**

1. **Full blood count:** A rise in white cell count will indicate an infection
2. **Urea and serum electrolyte:** Derangement may be seen with vomiting and diarrhea. Dehydration will be reflected in raised serum urea and creatinine.
3. **Serum amylase:** May be raised in small intestinal obstruction
4. **Metabolic acidosis:** It occurs due to combined effects of dehydration ketoacidosis and Loss of alkaline secretion. Very common in distal intestinal obstruction.

b. **Radiological investigation**

1. **X-ray:**

- It is essential to organize both erect and supine abdominal films in patients suspected of having intestinal obstruction.
- When obstruction occurs both fluids and gas collects in intestine.
- On the erect abdominal film more than three air fluid levels should be considered as abnormal.
- The number and distribution of fluid levels might also give information about the site of obstruction in the small bowel.
- In cases of mechanical obstruction there may be complete cut-off with no contrast passing beyond the point of obstruction.
- If there is free flow of contrast all the way to the rectum with no narrowing, colonic pseudo-obstruction is confirmed.

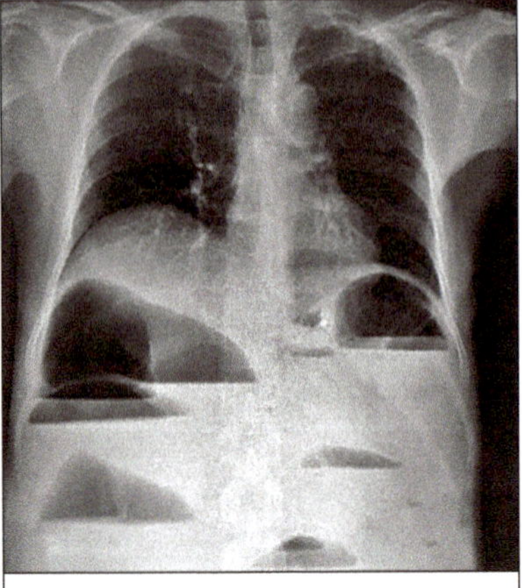

Plain X-ray of abdomen showing multiple air-fluid levels.

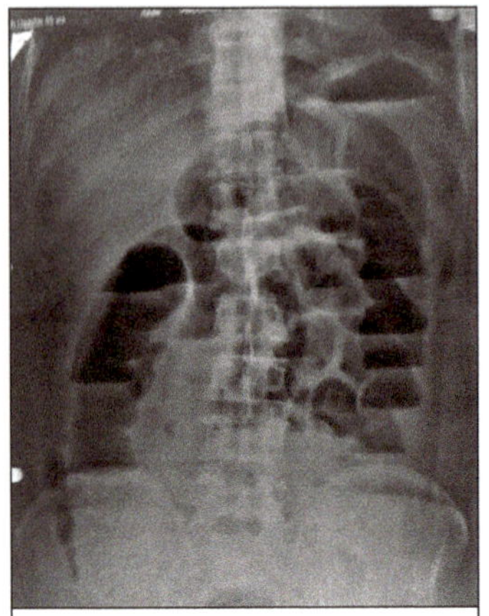

X-ray showing multiple air fluid levels suggestive of Intestinal obstruction

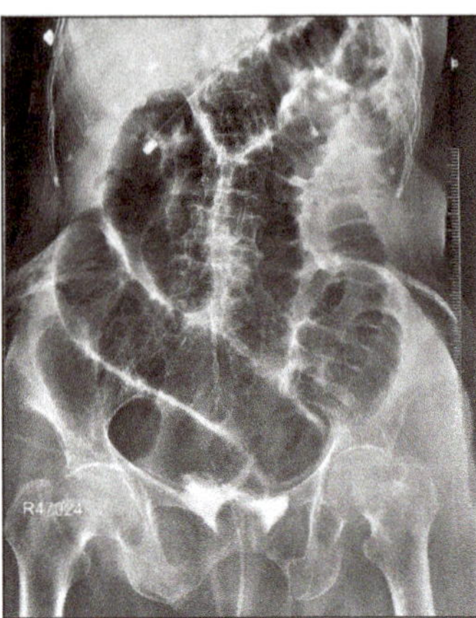

Supine view in patient with intestinal obstruction

2. **CT examination:**
   - Useful to identify the level of obstruction & whether the obstruction is partial or complete.
   - Useful in patients with a history of abdominal malignant disease, post surgical patients, and patients who have no history of abdominal surgery.
3. **Barium studies:** Useful to define the level of obstructed segment and degree of obstruction precisely.

14. **Management:**
   a. **Admission in ICU**
   b. **Nil per oral**
   c. **Analgesic and antipyretics**
   d. **Antiemetics:** May be administered if the patient is having vomiting.
   e. **Gastrointestinal drainage via a nasogastric tube**:
      1. Gastrointestinal drainage is done by the passage of Ryle tube.
      2. Aspiration with a nasogastric tube empties the stomach, reducing the risk of pulmonary aspiration of gastric content and minimizing further intestinal distension from preoperatively swallowed air
   f. **Fluid and electrolyte correction:** In intestinal obstruction there is a sodium and water loss, and therefore the appropriate replacement with ringer lactate solution or normal saline.
   g. **Broad-spectrum antibiotics are given prophylactically**
   h. **Treatment of underlying cause of obstruction**
      1. Patients with a partial intestinal obstruction may be treated conservatively with resuscitation and tube decompression alone.
      2. Surgical treatment is not needed in most of the cases of intestinal obstruction, if there are no obvious signs of strangulation or closed loop obstruction, such patient should be given a conservative trial for 48 to 72 hours and most patient resolve with conservative trial.

         This time should be used for adequate resuscitation and evaluation of the patient so that further line treatment can be planned.
      3. **Indications for early surgical intervention**
         - Obstructed external hernia
         - Clinical features suspicious of intestinal strangulation or closed loop obstruction
         - Obstruction in a 'virgin' abdomen not settling after conservative trial.
         - CT evidence of mass, non-palpable stricture, perforation
         - Signs of sepsis

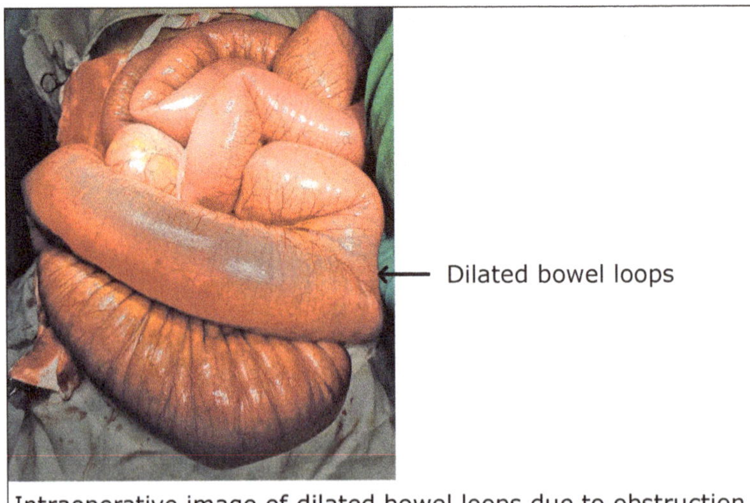

Intraoperative image of dilated bowel loops due to obstruction

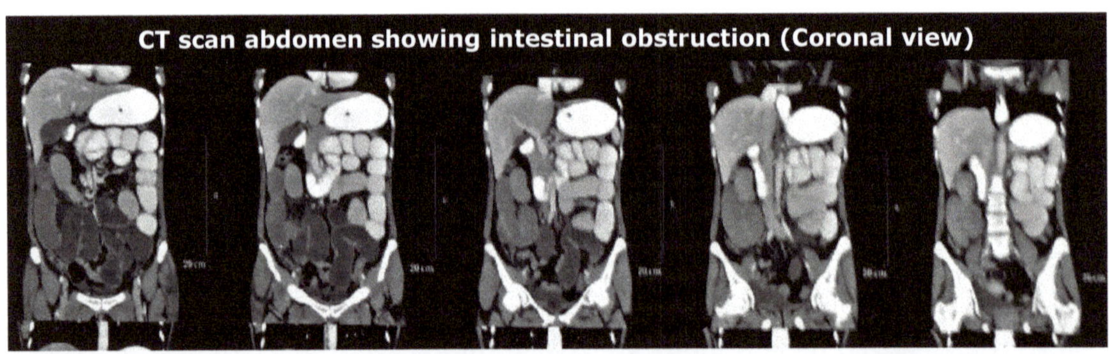

CT scan abdomen showing intestinal obstruction (Coronal view)

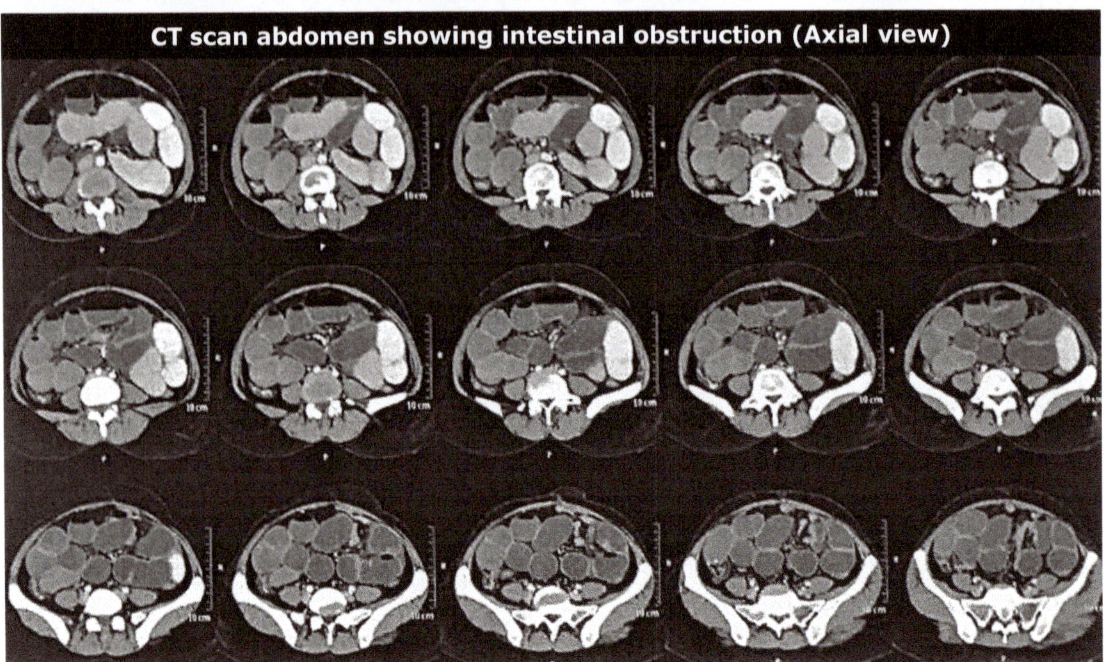

CT scan abdomen showing intestinal obstruction (Axial view)

4. **Principles of surgical intervention for obstruction in management of:**
    - The segment at the site of obstruction
    - The distended proximal bowel
    - The underlying cause of obstruction

15. **Complications:**
    a. **Sepsis**
    b. **Bowel ischemia**
    c. **Perforation**

16. **Common causes of obstruction and treatment:**

Volvulus	**Hernia**	**Adhesion**	**Intestinal atresia**
A loop of intestine twists around itself and the mesentery that supports it, resulting in a bowel obstruction	A hernia is the abnormal exit of tissue or an organ, such as the bowel, through the wall of the cavity in which it normally resides	Adhesions are fibrous bands that form between tissues and organs	Intestinal atresia is congenital malformation of the intestine due to defective development which is causing bowel obstruction
Caecal volvulus Twisting of caecal volvulus can lead to ischemia and needs resection. If viable, the volvulus should be reduced. Fixation of the cecum to the right iliac fossa **(Cecopexy)** **Sigmoid volvulus** Twisting of the sigmoid colon leads to ischemia Sigmoidoscopy is needed. In young patients, an elective sigmoid colectomy is required.	**Incarcerated hernia** An incarcerated hernia occurs when herniated tissue becomes trapped and cannot easily be moved back into place. An incarcerated hernia can lead to a bowel obstruction Surgery to release the herniated tissue and meshplasty Operated in emergency to avoid strangulation **Strangulated hernia** (when incarcerated hernial tissue develop ischemia due to vascular compromise leading to impending gangrene of tissue) Release the trapped tissue back into the abdominal cavity. Remove damaged tissue if needed and finally repair the hernia with tissue or anatomical repair	1. Initial conservative management(not given more than 72 hours) is based on intravenous rehydration and nasogastric decompression; occasionally, this treatment is curative 2. In some cases laparotomy is required. 3. Adhesiolysis with release or excision of band.	**1. Duodenal atresia** is corrected by a duodenostomy gastrojejunostomy 2. In most cases of **jejunal/ileal atresia,** the distal end of the dilated proximal small bowel is resected and a primary end-to-end anastomosis is done

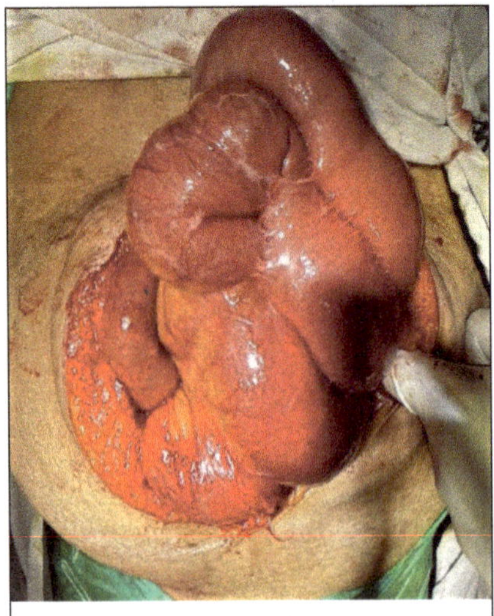

Interbowel adhesions

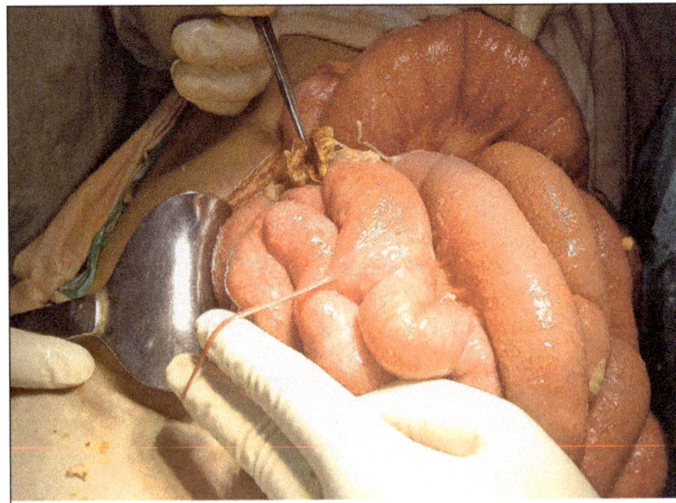

Intraoperative image showing adhesion band

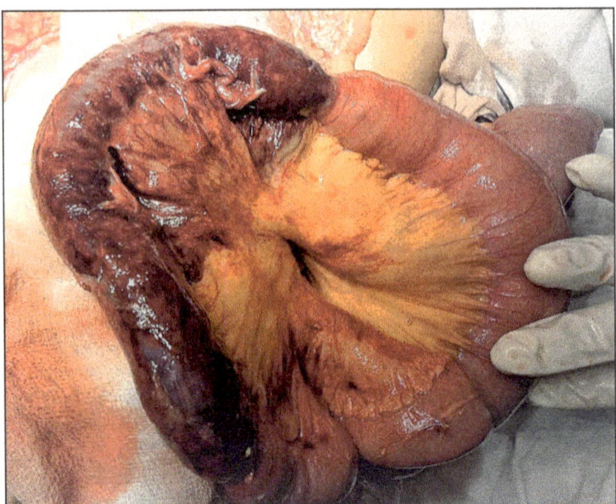

Intraoperative image showing strangulated bowel loop in hernia

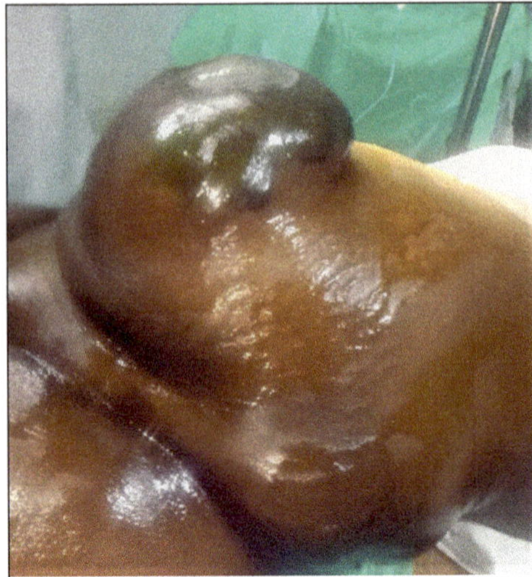

Strangulated ventral hernia with skin changes

PERITONITIS

1. An inflammation of the peritoneum (the lining of the inner wall of the abdomen and covering of the abdominal organs).
2. **Types of peritonitis**
   a. **Generalised**
      1. **Perforation**
         - Perforation of distal esophagus
         - Perforation of stomach due to gastric ulcer or gastric carcinoma
         - Perforation of duodenum (Duodenum ulcer)
         - Perforation of gallbladder (Cholecystitis)
         - Other causes of perforation (Appendicitis, inflammatory bowel disease, intestinal strangulation, colorectal carcinoma)

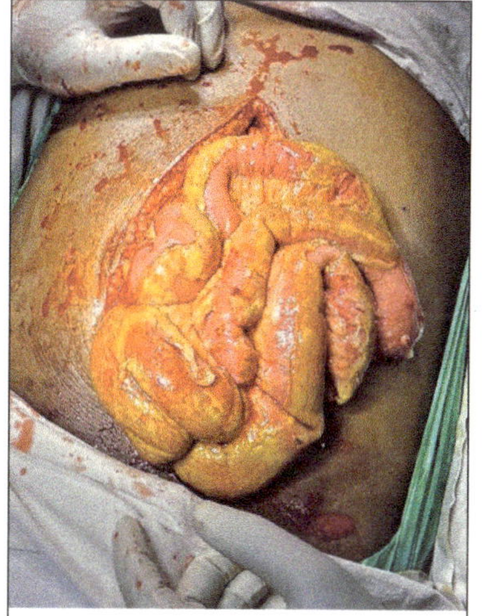

Bowel perforation with fecal peritonitis

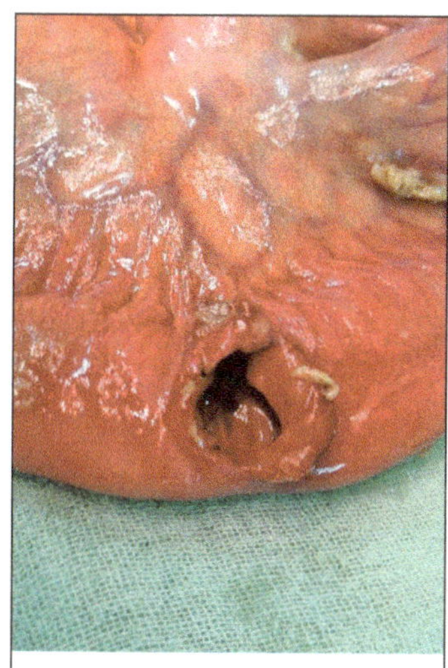

Bowel perforation

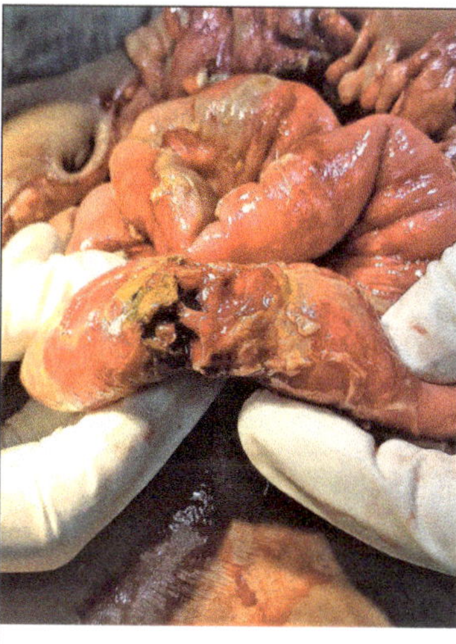

Intestinal perforation

      2. **Direct entry by operative handling**
      3. **Traumatic wound**
      4. **Intraperitoneal dialysis**
      5. **Through blood spread:** Septicemia or pyemia
   b. **Localised: Tuberculosis**
3. **Causes of peritoneal inflammation**
   a. **Bacterial**

1. **Gastrointestinal:** Perforation of bowel, spontaneous/transmural bacterial translocation, acute pancreatitis.
2. **Non gastrointestinal:** Pelvic inflammatory disease, torsion of ovary, surgical or perforative injury to the abdomen.

b. **Chemical:** Bile, barium

c. **Allergic:** Starch peritonitis

d. **Traumatic:** Operative handling

e. **Ischemic:** Vascular occlusion, strangulated occlusion

4. **Different paths for peritoneal infection**

a. **Gastrointestinal perforation:** Perforated ulcer, appendix, diverticulum

b. **Transmural translocation:** Ischemic bowel, pancreatitis

c. **Exogenous contamination:** open surgery, trauma, drains

d. **Female genital tract infection:** PID

e. **Hematogenous spread:** Septicemia

5. **Clinical features:**

a. **Symptoms:**

1. Abdominal pain
2. Anorexia, malaise, fever
3. Nausea, vomiting

b. **Signs**

1. Tachycardia, hypotension
2. Tenderness, Rebound tenderness
3. Guarding
4. Rigidity
5. Absent or reduced bowel sounds
6. Pain and tenderness on vaginal examination in pelvic inflammatory examination

c. **Signs and symptoms (Circulatory failure)**

1. Cold, clammy extremities
2. Sunken eyes
3. Dry tongue
4. Thready pulse

6. **Investigation:**

   a. **Radiological Investigation**

      1. **X-ray chest (PA view):** In perforation free Subdiaphragmatic gas

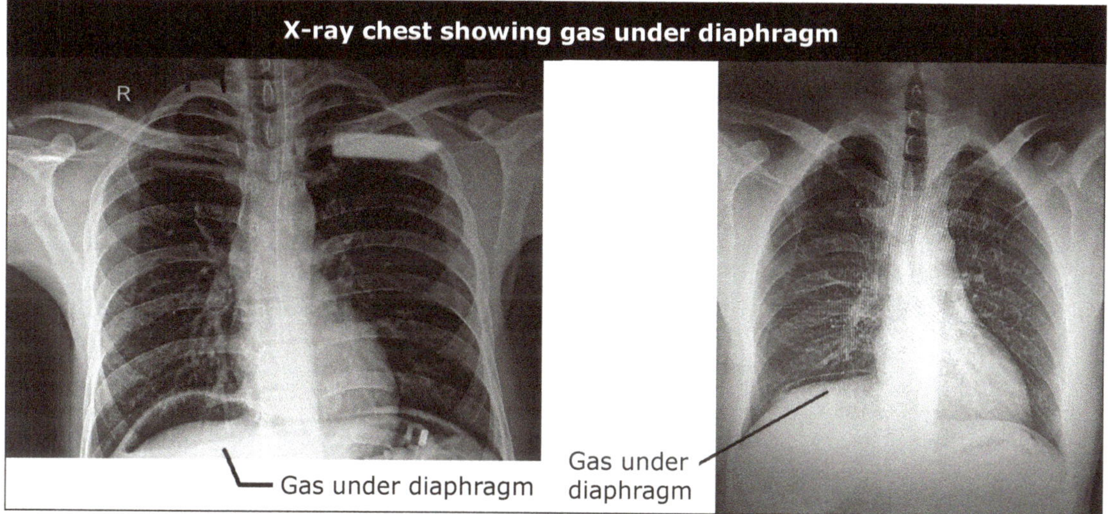

      2. **X-ray abdomen erect and left lateral:**

         Gas under the abdominal wall is more sensitive for diagnosis.

      3. **CT scan:** For differentiating the causes of peritonitis.

   b. **Laboratory investigation**

      1. Complete blood count
      2. Serum amylase, lipase (Pancreatitis)
      3. Serum electrolyte
      4. Renal functional test
      5. Arterial blood gas analysis
      6. Liver function test

7. **Management**

   a. **Correction of fluid and electrolyte imbalance:** In peritonitis, patients have hypovolemia with electrolyte imbalance.

      Monitor the fluid and electrolyte correction

      In shock inotropic support may be required

b. **Insertion of nasogastric drainage:** Allows drainage and aspiration of abdominal content until paralytic ileus is resolved.

c. **Urinary catheterisation:** To correctly measure the urinary output.

d. **Broad spectrum antibiotics:** Gram positive and gram negative organisms must be covered.

e. **Analgesia**

f. **Treatment of specific cause of peritonitis**

g. **Emergency exploratory laparotomy is often required in management of these patients.**

h. **If emergency surgery is not possible due to patient condition, consider putting drains under local anesthesia so that septic focus is reduced and once patients condition improve, can be taken up for surgey.**

8. Complications:

a. Septic shock

b. Acute renal failure

c. Multiorgan failure

d. Peritoneal abscess

RENAL CALCULI

1. Renal calculi is a common cause of severe lower abdominal pain and hence visit of patient visit to emergency department for pain relief.
2. The commonest urinary tract stones are calcium oxalate
3. Most of the stones which are < 5 mm will pass spontaneously
4. Larger stones may require procedures such as extracorporeal shock wave lithotripsy, ureteroscopy, or percutaneous nephrolithotomy.
5. **Etiology:**
   a. **Low urinary citrate excretion:** Citric acid keeps relatively insoluble calcium phosphate and citrate in soluble form.
   b. **Altered urinary solutes and colloids:**
      1. Dehydration concentrate urinary solutes until they precipitate
      2. Reduction of urinary colloids, which absorb solutes or mucoproteins, which are responsible for crystal and stone formation
   c. **Renal infection:** Favours formation of urinary calculi
   d. **Inadequate urinary drainage and urinary stasis:** Favours formation of urinary calculi
   e. **Prolonged immobilisation:** Causes a skeletal decalcification and increase in the urinary calcium favouring the calcium phosphate calculi.
   f. **Hyperparathyroidism:** Leading to hypercalcemia and hypercalciuria
6. **Types of renal calculi:**

Calcium oxalate	Triple phosphate	Urate stone	Cystine stones
Irregular with sharp projections The commonest urinary tract stone	Formed by the ammonia magnesium and calcium phosphate(struvite) and grows in alkaline urine infected with urea splitting bacteria	Multiple, uric acid stone Low urinary pH Hyperuricosuria Chronic metabolic acidosis	Congenital error of metabolism causes cystinuria
Abdominal pain Hematuria	Abdominal pain with hematuria, renal failure	Abdominal pain	Abdominal pain
Hard **Envelope shaped**	Smooth, dirty **Staghorn calculus**	Hard, smooth Pleomorphic crystals, usually **Diamond-shaped**.	Cystine stones are often multiple, are hard **Hexagonal shaped**
Radio-opaque	Radio-opaque	Radiolucent	Radio-opaque

7. **Clinical features:**

   a. **Pain:**

      1. It occurs in the most of persons of urinary calculi
      2. Renal pain occurs in the renal angle, the hypochondriac or both.
      3. Start from flanks & radiates to groin, penis, scrotum or labia as stone progresses down the ureter

   b. **Hematuria**

      It is commonly seen and small in amount

   c. **Oliguria and anuria:** Common in the obstruction

   d. **Pyuria:** Dangerous when develops in the obstruction

   e. **Nausea, vomiting:** Patient experience this visceral symptoms when the ureter is obstructed by a stone, the pressure in the proximal collecting system rises, with progressive distension

8. **Investigation:**

   a. **Complete blood count:** Leukocytosis may present

   b. **Metabolic panel:**

Serum chemistry
1. Calcium
2. Creatinine
3. Sodium
4. Potassium
5. Chloride
6. Bicarbonate
7. Phosphorus
8. Uric acid & cystine
9. Parathyroid hormone
10. 25-hydroxy-vitamin D

   c. **Renal function test: Serum creatinine, BUN**

   d. **Urinalysis:** Hematuria

   e. **Urine culture:** In UTI

   f. **Intravenous pyelography:** Establish the presence and position of calculus and the function of other kidney

   g. **Sonography**: Locating stones

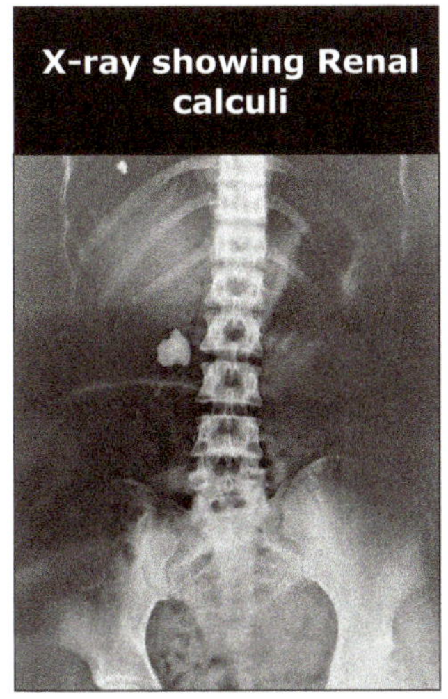
X-ray showing Renal calculi

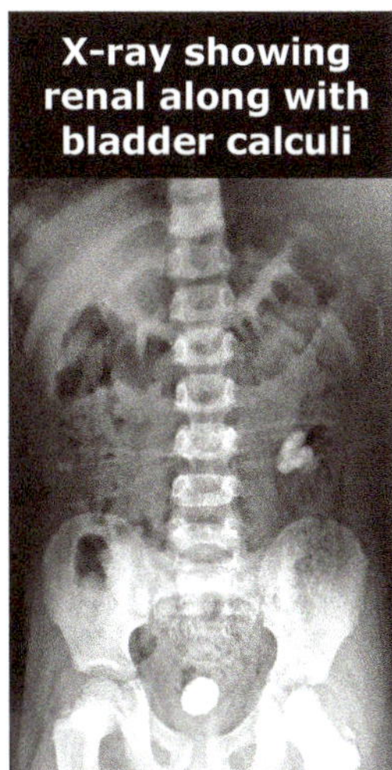
X-ray showing renal along with bladder calculi

h. **X-ray:** An opacity maintaining position relative to the urinary tract during respiration is likely to be a calculus.

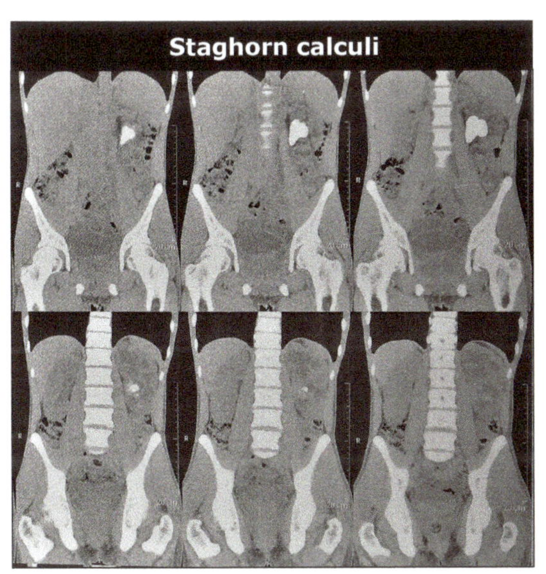
Staghorn calculi

i. **Non-contrast enhanced CT scan:** scan of the abdomen and pelvis is the preferred imaging study because of its superior compared with intravenous urography and plain radiography.

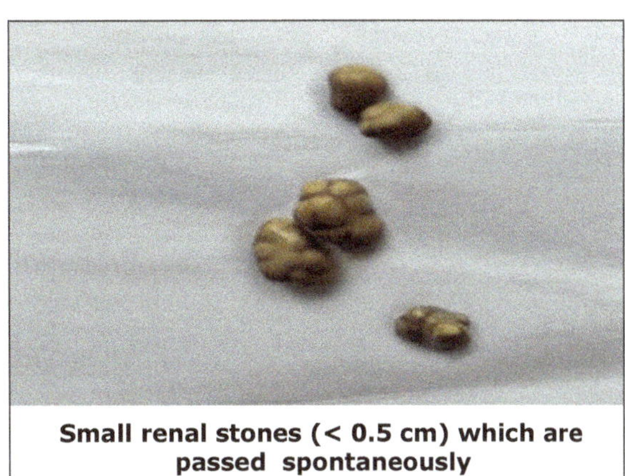
Small renal stones (< 0.5 cm) which are passed spontaneously

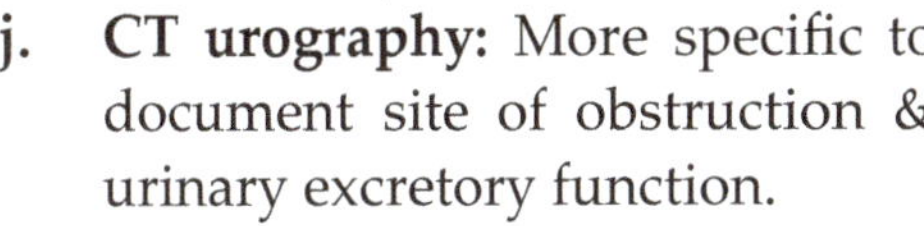

j. **CT urography:** More specific to document site of obstruction & urinary excretory function.

9. **Treatment:**

   a. **Conservative:**

      1. Calculi smaller than 0.5 cm pass spontaneously unless they are impacted.
      2. Hydrotherapy

   b. **Operative:**

      1. Most stones should be treated by minimal access and minimally invasive techniques
      2. Open operations are still needed when expertise not available or newer technology failed.
      3. **Modern methods:**
         - **Percutaneous nephrolithotomy:**
           i. Endoscopic removal of stones, fragmentation of larger stones is done by sonography, laser, electrohydraulic probe
           ii. Nephrostomy drain is placed in the kidney at the end of the procedure, which decompresses the kidney and allows repeated access, if necessary.
         - **Extracorporeal shockwave lithotripsy (ESWL):**
           i. Crystalline stones broken under impact of shock waves
           ii. Shock waves are targeted at stone by sonography or X-ray.
           iii. Stent is placed to drain the kidney and helps to pass the stone fragments
           iv. Impacted fragments are removed uretero scopically.
      4. **Open surgery:**
         - **Pyelolithotomy:** Indicated for stones in the renal pelvis
         - **Extended pyelolithotomy:** In this procedure incision is made in the renal calyces to remove staghorn calculi
         - **Nephrolithotomy:** This operative procedure is performed in a complex calculus branching into the most peripheral calyces
         - **Partial nephrectomy:** Done when a calculi in the lower calyx with infective damage to adjacent parenchyma

ACUTE SCROTUM AND ITS CAUSES

1. **Acute scrotum:** It is a spectrum of conditions affecting the scrotum and its contents that ranges from non serious musculoskeletal problems to emergency conditions such as Fournier's gangrene and testicular torsion that may require surgical intervention.
2. **Causes of acute scrotum:**
   a. **Traumatic causes:**
      1. Testicular rupture
      2. Intratesticular hematoma
      3. Hematocele

   b. **Infectious causes:**
      1. Acute epididymitis or epididymo-orchitis
      2. Acute orchitis
      3. Fournier's gangrene

   c. **Ischemic causes:**
      1. Torsion of testis or appendages
      2. Testicular infarction due to other vascular events
      3. Incarcerated/strangulated inguinal hernia with testicular involvement

   d. **Acute on chronic event:**
      1. **Hydrocele:** Rupture, hemorrhage, infection.
      2. **Spermatocele:** Rupture or hemorrhage
      3. **Testicular tumor:** Rupture, hemorrhage, infarction or infection
      4. **Varicocele**

   e. **Inflammatory causes:**
      1. Fat necrosis of scrotal wall
      2. Henoch -schonlein purpura of scrotal wall

TESTICULAR TORSION

1. **Definition:** Is a clinical condition whereby the testicle twists in such a way that its blood supply becomes compromised to ipsilateral testis.
2. Torsion of the testis is the most common genitourinary tract emergency.
3. Torsion of the testis occurs most frequently in early adolescence with a peak incidence at 14 years of age.

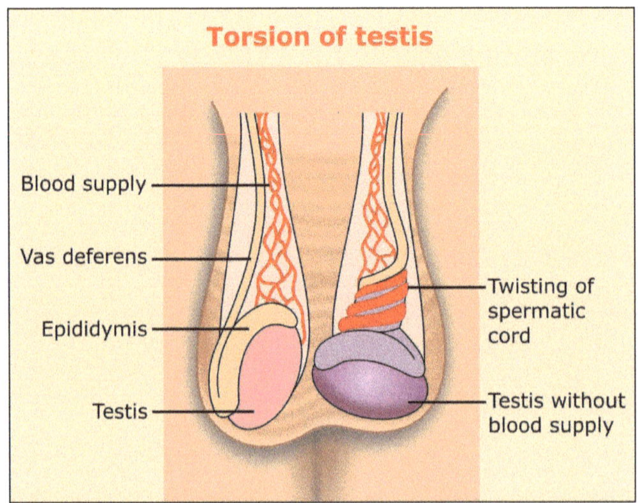

4. Although a few cases occur outside this age range.
5. If left untreated, the blood flow to the testicle ceases and the testicle dies.
6. Testicular salvage rate is higher if testicle is untwisted within 6 hours.
7. Normally testicular torsion is uncommon because the normal testis is anchored by gubernaculum and prevent rotation
8. **For the testicular torsion one of several abnormalities should present:**
   a. Inversion of testis is the most common predisposing cause.
   b. High investment of tunica vaginalis causes the testis to hang within the Tunica like clapper in the bell.
   c. Separation of the epididymis from the body of scrotum permits the testis torsion on the pedicle.
   d. In case of abnormalities mentioned above the spiral attachment of the cremaster favours rotation of testis around the vertical axis.
9. Straining on stool, lifting of heavy objects and coitus are all possible causes for testicular torsion.
10. Torsion may develop spontaneously in the sleep.

11. Pathophysiology:

a. As testicle rotates between the 90-180 degree the blood supply to testicle compromised and Complete torsion occurs when testicle twists >360 degree

b. Twisting of testicle → venous occlusion → engorgement → arterial ischemia → infarction of the testicle.

12. Types of torsion

a. Extravaginal torsion (Outside sack of tunica vaginalis):

1. Newborns without bell clapper anomaly
2. Poor attachment of testis to scrotal wall
3. Torsion at the level of external ring

b. Intravaginal torsion

1. More common
2. Occurs in the puberty or early adolescent
3. Bell clapper deformity

13. Clinical features:

a. Sudden agonising pain in the unilateral groin and lower abdomen.

b. Nausea, vomiting

c. Mild Fever

d. This condition is associated with activity, sports, trauma or awakening from sleep.

14. Physical examination:

a. Swollen, tender and high riding testis

b. Loss of cremasteric reflex

c. Abnormal transverse lie

d. Tenderness over scrotum

15. Investigation:

a. Doppler ultrasonography:

1. Diagnostic test of choice
2. To differentiate from other causes
3. Absence of testicular arterial flow confirms the torsion.

16. Treatment:

Surgical detorsion and orchiopexy

1. High suspicious of torsion then immediate surgical exploration

2. Prompt exploration, untwisting and fixation is the only way to save testis
3. Once the testis detorsed assess for the viability, if viable then fix it (orchiopexy).
4. If clearly necrotic then perform orchiectomy.
5. At the time of surgery, the surgeon must explore and fix the contralateral testis as anatomical predisposition is likely bilateral
6. Viability of testicle depend on degree of torsion and duration of torsion
7. If 24 hours or more elapse, testicular necrosis occurs in most of the cases.

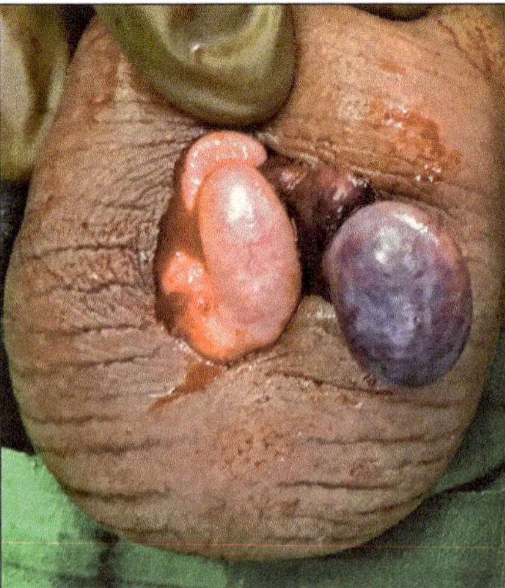

Torsion of testis: Left torsion testis with right normal testis

8. If surgical speciality is not immediately available manual detorsion can be attempted but generally avoided due to pain & risk of vasovagal shock.

17. Complications

a. Infertility
b. Pyocele
c. Testicular necrosis

FOURNIER'S GANGRENE

1. **Definition** Polymicrobial necrotising fasciitis of the perineal, perianal or genital areas of males.
2. Fournier's gangrene is a surgical emergency.
3. It is a form of necrotising fasciitis.
4. In this condition mixed infection of aerobic, anaerobic bacteria, Gram positive & gram negative organism are involved.
5. A fulminating inflammation of the subcutaneous tissues occurs, which results in endarteritis of the arterioles to the scrotal skin that results in gangrene.

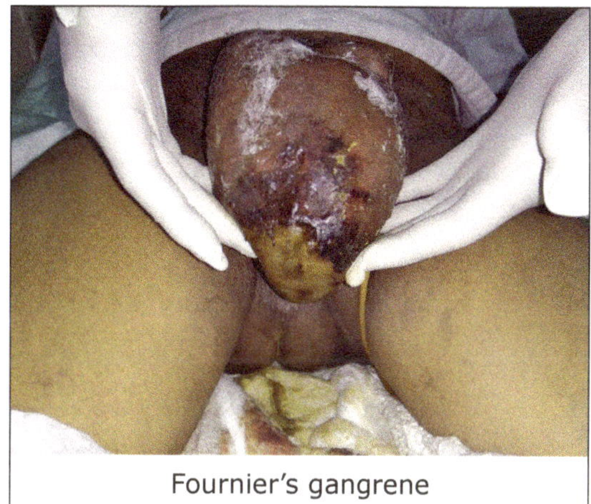

Fournier's gangrene

6. **Risk factors:**
   a. Diabetes mellitus
   b. Alcoholism
   c. HIV infection chronic steroid uses
   d. Malnutrition
   e. Malignancies
   f. Cirrhosis of liver
7. **Etiology:**
   a. It occurs in conjugation with sepsis of the testis, epididymis or perianal region
   b. It can arise following the minor injuries and procedures in perianal region
   c. An obvious cause is absent over half the cases.
8. **Pathophysiology:**

   Entry of bacteria → Fibroid coagulation of nutrient vessel → Decreased locally blood supply to skin → Decreased tissue O_2 tension → Growth of mixed type of organisms → Production of enzymes → Digestion of fascial barrier → Rapid spread of infection.
9. **Clinical features:**
   a. Begins with insidious onset of pruritus and discomfort of external genitalia
   b. Fever and lethargy present before 2-7 days before gangrene

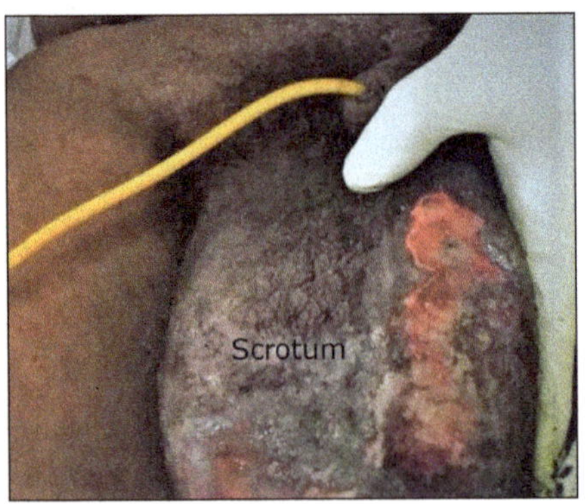

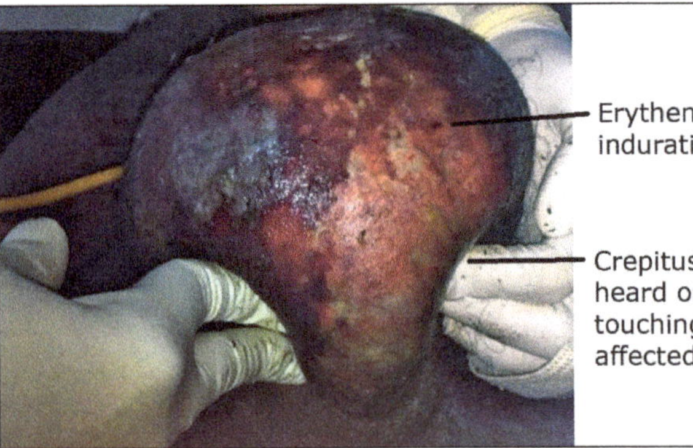

c. Proportional Pain and tenderness in the genitalia is hallmark.
d. Dusky appearance of overlying skin, subcutaneous crepitation, feculent odor
e. Obvious gangrene of a portion of genitalia
f. Purulent discharge from the wounds.
g. As gangrene develops pain subsides.

10. **Investigation:**
    a. Complete blood count
    b. Serum electrolyte
    c. BUN serum creatinine
    d. Blood sugar
    e. ABG
    f. Blood and urine culture and sensitivity
    g. Coagulation profile DIC
    h. Ultrasonography

11. **Treatment:**
    a. **Medical management:**
        1. Broad spectrum antibiotics to cover aerobic and anaerobic infection
        2. Tetanus prophylaxis
        3. Intravenous fluid resuscitation
        4. Other supportive measures in cases of systemic sepsis.

    b. **Surgical management:**
        1. Urgent surgical excision of the dead and infected tissue is essential
        2. Vacuum assisted dressing is applied over wound after infection has been controlled.
        3. Skin graft or flaps is often needed to reconstruct the defect.

EPIDIDYMO-ORCHITIS

1. **Definition:** Inflammation confined to the epididymis is called epididymitis and infection spreading to the testis is called as an epididymo-orchitis.
2. **Pathophysiology:**
   a. Epididymitis is commonly seen in sexually active young men occur from genital tract infections.
   b. In old age patient's common causes of epididymo-orchitis are urinary tract infections, reflux of urine into ejaculatory duct or urethral catheter.
   a. Infection of the urethra, prostate or seminal vesicle reaches epididymis via the VAS
3. **Clinical features:**
   a. Discomfort and pain in the epididymis, testicle or scrotum.
   b. Fever
   c. Tenderness to touch
   d. Epididymis and testicular swelling
   e. Scrotal wall appears red, edematous and shiny.
   f. **Positive Prehn's sign**: Pain relief with lifting the affected testicle, which points towards epididymitis.
4. **Investigation:**
   a. **Physical investigation**
   b. **Doppler ultrasound**
   c. **Blood investigation**
   d. **Urinalysis and culture**
5. **Treatment:**
   a. In Young men initial treatment with the doxycycline (100-200 mg daily) or quinolone.
   b. In older patient start with quinolone but if there is systemic sepsis start the intravenous antibiotics
   c. Scrotal support (MUST)
   d. Analgesics and antipyretics
   e. In urine analysis if a specific organism is isolated then choice of antibiotics is prescribed.
   f. Antibiotics should continue for at least 2 weeks or till the inflammation subsides

URINARY TRACT INFECTION

1. Infection in any part of the urinary tract i.e. kidneys, ureter, urinary bladder and urethra is called a urinary tract infection.
2. Urinary tract infection can be
   a. **Lower urinary tract infection: Urethritis and cystitis (Most common)**
   b. **Upper urinary tract infection: Acute pyelonephritis (Includes renal parenchyma and pelvis)**
3. Infection of the lower urinary tract without structural or functional abnormalities is called an uncomplicated UTI.
4. Infection in patients with underlying structural or functional abnormalities and/or impaired host defense obstruction to urinary flow are responsible for complicated urinary tract infection.
5. Asymptomatic bacteremia is used for patients with bacterial count of > 10 raised to 5 in urine samples without signs and symptoms suggestive for UTI.
6. Recurrent infection of the urinary tract leads to a considerable morbidity and also can cause life threatening septicemia and kidney failure.
7. **Etiology**
   a. **Bacteria:** E. coli (Most common), klebsiella, proteus, enterobacter sp.
   b. **Parasitic:** Hydatid cyst
   c. **Protozoal:** Trichomonas vaginalis
   d. **Helminth:** Enterobius
8. **Risk factors:**
   a. **Female Sex:**
      1. UTI is more common in women than men due to shorter urethra and closer to anus.
      2. In menopausal women: Loss of protective vaginal flora and vaginal atrophy responsible for recurrent urinary tract infection.
   b. **Sexual intercourse:** Sexually active persons are vulnerable for urinary tract infections
   c. **Diabetes:** High blood sugar is favourable environment for growth of pathogens
   d. **Urinary catheters:** Increases risk of infection
   e. **Spinal cord injury:** Because of voiding dysfunction
   f. **Vesicoureteric reflux:** An abnormal movement of urine from urinary bladder into ureter and kidneys (Main cause of UTI in children).
   g. **Prostatomegaly:** Incomplete voiding results in residual urine or urinary stasis, which can lead to increased risk of urinary tract infection.

9. Clinical features

a. High grade fever associated with chills (Acute pyelonephritis)
b. Flank pain
c. Suprapubic pain
d. Dysuria
e. Urgency
f. Frequency
g. Hematuria
h. Burning micturition
i. Oliguria
j. Associated symptoms: Vomiting, malaise, loss of appetite

10. Investigations

a. Complete blood count
b. Random blood sugar
c. Kidney function test
d. Urine routine, microscopy, culture and antibiotic sensitivity
e. Blood culture (Before starting antibiotic treatment)
f. Imaging: USG (KUB)/ CT scan (KUB)
g. Urodynamic study (To know how the bladder, sphincters and urethra holding and releasing urine)
h. Prostate specific antigen (CA prostate)

11. Treatment

Uncomplicated	**Complicated/acute pyelonephritis**	**Asymptomatic bacteremia**
Females: Tab. Nitrofurantoin monohydrate 100 mg BD for 5 days OR Tab. Cefixime 400 mg BD for 5 days **Males:** Tab. Ciproflox 500 mg for 7 days OR Tab. Nitrofurantoin monohydrate 100 mg BD for 5 days	INJ. Meropenem 1 gm TDS / imipenem 500 mg QID for 14 days. **OR** INJ. Piptaz 4.5 QID for 14 days.	Tab. Nitrofurantoin monohydrate 100 mg BD for 3 to 5 days **OR** Tab. Cefixime 400 mg BD for 3 to 5 days

TRAUMATIC TESTICULAR INJURY

1. Testicular trauma can occur in one or both testicles
2. The testis is damaged either by the blunt trauma or by penetrating trauma
3. Injuries can be simple as bruising or associated with significant intratesticular hematomas
4. Traumatic injury may cause rupture of tunica albuginea with very significant blood collection within the tunica vaginalis (Hematocele).
5. **Traumatic testicular injuries may cause:**
   a. **Testicular rupture:** Tear in the tunica albuginea resulting in extrusion of the testicular contents, including the seminiferous tubules
   b. **Intratesticular hematoma:** In intratesticular hematoma (ITH) blood collected within testis without rupture of the tunica albuginea following blunt scrotal trauma.
   c. **Contusion hematocele:** Hematocele occurs where there is blood collection between the layers of a sac that surrounds each testicle.
6. **Clinical features**
   a. Severe pain in scrotum
   b. Fever
   c. Redness
   d. Bruising
   e. Swelling
   f. Tenderness
7. **Investigation:**
   a. Physical examination
   b. Ultrasonography of testis
8. **Treatment:**
   a. **Supportive treatment**
      1. **Rest**
      2. **Scrotal support**
      3. **Analgesics and antipyretics**
   b. **Surgery management:**
      1. **In testicular rupture:** Testicular rupture is treated with surgery, though the procedure performed depends on the magnitude of the injury and the salvageability of the tissue.

2. **Intratesticular hematoma:**
   - **Severe pain and expanding:** Requires surgical exploration
   - **Mild to moderate pain and no expansion:** Observation with serial ultrasonography examination.
3. **Contusion hematocele:** In severe or non-resolving cases, surgical incision and drainage may be required.
4. If testis is non-salvageble then orchidectomy is to be considered.

GASTROINTESTINAL BLEEDING

1. It includes all forms of bleeding in the gastrointestinal tract, from the mouth to the rectum.
2. **Gastrointestinal bleeding is typically divided into two main types:**
   a. **Upper gastrointestinal bleeding**
   b. **Lower gastrointestinal bleeding.**
3. **Presentation of gastrointestinal bleed:**
   a. **Hematemesis:** It is defined as the vomiting of the fresh blood or either bright or coffee ground colored.
   b. **Melena:**
      1. It is a tarry black, sticky, foul smelling stool
      2. Usually occurs as a result of upper GI bleeding & bleeding occurs proximal to ligament of treitz.
   c. **Hematochezia:**
      1. Passage of red or maroon blood from the rectum
      2. It usually suggests bleeding from a source distal to the ligament of treitz.
      3. It can also occur from massive upper GI bleeds from esophagus, stomach and duodenum.
4. **Etiology:**
   a. **Upper GI bleed:**
      1. Duodenal ulcers
      2. Gastric ulcers
      3. Gastric erosion
      4. Esophageal varices
      5. Mallory weiss syndrome
      6. Gastric carcinoma
      7. Other causes like hemophilia, thrombocytopenia, rupture of aorta
   b. **Lower GI bleed:**
      1. Diverticular disease like diverticulitis
      2. Inflammatory bowel disease (IBD)

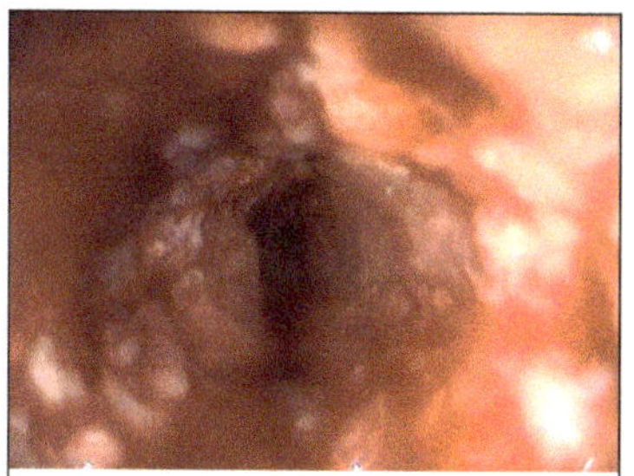

Upper GI endoscopy showing stricturing growth in mid esophagus

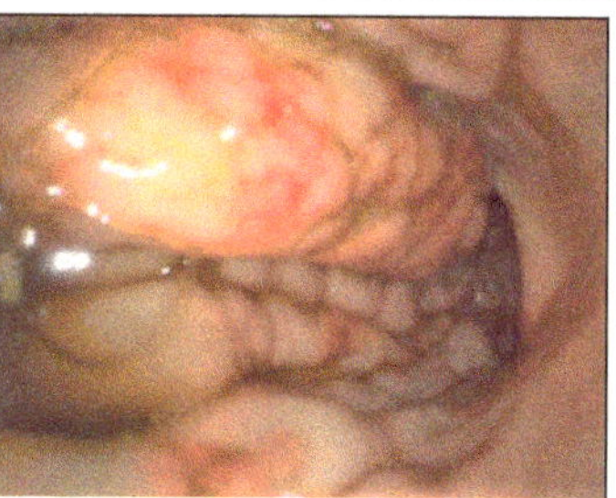

Gastroscopy showing proliferative growth in the body of stomach

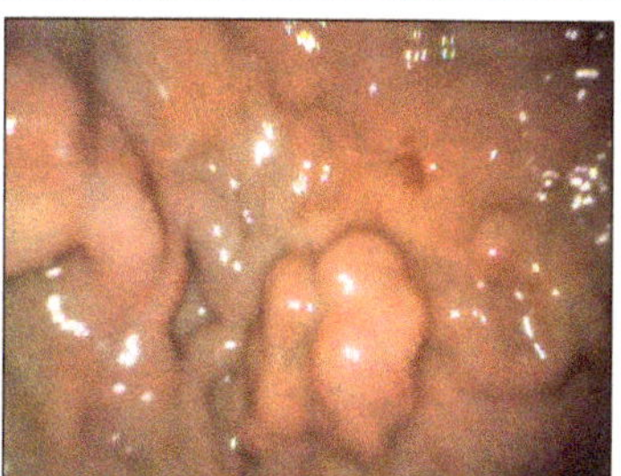

Upper GI endoscopy showing gastric varices

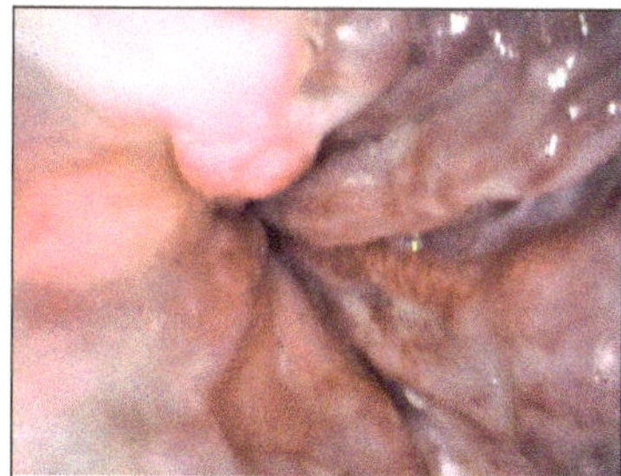

Upper GI endoscopy showing esophageal varices

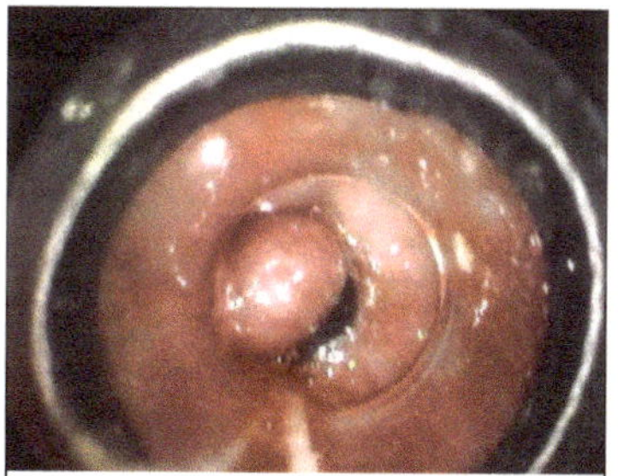

Endoscopic variceal band ligation

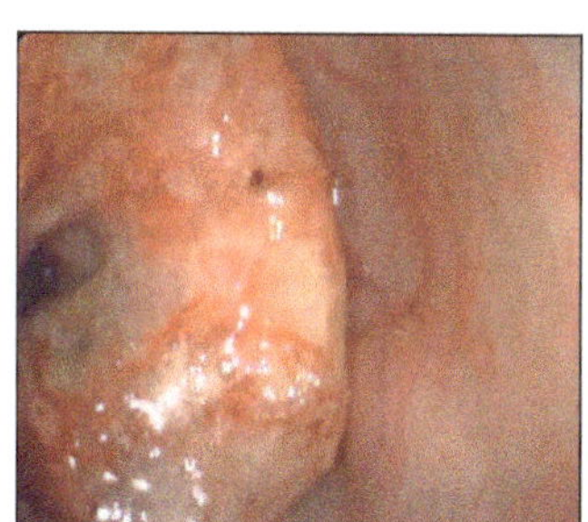

Colonoscopy image showing proliferative lumen occluding growth in rectosigmoid junction

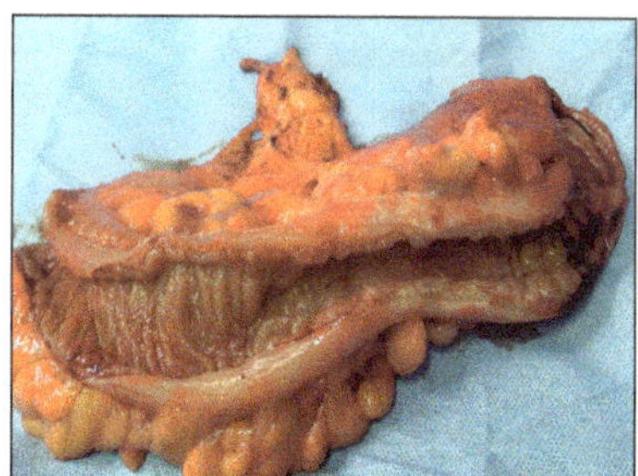

Segmental intestinal resection specimen showing features of Crohn's disease Bowel wall thickening, mucosal ulceration, cobble-stoning, mesenteric fat creeping.

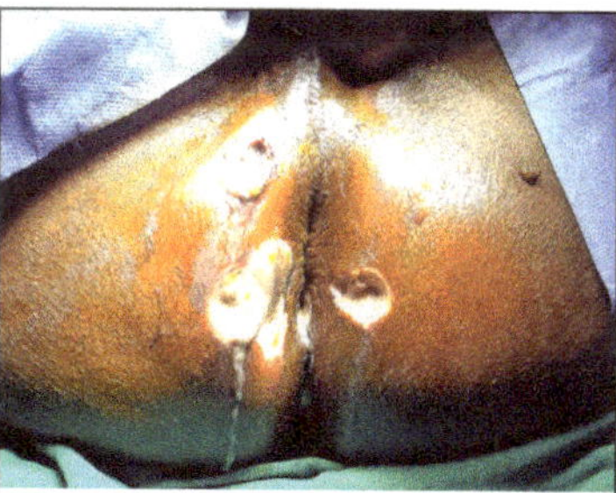

Peri-anal Crohn's disease

(Above images Courtesy Dr. Prashant Rao from the book Clinics in Surgical Gastroenterology)

3. Colon cancer
4. Neoplastic polyps
5. Internal hemorrhoids
6. Anal fissure

5. **Difference in between the upper and lower GI bleed:**

Features	Upper GI bleed	Lower GI bleed
Site	Above the ligament of treitz	Below the ligament of treitz
Presentation	Hematemesis/melena (Tarry stool)	Hematochezia
Nasogastric aspiration	Blood	Clear fluid
Bowel sounds	Hyperactive	Normal

6. **Assessment of blood loss:**

Blood loss	Clinical features
500 ML	No systemic signs except in the elderly and the anemic patients
1000 ML (20% reduction of blood volume)	Tachycardia, orthostatic hypotension, syncope, lightheadedness, nausea, sweating and thirst
2000 ML (40% reduction of blood loss)	Profound shock and possibly death.

7. **Management:**
   a. Initial assessment and start resuscitation
   b. Admit the patient
   c. Head raised to avoid the aspiration
   d. O_2 Administration
   e. Reassurance to the patient
   f. Secure two IV lines, start crystalloid solutions for resuscitation and send blood samples for grouping and cross matching.
   g. Assessment of blood loss by history and vitals for replacement of blood.
   h. **History:**
      1. **Regarding the color of vomitus or stool passed.**
      2. **Alcohol consumption history**: Alcohol causes mucosal damage
      3. **Anticoagulant therapy:** Warfarin, LMWH which affects the coagulation process
      4. **Coagulation disorders**
      5. **Liver diseases:** Alcoholic liver disorder

i. **Vital assessment:**
   1. Pulse rate
   2. Blood pressure
   3. SPO_2 saturation
   4. Capillary filling time
   5. Cold extremities

j. **Introduce the nasogastric tube:**
   1. Assessment of the quantity and the duration of bleed.
   2. Therapeutic cold water lavage till clear fluid aspirated but avoid hypothermia.

k. **Complete blood count**

l. **ABG**

m. **Blood grouping and cross matching to be done**

n. **Indication for blood transfusion**
   1. Acute or continuous blood loss
   2. Patient in shock (PR > 120; SBP < 100 mm of Hg; urinary output < 0.5 ML/kg/hr)
   3. Hb < 10 mg %
   4. PCV < 20

8. **Diagnostic testing:**

a. **Diagnostic endoscopy**

   Endoscopic diagnosis:
   1. Recent hemorrhage
   2. Predict risk of further bleeding and guide management decision
   3. Risk of further bleeding is present in following conditions
      - Active spurting
      - Non bleeding visible vessels
      - Active oozing
      - Adherent clot

- Flat pigmented spot
- Clean base (strong recommendation)

b. **Esophagogastroduodenoscopy:**

1. It has high diagnostic accuracy and therapeutic accuracy.
2. EGD should be performed in a hemodynamically unstable patient after proper resuscitation.
3. It benefits most of the patients having ongoing bleeding.
4. In stable patients it is performed electively

c. **Colonoscopy:** Performed after emptying of bowel in clinically stable patients

d. **Anoscopy:** Anoscopy is used to diagnose hemorrhoids, anal fissures (tears in the lining of the anus), and some cancers.

e. **Capsule endoscopy:** A procedure used to record internal images of the gastrointestinal tract for use in diagnosis

No therapeutic interventions possible.

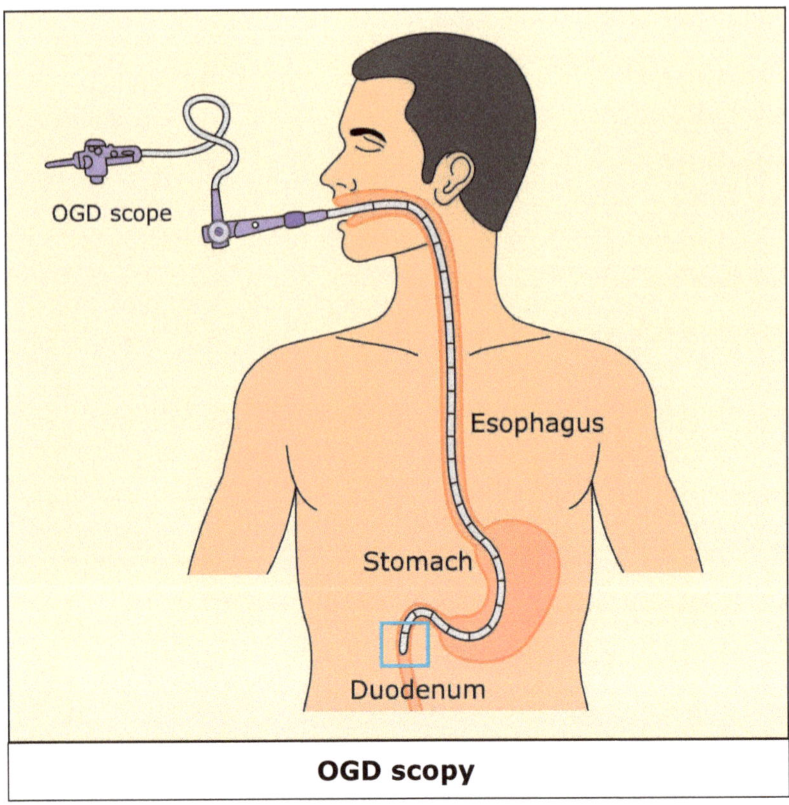

OGD scopy

9. Management

A. Non variceal bleeding, upper GI bleeding:

1. Peptic ulcer disease	**1. Medical management:** a. Already discussed in previous topic **2. Endoscopic management:** a. Endoscopic options include epinephrine injections, heater probes and coagulation as well as the application of clips. b. In the rebleeding ulcer a second attempt of endoscopic management can be attempted, if fails then urgent surgical intervention required. **3. Surgical management:** a. Only few patients with bleeding ulcers require the surgical intervention b. Forrest classification, size and location of ulcer is very important indicator of rebleeding 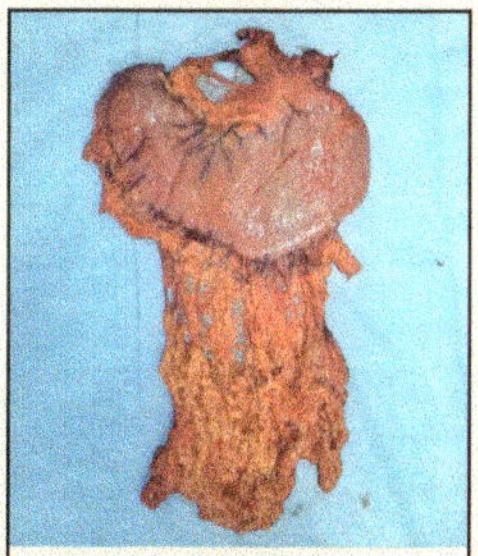 **Surgical options:** **1. Vagotomy/highly selective vagotomy** **2. Gastrectomy** **3. Graham's patch:** Piece of omentum is used to close the perforation **4. Suture ligation of gastroduodenal artery** **5. Under running an ulcer** **6. Antrectomy:** removal of entire antrum, eliminate gastric phase **7. Vagotomy plus antrectomy;** eliminate both cephalic and gastric phase **8. Pyloroplasty:** widen the lower part of stomach i.e pylorus **9. Duodenotomy:** perform an anterior longitudinal duodenotomy extending across the pylorus to the distal stomach Total gastrectomy specimen (Courtesy Dr. Prashant Rao from the book Clinics in Surgical Gastroenterology)
2. Mallory-weiss tears	1. Mucosal tear and submucosal tear that occurs near the gastroesophageal junction. 2. In most of cases only supportive therapy is needed 3. Local Endoscopic therapy with injection or electrocoagulation 4. Endoscopic therapy fail, then angiographic embolization with gelatin sponge 5. If these maneuvers fail then operative management is required.
3. Stress gastritis	Cushing's ulcer occurs due to head injury and curling ulcer occurs due to burn. **1. Medical therapy:** Already discussed in previous topic **2. Surgical options:** Vagotomy and pyloroplasty with oversewing of the hemorrhage or near total gastrectomy

(Continued)

4. Esophagitis	It occurs due to repeated exposure of acidic gastric secretion to mucosa in GERD and which may lead to upper GI bleed. 1. Various infections also cause esophagitis, particularly in immunocompromised patients. 2. Acid suppression therapy is important. 3. Endoscopic therapy. 4. Surgery is rarely required.
5. Malignancy	1. Upper GI tract malignancy is usually associated with chronic anemia or occult blood in stool 2. Malignant ulcerative lesions have persistent bleeding. 3. Surgical, chemotherapy and radiations are treatment options.
6. Dieulafoy lesion	1. Dieulafoy lesions are vascular malformation found primarily along the lesser curvature of the stomach, but can occur anywhere in the gastrointestinal tract 2. Initially endoscopy is used to control the bleeding. 3. If the endoscopic therapy fails, angiographic coil embolization can be successful. **4. Surgical intervention:** In some cases may be required if above therapy fails to control bleeding. Partial gastrectomy if source of bleeding is not identified.
7. Gastric anal vascular ectasia (GAVE)	1. It is also called a **watermelon stomach.** 2. Acute hemorrhage is rare in this condition 3. Endoscopic surgery in the persistent bleeding by Argon plasma coagulation. **4. Surgical management:** Who fail to respond to endoscopic therapy should be considered for antrectomy.

B. Variceal bleeding: Discussed in medicine emergency

10. Lower GI bleeding management:

Diverticular disease	1. Diverticula are the most common cause of significant lower GI bleed 2. The best method of diagnosis and treatment is colonoscopy **3. Treatment:** If the bleeding diverticulum is identified then epinephrine injection used to stop bleeding 4. Electrocautery can also be used 5. Endoscopic clips are also a good option. 6. If the above methods fails then Angiography with embolization can be considered.

(Continued)

Neoplasia	1. In colorectal carcinoma there is no significant lower GI bleeding. 2. The bleeding is usually painless, intermittent and less in nature. 3. Mostly patient present with iron deficiency anemia, weight loss ,anorexia. 4. Gastrointestinal stromal tumors can be associated with massive hemorrhage. 5. Polyps can also cause bleeding and it can be treated with endoscopic therapy. 6. The best diagnostic procedure is colonoscopy.
Anorectal disease	1. The most common cause of anorectal bleeding are internal hemorrhoids, anal fissure. 2. The bleeding is bright red colored and less in amount. **In internal hemorrhoids:** Painless bleeding occurs in hemorrhoids **3. Treatment:** Stool bulking agents, encourage more water intake, stool softener and high fiber diet. 4. Other treatment options: Sclerosing injections, rubber band ligation, infrared coagulation 5. If above measure fails then the surgical hemorrhoidectomy may be needed **In anal fissure:** 1. Produce painful bleeding after a bowel movement. **2. Treatment:** Stool bulking agents (Psyllium, ispaghula, wheat bran) increased water intake, stool softeners and topical nitroglycerine ointment or diltiazem to relieve sphincter spasm and to promote healing. 3. A careful investigations are required to rule out the cancer.
Colitis	**Ulcerative colitis:** Mucosal disease start distally in rectum and extends proximally in the entire colon **1. Clinical features:** Bloody bowel movements, crampy abdominal pain and tenesmus (Persistent urge to evacuate the bowel). **2. Diagnosis:** Careful history and flexible endoscopy with biopsy **3. Treatment:** Medical therapy with steroids, 5 aminosalicylic acid compounds (Mesalamine) and immunomodulatory agents (azathioprine, methotrexate) and supportive care **4. Surgical:** Done in the toxic colon or hemorrhage that is not controlled by medical management. **Crohn's colitis:** **1. Clinical features:** Guaiac positive diarrhea, mucus filled diarrhea but not associated with bright blood 2. It can affect entire GI tract 3. It is characterized by skip lesions, transmural thickening of bowel wall and granuloma formation. **4. Diagnosis:** Endoscopy and contrast study **5. Treatment:** Medical therapy with steroids, 5 aminosalicylic acid compounds and immunomodulatory agents and antibiotics

(Continued)

	Infective colitis: Causes bloody diarrhea (e.g. E. coli, salmonella, shigella, clostridium difficile) 1. **Clinical features:** Bloody diarrhea, foul smelling diarrhea, if patient is treated with prior antibiotics and hospitalization. 2. **Diagnosis:** History and stool culture 3. **Treatment:** Supportive care and oral or intravenous metronidazole or oral vancomycin plus probiotics. **Ischemic colitis:** 1. Mesenteric ischemia can be secondary to either acute or chronic arterial or venous insufficiency. 2. Predisposing factors include pre-existing cardiovascular disease, recent abdominal vascular surgery, hypercoagulable states. 3. **Clinical features:** a. Abdominal pain, bloody diarrhea b. Marked leukocytosis, fever, tachycardia, acidosis and features of peritonitis indicate ischemia that requires urgent surgical intervention. c. Excessive abdominal pain without obvious clinical findings may suggest ischemia. d. Complete obstruction of the vessel will lead to gangrene and necrosis of colon. 4. **Diagnosis:** a. CT scan shows thickened bowel wall. b. CT angiography will show the site of obstruction. c. Confirmed with flexible endoscopy. 5. **Treatment:** **a. Supportive care:** Bowel rest, intravenous antibiotics, cardiovascular support. b. In most cases the transient ischemia is self limited and resolved without incident, although some patients develop a colonic stricture. **c. Surgery:** • Surgery is required in few cases of progressive ischemia and gangrene • Resection of ischemic segment of intestine with creation of an enterostomy. • Early cases or transient cases respond well to interventional angioplasty.

SKIN AND SOFT TISSUE INFECTION

1. **Soft tissue** includes the tissues that connect, support, or surround other structures and organs of the body.
2. Soft tissue includes skin, subcutaneous tissue, tendons, ligaments, fascia, skin, fibrous tissues, fat, and synovial membranes (which are connective tissue), and muscles, nerves and blood vessels (which are not connective tissue)
3. Skin and soft tissue infections (SSTIs) involve microbial invasion of the skin and underlying soft tissues.
4. They have variable presentations, etiologies and severities.
5. Skin and Soft tissue infections can be localised or spreading.
6. This infections can be necrotising or non necrotising.
7. Spreading necrotising soft tissue infection constitutes life treating surgical emergencies.
8. **They are generally classified into two categories:**
   a. **Purulent infections (e.g., furuncles, carbuncles, abscesses)**
   b. **Nonpurulent infections (e.g., erysipelas, cellulitis, necrotizing fasciitis).**
9. **Purulent infections:**
   a. **Abscesses:**
      1. A collection of pus that has been formed within tissue or body.
      2. Abscesses may occur in any kind of tissue but most frequently on the skin surface (where they may be superficial pustules (boils) or deep skin abscesses) also occur in the liver, lungs, brain, teeth, kidneys and tonsils.
      3. Abscess contains hyperosmolar material that draws in fluid due to which we fill pain due to increased pressure.
      4. Wound abscess may discharge spontaneously by tracking to the surface.
      5. **Causes**
         - Abscesses are caused by a bacterial infection, parasites or foreign substances.
         - Bacterial infection is the most common cause
         - Predominantly pyogenic organism are involved e.g. staphylococcus aureus
         - Cold abscess occur due to TB lymphadenitis
      6. **Classical symptoms of inflammation:**
         - Pain (Dolor)
         - Swelling (Tumor)

- Redness (Rubor)
- Heat (Calor)
- Loss of function (Functio laesa)

7. **Investigation**
   - **X-ray:** If suspecting foreign body
   - **Sonography:** Imaging in the emergency department can help in diagnosis and to understand extent of infection in deeper tissues.
8. **Treatment**
   - Incision and drainage
   - **Antibiotics:** Depends on severity, location of abscess and type of microorganisms involved.
   - Analgesics and antipyretics
   - Warm compresses and elevation of the limb may be beneficial for a skin abscess.
   - In case of cold abscess non dependent aspiration of purulent material is done (To prevent formation of sinus tract).

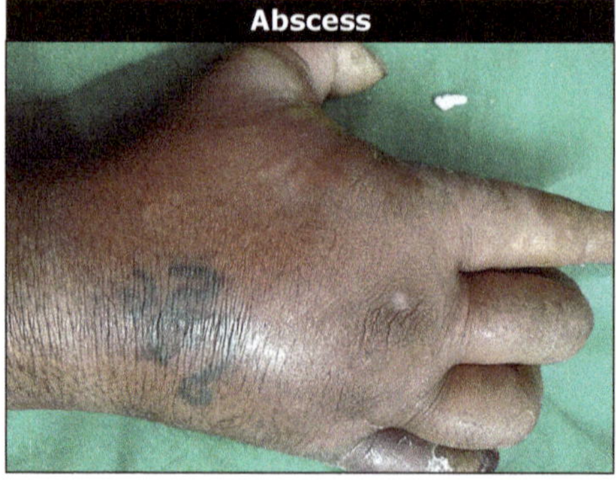

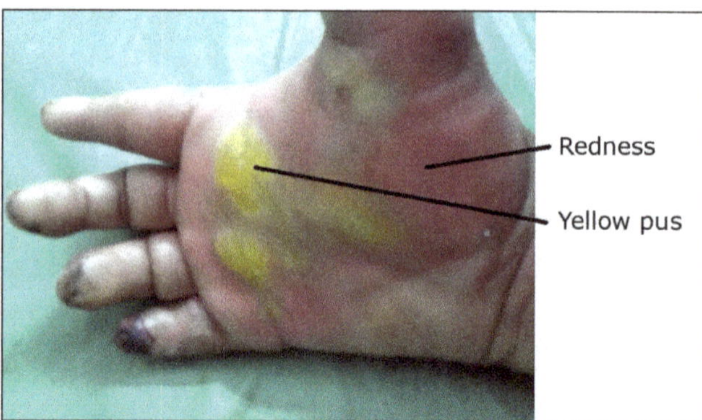

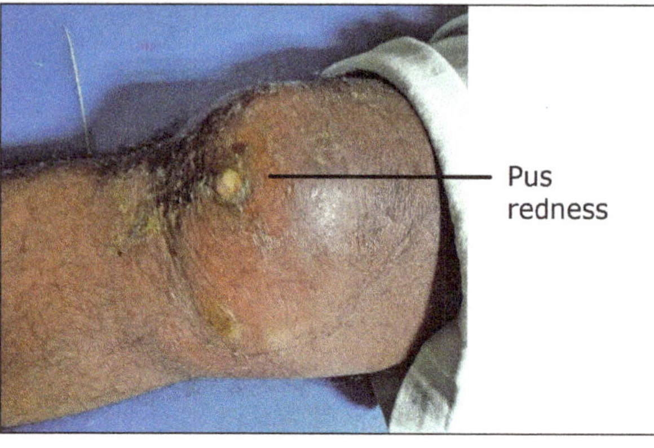

b. **Furuncles (common boil) and carbuncles**

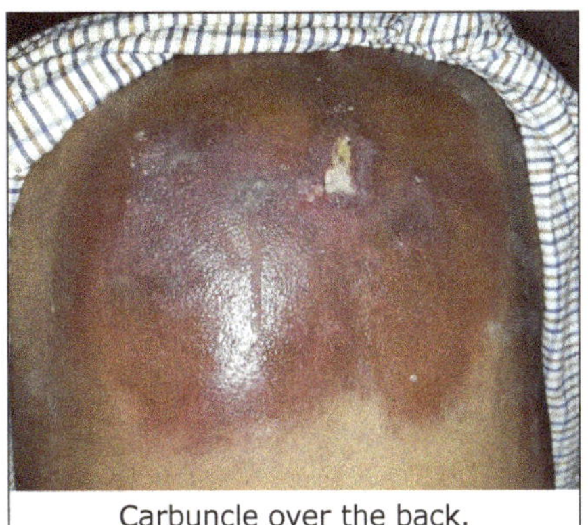

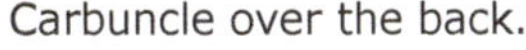

Carbuncle over the back.

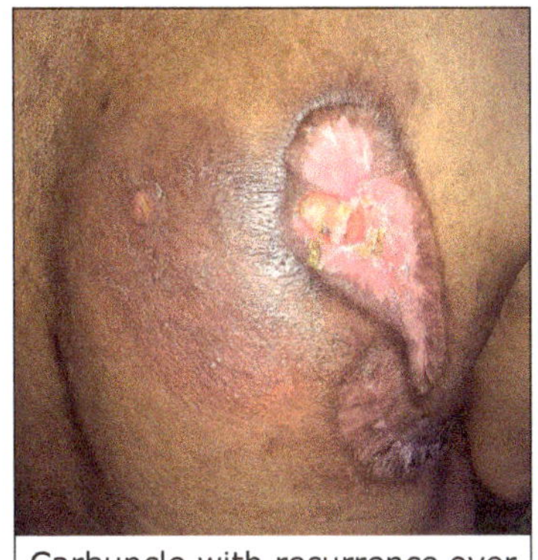

Carbuncle with recurrence over the back.

1. Furuncle and carbuncles two different clinical forms of deep folliculitis that involves in deep dermis and subcutaneous fat.
2. Furuncle involves single hair follicle
3. Carbuncle occur when the furuncle spread to multiple follicles & surrounding subcutaneous tissue.
4. Staphylococcus is the usual causative organism.
5. Furuncles commonly present on axillae, buttocks, perianal region, thighs and face
6. For carbuncles common site is nape of neck other sites are back of trunk and proximal extremities
7. On inspection the carbuncle looks small externally but on palpation we feel that a larger area of infection is involved internally
8. **Predisposing factors**
   - Poor hygiene
   - Excessive sweating
   - Uncontrolled diabetes mellitus
   - Occlusive clothing
9. **Diagnosis:**
   - Characteristic morphology of lesion is diagnostic.
10. **Treatment**
    - Oral NSAIDs
    - Systemic antibiotics
    - Culture and sensitivity testing for specific antibiotics therapy.
    - Surgical desloughing
    - After surgical desloughing regular dressing of ulcer with antiseptics and granulation forming agents
    - Skin grafting may be needed for larger defect.

10. **Non purulent infections**

   a. **Erysipelas**

      1. A superficial skin infection with atypical skin rash, commonly develops the legs, toes, face, arms and fingers
      2. The most common cause is Group A streptococcal bacteria especially streptococcus pyogenes
      3. Usually associated with breach in skin or wound
      4. Affected area is tender, erythematous & edematous
      5. This disease is most common among the elderly, infants and children.
      6. **Risk factors**
         - Immune deficiency
         - Diabetes
         - Chronic alcoholic
         - Skin ulceration
         - Fungal infections
         - Impaired lymphatic drainage (e.g., after mastectomy, pelvic surgery, bypass grafting)
      7. **Clinical features:** Fever with chills, characteristic skin rash, headache, nausea
      8. **Diagnosis:** Appearance of well-demarcated rash and inflammation
      9. **Treatment:**
         - Depending on the severity, treatment involves either oral or intravenous antibiotics
         - Analgesics and antipyretics
         - Supportive therapy
         - Complete blood count for leukocytosis
         - Culture and sensitivity of swab for specific antibiotic therapy
         - Debridement may be needed if spreading or skin turns gangrenous.

   b. **Cellulitis**

      1. Bacterial infection of skin and subcutaneous tissue that is more generalised than erysipelas.
      2. Usually associated with broken skin or preexisting ulceration
      3. Cellulitis is characterised by expanding area of erythematous or edematous tissues
      4. Commonest organism involved is streptococcus

5. **Clinical features:**
   - Fever
   - Malaise
   - Pain
   - Leukocytosis on complete blood count
   - In some patients, clinical features of septic shock may develop such as tachycardia, tachypnea, hypotension, cold clammy skin, altered mental status

6. **Treatment**
   - **Initially high dose broad spectrum antibiotics are started**
   - **Blood and skin cultures are taken for sensitivity to start specific antibiotic therapy.**
   - **Elevation of the affected extremity, glycerol & MGSO4 dressing**
   - **Analgesics and antipyretics**
   - Debridement & desloughing with fasciotomy (If indicated) of the affected part followed by regular dressing.

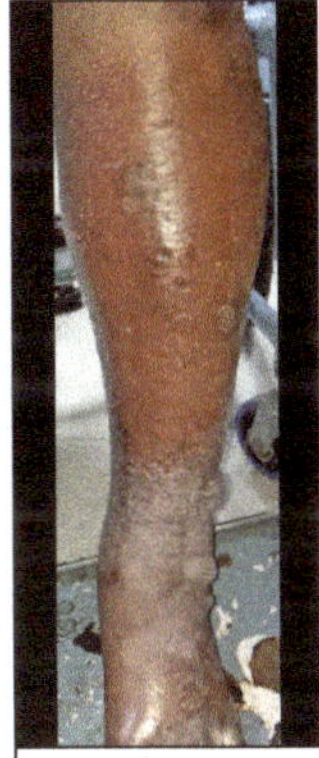
Cellulitis with blisters

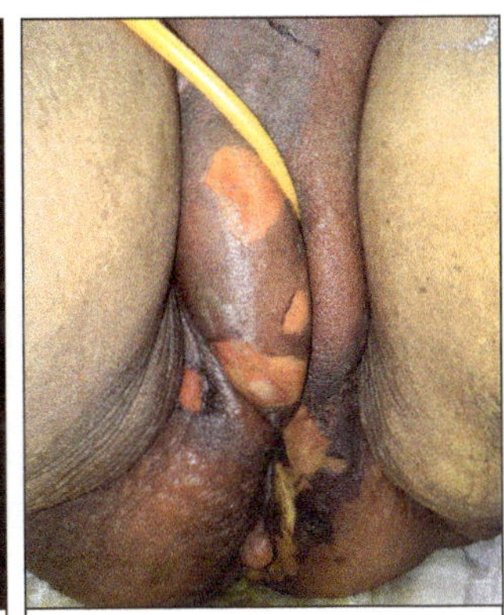
Perineal cellulitis

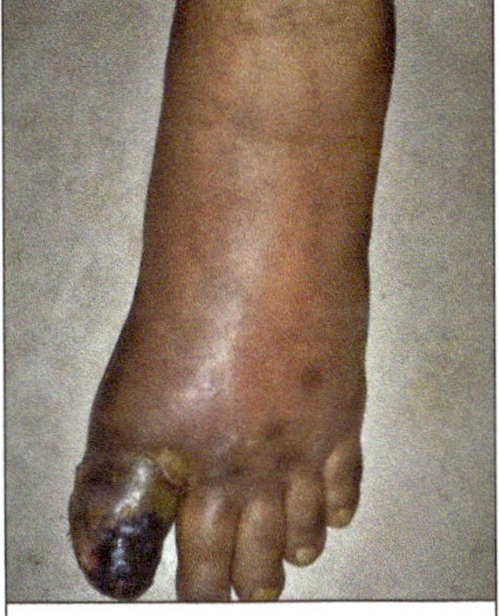
Cellulitis of left foot showing gangrene of distal toe with sloughing of skin associated with swelling & redness over the foot with necrotic patches

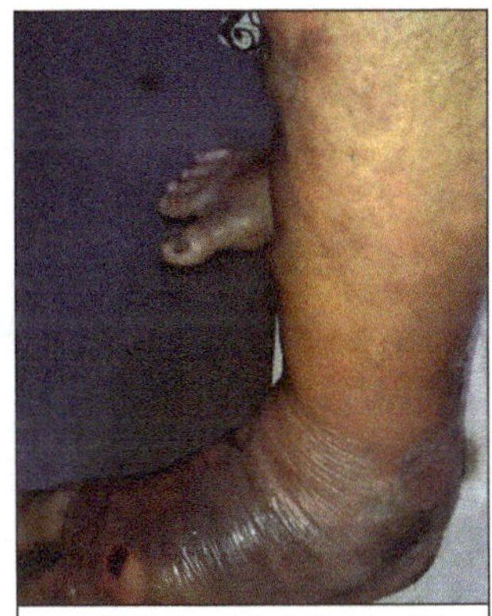
Cellulitis of left foot with necrotic patches

   - Consider arteriovenous doppler of affected limb to rule out deep venous thrombosis, peripheral vascular disease as these may prevent healing & further worsen the condition.
   - Operative management for cellulitis should be kept as last option in presence of DVT.

c. **Necrotising fasciitis**

1. A type of rapidly spreading skin and soft tissue infection involving necrosis of fascia and subcutaneous tissues
2. Most commonly a streptococcus species in combination with staphylococcus, E. coli, pseudomonas, proteus, bacteroides, clostridia.
3. Most commonly occur in lower extremities
4. The infection process rapidly spread along the muscle fascia, suprafascial plane and subcutaneous tissue
5. Patient gives history of trauma or infection
6. Patient rapidly progress to septic shock, so this is a surgical emergency
7. **Clinical features:**
   - Fever
   - Malaise
   - Edema stretching beyond the visible erythema
   - Texture of skin becomes woody
   - Leukocytosis on complete blood count
   - Signs of sepsis

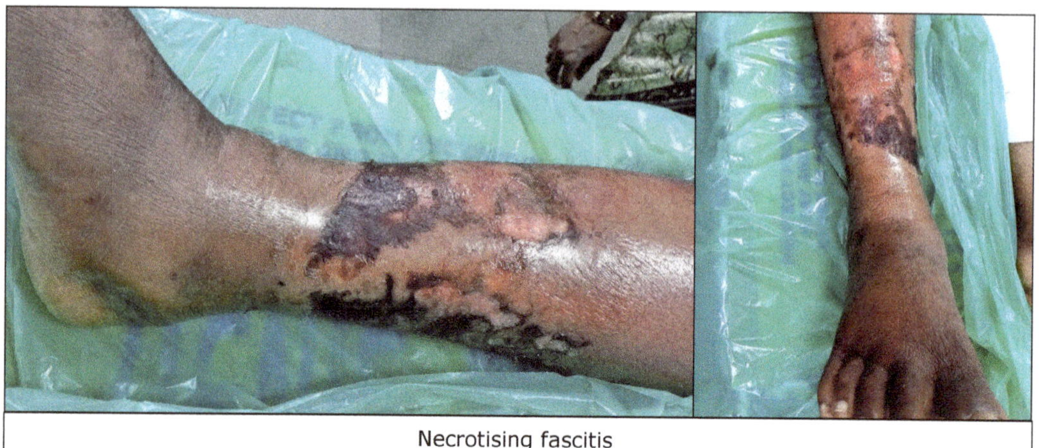

Necrotising fascitis

8. Management:
   - **Hospitalisation**
   - **Monitor pulse, Blood pressure, leukocyte count**
   - **Patient resuscitation with intravenous fluids and other supportive measures**

- **Symptomatic treatment:** analgesics and antipyretics
- **Initially, high dose broad spectrum antibiotics are started and then specific antibiotics are given as per culture & sensitivity report.**
- **Some patients may require ionotropic, respiratory support in management of septic shock.**
- **Surgical management:** Diseased area should be debried as soon as possible until viable healthy bleeding tissue is reached followed by regular dressing.

BURN

1. A burn is a type of injury to skin, deeper tissues
2. Most burns are due to heat from hot liquids, solids, or fire
3. Majority of burns in children are scald burns which are caused by accidents with kettles, pans, hot drinks and bath water.
4. Most electrical and chemical injuries occur in adults are accidental.
5. Cold and radiation are very rare causes of burns.
6. **Etiology of burn:**
   a. **Dry heat**
   b. **Flame burn**
   c. **Electrical burn**
   d. **Chemical burn (Acid or alkali)**
   e. **Ionizing radiation**
   f. **Frostbite (Cold injury)**
7. **Classification of burn:**

Type	Layer involved	Appearance	sensation
1st degree [Superficial burn]	Localized to Epidermis	Red skin without blisters	Painful
2nd degree [Superficial partial thickness	Burn involve epidermis and superficial dermis i.e. papillary	Redness with clear blisters, blanches with pressure	Very painful
2nd degree [Deep partial thickness]	Burn involve epidermis and extend into deep dermis i.e. reticular	Yellow or white	Discomfort
3rd degree [Full thickness]	Extend through entire dermis	White or brown without blanching	Painless
4th degree	Extend through entire skin and into underlying fat, muscle and bone	Black, charred with eschar	Painless

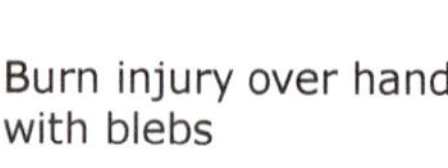
Burn injury over hand with blebs

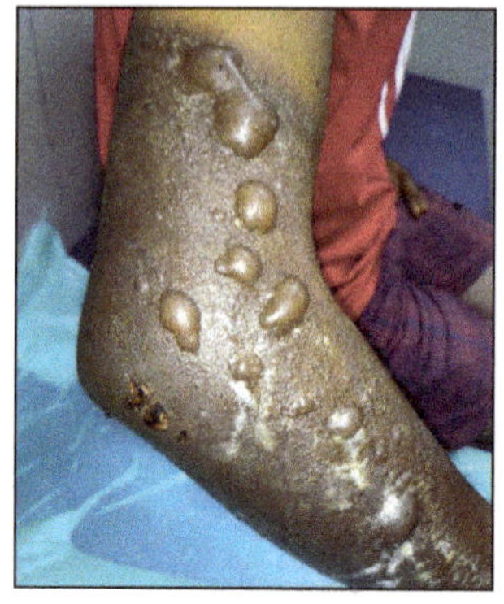

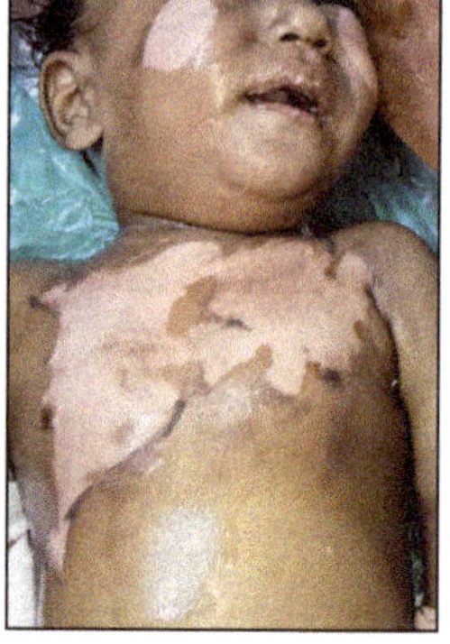
Child with superficial burn injury

8. **Assessment of burn:**

   a. **Assessment of size of burn:**

      1. Burn size should be assessed carefully & during assessment soot and debris should be washed.
      2. During assessment, care should be taken to avoid hypothermia.
      3. Outside the hospital rough guide to assess the TBSA by using RULE OF NINE.
      4. In small or patchy burns the best way to measure the burn't BSA is patient's whole hand [Digits and Palm] which represents 1% of TBSA.
      5. Accurate way of measuring the size of burn is by using Lund and browder chart which maps out the percentage of TBSA based on sections of our anatomy

   b. **Assessment of depth:**

      1. We can understand depth of burn with the help of comes history of burn (Cause of burn, contact period with etiological agent, first aid).
      2. The burning of human skin depends on temperature and contact period with etiological agent.

Different Causes of burn	**Probable depth of burn**
Scald Burn (With hot liquid)	Superficial, In the absence of good first aid deep dermal patches can occur
Flame burns (Superheated and oxidized air)	Mixed deep dermal and full thickness
Electric contact burn (Electric current through tissue)	Full thickness.
Alkali burn including cement (Noxious effect)	Often deep dermal or full thickness
Acid burn (Noxious effect)	**Weak concentration:**.Superficial **Strong concentration:** Deep dermal.

9. **Management of burn**

   a. **Prehospital care:**

      1. **Stop the burning process:** stop, drop and roll is a good method of extinguishing fire.
      2. **Cool the burn wound (Avoid ice cold water):** Immediately after burn pour the room temp water on the burn wound to minimize a depth of injury.
      3. **Give analgesia**
      4. **Give O_2:** If history of patient trapped in fire of enclosed space then O_2 administration is required especially in altered consciousness.
      5. **Elevation:** Elevation of burn limb avoids the swelling and discomfort.
      6. Remove constrictive clothings like tight shirt, pants, or metal rings or any thing restricting blood supply and respiration.

7. Remove jewellary like rings, bangles, chains as once edema sets in it is difficult to remove this and due to this vascular compromise and gangrene can occur.

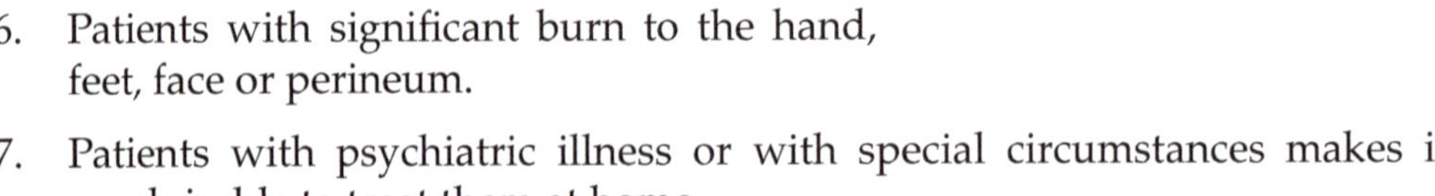

Burn injury over hand with ring causing vascular compromise in ring finger

b. **Admission criteria:**

1. Suspected airway or inhalational injury.
2. Any burn which requires fluid resuscitation.
3. Any burn which requires surgery.
4. All electrical and chemical burn or any mild cases of electrical/chemical burn with high potential of complications.
5. Any burn patient of extremes of ages.
6. Patients with significant burn to the hand, feet, face or perineum.
7. Patients with psychiatric illness or with special circumstances makes it unadvisable to treat them at home.

c. **Hospital care:**

1. **Principles of management burn as per ATLS (ABCDEF):**

- **Airway control**
  - i. In airway burn which leads to swelling of the airway and may cause complete occlusion of the upper airway.
  - ii. Early elective intubation is safest, as emergency crico thyroidectomy may be required, if there is delay in the intubation due to delayed diagnosis of airway burn
  - iii. Airway injury is always suspected in patients with facial burn.
  - iv. Symptoms of laryngeal edema includes change in voice, stridor, anxiety and difficulty in breathing
  - v. Upper airway obstruction may develop rapidly so needs continuous monitoring of patient is required.
- **Breathing**
  - i. History of patient traped in the fire, soot in the nose, increase in respiratory rate and efforts, decreased oxygen saturation indicate the inhalation injury.
  - ii. Warm humidified O_2, nebulisation, physiotherapy is very useful.
  - iii. Arterial blood gas analysis, respiratory rate monitoring and chest X-ray should be done to see the progress of inhalation injury.

iv. If condition deteriorates then positive pressure ventilation, intubation will be needed.

- **Fluid resuscitation:**

  i. Principle of fluid resuscitations is to provide sufficient circulation not only to perfuse essential organs like brain, kidney and gut but also to the peripheral skin especially damaged skin.

  ii. If oral fluid is recommended then salt must be added to oral fluid. Fluid requirement can be calculated by standard formulas.

  iii. Most common fluid used in resuscitation includes ringer lactate/ hartmann's solution & other solutions used are fresh frozen plasma (FFP), albumin and hypotonic saline.

  iv. Most commonly used formula for fluid resuscitation is **parkland regimen:** 4 X TBSA X WEIGHT(KG)= Volume of fluid in ML

    a. Half of this volume given in 1st 8 hours

    b. Second half in the next 16 hours.

  v. Other regimens used for fluid resuscitation includes:

    a. Evans formula

    b. Muir and barclay

    c. Modified brooks formula: 1.5 mL/kg per % TBSA burn

  vi. Most commonly used colloid based formula is

  Muir and barclay:

    a. 0.5 X % TBSA X weight (kg) = one portion

    b. Periods of 4 hours/4 hours/4 hours for the first 12 hours, 6 hours/6 hours between 12 and 24 hours and 12 hourly respectively.

    c. One portion should be given in each period.

- **Monitoring of fluid resuscitation:**

  i. Monitoring of resuscitation is based on urinary output

  ii. Output should be between 0.5 ml and 1.0 ml/kg/hour

  iii. Hematocrit measurement is a useful tool in confirming suspected under or over hydration.

- **Other management in the treatment of burn patient:**

  i. Analgesia: NSAIDs in superficial burns and IV opiates are used for large and very painful burns.

ii. **Energy balance and nutrition:** Burn patients should start feeding within 6 hours to reduce gut mucosal damage and patient need extra feed

iii. **Escharotomy:**

a. Circumferential full thickness burns to the limbs require emergency surgery to relieve pressure inside a compartment and to improve blood supply.

b. The tourniquet effect due to burn treated by incising the whole length of full thickness burns in the mid axial line to avoid damage to major nerves.

- **Control of infection:**

i. Patient with major burns are immunocompromised so they are more vulnerable to infections.

ii. Pathogenic and opportunistic bacteria (Pseudomonas) and fungi enter via the burn wound, catheter and via IV line.

iii. Sterile precautions must be rigorously used.

iv. Swab for culture should be taken regularly.

v. Appropriate antibiotic (Topical & systemic agents) should be started as per culture report.

vi. Proper nursing care

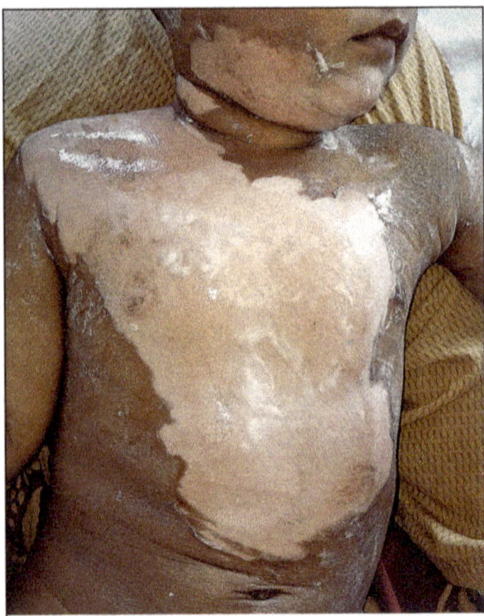

Burns child with collagen dressing

- **Physiotherapy:** Reduces swelling and improves the final outcomes of patients.
- **Psychological support**

2. **Wound management:**

- **Dressing:** The key lies in the dressing that it is easy to apply, non painful, reduces pain, simple to manage and locally available.
- **Types of methods:**

i. **Open method:** Silver sulfadiazine application without dressing commonly used in burns of face, head and neck.

ii. **Closed method:** Dressing done to protect the wound and soothe.

Depth of burn	Type of dressing
First-degree wounds	No dressing and are treated with topical antibiotics
Second-degree wounds	Daily dressing changes with topical antibiotics, cotton gauze, and bandage. Or temporary biological or synthetic covering
Deep second-degree and third-degree wounds	Initial dressings to hold bacterial proliferation till excision and grafting for sizable burns.

- **Complications**
  i. Bacterial infection, which may lead to sepsis
  ii. Fluid loss leads to hypovolemia.
  iii. Hypothermia
  iv. Breathing problems due to inhalation of smoke particles.
  v. Scars or ridged areas caused by an overgrowth of scar tissue (keloids)
  vi. Bone and joint problems, such as when scar tissue causes the shortening and tightening of skin, muscles or tendons (contractures)
  vii. Hypoproteinemia due to protein loss from the exudative fluid.

DEEP VENOUS THROMBOSIS

1. **Definition:** Formation of a blood clot within the venous system and may occur in the superficial system usually described as (superficial thrombophlebitis) or deep system (deep venous thrombosis or DVT).
2. Venous thrombosis of the deep veins of the leg may cause pulmonary embolism/ sudden death.
3. **Etiology:** Three factors described by virchow for the development of venous thrombosis are as follows:
   a. **Changes in vessel wall (Endothelial damage)**
   b. **Prolonged stasis (Which is diminished blood flow through the veins)**
   c. **Coagulability of blood (Thrombophilia)**
4. **Risk factors for venous thrombosis:**

Patients factors:	**Abnormalities of thrombosis and fibrinolysis**	**Disease or surgical procedure:**
1. Advanced age 2. Obesity 3. Tobacco use 4. Varicose veins 5. Intravenous drug abuse. 6. Prolonged Immobilization (Paralysis, spinal cord injury) 7. Pregnancy 8. Puerperium 9. High dose estrogen therapy 10. Previous history of deep vein thrombosis or pulmonary embolism 11. Thrombophilia	1. Factor V Leiden mutation 2. Antithrombin III deficiency 3. Prothrombin gene mutation 4. Protein C deficiency 5. Protein S deficiency 6. Homocysteinemia 7. Antiphospholipid syndrome 8. Lupus antibody 9. Anticardiolipin antibody	1. Malignancy 2. Trauma or surgery, especially of pelvis, hip and lower limb 3. Paralysis of lower limbs 4. Infection e.g. Covid 19 infection 5. Recent myocardial infarction (Arrhythmias) 6. Inflammatory bowel disease 7. Nephrotic syndrome 8. Antibody or lupus anticoagulant

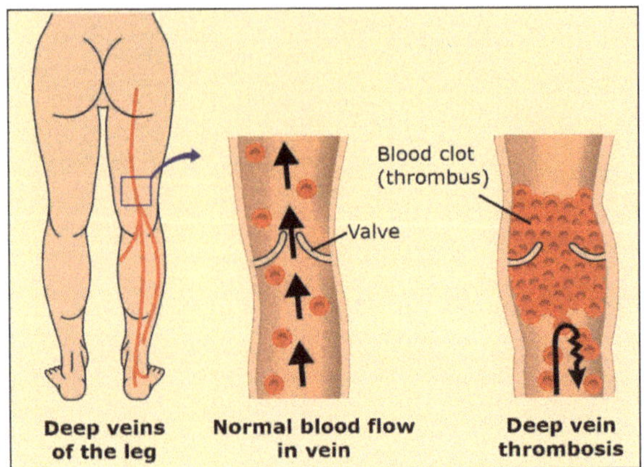

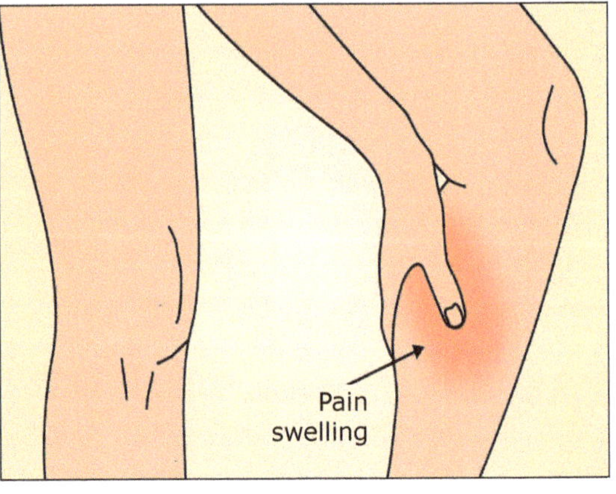

5. **Clinical features:**

   a. Calf pain (Usually unilateral)

   b. Tenderness over the course of deep vein (Femoral artery or popliteal vein)

   c. Low grade pyrexia

   d. Mild pitting edema of ankle

   e. Stiff calf and dilated superficial veins (In delayed case swelling and tenderness of entire limb occurs)

   f. **In case of pulmonary emboli:** Pleuritic pain, hemoptysis, Cyanosis, dyspnea, raised neck veins, a fixed split second heart sound and pleural rub

   g. **Phlegmasia cerulea dolens:** Painful blue inflammation of leg

   h. **Phlegmasia alba dolens:** Painful white inflammation of leg

   i. **Homan's sign:** Calf pain on flexion of knee and dorsiflexion of ankle

   j. **Moses sign:** Pain with calf compression against the tibia

6. **Test and diagnosis:**

   a. **Blood test:**

      i. **D -DIMER:** Almost all the patients having severe DVT have elevated blood levels of a clot dissolving substance called D-dimer.

      ii. Blood tests for clotting disorders like PTINR, BT, CT

   b. **Sonography (Duplex with color doppler):** Filling defect in flow and lack of compressibility indicate the presence (Duplex compression examination) of a thrombosis.

      This is accurate and reliable for femoral and popliteal clots but less certain in tibial vein clots.

   c. **Ascending venography (Rarely done nowadays)**: Which shows a thrombus as a filling defect

   d. **MRI scan:** Magnetic resonance venography is now as accurate as contrast venography

   e. **CT Scan chest with angiography:** Definitively diagnose a pulmonary embolism as a filling defect in pulmonary arteries

7. **Modified Wells criteria for predicting deep vein thrombosis (DVT)**

Variables for prediction	Score
Bedridden for more than three days or surgery in the last 4 weeks	1
Lower limb trauma or surgery or immobilisation in a plaster cast	1
Localised tenderness along the line of femoral or popliteal veins	1
Entire limb swollen	1
Calf > 3 cm larger circumference than the other side (Measure 10 cm below the tibial tuberosity)	1
Pitting edema confined to symptomatic leg	1
Dilated collateral superficial veins (not varicose veins)	1
Previous documented history of DVT	1
Malignancy (including treatment up to 6 months ago)	1
Alternative diagnosis more likely than DVT	-2

Probability of DVT	Score
Low probability of DVT	-2 to 0
Moderate probability of DVT	1-2
High probability of DVT	> 2

8. **Differential diagnosis:**

   a. **Deep venous thrombosis:**

      1. A calf muscle hematoma
      2. A ruptured plantaris muscle
      3. Ruptured baker cyst (a swelling in the popliteal space, the space behind the knee)
      4. Thrombosed popliteal aneurysm
      5. Arterial ischemia

   b. **Pulmonary embolism:**

      1. Myocardial infarction
      2. Pleurisy
      3. Pneumonia

9. **Treatment:**

   a. **Anticoagulant therapy:**

      1. **Lower molecular weight heparin**

         - LMWH /Heparin Should be started within 24 hours
         - Dose of LMWH: 0.6 mg BD Subcutaneously
         - Dose of heparin: 5000U IV bolus f/b 18 Units/kg/hr & maintain PTT between 60-80 sec.
         - If patient is sensitive to heparin induced thrombocytopenia give fondaparinux and bivalirudin

      2. **Warfarin**

         - Should be started on the same day of heparin
         - Maintain INR between 2-3
         - Continue warfarin for 3 months or longer depending upon the risk factor or recurrence.

      3. **Novel oral anticoagulant (NOAC)**

         - Example: Rivaroxaban & Dabigatran are alternative medications to warfarin in high risk patients.

   b. **Inferior Vena Caval filter /Umbrella filter**

      1. It is used when patient has bleeding risk
      2. Umbrella filter placed in inferior vena cava to prevent migration of clot higher up (To prevent pulmonary embolism)

   c. **Thrombolysis:**

      1. Thrombolysis should be considered in patients with an iliac vein thrombosis, especially if they are seen early and the limb is extremely swollen.
      2. Tissue plasminogen activator is used in thrombolysis.
      3. In some cases, venous stents are used to improve blood flow to limb specially in thrombus of iliac region.

   d. **Surgical venous thrombectomy: Rarely done nowadays.**

10. **Complications of DVT and its management**

    a. **Pulmonary Embolism**

       1. **Anticoagulation therapy**
       2. **Continuous monitoring of patient**

3. **Thrombolysis**
4. **Radiologically guided catheter embolectomy**

b. Post thrombotic Syndrome (PTS)

1. PTS can be prevented with thrombolysis, endovenous thrombectomy & stenting
2. ⅔ rd patient of DVT develops PTS
3. **Treatment:**
   - **Lifelong compression**
   - **Venous recanalisation**
   - **Stenting**
   - **Venous bypass**

Section 2

Ear, Nose and Throat Emergencies

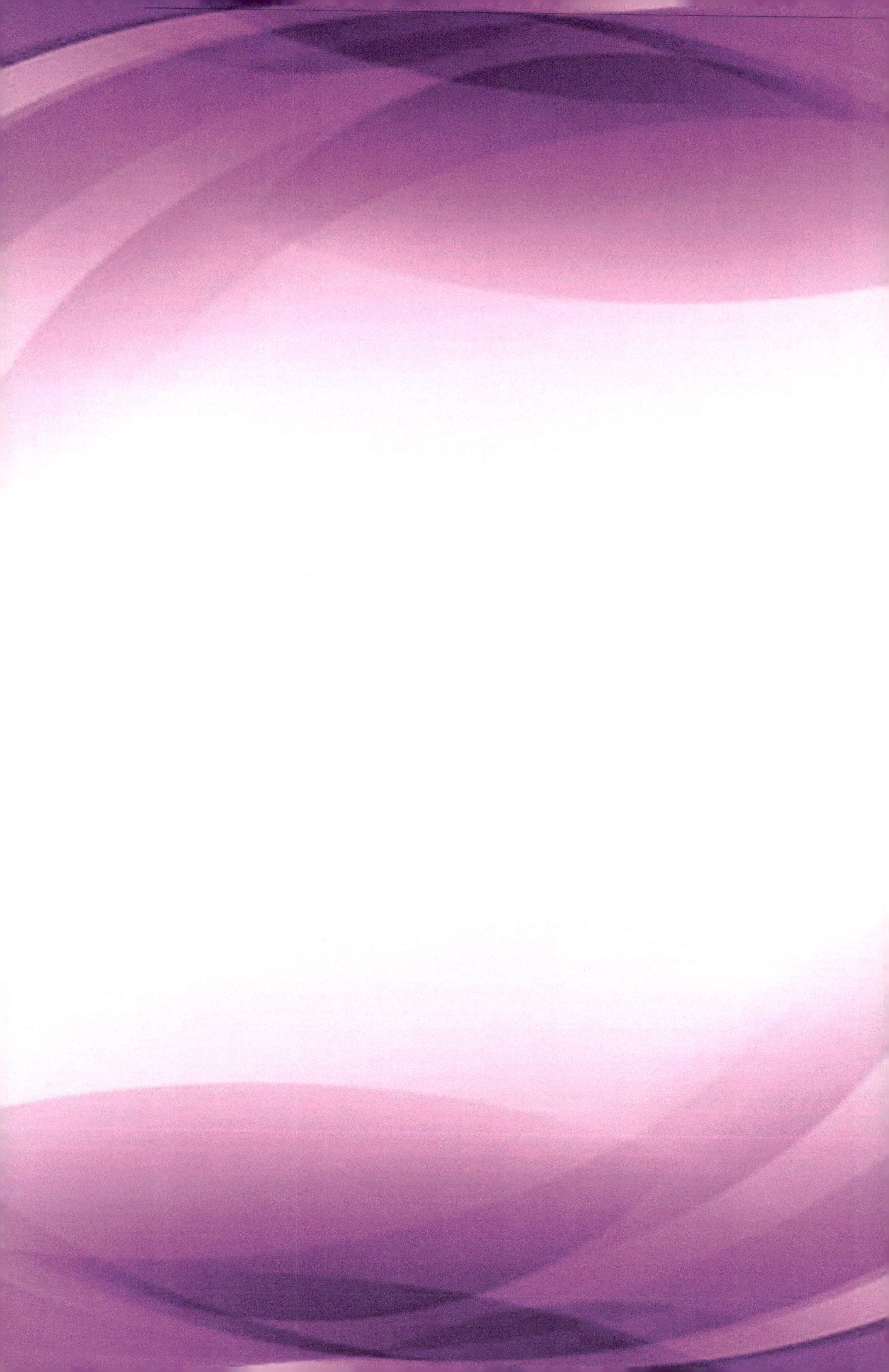

CHAPTER

2 Ear, Nose and Throat Emergencies

EXAMINATION OF EAR, NOSE AND THROAT

Ear	Nose and paranasal sinus	Oral cavity	Throat (Pharynx and Larynx)
Physical examination	**Physical Examination**	**Physical examination:**	**Physical examination:**
1. External ear a. Size, shape and position of pinna b. Swelling, ulcer, scar, sinus and fistula c. Palpation: tenderness, raised temperature, pain on movement of pinna.	**1. External nose** a. Nasal bridge deformity, scars, ulcers, sinus, swelling, broadening of nose. b. Crepitations or tenderness on palpation.	**1. Lips** Ulcers, growths, swelling, crusts, scars, vesicles, cleft lips **2. Buccal mucosa** Ulceration, swelling or growth, leukoplakia, erythroplakia, pigmentation, atrophy, submucous fibrosis	**1. Nasopharynx** Anterior rhinoscopy, posterior rhinoscopy, digital examination and endoscopy **1. Discharge** **2. Crusting** **3. Mass** **4. Bleeding**

(Continued)

Ear	Nose and paranasal sinus	Oral cavity	Throat (Pharynx and Larynx)
2. External auditory canal a. Size of meatus b. Content of lumen c. Swelling **3. Tympanic membrane** a. Color b. Position (Retracted, protruded) c. Surface d. Thickness and transparency e. Mobility **4. Middle ear mucosa and its contents** Examined through the perforation, transparent TM or on surgical exploration **5. Mastoid region (swelling)** **6. Eusthachian tube examination** Posterior rhinoscopy, valsalva maneuver, eustachian catheterization **7. Facial nerve (UMN/LMN)** **FUNCTIONAL EXAMINATION** **1. Auditory function** a. Voice test b. Tuning fork test **2. Vestibular function (For Vertigo)**	**2. Anterior rhinoscopy** Nasal cavity and secretions, position of nasal septum, floor of nose, swelling of turbinates, properties of mucosal surface, Ulceration or presence of foreign body, mass. **3. Posterior rhinoscopy** Posterior margin of septum, posterior choanae, posterior ends of turbinates nasopharynx **FUNCTIONAL EXAMINATION** **1. Patency of nose** Spatula test / cotton-wool test **2. Sense of smell** Clove oil, essence of rose, coffee **PARANASAL SINUSES:** 1. Inspect for swelling over PNS, skin changes, lid edema, conjunctival congestion, proptosis. 2. Palpate frontal, maxillary and ethmoidal sinus simultaneously 3. Transillumination test	**3. Teeth and gums** Loose teeth, caries, number of teeth, misaligned teeth & Gums: redness, ulceration, swollen or growth **4. Hard palate** Cleft or high arched palate, ulcers or growth, selling, oronasal fistula, bony growth **5. Anterior two-third tongue** Macroglossia, deviation or protrusion, color, ulcers, fissures, red/white lesions, proliferative growth **6. Floor of mouth** Swelling, ulcers, scars, tongue tie	**2. Oropharynx** **a. Tonsils** Size, symmetry, membranes, ulcers, bulging mass and tonsillar pillars **b. Soft palate** Redness, swelling, bulge, vesicles, ulcers/growth, notch, fibrosis, cleft palate and uvula (position and surface) **c. Posterior pharyngeal wall** Swelling, ulcers/ growth, crusting and Post nasal purulent drip **d. Base of tongue and vallecula** Swelling (solid or cystic), ulceration, color of mucosa, veins, lingual thyroid **3. Laryngopharynx and larynx examination (By laryngoscopy):** It includes examination of hyoid bone, thyroid cartilage, thyroid notch, cricoid cartilage and tracheal rings **Examine** a. Redness b. Swelling or bulging c. Contour, widening or displacement of larynx d. Movement of larynx on deglutition and breathing (Present or absent) **e. Post laryngeal crepitation** (Present or absent)

EAR TRAUMA

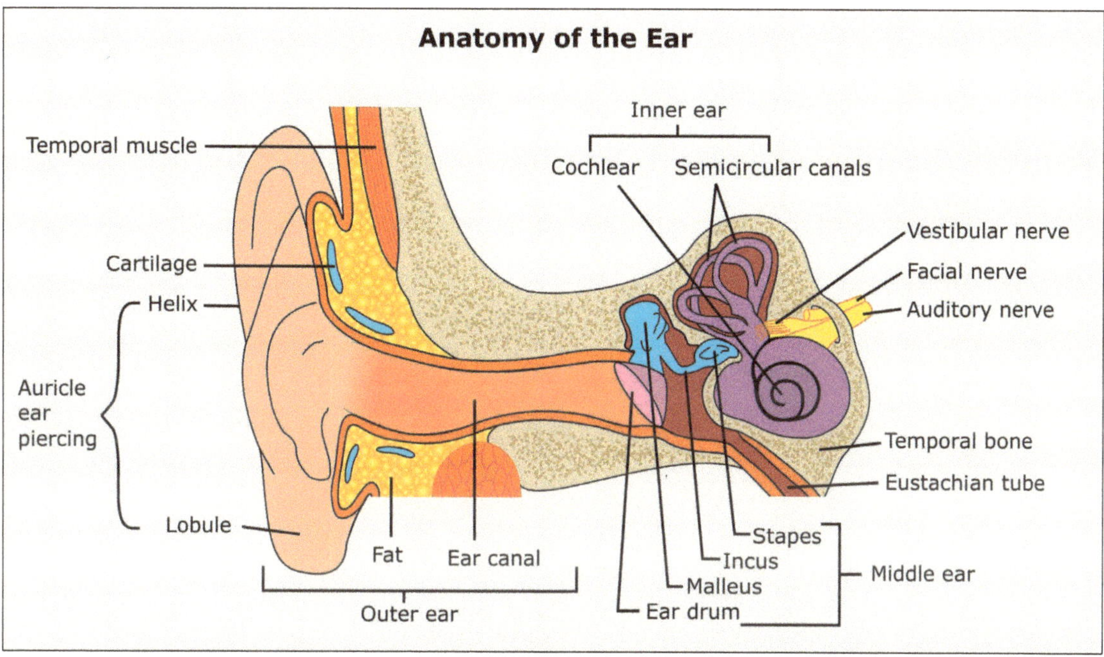

1. Traumatic injury to ears can occur in a number of ways
2. Most common causes of ear injuries are a slap to the ear, an ear bud injury, a severe blow to the head from falling off a bicycle or having a motor vehicle accident, loud noise, blast injury.
3. Trauma may lead from minor to severe injuries, which may need emergency management
4. **Traumatic injuries of the ear includes:**

   A] External ear:

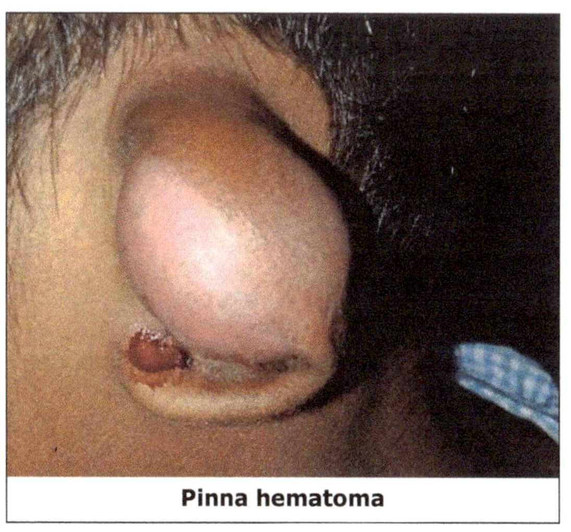

Pinna hematoma

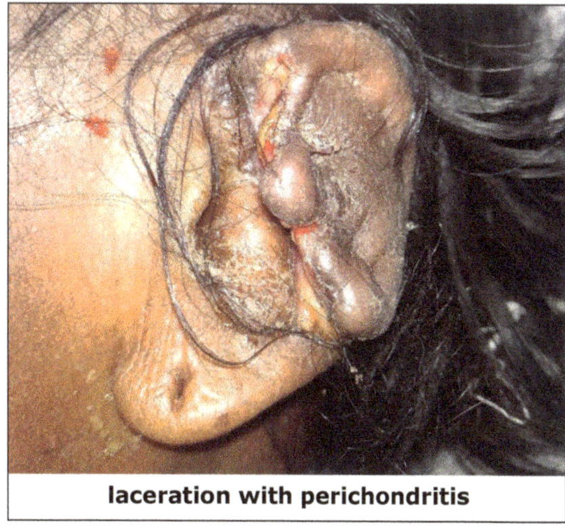

laceration with perichondritis

1. Avulsion of pinna
2. Lacerations of auricle
3. Hematoma of auricle
4. Laceration of external auditory canal
5. Traumatic rupture of tympanic membrane: Due to hair pins, needles, matchstick, unskilled instrumentation, open handed slap, blast and forceful valsalva, diving, water sports and forceful syringing.

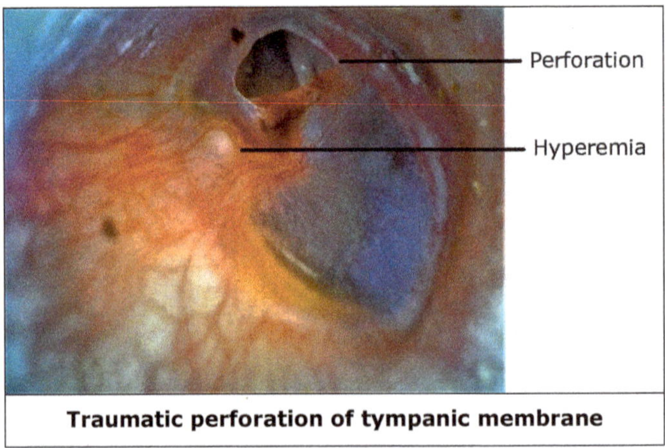

Traumatic perforation of tympanic membrane

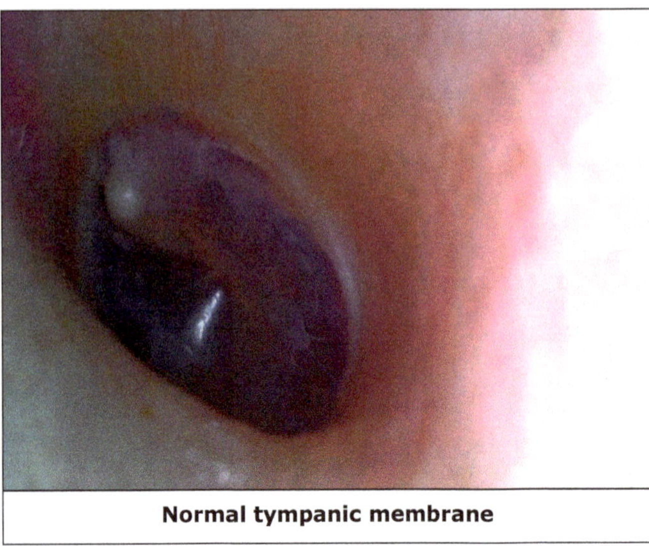

Normal tympanic membrane

B] Middle ear:

1. Hemotympanum
2. Otitic barotrauma

C] **Inner ear:**

Audiovestibular system injury

5. **Symptoms of ear trauma**

A] **Symptoms of an outer ear trauma include:**

1. Bleeding from ear.
2. Pain and tenderness of ear
3. Redness / pinna swelling
4. Hematoma over the pinna
5. Bruising of the ear.

B] **Symptoms of middle ear injury:**

1. Dizziness/vertigo with or without nausea or vomiting
2. Bleeding from ear canal
3. Hearing loss
4. Earache
5. Ear fullness
6. Tinnitus

C] **Symptoms of inner ear:**

1. Vertigo (Patient feels that room is spinning) with or without nausea or vomiting
2. Hearing loss

6. **Management:**

Types of ear trauma	Management
Laceration of pinna	Perichondrium is stitched with absorbable suture. Stripping of perichondrium from cartilage must be avoided as its result in avascular necrosis The fine nonabsorbable sutures are used for the skin closure Broad spectrum antibiotics are prescribed.
Avulsions of pinna	When pinna remains attached to the head by a small skin pedicle then primary reattachment is usually successfully done Completely avulsed pinna can be reimplanted by micro vascular surgery or Skin of the avulsed segment of pinna is removed and cartilage of ear pinna implanted under the postauricular skin for later reconstruction

(Continued)

Types of ear trauma	Management
Hematoma of auricle	Aspiration of hematoma under aseptic conditions Prophylactic antibiotics Pressure dressing Packing of all concavities of the auricle to prevent reaccumulation of blood Incision and drainage is required when aspiration fails Pressure applied by dental rolls which are tied with through and through sutures/pop cast
Minor lacerations of EAC	They heal without complications
Major lacerations of EAC	Managed surgically to avoid stenosis of the canal.
Perforation of tympanic membrane	Conservative management The edge of perforation is repositioned and advised patients to keep ear dry and follow up regularly. If not healing after conservative management then go for definitive surgery.
Otitic barotrauma Inability to ventilate middle ear due to abnormal dysfunction of ET Occurs in rising ambient pressure (descent in flight /scuba diving)	Repeated valsalva maneuver, yawning, swallowing Steroids Analgesic Decongestant and mucolytics Myringotomy with grommet insertion in refractory cases.
Hemotympanum Hemotympanum is often the result of basilar skull fracture	Skull fractures usually heal on their own but rule out other cranial nerve involvement. Several complications can occur after fracture so management of complications are necessary If you have CSF leaking then you're at a higher risk of developing meningitis.
Inner ear trauma	Hearing aid Cochlear implants
Fracture of temporal bone	Fracture of temporal bone may be longitudinal, transverse or mixed Facial palsy seen mostly in transverse temporal bone fracture. If paralysis is immediate then surgery requires urgently to decompression or re-anastomosis of cut ends of nerve or cable nerve grafts If Delayed paralysis then conservative management is required.

EPISTAXIS

1. Epistaxis is defined as acute hemorrhage from the nose.
2. It is a frequent emergency department (ED) complaint and often causes significant anxiety in patients

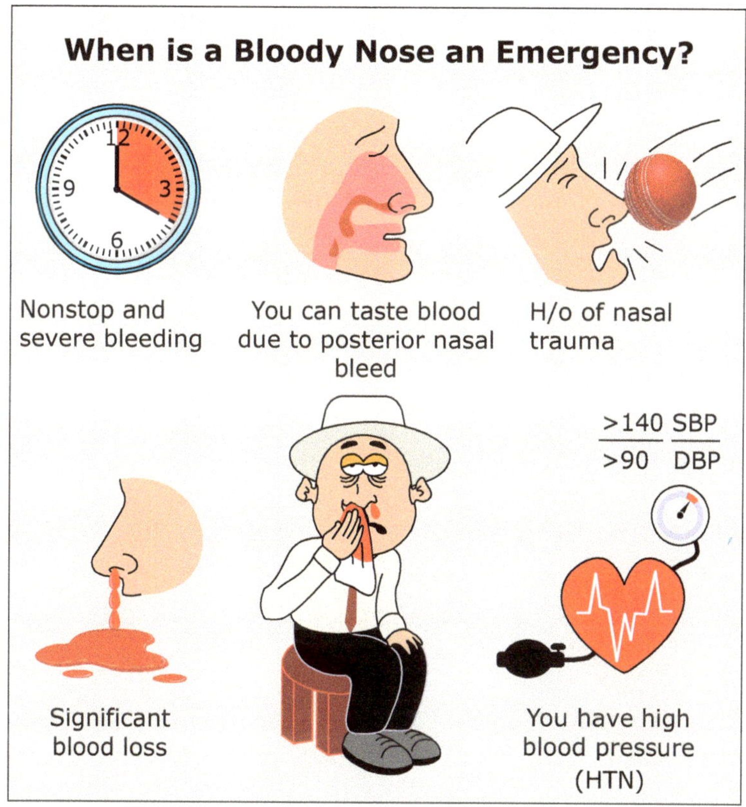

3. We should try to find its local and systemic causes.
4. **Causes of epistaxis:**

Local causes	General causes
1. Trauma: Finger nail injury, nasal injury by accident, head injury, violent sneezing 2. Infection: Rhinosinusitis, vestibulitis, sinusitis, adenoiditis, rhinosporidiosis, granulomatous lesions.	**1.** Cardiovascular: Hypertension, congestive heart failure, mitral stenosis, eclampsia of pregnancy **2.** Hemopoietic: Thrombocytopenia, leukemia, aplastic anemia, coagulopathy, hemophilia. **3.** Nutritional: Malnutrition Vit. A, D, C, E and K deficiency.

(Continued)

Local causes	General causes
3. Environmental: Dry environment High altitude, sudden decompression, chemicals, pollution. 4. Neoplasm: A] Benign: Hemangiomas, Inverted papillomas, Juvenile Angiofibroma, AV malformation. B] Malignant: Adenocarcinoma, epidermoid carcinoma, olfactory neuroblastoma. 5. Drugs: Excessive nasal decongestant use, sniffing of cocaine.	**4.** Liver diseases: Hepatic cirrhosis leads to deficiency of clotting factors **5.** Blood vessels: Arteriosclerosis, collagen disease. **6.** Kidney diseases: Chronic nephritis and renal failure **7.** Drugs: Anticoagulant therapy, NSAIDs **8.** Acute infection: Malaria, dengue, typhoid, influenza, measles with thrombocytopenia.

5. **The Common cause of nosebleeding:**

   A] **Children:** Repeated fingernail trauma.

   B] **Elderly:** Hypertension, atherosclerotic changes and malignancy

6. **Little's area /kiesselbach's plexus** is the most common site of nose bleeds in children and young adults.

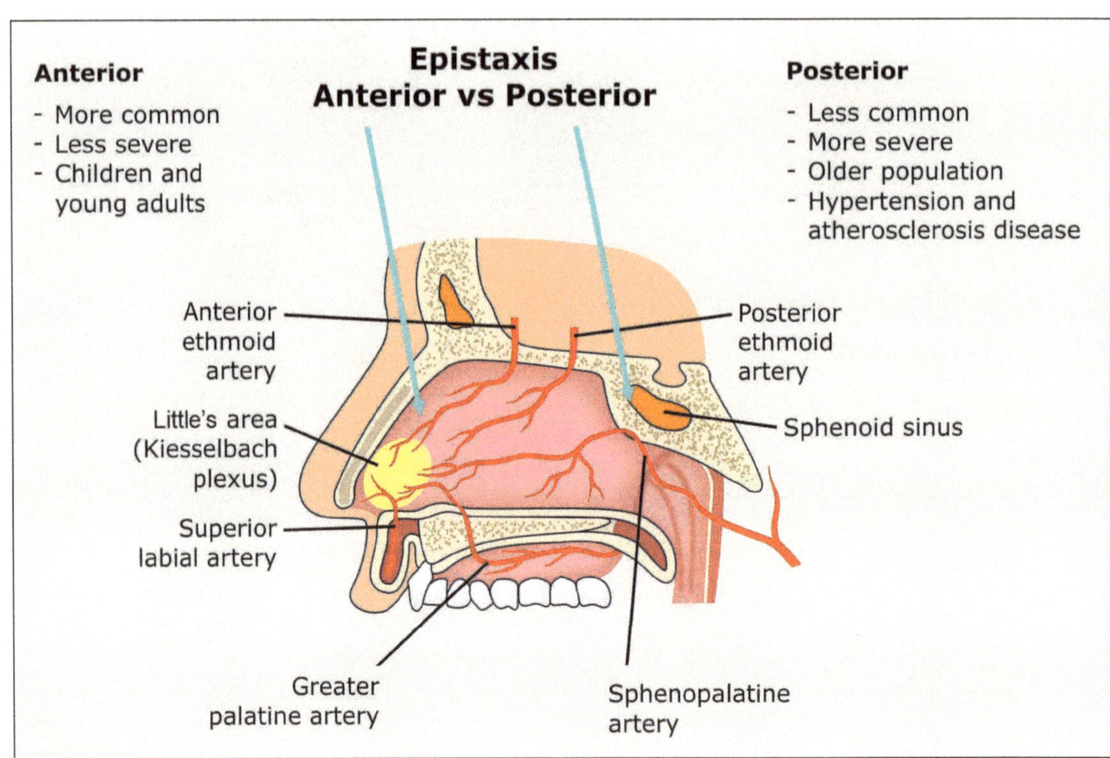

7. **Difference between anterior and posterior nasal bleeding**

	Anterior	**Posterior**
Incidence	More common	Less common
Common sites	Little's area	Posterosuperior part of nasal cavity
Localization of bleeding	Easy	Difficult
Common age group	Children and young	Elderly people (after 40 years)
Common cause	Trauma	Arteriosclerosis and hypertension
Nasal endoscopy	Not required	Required
Severity	Mild bleeding Easy to manage in OPD by pinching nose or anterior nasal packing	Severe bleeding difficult to manage in OPD May require operation theatre for Mx

8. **Management of nasal bleeding:**

A] General measures:

1. **Initial first aid:**

a] Pinch the nose with thumb and index finger for 5 min.

It usually stops the bleeding from the Little's area

b] Use decongestant nasal drops

c] Cold compresses over the nose results in reflex vasoconstriction which helps to stops bleeding

d] Use Trotter's method: Patient is made to sit and lean a little forward over a basin to spit any blood and breath quietly from mouth.

2. **Assessment of blood loss and adequate replacement: Assess the blood loss directly by** spitting and vomiting and replace the loss.

3. **Monitoring of vitals:** For hemodynamic stability.

4. **Antibiotics:** In case of infection and nasal packing.

5. **Investigations:**

a] Complete blood count, BT and CT, PT-INR

b] Blood grouping and cross match

c] Radiological: X-ray, CT, MRI and angiography.

B] Measures to stop bleeding

1. **Nasal cautery:**

a] Chemical cautery

b] Electrocautery

2. **Anterior nasal packing:**

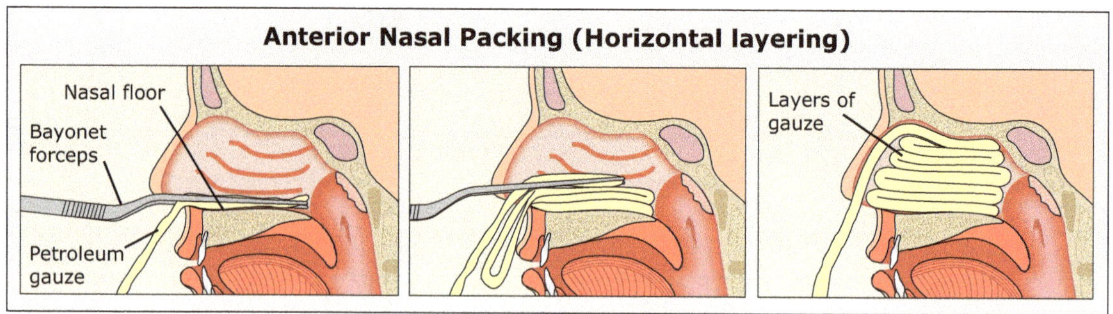

Under local anesthesia

a] **Indication:** Done in anterior nasal bleeding, firstly cauterization of bleeding area is tried and if profuse bleeding is present and site of bleeding cannot be localized, anterior nasal packing is done.

b] **Method:** One meter long ribbon gauze, which is soaked in liquid paraffin is used to pack the nasal cavity by layering.

c] Pack can be removed after 48 hours.

3. **Posterior nasal packing:**

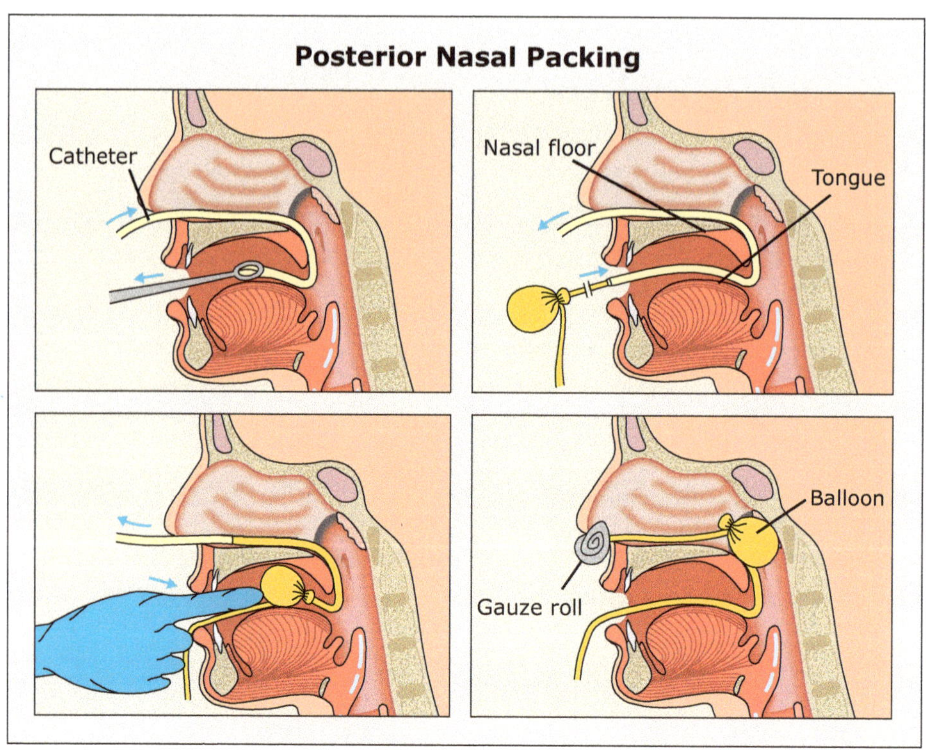

a] **Indications:** When cauterization fails and posterior bleeding site is not visualized.

b] **Done by using:** 1. Gauze 2. Foley's catheter 3. Nasal sponge 4. An inflatable nasal balloon catheter.

4. **Arterial embolisation:** Done in refractory cases of epistaxis.

   Method: First diagnostic angiography of bilateral carotid system is done

   Catheter is inserted into the internal maxillary artery for embolization.

   Gelfoam and or polyvinyl alcohol particles are used for embolization.

5. **Arterial ligation:** Ligation of external carotid artery and maxillary artery.

6. **Surgical methods:** Endoscopic sphenopalatine artery ligation or external carotid artery ligation

NASAL BONE AND SEPTUM FRACTURE

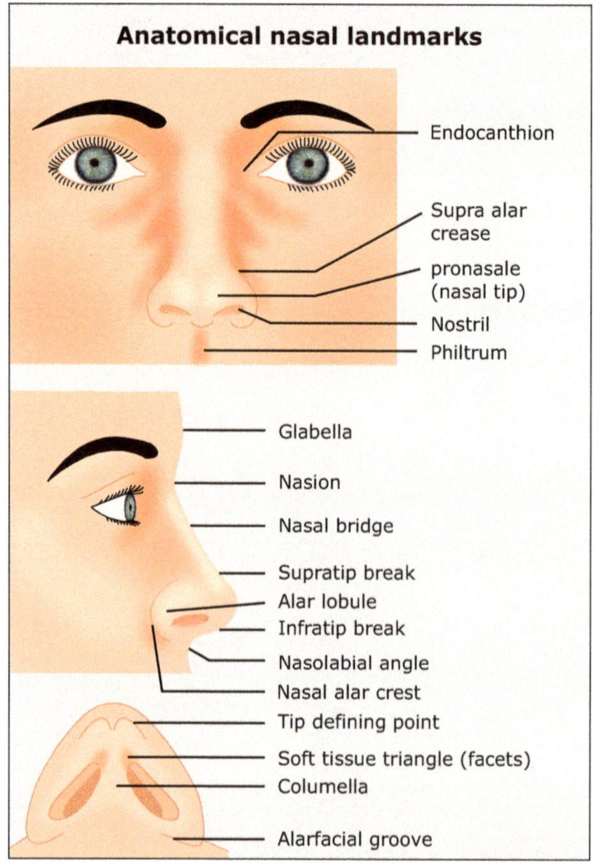

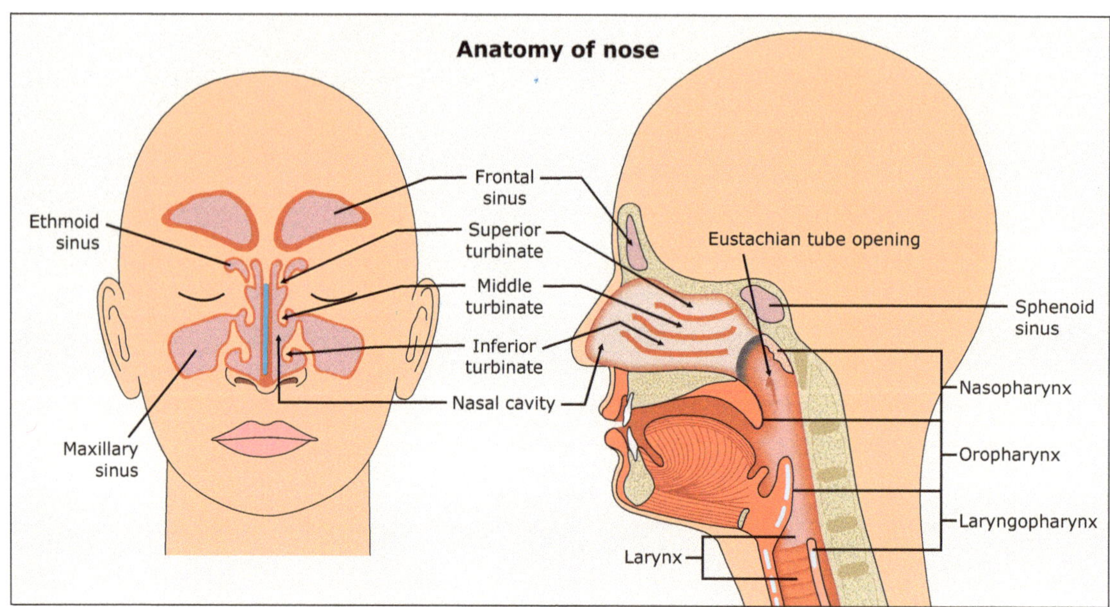

1. A nasal fracture, commonly referred to as a broken nose.
2. A fracture of one of the bones of the nose may occur after trauma..
3. The most common causes of fracture are assault, sports related injury, falls and motor vehicle collision.
4. Nasal bone fractures are the third most commonly fractured bone of the body.
5. It can also involve nasal septum which may be bucked, dislocated or fractured into several pieces.
6. Septal hematoma can occur after trauma to the nose which has to be drained urgently.

NASAL BONE FRACTURE

1. Direction and the magnitude of traumatic force is responsible for determining the depth and type of injury.
2. **There are two types of nasal fractures:**

   A] Depressed (Frontal blow)

   B] Angulated (Lateral blow)

   A] Depressed:

   1. A frontal blow to the nose can cause an open book fracture, where the nasal septum collapses and nasal bone spreads out.
   2. Greater force over the nose may result in a comminuted fracture of nasal bones along with frontal processes of the maxilla which flatten and widen the nasal dorsum.

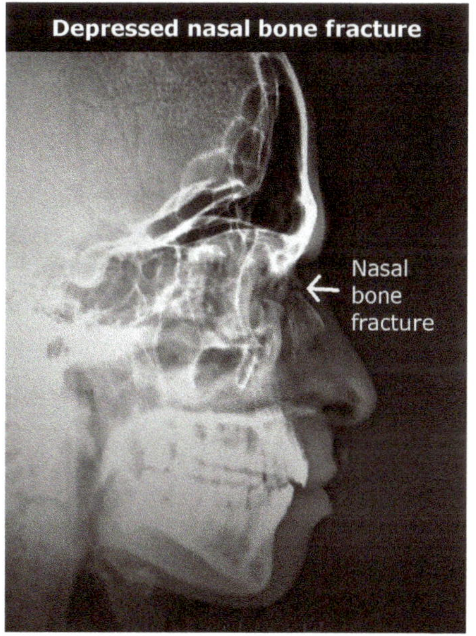

   B] Angulated:

   1. In angulated fracture, lateral blow causes depression of nasal bone or fracture of nasal bone or septum .
   2. This results into a deviation of nasal bridge.

3. **Signs and symptoms:**
   1. Epistaxis (Anterior or posterior)
   2. Pain

3. Nasal deformity (Depressed/flattening from the front or side) and nasal pyramid deviation.
4. Swelling becomes visible within a few hours and hides the effect
5. Periorbital ecchymosis (Purple colored diffuse bruising appears due to collection of blood into the skin).
6. Difficulty in breathing due to nasal obstruction
7. Septal deviation
8. Tenderness, crepitus and mobility of fractured segments.

4. **Diagnosis:**
   1. **Clinical:** Usually by clinical findings
   2. **X-ray:** Useful for documenting a medicolegal case.
5. **Treatment:**
   1. **Emergency management:**
      a. Elevation of head
      b. Cold compresses to reduce edema
      c. If active bleeding is present, control the active bleeding.
      d. Analgesics and decongestant nasal drops
   2. **Surgical management:**
      a. Surgery can be done after edema subsides as the edema not only hides the deformity but also interferes with reduction.
      b. Ideal time for reduction is either immediate before swelling or after swelling get subsides i.e. 5-7 days later.
      c. The reduction should be done within 2 weeks as after this time period fracture heals.
      d. Before reduction of the nasal bone fractures are must look for a septal hematoma and drain it as it may result into a septal abscess, septal perforation or saddle bone deformity.

A] **Closed reduction:** Digital reduction or with the help of instruments.

B] **Open reduction:** It is needed in some cases where closed method fails or having septal injury or deformity.

C] **Healed nasal deformity is corrected by rhinoplasty and septorhinoplasty.**

FRACTURE OF NASAL SEPTUM

1. Facial trauma from the front, side or downward direction may result in fracture of the nasal septum.
2. Nasal septum can get bucked and fractured vertically and horizontally or may crush into pieces.
3. **Types:**

   A] Jarjavay fracture:

   1. It results from a blow from the front.
   2. A fracture that runs horizontally across the septum.
   3. The horizontal fracture starts just above the anterior nasal spine and runs backwards and parallel and above the junction of septal cartilage with the vomer.

   B] Chevallet fracture:

   1. This type of fracture results from a blow from below
   2. It is a vertical fracture and it starts from anterior nasal spine of maxilla and runs upwards towards the direction of junction of bony and cartilaginous nasal dorsum.

4. **Treatment:**
   1. They need urgent treatment
   2. Hematoma to be drained at the earliest as it may result into septal abscess.
   3. Reposition of the dislocated septal cartilage and fractured segments of septum and it should be supported between mucoperichondrial flaps
   4. The mattress sutures are taken and nasal packing is done.

5. **Complications:**
   1. Deviation of the cartilaginous nose
   2. Asymmetry of nasal tip, columella and the nostril.
   3. Septal hematoma and nasal synechia.

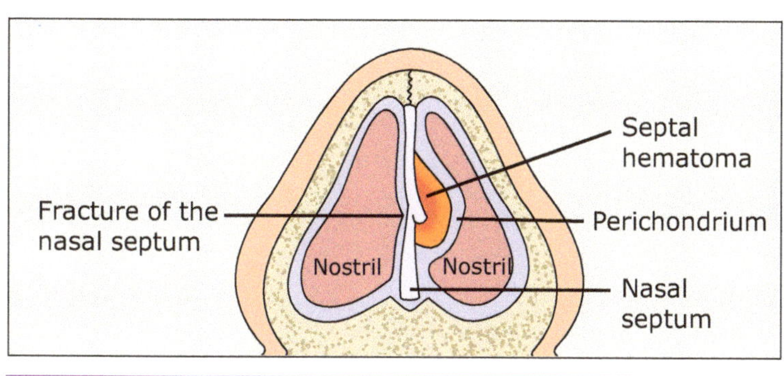

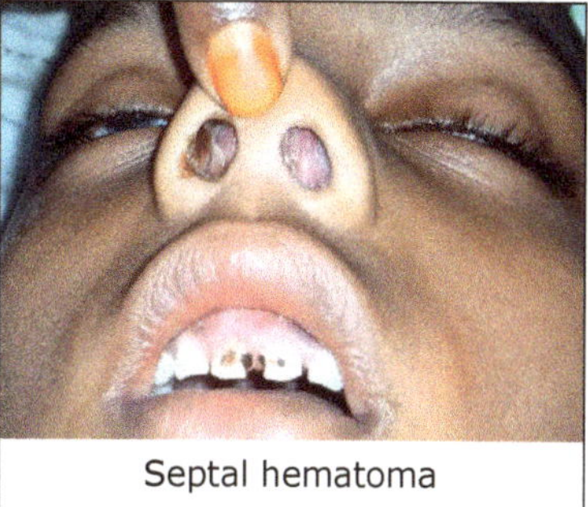
Septal hematoma

NASAL FOREIGN BODY

1. Nasal foreign bodies are a common cause in children to visit the emergency department.
2. Child may place foreign objects into their mouth, nose, or ears as a result of their curiosity or it may go accidentally while playing.

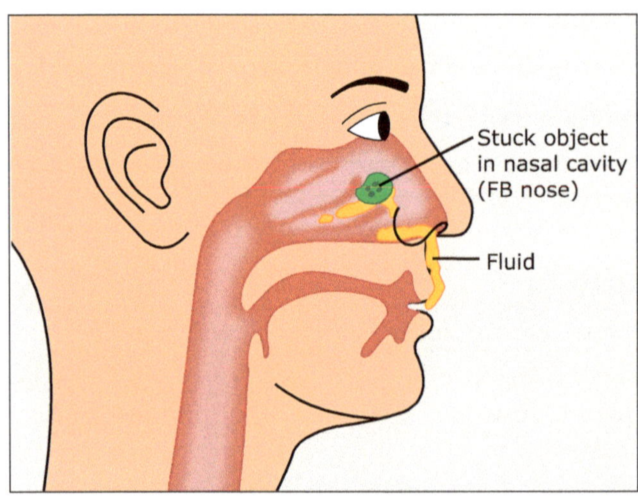

Nasal foreign body

3. Most of the nasal foreign bodies are harmless, but this can create choking, and serious injuries or infections depending on the foreign body.
4. **Common items that children put in their noses include:**
   a. Small toys
   b. Cotton
   c. Cloths, paper
   d. Pieces of eraser
   e. Tissue
   f. Clay (used for arts and crafts)
   g. Food
   h. Pebbles
   i. Dirt
   j. Paired disc magnets
   k. Button batteries
   l. Usually lodge in the floor of the anterior or middle third of the nose.

5. **Signs and symptoms:**
   1. **Breathing difficulty**
   2. **Discharge from nose:** Drainage may be clear, gray, or bloody. Nasal discharge with a bad odor may be the sign of an infection.

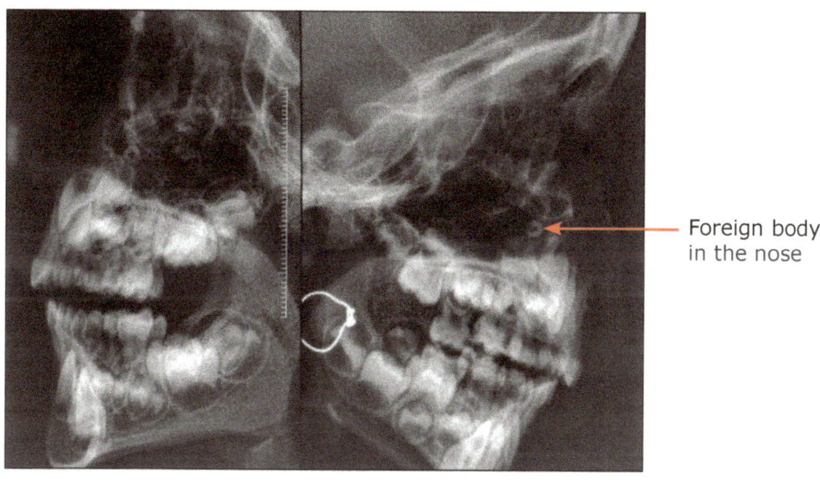

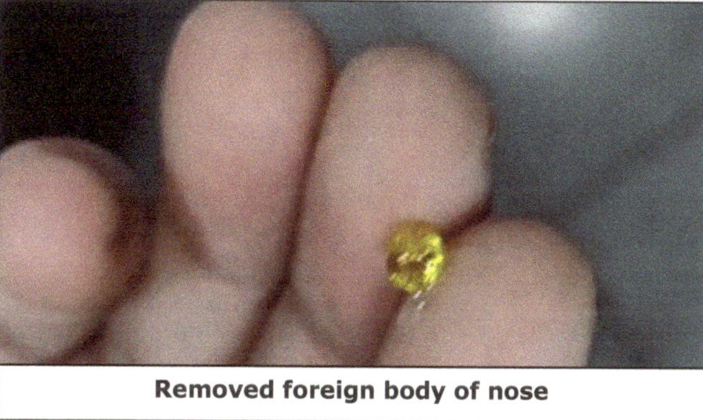

Removed foreign body of nose

6. **Management:**
   1. **For good visualization:** Use head lamp and nasal speculum
   2. Topical anesthetic (spray or drops) inside the nose to slightly numb the area.
   3. To remove cloth, cotton or paper alligator forceps is used.
   4. Other hard foreign bodies are removed by grasping them with bayonet forceps or kelly's clamp.

      In some cases we can remove them by going behind the foreign body with the help of ear curette, single sin hook or right angle hook.
   5. Other instrument useful in nasal foreign body removal includes vectis/jobson horn ring curette/ET catheter

LIP, TONGUE AND CHEEK LACERATION

Lip	**Tongue**	**Cheek**
Due to Road traffic accidents, physical assaults, bite (human or animal)	Due to seizures, road traffic accidents	Due to animal bite, physical assaults or sports, road traffic accidents
1. Proper surgical toilet by irrigation preferably with normal saline 2. Debridement of devitalized tissue 3. Inspect for foreign body 4. Primary closure of wound except in high risk cases 5. Antibiotic therapy (amoxicillin + metronidazole) 6. Tetanus and rabies immunisation as per history 7. Maintain oral hygiene	1. Wound assessment to know whether the sutures are required or not a. Laceration or avulsion which are small do not require repair as the tongue has the ability to bulk up by hypertrophy. b. Lacerations that involve large flaps, through and through injury or active bleeding needs repair. c. Position of laceration also important for management 2. Tip or lateral edge tissue loss will not cause permanent deficit as tongue bulk up via hypertrophy 3. Injury at the base of tongue is problematic as there is a hypoglossal nerve 4. Inspect for retained foreign bodies 5. For large laceration layered suturing is required 6. Use absorbable suture material (vicryl or chromic catgut) 7. Antibiotic therapy 8. In complex laceration take help of otolaryngologist or oral maxillofacial surgeon 9. Maintain oral hygiene	1. Examine the size, depth (through and through) and also examine test facial nerve and its branches 2. Small mucosal lacerations do not require repair, they heal by its own. 3. In complex laceration take help of otolaryngologist or oral maxillofacial surgeon 4. In Large laceration Do copious irrigation to remove debris or bacteria and Close with 5.0 monofilament absorbable sutures 5. Through and through sutures Close layer by layer from oral mucosa to towards skin, which should be followed by copious irrigation of wound to remove debris and bacteria 6. Appropriate antibiotic cover 7. Tetanus and rabies immunisation as per history 8. Maintain oral hygiene

ACUTE EARACHE / OTALGIA

1. Otalgia refers to pain in and around the ear.
2. Many patients in emergency department present with acute ear pain (otalgia)
3. For the treatment of otalgia, it is essential to find its cause (systemic or local).

Etiology:

1. **Primary otalgia:** Ear is the source of the pain

   Pain in and around the ear can be caused by trauma, inflammation and neoplasm.
2. **Secondary otalgia:** When the ear is not the source of the pain.

   The secondary otalgia is referred from the head and neck regions, which is innervated by the nerves that also supply the ear.

A] Local causes:

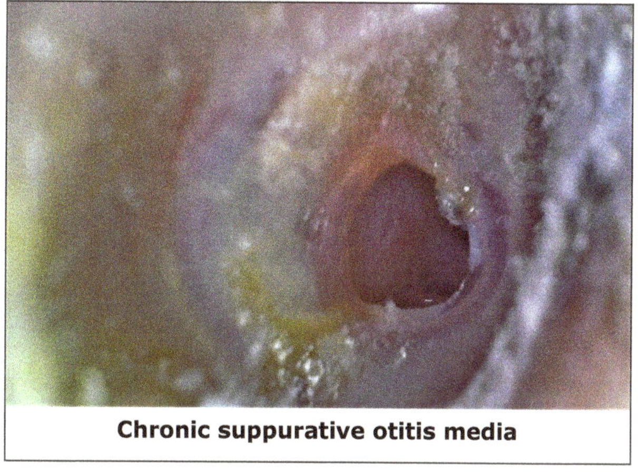

Chronic suppurative otitis media

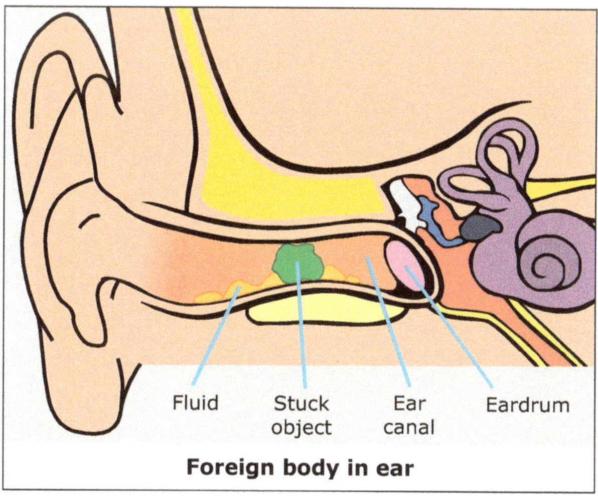

Foreign body in ear

1. **Intracranial complication of otitis media:** Extradural abscess
2. **Auricle:** Skin lesion, perichondritis/chondritis, trauma.
3. **External auditory canal (EAC):** Furuncle, impacted wax, foreign bodies mostly insects, trauma, otitis externa, otomycosis, herpes zoster oticus
4. **Middle ear:** Acute otitis media, eustachian tube obstruction, mastoiditis, cholesteatoma, barotrauma and malignancy of middle ear.

B] Secondary causes:

1. **Dental or periodontal diseases:** Tooth caries, apical abscess, impacted molar malocclusion, erupting dentition in children.
2. **Oral cavity:** Infections, trauma, aphthous ulcer or malignant ulcers
3. **Salivary glands:** Parotid and submandibular inflammatory and malignant disease.
4. **Temporomandibular joints:** Osteoarthritis, recurrent dislocation, malocclusion, bruxism
5. **Nose and paranasal sinuses:** Trauma, infection, tumors
6. **Thyroid:** Thyroiditis
7. **Nasopharynx:** Infection and tumors
8. **Oropharynx:** Acute tonsillitis, peritonsillar abscess, ulcers
9. **Vallecula, larynx, laryngopharynx, esophagus:** Ulcerative lesions, malignancy
10. **Esophagus:** Hiatus hernia with GERD
11. **Cardic:** Coronary artery diseases, aneurysm of great vessels
12. **Cervical Spinal:** Cervical spondylosis, arthritis, caries spine
13. **Peri-auricular lymphadenopathy:** Scalp or neck infections.
14. **Neuralgia:** Trigeminal, Glossopharyngeal, Sphlenopalatine
15. **Headache**
16. **Bell's palsy**
17. **Herpes zoster oticus**
18. **Psychogenic:** If no any cause has been discovered then pain will be functional in origin but the patient should be kept under observation for re-evaluation.

History:

1. **Onset**
   a. **Sudden:** Acute otitis media, furunculosis, otitic barotrauma
   b. **Gradual:** Otitis externa secondary to CSOM, malignant otitis externa,
2. **Duration**

   Short duration: ASOM, perichondritis of ear pinna.

   Long duration: Malignancy
3. **Nature of pain**

   Dull pain: Eczematous otitis externa, secretory otitis media, impacted wax

   Sharp pain: Furunculosis, otitic barotrauma

   Throbbing pain: ASOM
4. **In case of ruptured tympanic membrane:** Pain relieved when discharge starts from the ear.
5. **Symptoms associated with primary and secondary otalgia:**

Primary otalgia	Secondary otalgia (Referred otalgia)
Ear discharge	Dysphagia/odynophagia
Hearing loss	Neck swelling /goiter
ear fullness	Sore throat with fever
vertigo	Nasal discharge
Tinnitus	Dental disease
Swelling of pinna or surrounding area	Hoarseness of voice
Trauma, foreign body in ear	Pain on chewing /trismus (TMJ dysfunction)

6. **Associated symptoms with otalgia:** Fever, headache, vomiting, convulsions.
7. **Cardiac history**
8. **GI history**
9. **Dental history**
10. **Cervical spine history**
11. **Past history:** Ear surgery

Physical examination:

1. **Ear, nose, throat, head and neck examination**
2. **Dental examination:** Look for caries, malocclusion, absent dentition.

3. **Craniomandibular:** Palpate TMJ joint and pterygoid muscle
4. **Cervical spine examination:** Mobility and tenderness
5. **Neurological examination:** Especially V, VII, IX and X

Investigations:

1. **Flexible fiberoptic examination of nose, pharynx and larynx**
2. **Esophagogram**: For hiatus hernia
3. **X-ray cervical spine**: Cervical spondylosis
4. **X-ray of TMJ joint and styloid process**
5. **Orthopantomogram (OPG)**: For caries of tooth

Management of primary otalgia:

Diseases of external ear	Definition	Clinical features	Management
Otitis externa	Inflammation of EAC(external auditory canal)	Otalgia and otorrhea **In severe cases** Regional lymphadenopathy and periauricular cellulitis	**Aural toilet** **Acidification** of EAC **Topical antibiotics** (quinolone antibiotic drops e.g. oflox, ciproflox) **Oral antibiotics**
Otomycosis (aspergillus niger and candida albicans)	Fungal infection of ear	Intense itching, ear pain and discomfort Watery discharge with musty odor ear blockage	**Dry ear** **Antifungal agents** Povidine iodine, 2% salicylic acid in alcohol for 1 week. **In aspergillus niger** Acetic acid drops and gentian violet painting is effective **In candida albicans** Clotrimazole, nystatin solutions or cream are effective **Antibiotics / steroid drops in case** secondary bacterial infection
Furunculosis	Staphylococcal infection of hair follicle	Severe pain and tenderness Small Nodular swelling proceeds to fluctuating Painful jaw or pinna movement periauricular lymphadenopathy	**Oral antibiotics** for antistaphylococcal infection **Analgesics, Local heat 10% ichthammol glycerin wick, Incision and drainage** in case of abscess.

(Continued)

Diseases of external ear	Definition	Clinical features	Management
Herpes zoster oticus (Ramsay-Hunt syndrome) **Caused by the Varicella -zoster virus**	Peripheral facial nerve palsy accompanied by an **erythematous vesicular rash on the ear** (zoster oticus) or in the mouth	Unilateral facial palsy Painful vesicles with erythematous base appears in the canal and cochlea, behind the pinna and or soft palate	**Antiviral therapy:** Tab acyclovir 800 mg 5 times a day or famcyclovir 500 mg TDS or valacyclovir 1 gm TDS for 7 days **Tab prednisone** begins usually with 1 mg/kg then tapers the dose. **Topical antibiotic /steroid ear drops** **Eye care**
Impacted ear wax	Secretions of sebaceous and ceruminous gland with desquamated epithelial cells and keratin forms wax	Hearing loss or sense of blocked ear Tinnitus and dizziness Earache Wax granuloma formation Reflex cough due to stimulation of auricular branch of vagus nerve	**Wax softening agents:** 5% sodabicarb in equal parts of glycerin and water Liquid paraffin Olive oil Paradichlorobenzene **Wax removal by instruments:** Cerumen hook, scoop, Jobson-Horne probe, wax hook and vectis
Foreign body ear **Types of foreign bodies:** **A] Non living** 1. **Hygroscopic:** Grain seeds: peas, rice, wheat 2. **Non hygro-scopic:** chalk, matchstick, cotton swab sponge, paper. **B] living:** insects Mosquitoes, cockroaches, ants	**Features of foreign body:** **Vegetable foreign bodies** swell up with time and get impacted in the ear canal, they may result in suppuration **Living foreign body:** In this cases patients have severe pain and irritation due to its movement in ear	**Treatment:** 1. **Antibiotics:** Antibiotics used to control the infection and edema. 2. **Ear drops:** Glycerine and absolute alcohol drops used in hygroscopic foreign body to shrunk 3. **Removal of foreign body:** Best to remove under operative microscope Soft and irregular like cotton, paper, sponge removed by forceps Smooth objects and seed grains removed by syringing	Wax hook is passed beyond the foreign body then removed outside against the either floor or posterior wall. Insects are killed by the instilling oil, chloroform or water and then removed. In uncooperative children the foreign bodies are removed under general anesthesia Postaural incision may be needed to remove foreign body impacted deep inside the external acoustic meatus, gone deep inside middle ear. **Complications:** Secondary infection Injury to middle ear structure and tympanic membrane

ACUTE OTITIS MEDIA

Acute otitis media	**Clinical features: as per stages:**	**C] Suppuration:**	**Management:**
An acute pyogenic inflammation of the middle ear cleft, which includes the eustachian tube, middle ear, attic, aditus, antrum and mastoid air cells **Complications:** 1. **Intracranial:** Meningitis, brain abscess, subdural empyema, epidural abscess, or sinus thrombosis 2. **Extracranial:** Mastoiditis, postauricular abscess, petrous apicitis, labyrinthine fistula, facial nerve paralysis, or acute suppurative labyrinthitis	**A] Tubal occlusion:** 1. **Symptoms:** Mild deafness, ear fullness, ear pain, no fever 2. **Signs:** Retracted tympanic membrane loss of cone of light Conductive hearing loss **B] Pre-suppuration:** **Symptoms:** Marked earache (throbbing pain), high grade fever, tinnitus **Signs: on otoscope:** Cart wheel appearance of the tympanic membrane, Conductive hearing loss on tuning fork test, Loss of cone of light	**Symptoms:** Excruciating pain, increasing deafness, rising fever, vomiting, even convulsions **Signs:** **Yellow spot on TM,** tenderness on mastoid antrum, clouding of air cells in X-ray of mastoid **D] Resolution:** **Symptoms:** Otorrhea (initially blood tinged later becomes purulent), ear pain and fever subside **Signs:** Perforation of pars tensa usually in anteroinferior quadrant	**Antibiotics:** Till the tympanic membrane and hearing becomes clear. First line of antibiotics is amoxicillin, ampicillin **If allergic to penicillin:** cefaclor, cotrimoxazole and erythromycin 5 day or 10-14 days course. **Decongestant: (Oral or nasal)** To relieve ET edema and promote ventilation of middle ear.(xylo or oxymetazoline, pseudoephedrine) **Analgesics and antipyretics:** Relieves Pain and fever **Ear drops and aural toilet:** Quinolone /steroid ear wick/ drops **Dry local heat:** It relieves pain.

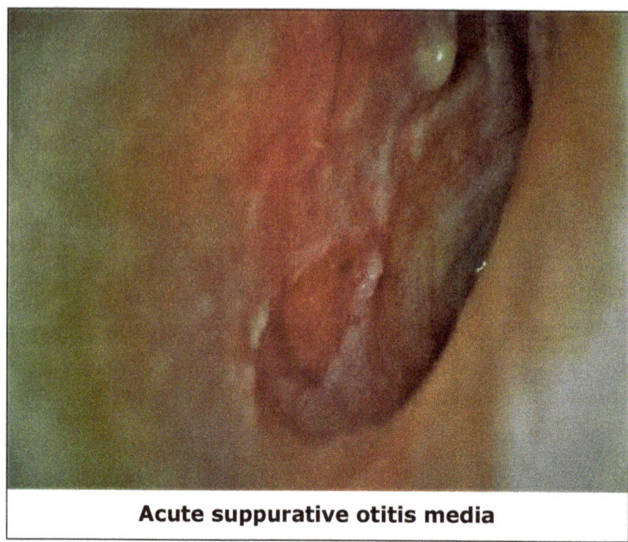

Acute suppurative otitis media

ACUTE MASTOIDITIS

1. It is an inflammation of the mucosal lining of the antrum and the mastoid air cell system.
2. Acute mastoiditis usually accompanies or follows acute suppurative otitis media.
3. **Clinical features**
   a. **Symptoms:**
      1. Patient appears ill and toxic
      2. Pain behind the ear
      3. Fever: Mild fever in adults and high grade in children.
      4. Ear discharge: Mucopurulent or purulent discharge
   b. **Signs:**
      1. Mastoid tenderness
      2. Swelling over the mastoid
      3. Hearing loss: Conductive type of hearing loss is always present
      4. In most of cases a small perforation is seen in the pars tensa portion of the tympanic membrane but in a few cases the tympanic membrane remains intact.
4. **Investigations:**
   a. **Complete blood count:** Polymorphonuclear leukocytosis is seen
   b. **ESR:** Raised
   c. **Ear swab:** For culture and sensitivity
   d. **X-ray mastoid:** Clouding of air cells due to collection of exudate in them
   e. **Non contrast CT scan of temporal bone:** Will show the fluid in the mastoid air cell and reveal bony breakdown.
5. **Treatment**
   a. **Hospitalisation**
   b. **Antipyretics and maintain hydration**
   c. **IV Antibiotics:** Starts with broad spectrum antibiotics and specific antibiotic therapy as per culture and sensitivity report.
   d. **Myringotomy:** When pus is under tension it is relieved by wide myringotomy.
   e. **Cortical mastoidectomy**

CHOLESTEATOMA

Cystic structure filled with desquamated squamous cell debris in the middle ear (skin in the wrong place) **Pathogenesis of acquired cholesteatoma:** **1. Wittmaack's theory:** Invagination theory **2. Ruedi and lange theory (basal cell hyperplasia)** **3. Habermann's theory (epithelial invasion or migration theory)**	**Types:** **A] Congenital:** It arises from the embryonic epidermal cell rests entrapped in the middle ear cleft or temporal bone. **Primary:** Neither a history of a pre-existing tympanic membrane perforation nor otorrhea **Secondary:** Pre-existing perforation of pars tensa which is usually posterosuperior marginal perforation or sometimes large central perforation **B] Acquired:** They are the most common of cholesteatomas and result from AOM and otitis media with effusion.	**Clinical features:** **Symptoms:** Ear discharge persistent malodorous ear discharge is usually purulent and scanty in amount. **Slowly progressive hearing loss:** Conductive hearing loss, sensorineural elements may be added to hearing loss. Hearing normally means the ossicular chain is intact. **Symptoms of sequelae:** Pain, vertigo, facial palsy, headache, vomiting, ataxia and fever.	**Diagnosis:** Physical and functional examination of the ear Temporal bone X-ray CT scan may help to rule out other, often more serious causes for the patient's clinical presentation **MRI scan:** helps in planning of surgery. **Treatment:** **C**ontrol infection with oral antibiotic drugs or local antibiotic ear drops. **C**lear ear discharge **A**ural toilet **Standard treatment is to surgically remove the growth.** **Types of surgery:** **Canal wall up** **Canal wall down**

PERITONSILLAR, RETROPHARYNGEAL ABSCESS AND LUDWIG'S ANGINA

	Clinical features	Management
Peritonsillar abscess (Quinsy) collection of pus in the peritonsillar space	**Symptoms:** Unilateral sore throat, Otalgia, foul breath, hot potato speech, odynophagia(drooling of saliva from angle of mouth), fever, general symptoms-malaise, nausea, constipation. **Anterior pillar** - swelling and congestion **Tonsils** - enlarged **Uvula** - swollen, edematous and pushed to the opposite side **Torticollis** - neck is tilted towards side of abscess	**A] Medical:** 1. Hospitalization 2. Antibiotics covering both aerobic and anaerobic 3. Analgesics and antipyretics 4. Oral hygiene 5. IV fluids **B] Surgical:** 1. Incision and drainage of abscess 2. Interval tonsillectomy
Retropharyngeal abscess (Commonly seen in patients with age of <3 years)	**Symptoms:** **S**tridor **D**ysphagia and respiratory distress **C**roupy cough **T**orticollis (Head becomes persistently turned to one side) **U**nilateral bulging in posterior pharyngeal wall on one side of midline **Diagnosis:** X-ray soft tissue neck lateral view CT scan	**A] Medical:** 1. Hospitalization 2. Antibiotics covering both aerobic and anaerobic 3. Analgesics and antipyretics 4. IV fluids to correct dehydration. **B] Surgical:** **1. Incision and drainage** of abscess and prevent aspiration of pus while drainage **Tracheostomy:** In large abscess causing respiratory distress and laryngeal edema
Ludwig's angina: Deep cellulitis around the submandibular gland and floor of mouth and deep neck fascia	**S**ubmandibular swelling: Pain, red, warm and tender **S**welling or tenderness of submental or submaxillary space (If involved) **L**aryngeal edema may occur **S**wollen tongue which is pushed upwards & backwards threatening the airway patency **G**eneral manifestations of toxemia	**A] Medical:** 1. Hospitalization 2. Antibiotics covering both aerobic and anaerobic 3. Analgesics and antipyretics 4. IV fluids **B] Surgical:** Urgent drainage through submental incision, which deepened to allow division of mylohyoid muscle **C] Tracheostomy** if airway is endangered

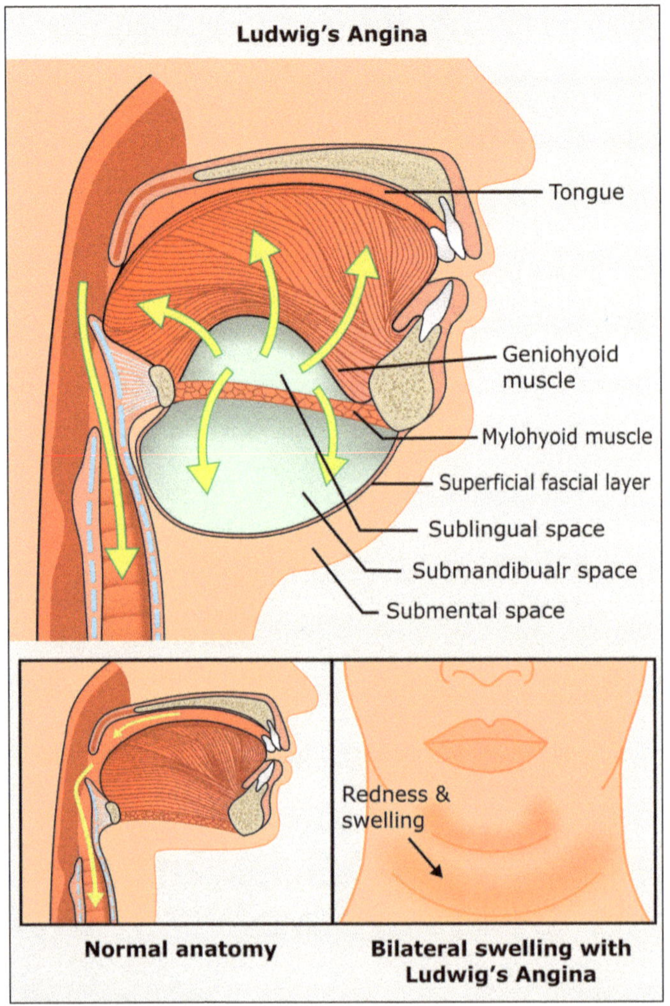
Ludwig's Angina
Tongue
Geniohyoid muscle
Mylohyoid muscle
Superficial fascial layer
Sublingual space
Submandibualr space
Submental space
Redness & swelling
Normal anatomy
Bilateral swelling with Ludwig's Angina

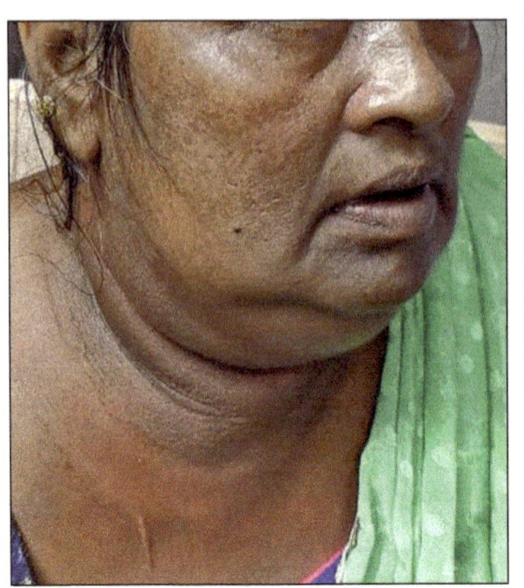

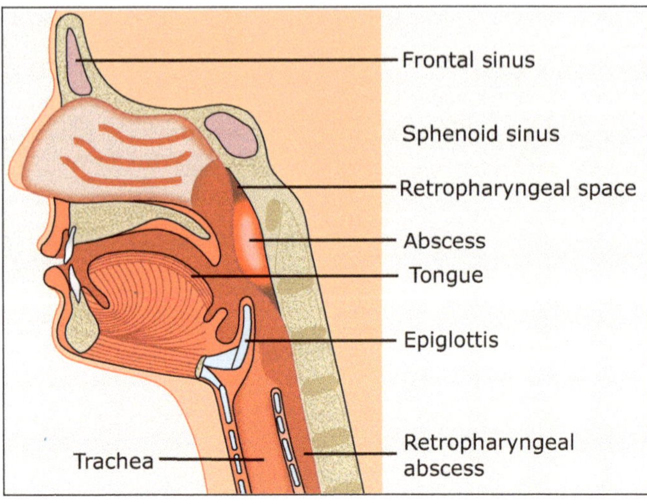
Frontal sinus
Sphenoid sinus
Retropharyngeal space
Abscess
Tongue
Epiglottis
Trachea
Retropharyngeal abscess

INHALED FOREIGN BODY

1. Accidentally the patient inhales the organic or non organic foreign body.
2. This objects can enter in the trachea through the mouth or nose.
3. If foreign body enters the airways then it may cause choking.
4. Depending on the size, nature, a foreign body may lodge into the larynx, trachea or bronchi.
5. A large foreign body cannot pass below the glottis and get lodged in the subglottic space and a small foreign body can pass down into the trachea or bronchi.
6. Sharp foreign bodies like fishbone, needles, pins FB get stuck into the larynx or tracheobronchial tree.
7. Predisposing factors include age, unconscious adults, disturbed swallowing (coughing, laughing, talking, crying), paralysis of the pharynx and larynx due to lesions of IX and X cranial nerve.
8. **Depending on the nature of FB the patient will have the symptoms:**
    a. **Non irritating FB:** Metallic items, glass, plastic remain nonsymptomatic for a long time.
    b. **Irritating FB:** Vegetables (seeds, beans, peanuts) swell with time and cause irritation of tracheobronchial tree so edema and congestion occurs which causes airway obstruction.
9. **The obstruction is classified as:**
    a. **A partial obstruction**
    b. **Complete obstruction.**
10. **Signs of partial obstruction:** Choking with drooling of saliva, stridor, and the patient maintains the ability to speak.
11. **Signs of complete obstruction:** Choking with inability to speak or cough, and associated with cyanosis.

12. **Clinical features:**

Laryngeal FB	**Small FB:** Throat discomfort, stridor, dyspnea, hemoptysis, hoarseness of voice, croupy cough **Large FB:** Patient gets cyanosed and dies.
Tracheal FB	**F**oreign bodies in the trachea are relatively uncommon. **R**espiratory distress is much more marked than in cases of a foreign body in the bronchus. **I**rritating cough, an audible flap, tracheal flutter and an asthmoid wheeze. **T**hud, flap and flutter sounds are produced by the movement of the foreign body inside the tracheal lumen during respiration.
Bronchial FB	**I**rritating cough with pain on the affected side. **F**ever and fetid sputum develop when there is secondary infection. **F**oreign bodies in the right bronchus are twice as common as those in the left **O**bstruction can lead to emphysema, atelectasis **F**oreign bodies in the bronchus rarely cause acute respiratory distress and air hunger and cyanosis are not marked.

13. **Diagnosis:**

    1. **X-ray:** Soft tissue neck PA and lateral view in extended position

       Chest PA and lateral view at the end of inspiration and expiration

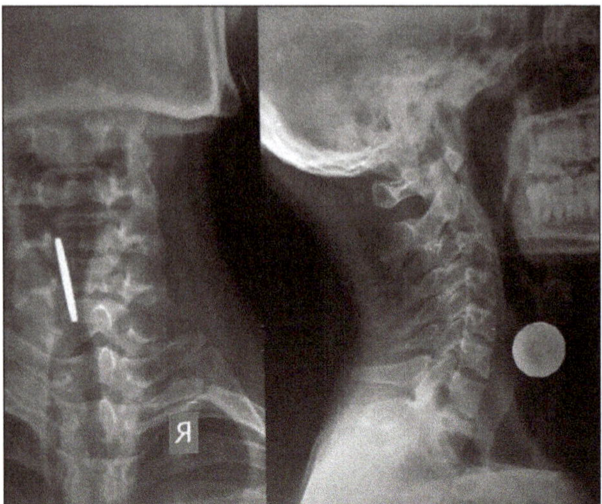

    2. **Fluoroscopy/videofluoroscopy**
    3. **Bronchograms**
    4. **CT scan with virtual bronchoscopy**
    5. **Laryngoscopy and bronchoscopy:** Diagnostic and therapeutic

14. **Management:**
    1. **Antibiotics: for infection**
    2. **Steroids**
    3. **Oxygen administration**
    4. **For laryngeal foreign body:** A) Cricothyrotomy or emergency tracheostomy
       B) Direct laryngoscopy or laryngofissure
    5. **For tracheal and bronchial foreign body:** Bronchoscopy done under general anesthesia
15. **Complications:**
    1. Inflammation of the airway walls or lung abscess from a foreign body remaining in the airway
    2. Pneumonia in the same lung field

INGESTED FOREIGN BODY

1. Children are the most common patients presenting to emergency departments with an esophageal foreign body.
2. FB may be lodged in the tonsil, base of tongue, vallecula, pyriform fossa or esophagus
3. Examples of common foreign bodies which lodges in esophagus are coin, piece of meat, chicken bone, teeth, safety pin and marble piece
4. The most common site of impaction of fish bone is palatine tonsil.
5. **Risk factors for foreign body ingestion in the esophagus are:**
   a. **Children (They have a tendency to put anything in mouth),**
   b. **Lack of tactile sensation while chewing**
   c. **Narrowed esophageal lumen (Stricture and carcinoma)**
   d. **High risk conditions: Unconscious patient, under alcohol intoxication, seizures**
   e. **Psychotic persons (Attempt to commit suicide)**
6. **Clinical features:**
   a. History of initial choking or gagging
   b. Discomfort or pain in the lower part of the neck
   c. Dysphagia
   d. Respiratory distress in children due to upper esophagus FB
   e. Odynophagia
   f. Blood-stained saliva
   g. Substernal pain or epigastric pain due to esophageal spasm.
7. **Investigation:**
   1. X-ray soft tissue neck and chest posteroanterior view and lateral view
   2. Esophagoscopy

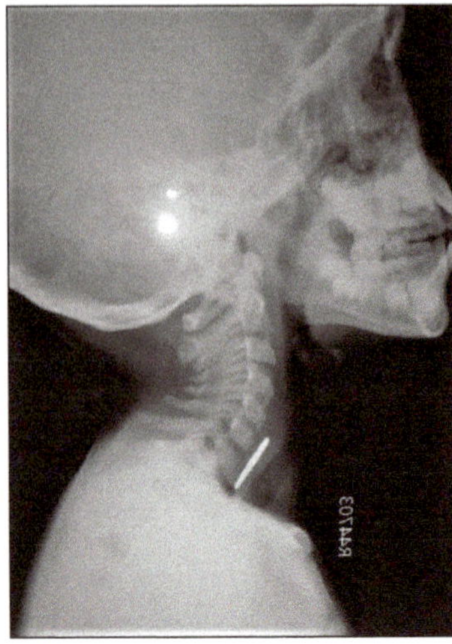

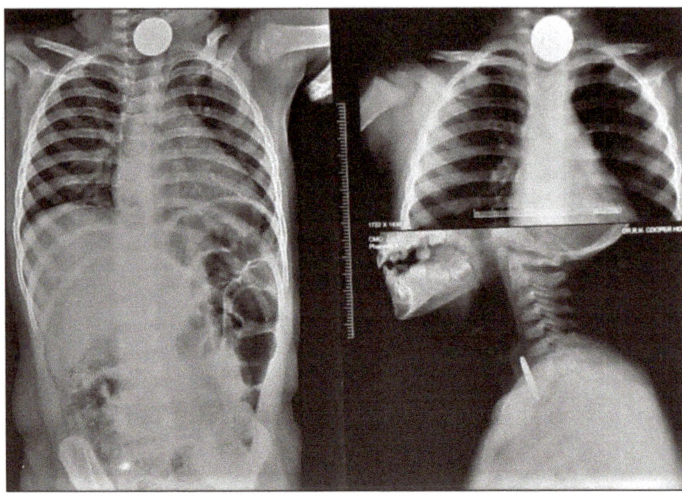

8. **Management:**
    1. **Esophagoscopy:** Most common and preferred modality of treatment for removal of FB under general anesthesia or topical anesthesia.
    2. **Rigid esophagoscopy:** Any type of FB can be removed under general anesthesia.
    3. **Cervical Esophagostomy:** For FB impacted above the thoracic inlet.
    4. **Transthoracic Esophagectomy:** For FB impacted into thoracic esophagus, chest is opened at an appropriate level.
    5. An FB which reaches the stomach may pass through the rest of gastrointestinal tract without difficulty

       Patient should take normal diet, examine the stool everyday

       Don't give purgatives to hasten the passage
    6. **Operative intervention required into following situations:**

       A] Pain and tenderness in abdomen

       B] No progress of FB on serial X-rays taken in intervals

       C] In children (< 2 years), FB > 5 cm long usually does not pass through the turns of the duodenum

       D] Patients having pyloric stenosis.

       E] Sharp foreign body with perforation or likely to penetrate or get obstructed.
9. **Complications:**
    1. Perforation of esophagus by the sharp objects may lead to mediastinitis, pericarditis or empyema.
    2. Ulceration and stricture
    3. Respiratory obstruction
    4. Tracheoesophageal fistula
    5. Periesophageal cellulitis and abscess

BELL'S PALSY

1. The most common form of facial paralysis is Bell's palsy
2. It is defined as the acute onset idiopathic, peripheral facial paralysis or paresis
3. Risk of Bell's palsy is more in diabetic (Angiopathic) and pregnant women (Retention of fluids)
4. It usually affects just one side of the face
5. Symptoms appear suddenly
6. **Etiology:**

   A] **Viral infection:** Most evidence supports the viral etiology of herpes simplex, herpes zoster or Epstein-Barr virus.

   B] **Vascular ischemia:** e.g. Primary (cold, emotional stress), secondary (results of primary ischemia which leads to increased capillary permeability leading to exudation of fluids and compression of microcirculation of nerve.

   C] **Hereditary:** Positive family history

   D] **Autoimmune disorders:** T- lymphocyte changes seen in Bell's palsy cases.

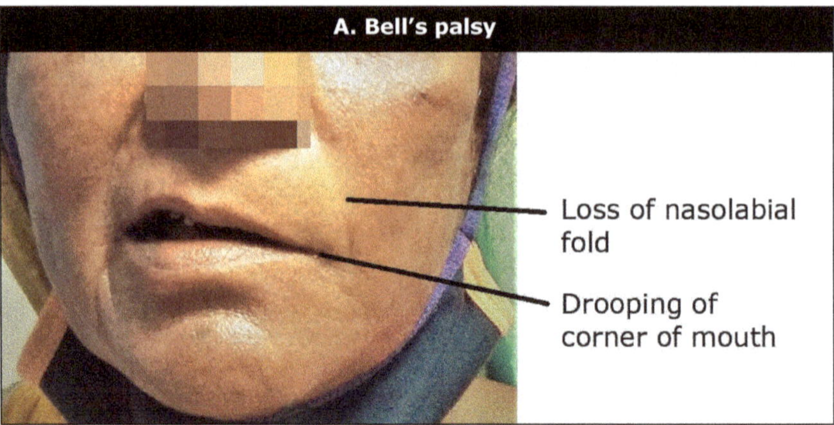

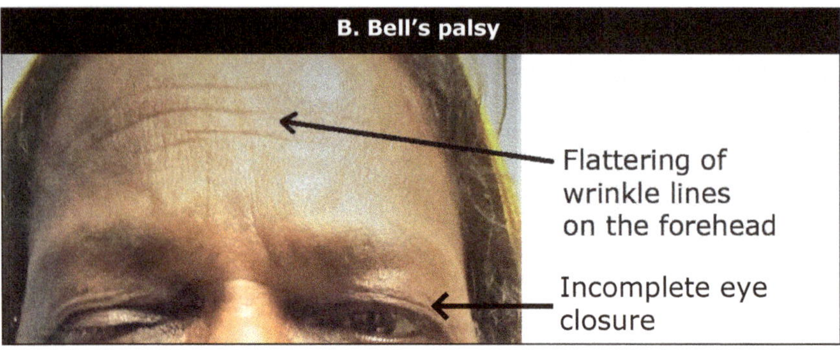

7. **Clinical features:**

   a. The early symptoms of Bell's palsy

      1. A mild fever

      2. Pain behind the ear

      3. A neck stiffness

      4. Weakness and/or stiffness on one side of the face.

      5. Maximal weakness occurs mostly by 48 hours after onset of symptoms.

   b. One sided facial weakness hence becomes asymmetrical

   c. Inability to close the eyes

   d. Bell's phenomenon (While closing eye eyeball turns up and out)

   e. Saliva dribles from the angle of mouth

   f. Tears flow down from eye (Epiphora)

8. **Diagnosis:** The diagnosis of Bell's palsy can usually be made clinically in patients based on the following findings:

   a. Typical presentation

   b. No risk factors or No other symptoms for causes of facial paralysis

   c. No herpes zoster infection of the external ear canal

   d. A normal neurologic examination other than the facial nerve.

9. **Treatment**:

   A] General:

      1. Reassurance

      2. Relief of ear pain by analgesics

      3. Eye must be protected against exposure keratitis with the help of artificial tear drops, soft eye pads .

      4. Physiotherapy or massage of the facial muscles

      5. Psychological support to the patient.

   B] Medical management:

      1. **Steroids:**

         - Prednisolone is the drug of choice

- If patients present within 1 week, the adult dose of prednisolone is 1 mg/kg/day (60-80 mg) divided into morning and evening doses for 5 days.
- Patient is seen on the 5th day and if paralysis remains incomplete or is recovering, dose is tapered during the next 5 days.
- If paralysis remains complete on the 5th day, the same dose is continued for another 10 days and thereafter tapered in the next 5 days (total 20 days).

2. **Antiviral agents:** Valacyclovir (1000 mg daily for 5–7 days) or acyclovir (400 mg five times daily for 10 days)

   Combination therapy with prednisone plus valacyclovir might be better than prednisolone alone.

C] **Surgical management:** Nerve decompression surgery relieves pressure on the nerve fibres and thus improves microcirculation of the nerve.

TRISMUS

a. **Trismus:** Uncontrolled inability to open the mouth or jaw

b. **Etiology**

Intraarticular	Extra Articular
1. Ankylosis 2. Arthritis synovitis 3. Pathology of meniscus	1. Infection: Dental infections, tonsillitis, tetanus, 2. Trauma: # or dislocation of mandible or zygomatic arch 3. Dental treatment related: Tooth extraction, local anesthetic injection 4. TMJ problem: Myofascial muscle spasm, internal derangement. 5. Neoplasm: Primary and secondary tumors of epipharyngeal and parotid region, jaw joints Submucous fibrosis Myositis ossificans 6. Drugs: Phenothiazine, succinylcholine, tricyclic antidepressant, metoclopramide 7. Radiotherapy: Osteoradionecrosis, post radiation fibrosis 8. Congenital 9. Miscellaneous: Hysterical

c. **History, examination and investigation:**

1. **History:**
    a. Onset, nature, progression and relieving factors
    b. Dental treatment, trauma, medical conditions, radiotherapy or drug intake
    c. Inquire about pain in neck, shoulder, back muscles and joints
    d. Inquire about sleep bruxism (clenching, grinding, tooth tapping)or daytime parafunction (clenching, gum chewing, finger nail biting)
2. **Examination**
    a. Facial symmetry
    b. Measure mouth opening and lateral range of jaw motion
    c. Palpate the masticatory muscles
    d. Check tenderness, uncoordinated movement, clicking sound and crepitus at TM Joint
    e. Dental examination (Caries, inflammation)
3. **Investigation**
    a. Periapical radiograph

   b. Panoramic radiograph
   c. CT scan TM joint
   d. MRI scan
   e. Axiography

d. **Treatment**

1. **Heat therapy:** Moist hot towel over affected area for 15-20 min.
2. **Medical therapy:**
   a. **A**spirin is usually adequate for pain, sometimes narcotic analgesia for intense pain
   b. **B**enzodiazepines for muscle relaxation (Diazepam 2.5-5 mg)
   c. **A**ppropriate antibiotics in case of infection
   d. **B**otulinum injections
3. **Physiotherapy:** For opening or closing of mouth
4. **Trismus appliances:** Used in combination with physiotherapy
5. **Surgery:** Rarely required

VERTIGO

1. Vertigo is a type of dizziness.
2. It is a symptom where a person feels that they or the objects around them are moving when they themselves are not moving.
3. It occurs most commonly due to vestibular cause.
4. Dizziness is a common term used by the patient for describing the symptoms like vertigo, confusion, blurring of vision, lightheadedness, gait disturbance.
5. **Vertigo is classified into either peripheral or central depending on the location of the dysfunction:**

   A] **Peripheral:** It includes dysfunction of labyrinthine, vestibular, visual or somatosensory.

   B] **Central:** Dysfunction in central nervous system after entrance of vestibular nerve in brainstem and involve vestibulo-ocular, vestibulo-spinal and other central nervous system pathways.

   C] **Other:** Psychogenic vertigo
6. **Vestibular disorder:**

Peripheral disorder	Central disorder
I] Labyrinthine and vestibular causes	
Benign paroxysmal positional vertigo (BPPV)	**Brainstem ischemia / infarction, embolism, hemorrhage**
Meniere's disease	**Transient ischemic attack**
Vestibular neuronitis	**Multiple sclerosis**
Labyrinthitis	**Vertebrobasilar insufficiency**
Vestibulotoxic drugs e.g. gentamicin, tobramycin, netilmicin	**Acute cerebellitis**
Cerebro pontine angle tumors e.g. Acoustic neuroma, meningioma, cyst	**Neoplasm of brainstem & IV ventricle**
Syphilis	**Basilar migraine**
Head injury	**Epilepsy**
II] Visual causes (Incorrect or new spectacles, extraocular paresis)	**Cervical vertigo**
III] Somatosensory causes (Peripheral neuropathy, myelopathy)	

7. Careful history from the patient taken focused on meaning of dizziness to patient as dizziness is a symptom used to describe various complains

8. **When the meaning of dizziness is uncertain then the following tests may be helpful:**

   A] **Rotational test:**

   Rapid rotation and abrupt cessation of movement in a swivel chair this is a simplest provocative test for vestibular dysfunction, this test always induces the vertigo.

   B] **Valsalva maneuvers:** Exacerbate vertigo in patients with cardiovascular disease.

   C] **Check for orthostatic hypotension:** Duplication of symptoms during orthostatic hypotension indicate cerebral ischemia.

9. **If patient history is related to true vertigo then we have to understand whether the cause is peripheral or central**

Features	Peripheral	Central
Onset	Rapid	Gradual
Nystagmus	Combined horizontal, torsional Inhibited by fixation of eye No changes with gaze changes Decreases with several days	Purely vertical, horizontal or torsional Not inhibited by the fixation of eye Changes with change in the gaze.
Imbalance (postural instability)	Mild to moderate	Severe
Severity of vertigo	Intense	Less intense
Nausea and vomiting	May be severe	Mild to moderate
Tinnitus and /or hearing loss	Often present	Usually absent
Neurological dysfunction	Rare	Common

The most common diseases that result in peripheral vertigo are Benign paroxysmal positional vertigo, Labyrinthitis, Meniere's disease.

Benign paroxysmal positional vertigo	Patient have episodes of vertigo with movement and in between these episodes patient is normal. The episodes of vertigo should last less than one minute. In BPPV, Dix-hallpike test produces nystagmus
Meniere's disease	In this condition patient have tinnitus, hearing loss and episode of vertigo last for > 20 minutes
Labyrinthitis	Onset of vertigo is sudden and the nystagmus occurs without movement.

10. **A central cause can be suspected in elderly patients with positive history of hypertension, ischemic heart disease, cerebrovascular accident, smoking**

Vertebrobasilar insufficiency	Vertigo is abrupt in onset, last several minutes It is associated with nausea and vomiting, other neurological symptoms like difficulty in swallowing, limb weakness, visual disturbances, diplopia due to ischemia of other areas of the brain.
Basilar migraine	Patient have occipital headache,visual disturbances, diplopia and severe vertigo . Migraine which is abrupt in onset and may last for 5-60 min. It is common in adolescent girls and having strong menstrual relationship. Patients with positive family history.
Cerebellar disease	Acute cerebellar disease may cause severe vertigo, vomiting and ataxia.

11. **Test used for evaluation of vertigo:**

A] **Caloric reflex test:** This is a test of the vestibulo-ocular reflex that involves irrigating the ear with cold or warm water or air into the external auditory canal and normally it induces nystagmus.

1. A decreased response to this test indicates vestibular disorder
2. Inability to have nystagmus with ice cold water indicates dead labyrinthine.

B] **Visual fixation:** After fixating eye the intensity of nystagmus and velocity is increased in the patient with peripheral vestibular lesions

C] **Auditory testing:** In patients with hearing loss, tinnitus or other auditory symptoms.

D] **MRI scan:** To determine central cause of vertigo

12. **Management:**

A] **To abolish the vertigo:** Bed rest and vestibular suppressant drugs.

1. **Anticholinergics:** Hyoscine hydrobromide (Scopolamine)
2. **Anticonvulsants:** Topiramate or valproic acid for vestibular migraines
3. **Antihistamines:** Betahistine, dimenhydrinate, or meclizine
4. **Tranquiliser with GABA - ergic effects**: Diazepam
5. **Calcium channel antagonists:** Cinnarizine

B] **Vestibular rehabilitation:** After termination an acute attack vestibular exercises should begin and vestibular suppressants should be avoided because dizziness is required for compensation.

C] Definitive treatment of underlying cause of vertigo

Meniere's disease	Low salt diet, diuretics
Migraine	Anti-migraine
Vertebrobasilar insufficiency	Antiplatelets
Transient ischemic attack	Anticoagulation
Autoimmune inner ear disease	Steroids and immunosuppressant agents
Syphilitic labyrinthitis	Antibiotics and steroids

Section 3

Ophthalmology Emergencies

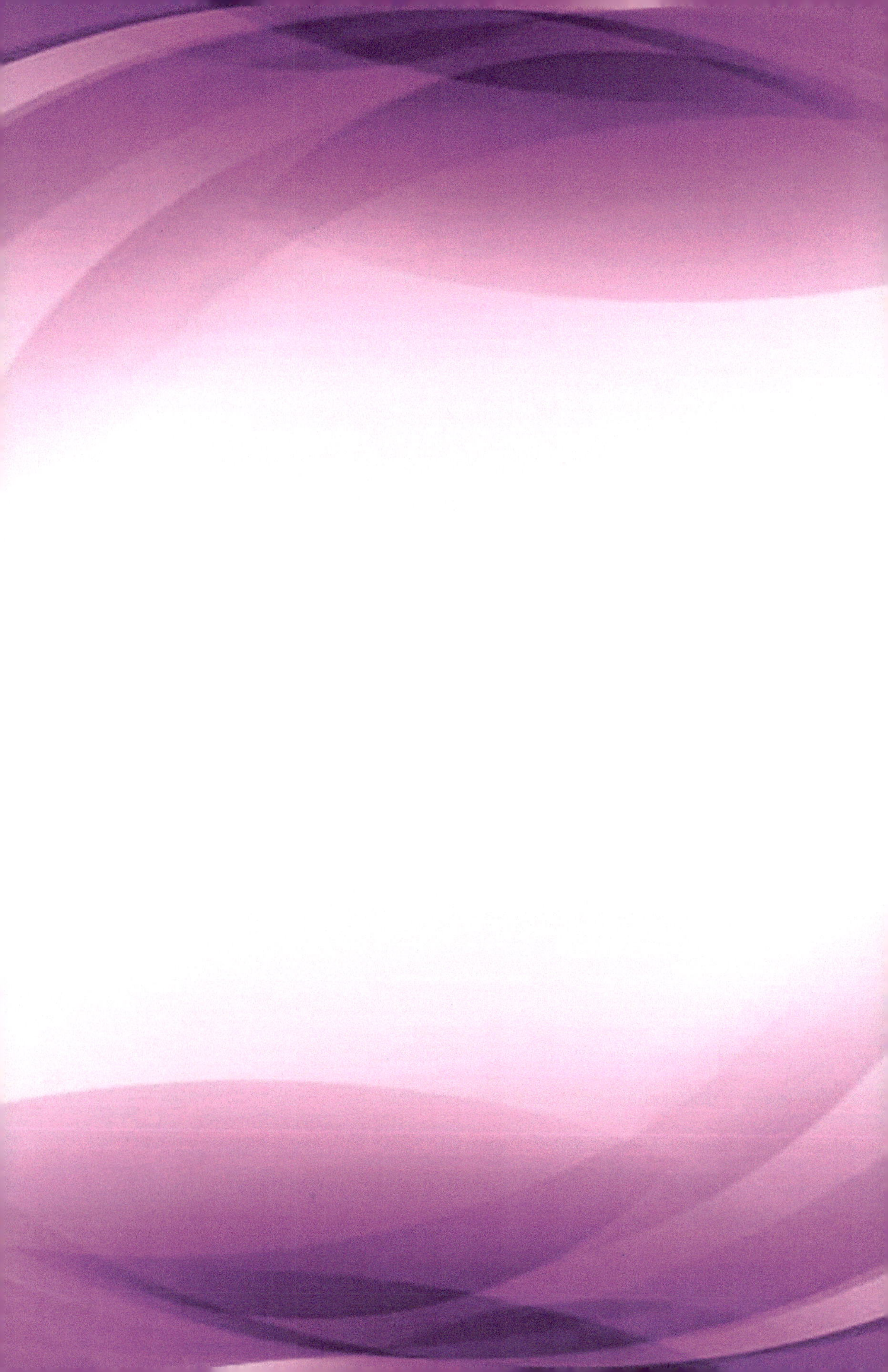

CHAPTER

3 Ophthalmology Emergencies

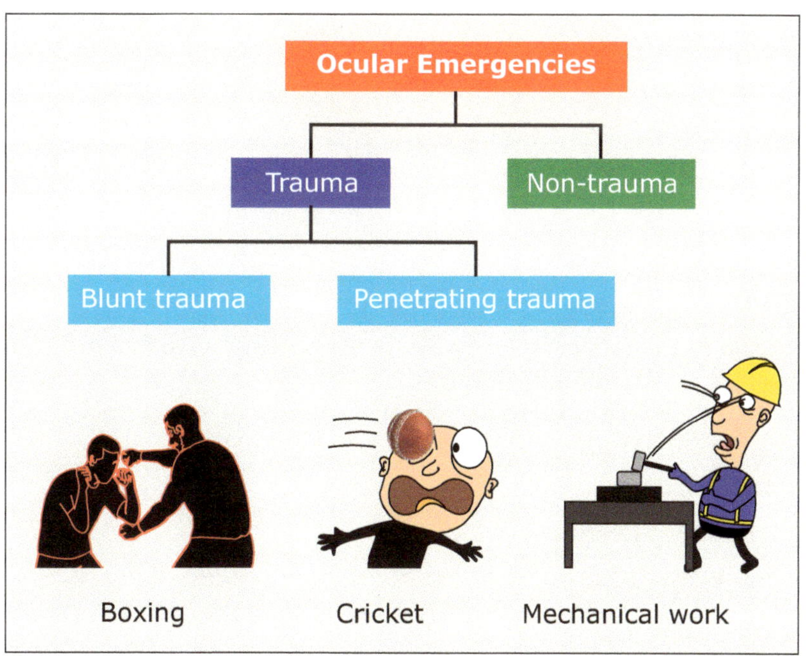

OCULAR EXAMINATION

a. **History**

1. **Take full ophthalmic history (Onset, duration and progress)**
    a. Which eye is affected?
    b. Both eyes are affected?
    c. Time span of developing symptoms
    d. Are there flashing lights or floaters
    e. Previous ophthalmic history and treatment
    f. Medical and drug history
    g. Family history (e.g. glaucoma)

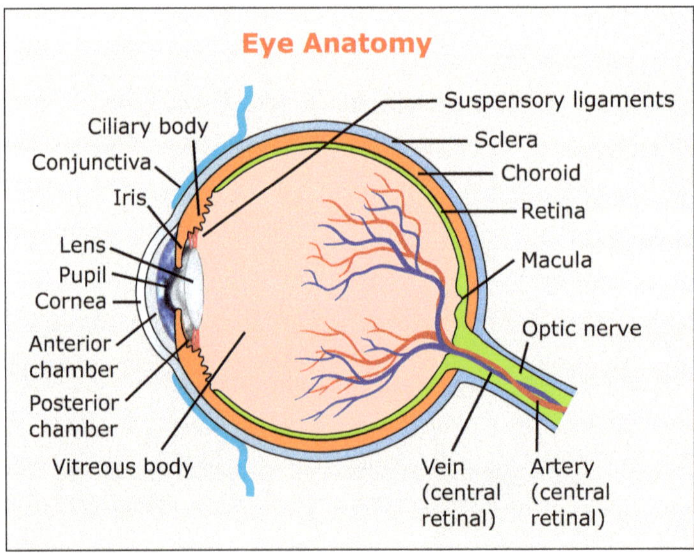

b. **Visual acuity**

Always measure visual acuity of patients presenting with eye problems (failure to document may constitute negligence)

c. **Pupillary reaction**

d. **Eye movement**

1. **Check the eye movements**
2. **Ask about diplopia**
3. **Look for nystagmus**

e. **Visual fields**

f. Direct assessment: Look for inflammation or foreign body

g. Fundoscopy

   1. First check red reflex

   2. Decreased red reflex is seen in the patients with vitreous hemorrhage, cataract etc.

   3. Examine the optic disc

   4. Look for retinal hemorrhage, vessels abnormalities

h. Slit lamp examination

   To examine in detail conjunctiva, cornea and anterior chamber

i. Intraocular pressure measurement

j. Temporal arteries: If a patient is having tenderness on palpation of the temporal arteries then there is a possibility of temporal arteritis.

EYELID TRAUMA

PERIOCULAR HEMATOMA (BLACK EYE)

1. Black eye is the most common blunt injury to the eyelid or face.
2. It is bruising around the eye commonly due to an injury to the face rather than to the eye.
3. The name "black eye" is given due to the color of bruising i.e black.
4. It is due to collection of blood in subcutaneous tissue from broken vessels and capillaries.
5. In most of the times black eye injuries are not serious in nature .
6. However, it is necessary to rule out other associated serious condition occurring due to blunt trauma to the globe like:
    a. **Hyphema** (Bleeding within the anterior chamber of eye, is serious and can reduce vision and damage the cornea)
    b. **Orbital wall fractures & basal skull fracture**
    c. **Retinal injuries**
7. Skull base fracture also gives a characteristic bilateral ring like hematomas **(Panda eyes)**

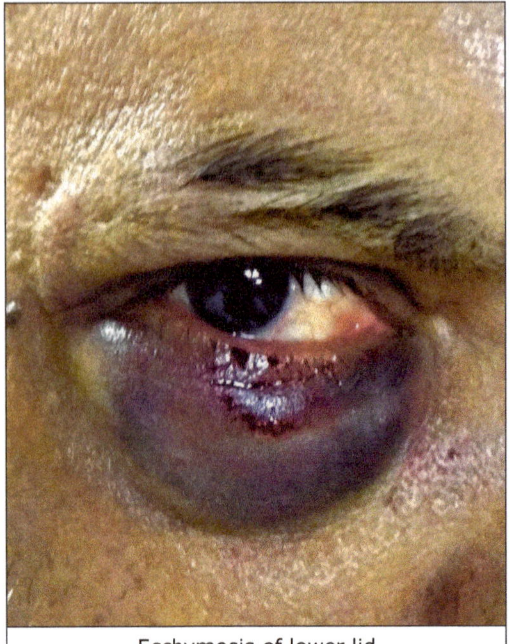

Ecchymosis of lower lid

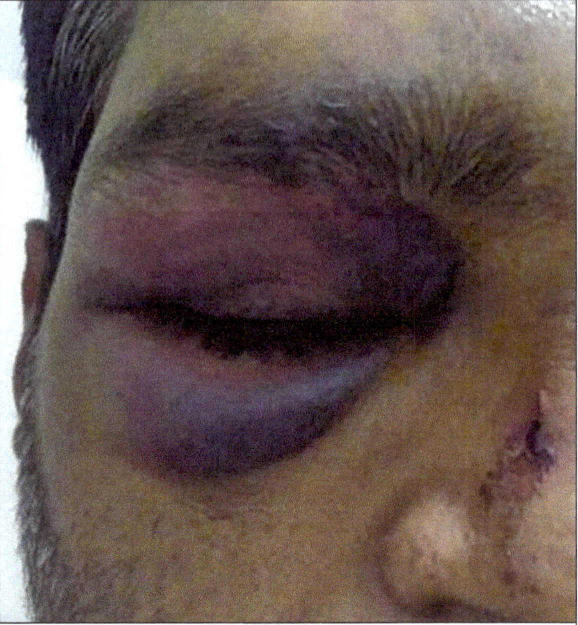

Ecchymosis of upper & lower lid (post trauma)

8. **Treatment:**
   a. Applying an ice pack will keep down swelling and reduce bleeding by constricting the capillaries.
   b. Analgesic drugs (painkillers) can be administered to relieve pain.

LID LACERATION

1. Traumatic eyelid laceration cases are also more common in emergency department
2. In the presence of a lid laceration, careful examination and wound exploration is necessary to exclude associated corneal and globe injuries.
3. It is commonly caused by trauma by sharp or blunt objects.
4. Simple superficial horizontal lacerations may be repaired by the Emergency Physician
5. **The following eyelid lacerations should be repaired by an ophthalmologist:**
   a. Trauma associated with ptosis, tarsal plate or levator palpebrae muscle involvement
   b. Canalicular tear (Injury near medial canthus)
   c. Lacrimal duct or sac involvement
   d. Laceration involves full thickness of lid (or "through and through" laceration)
6. **Procedure:**
   a. Position patient: supine position
   b. Tetanus toxoid 0.5 ml IM (As per immunisation status)
   c. May use topical anesthetic to instill in each eye.
   d. Use a protective scleral shell over the affected eye.
   e. Irrigate surrounding skin and clean with a povidone-iodine solution.
   f. Sterile drapes are used to isolate the area.
   g. Remove any foreign body or particulate matter, if present.
7. Administer local subcutaneous anesthetic (2% lidocaine with 1: 100, 000 epinephrine) for anesthesia

Types of lacerations	Management
Superficial lacerations	Sutured with non absorbable suture material like silk or nylon
Lid margin lacerations	Initially tarsal plate is approximated with the help of vicryl 6-0 and then lid margin with silk or nylon 6-0.
Lacerations with mild tissue loss	Prevents direct primary closure. Can usually be managed by performing a lateral cantholysis for orbital compartment syndrome. (Surgical exposure of the lateral canthal tendon)
Lacerations with extensive tissue loss	Requires major reconstructive procedures.
Canalicular lacerations	Repaired within 24 hours, with silicone tubing if both canaliculi are involved, or monocanalicular stent if only one canaliculus is involved.

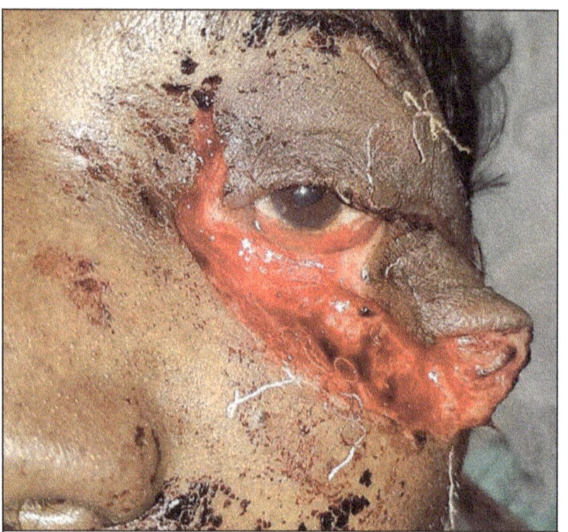

Contused lacerated wound lid including canaliculi (Pre-operative)

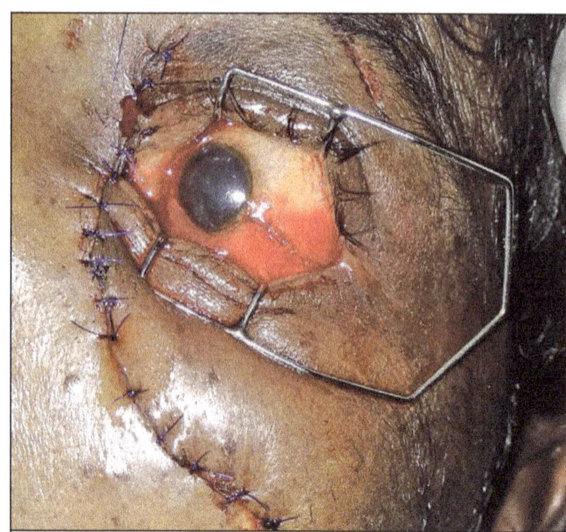

Sutured contused lacerated wound (post-operative)

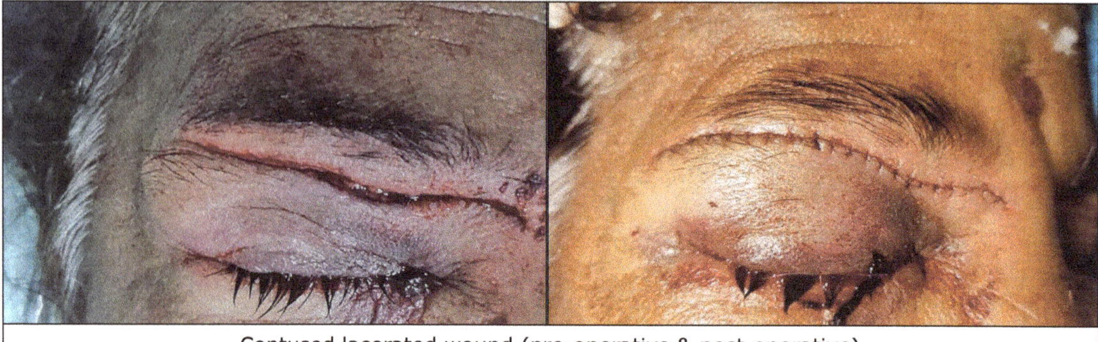

Contused lacerated wound (pre-operative & post-operative)

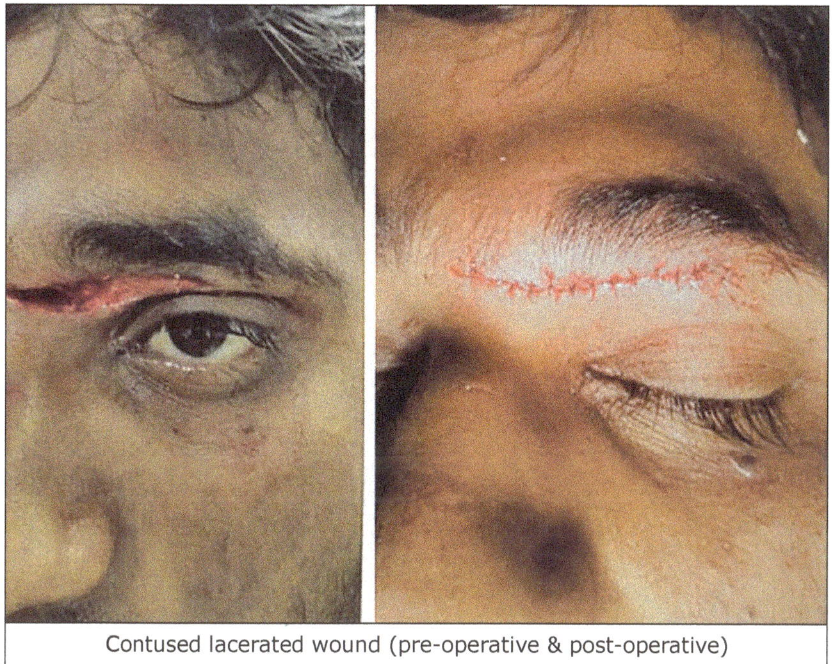

Contused lacerated wound (pre-operative & post-operative)

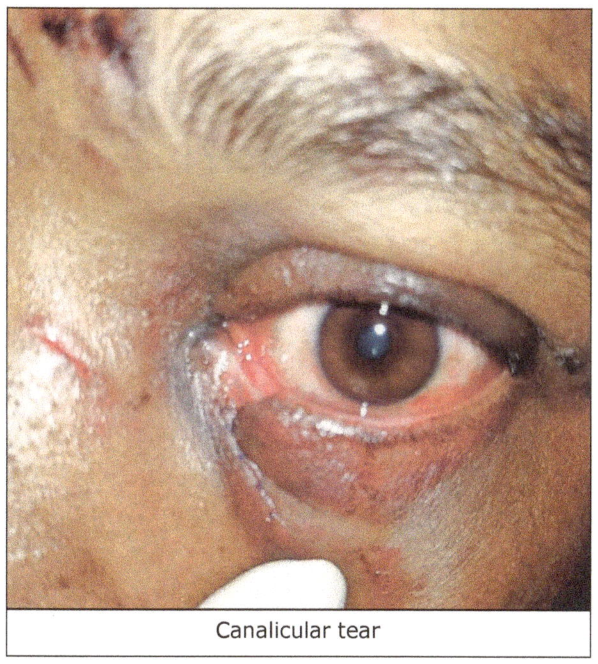

Canalicular tear

ORBITAL TRAUMA

1. Blow-out fractures of the orbit are caused by a large object that is greater in diameter than the orbital aperture (about 5 cm) which is usually by the blunt objects such as cricket ball or a tennis ball
2. The object transmits force into the orbit, which is then reflected back.
3. Orbital opening is blocked by the object so that the back force is directed at the orbital walls thereby damaging the thinner walls
4. Bones of the lateral wall and the roof are usually able to withstand such trauma but the thinnest medial wall and inferior (floor) wall get fractured.
5. Most commonly orbital floor blowout fracture occurs, but it can also affect the medial wall of the orbit.
6. Following points must be assessed in orbital injury:
   a. **Visual acuity**
   b. **Anterior chamber**
   c. **Integrity of globe**
   d. **Pupil shape and reactivity**
   e. **Extraocular movement (9 gazes)**
   f. **Posterior segment examination**
7. **Clinical features:**
   a. Orbital pain
   b. Nausea and bradycardia due to oculocardiac reflex (Due to traction applied to extraocular muscles and compression of eyeball)
   c. Subcutaneous emphysema
   d. Enophthalmos (Prolapse of orbital contents into maxillary and or ethmoidal sinuses)
   e. Limitation of eye movement (Restricted gaze suggests orbital Fracture with entrapment)
   f. Abnormal pupil size and reactivity
   g. Diplopia
   h. Photophobia
   i. Decreased visual acuity.

8. **Evaluation**
   a. **Slit lamp examination** (For Abrasion, Laceration, foreign body, Ulceration, Hyphema, Hypopyon, Traumatic Iritis, Lens dislocation, globe injury).
   b. **Non contrast CT face or orbit.**
   c. **Ocular ultrasound** if no open globe injury.
9. **Management: Depends on specific injury**
   a. **Orbital floor fracture:**
      1. **Symptoms and signs**
         i. **Pain, local tenderness**
         ii. **Diplopia:** On vertical eye movements.
         iii. **Enophthalmos:** May be associated with the severe fracture.
         iv. **Periocular signs: Black eye**, edema and sometimes subcutaneous emphysema.
         v. **Visual function:** Especially acuity, should be recorded and monitored in the acute situation.
         vi. In orbital floor fracture if infraorbital nerve is damaged then it will result into anesthesia/dysesthesia in its region of distribution.
         vii. **Ocular damage:** Careful examination of the globe to rule out the following conditions:
            - Hyphema (Collection of blood inside the anterior chamber of the eye)
            - Angle recession tear between the circular and longitudinal fibers of the ciliary body
            - Retinal dialysis (A **tear** of **the retina** from its insertion at the ora serrata)
         viii. **Tomography:** To document muscle involvement
         ix. **Hess chart**
      2. **Diagnosis:**
         i. **Radiograph (Water's view radiograph)** Shows polypoid mass herniated from the floor into the maxillary antrum, classically known as **Teardrop sign**, as it usually is in the shape of a teardrop.
         ii. **CT scan:** CT scan with axial and coronal view is the optimal study of choice for orbital fractures.

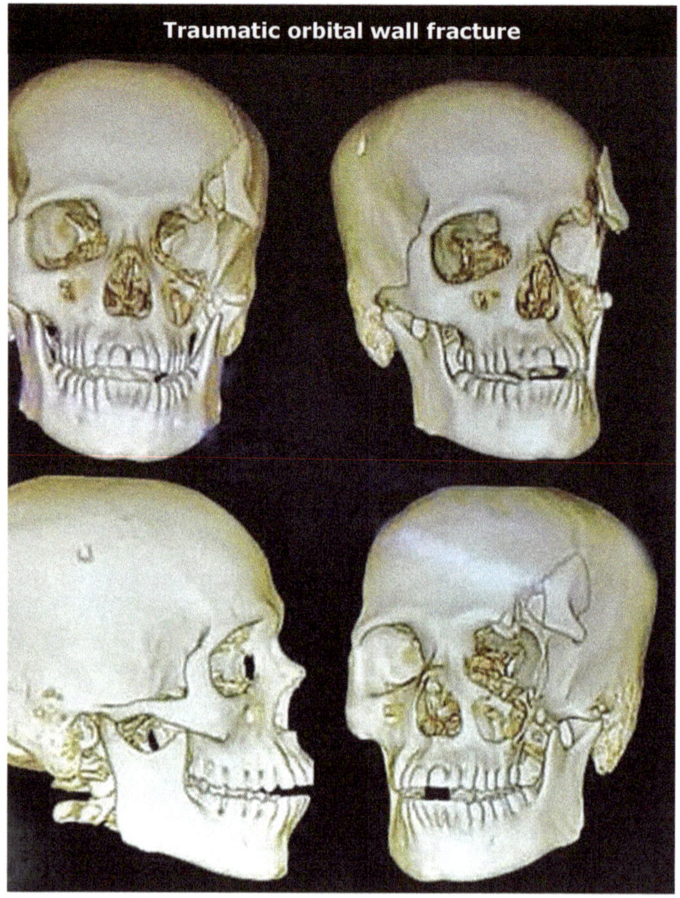

3. **Treatment:**

   i. Oral antibiotics

   ii. Ice packs application and use nasal decongestants

   iii. Systemic steroids are indicated if there is optic nerve compromise due to severe orbital edema.

   iv. The patient should be instructed not to blow his or her nose, as it may result in forcing infected sinus contents into the orbit.

   v. Surgical Indication:

   - Large fractures need early repair, preferably within 2 weeks after injury, as these fractures cause substantial muscle dysfunction due to entrapment of the tissue.
   - Fractures with entrapment of orbital contents
   - Marked enophthalmos.

b. Medial wall fracture

1. Medial wall fractures can occur alone or as part of a complex fracture
2. In patients with good extraocular motility, minimal diplopia and no significant enophthalmos (i.e. < 2 mm and cosmetically acceptable), conservative management is adequate.
3. **Surgical repair done :-** If the patient has symptomatic diplopia and positive forced duction test or large fracture causing latent enophthalmos. In this case repair is done within 2 weeks of initial trauma because fibrosis and scarring make delayed repair difficult.
4. Treatment involves release of incarcerated tissue and repair of the bony defect.

c. Roof fracture

1. Roof fracture is mostly associated with other orbital fracture but isolated orbital roof fractures in adults are uncommon
2. In children, mild grade trauma can result into fracture.
3. The frontal sinus is often involved.
4. In this type of fracture always examine for CSF leak, as it carries risk of meningitis.
5. Reconstructive surgery is needed in patients with downward displacement of fracture fragments.
6. If signs of muscle entrapment (e.g. levator dysfunction) are seen, surgery may be required.

d. Lateral wall fracture

1. Commonly seen with zygomatic malar complex (ZMC) fractures
2. Lateral wall fracture is not commonly involved in facial trauma as it is more solid and usually associated with extensive force trauma.
3. Non-displaced or mildly displaced fracture may be managed conservatively without surgical repair.
4. If the displaced lateral wall fracture causes visual loss, ocular motility disturbance, enophthalmos or flattening of the malar eminence, fracture repair is indicated.

OPEN GLOBE INJURY

a. Open globe injuries involve a full thickness injury of the eye ball .

b. The most frequent causes are physical assault, domestic and work place accidents, road traffic accidents, and sports related.

c. **Mechanism of injury:** Blunt or penetrating trauma.

d. Penetrating trauma may occur from bullet, knife, needles, screwdriver, nails etc.

e. In open globe injury there are more chances of introduction of infection into the globe which is the most dreaded complication.

f. Post traumatic iridocyclitis is a common sequel to a perforative wound.

g. Suspect for globe penetration in patient with any puncture or laceration injury to the eyelid or periorbital area.

h. During a globe rupture, the outer covering/layers of the eye are completely ruptured and the vitreous and/or aqueous humour drain through the site of rupture, causing the eye to 'deflate'.

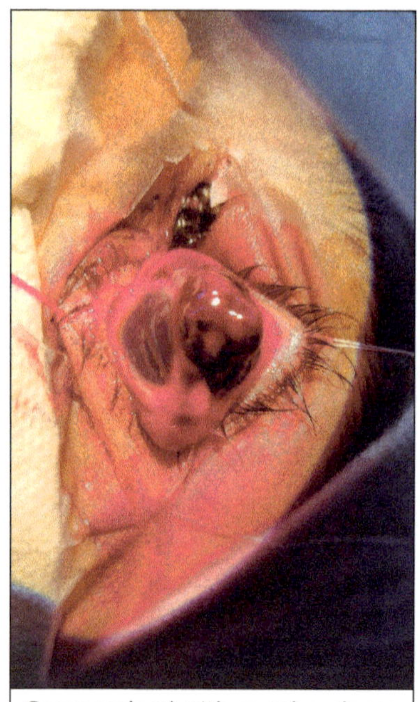

Corneoscleral with uveal prolapse (pre-operative)

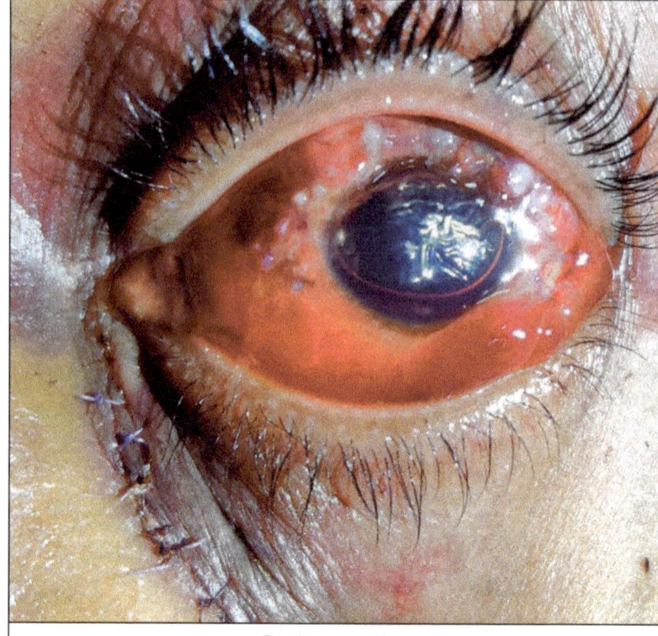

Post-operative

i. **It includes**

1. **Globe rupture:** It is a full-thickness wound caused by blunt trauma and globe ruptured occur at its weakest point and it is an inside-out injury.

2. **Globe laceration:** It is a full thickness wound caused by sharp object or direct impact of object.

   It includes:

   a. **Penetrating injury:** Penetrating injury has a one full-thickness wound, usually caused by a sharp object, without an exit wound.

   b. **Perforation injury:** Perforation injury has two full-thickness wounds, one is caused by entry of object and another caused by exit of object (Through and Through injury) e.g. Missile injury.

j. **Clinical features**

1. **Symptoms:**

   a. Pain

   b. Decreased vision (Sudden onset)

   c. Loss of vitreous fluid

   d. Patient gives h/o trauma commonly during hammer work, fall or sharp objects entering globe

2. **Signs**

   a. Full thickness scleral/corneal conjunctival lacerations

   b. Severe subconjunctival hemorrhage

   c. A shallow or deep anterior chamber

   d. Lens material or vitreous in anterior chamber of eye

   e. Foreign body tract or new cataract in lens (Traumatic cataract)

   f. Limitation of extraocular motility

   g. Loss of red reflex (Vitreous hemorrhage, retinal detachment)

   h. Intraocular content outside the globe

   i. Iridodialysis (Separation or tearing away of the iris from its attachment to the ciliary body)

   j. Cyclodialysis (A separation of the ciliary body from the scleral spur, creating a direct connection between the anterior chamber and the suprachoroidal space).

   k. Dislocated or subluxated lens

k. **Diagnosis:**

1. **Penlight**
2. **Indirect ophthalmoscope**

3. **Slit lamp examination with gentle manipulation**
4. **Traumatic history**
5. **CT scan orbit:** With thin cuts to evaluate the radio-opaque intraocular foreign body, orbital fracture

I. **Management:**

1. Bed rest
2. Place Fox shield
3. Antiemetics (Cardio-ocular reflex causes vomiting)
4. Analgesic for pain relief.
5. Intravenous antibiotics
6. Injection tetanus toxoid 0.5 ml IM (if not up to date)
7. **Eye drops with preservatives and eye ointments are best avoided in open globe injury.**
8. **Surgical exploration:** Globe exploration should be performed in suspected penetrating trauma
9. **Vitrectomy** is performed in
   a. Vitreous hemorrhage with an intraocular foreign body
   b. Retinal detachment
10. If vitrectomy not required then, closure of the open globe is done primarily
11. After primary closure, patients should be followed up for examination and ultrasound to identify & manage posterior segment complications, if any.

CLOSED GLOBE INJURY

a. The extent of ocular damage depends on the severity of trauma.

b. The corneoscleral wall of the globe is intact in closed globe injuries.

c. Mostly limited to either the anterior or posterior segment

d. Blunt trauma commonly results in more obscure long-term effects

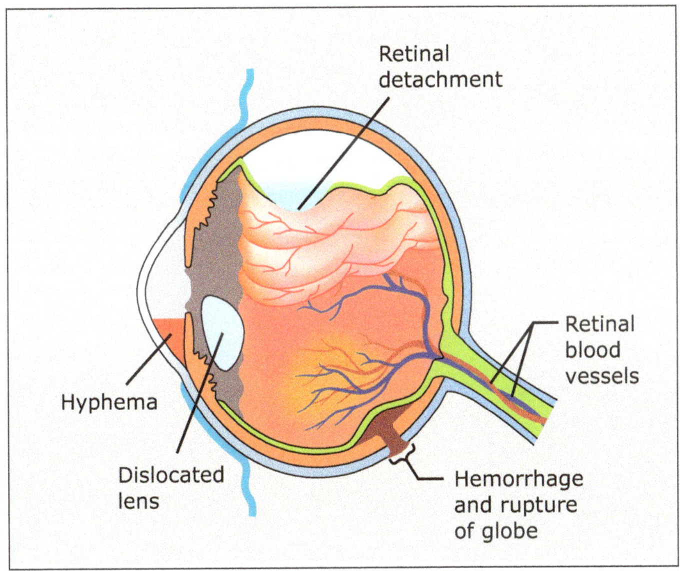

e. **It includes:**

1. **Partial thickness wound of eyewall**
2. **Contusion (no eye wall wound)**

f. **Causes:**

1. Sporting balls (e.g. cricket ball, tennis ball, shuttlecock)
2. Blunt trauma in a fistfight
3. Other high speed flying objects.

g. **It includes following injuries**

1. **Conjunctiva:**
   a. Subconjunctival hemorrhage
   b. Conjunctival abrasion
2. **Cornea:**
   a. Corneal abrasion

3. **Anterior uvea:**
   a. Hyphema
   b. Tears of the iris sphincter and iridodialysis
   c. Angle recession and cyclodialysis
4. **Lens:**
   a. Rosette cataract
   b. Dislocation of the lens
   c. Rupture of the anterior or posterior capsule
5. **Vitreous Hemorrhage**
6. **Choroid:**
   a. Choroidal rupture
   b. Suprachoroidal hemorrhage
7. **Retina:**
   a. Retinal or subretinal hemorrhage
   b. Retinal edema/**Berlin's edema/Commotio retinae** (Retinal whitening associated with trauma related retinal edema)
   c. Retinal detachment
   d. Retinal dialysis
   e. Macular edema or hole
8. **Optic nerve:**
   a. Optic nerve avulsion
   b. Hemorrhage of the optic nerve sheath

SUBCONJUNCTIVAL HEMORRHAGE

1. Subconjunctival hemorrhage is due to the rupture of small vessels.
2. This may occur spontaneously in elderly people with fragile vessels or those with hypertension or after local ocular trauma or ophthalmic surgery
3. Violent coughing, powerful sneezing, straining action can cause rupture of small blood vessels of eye
4. Recurrent cases of subconjunctival hemorrhage needs further investigations for bleeding disorders or leukemia.
5. Sub conjunctival hemorrhages also result from heavy or sustained pressure on the thorax and abdomen, as in persons squeezed in a crowd or by machinery.
6. The blood gradually gets absorbed within 1 to 3 weeks without treatment.

7. If mild ocular irritation is present, artificial tear drops can be prescribed four to six times a day
8. Tab vitamin C (500 gm) TDS is prescribed.

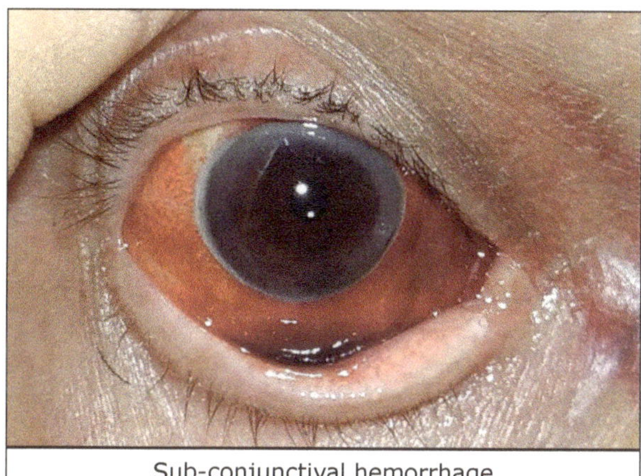
Sub-conjunctival hemorrhage

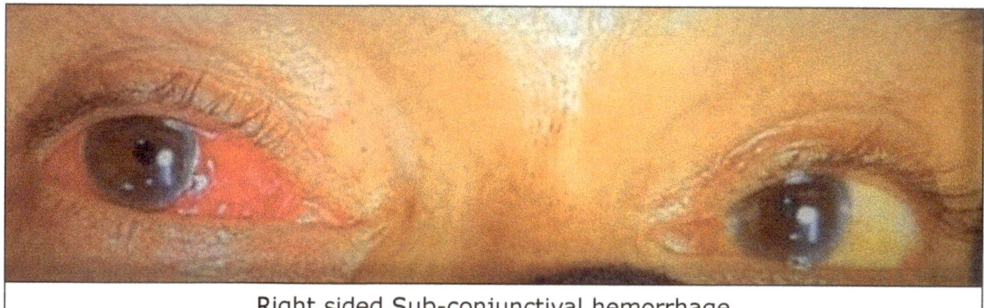
Right sided Sub-conjunctival hemorrhage

WOUNDS OF CONJUNCTIVA

1. **Signs and symptoms:**
    a. Redness
    b. Foreign body sensation
    c. Mild pain
    d. History /mechanism of ocular trauma
2. **Investigation:**
    a. **Complete eye examination:** complete exploration of sclera under the conjunctival laceration to rule out scleral laceration or sub conjunctival foreign body and open globe injury

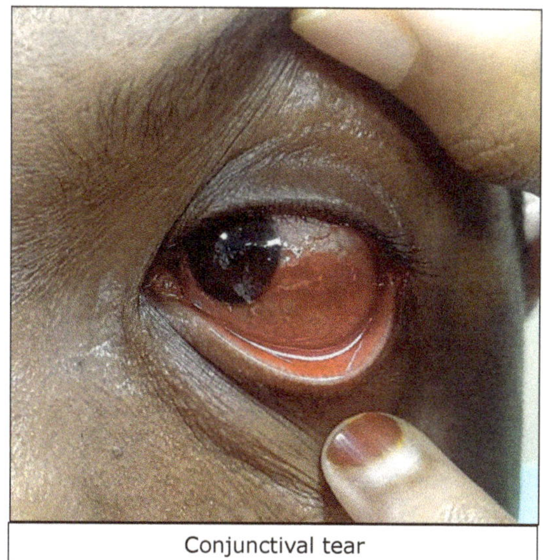
Conjunctival tear

b. **CT scan orbit without contrast:** Performed if associated with more severe injury to rule out intraocular or intraorbital foreign body

c. **B scan:** It is better avoided in open globe injury, so as to avoid pressure on the globe as it can further increase complication

   However, gentle B scan can be performed in certain traumatic cases e.g. traumatic endophthalmitis.

d. In the case of a suspected ruptured globe the exploration is done under general anesthesia in an operative room specially in children.

3. **Treatment:**

   a. **Antibiotic ointment:** Erythromycin, bacitracin, chloramphenicol/polymyxin B.

   b. Most of the conjunctival laceration heal without surgical repair.

   c. Suturing is done if the laceration is large in size.

WOUNDS OF CORNEA

1. **Types of corneal injuries**

   a. Partial thickness

   b. Full thickness

2. **Signs and symptoms:**

   a. Diminution of vision

   b. Photophobia

   c. Pain

   d. Congestion

3. **Investigation:**

   a. **Visual acuity**

   b. **Examination of eye on slit lamp**

   c. **Seidel test:** Positive in non sealed full thickness corneal tear

   d. **Examination of eyelid and adnexa**

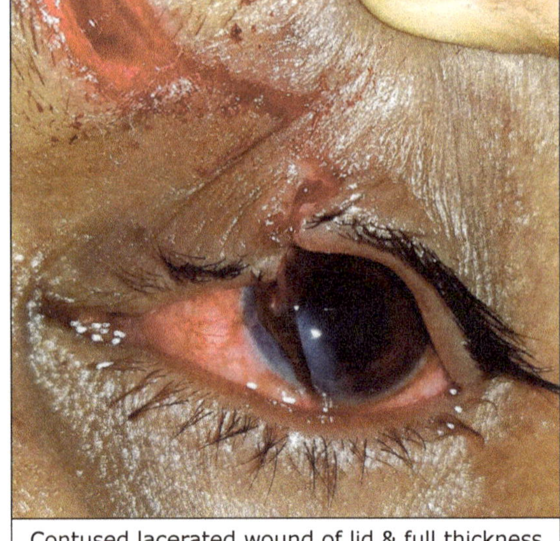

Contused lacerated wound of lid & full thickness corneal tear

4. **Treatment:**

   Partial thickness

   1. Cycloplegic eye drops (atropine 1%, homatropine 0.5%)

2. Topical Antibiotic (Polymyxin B/bacitracin ointment, Fluoroquinolone drops e.g. moxifloxacin, gentamicin)
3. Preservative free lubricant drops
4. When the wound is not full thickness or only approaching full thickness in a very small area the flap can be kept well apposed in its correct anatomical location without suture
5. If the flap is displaced, it has to be repositioned and secured with sutures.
6. If suturing required then tightness and number of sutures should be just enough to hold the flap in place.
7. Tetanus toxoid if not updated.

Full thickness

These require surgical repair in the operating room with 10-0 nylon sutures.

TRAUMATIC CATARACT

a. A traumatic cataract occurs secondary to trauma to the eye.
b. Trauma (Penetrating or blunt) disrupts and causes damage to lens fibers .
c. The morphology of a classic traumatic cataract is referred as a rosette or stellate type
d. If not aspirated at earliest may lead to serious complications

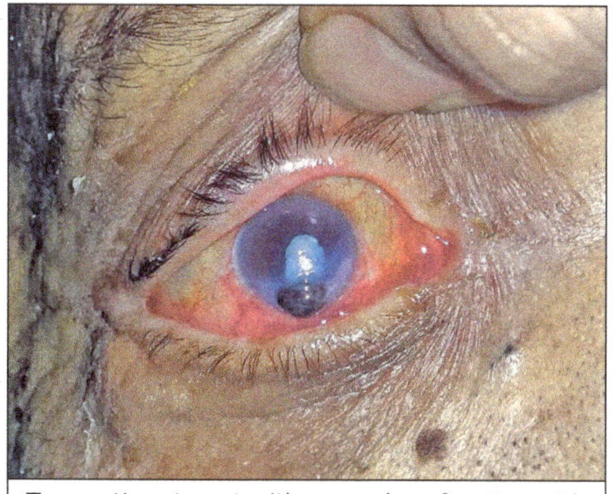

Traumatic cataract with corneal perforation with uveal prolapse

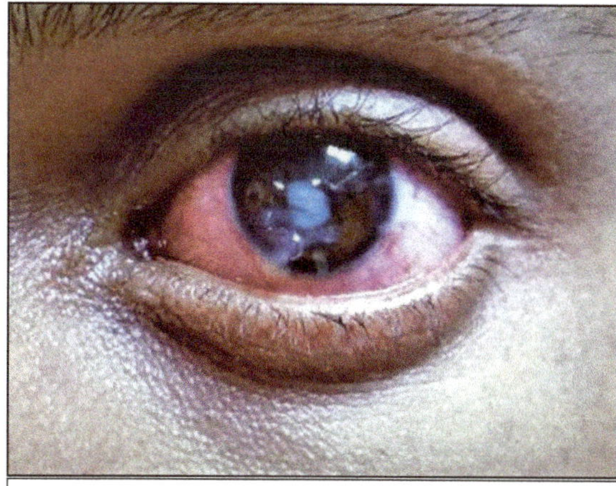

Traumatic cataract

Clinical features

1. History of trauma to eye
2. Defective vision of sudden and profound nature
3. Pain and redness of eye
4. Photophobia
5. Watering of eye

Treatment

Plan for cataract surgery with IOL implantation later

HYPHEMA

a. It is a hemorrhage in anterior chamber

a. Commonly caused by blunt ocular injury.

b. Bleeding occurs typically from the iris root or ciliary body

c. In hyphema, characteristically, the blood settles inferiorly in anterior chamber with a resultant fluid level except when hyphema is total (Eight ball hyphema).

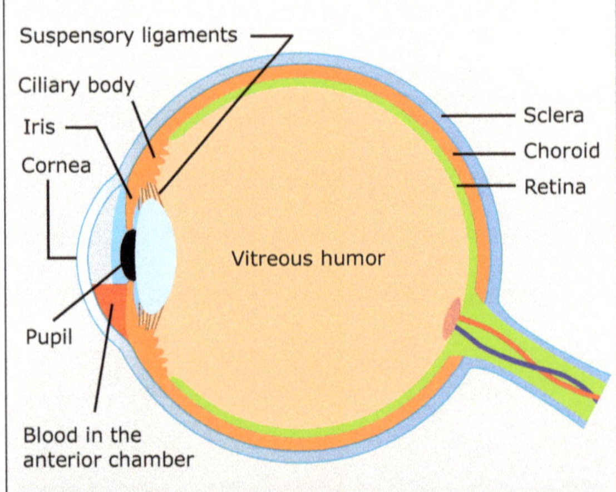

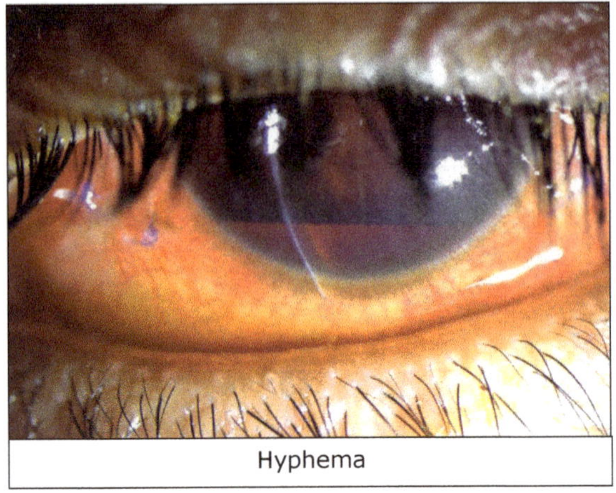
Hyphema

d. Treatment

1. **Bed rest**
2. **Head elevation**
3. **Topical corticosteroids** (prednisolone 1%, dexamethasone 0.5%): Reduce the inflammation
4. **Topical cycloplegic agents:** relieve ciliary spasm or photophobia.
5. **Intraocular pressure management:** Systemic carbonic anhydrase inhibitors and hyperosmotic agents (acetazolamide or mannitol) may be required if topical management fails to control the pressure.
6. If the above management fails then surgical interventions are required.

SCLERAL INJURY

1. Scleral wounds more than 3–4 mm posterior to the limbus are sutured completely after a thorough exploration.
2. They are also treated with surrounding cryo-applications.

VITREOUS HEMORRHAGE

1. Trauma is also a leading cause of vitreous hemorrhage
2. Due to traumatic injury retinal vessels bleed into vitreous which leads to vitreous hemorrhage.
3. **Diagnosis:**
    a. Ophthalmoscopy
    b. Intra ocular pressure (IOP)
    c. B scan ultrasonography
4. **Management:**
    a. Rest
    b. Propped up position
    c. Tab vitamin C 500 mg qds.
    d. Vitrectomy is performed urgently if associated with other traumatic complications like retinal detachment, intraocular foreign body, macular hole
    e. In absence of above traumatic complication watchful waiting is done on an outpatient basis.

FOREIGN BODY

1. Foreign body may be corneal, conjunctival or intraocular
2. The most common foreign bodies in the cornea are pieces of metal or rusty objects.
3. Other common foreign body includes dust, dirt, contact lenses, sand, cosmetics
4. FB like small particles of dust, sand, metals are responsible for corneal or conjunctival injuries such as abrasions.
5. Some foreign bodies drain into a lacrimal drainage system and some get attached to superior tarsal conjunctiva and produces abrasions over cornea in vertical direction with closure of eyelid.
6. **A foreign body entering the eye may cause damage to the eye in one of the following three ways:**
   a. **By mechanical effects**
   b. **By the introduction of infection**
   c. **By specific action (chemical or otherwise) on the intraocular tissues.**
7. **Always keep in mind the possibility of intraocular foreign body**
8. **Signs and symptoms:**
   a. **Foreign body sensation**
   b. **Watering of eye**
   c. **Redness of eye**
   d. **History of trauma**
9. **Diagnosis:**

   Local anesthetic drops are used only for eye examination and for doing procedure.
   a. **Visual acuity**
   b. **Slit lamp examination:** Determine the position and depth of the foreign body and also to examine entry wounds.
   c. Dilate the eye to examine the posterior chamber for intraocular foreign body
   d. **B scan**
   e. **CT scan:** Intraocular foreign body or orbital fracture.
   f. **Ultrasonographic biomicroscopy**: For suspected intraocular foreign body in angle.

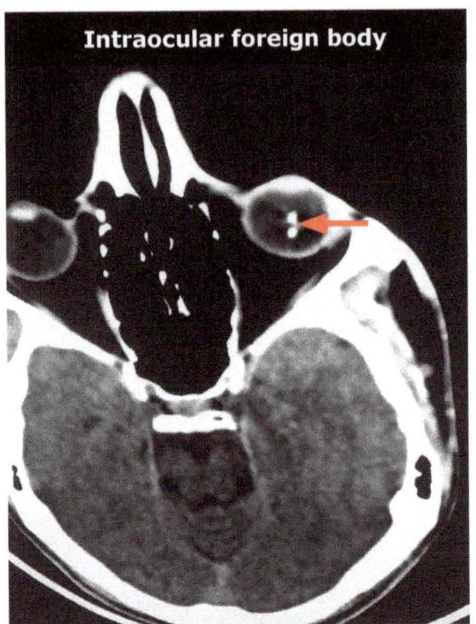

10. **Treatment:**

A] Corneal foreign body:

a. Apply topical anesthesia (Proparacaine 1%)

b. Remove the corneal foreign body with a small gauge needle (26G, 30G), foreign body spud, fine forceps.

c. Multiple foreign bodies can be removed more easily by irrigation with sterile neutral pH solutions.

d. Measure the size of epithelial defect caused by the foreign body.

e. Treat the defect as corneal abrasion with topical lubricants and antibiotics and/or eye patching.

f. If there is a full thickness involvement of cornea by foreign body then exploration and removal is done in an operative room.

g. Perform Seidel test to ensure removal did not perforate cornea

h. Irrigate eye profusely with normal saline post-removal

i. Consider cycloplegics (e.g. Cyclopentolate or homatropine) for significant photophobia

j. Consider topical antibiotics (Polymyxin B /bacitracin ointment, Fluoroquinolone drops e.g. Moxifloxacin, gentamicin) for corneal involvement.

k. Inform the patient to meet urgently if there is worsening of symptoms

B] Conjunctival foreign body:

a. Remove foreign body under topical anesthesia

b. Multiple loose superficial foreign body can be often removed with balanced salt solution (BSS) irrigation

c. Foreign body can be removed by cotton-tipped applicator soaked in topical anesthetic or with fine forceps

d. For a deeply embedded foreign body, removal can be done using a cotton tipped applicator soaked in 2.5% phenylephrine to reduce the bleeding from conjunctiva.

e. In some cases conjunctival excision may be required.

C] Intraocular foreign body:

a. A detailed history is a very important aspect of IOFB injuries to find a clue about the nature of the IOFB and for medico-legal aspects

b. Intraocular mechanical effect depends on the size, velocity & type of foreign body.

c. Patients may not complain of vision loss or severe pain, but a small entry wound can be found on careful examination.

d. Determining the nature and size of IOFB is very important for planning the management.

e. A complete examination of both eyes is necessary, even if the other eye is asymptomatic.

f. Localization of the IOFB is the prime aspect of management.

g. Whether the IOFB is in the eye (anterior or posterior) or in the orbit.

h. **Investigation:**

   i. **Plain X-ray:** Useful in radio-opaque foreign bodies only and will not detect radiolucent IOFBs such as wood or glass.

   ii. **Computed tomography scan:** Provides much more reliable information regarding the size, shape and localization of the foreign body.

   iii. **Ultrasonography:** Useful in determining the extent of the intraocular damage, determining the presence of a retinal detachment, double perforation, as well as in detecting foreign bodies nature and shape

   iv. **MRI scan:** Not used in suspected metallic IOFB.

i. **Treatment:**

   i. Protection of the globe with a shield

   ii. Avoiding any pressure over the globe

   iii. Tetanus toxoid as per immunisation status

   iv. A delay in management may be complicated by infection.

   v. Broad-spectrum antibiotic prophylaxis

   vi. Forceps (Basket forceps, IOFB forceps) may be used for removal of foreign bodies.

   vii. Definitive treatment is surgery.

CHEMICAL INJURY OF EYE

a. Ocular chemical burns are common and serious emergencies that require immediate evaluation and management.

b. Chemical injuries are most commonly caused due to lime chuna, fertilizers, holi colors, floor cleaner etc.

c. In most of cases injury is accidental and in some cases it is due to assault.

d. Majority of accidental burns occur at the workplace.

e. It occurs mostly in the person who works in chemical industries, laboratories or factories.

f. Alkali burns are more common as compare to acid burns, since alkalis are more widely used both at home and in industry.

g. The severity of a chemical injury depends on the properties of the chemical, which area of ocular surface affected and duration of exposure.

h. Acid injury is less severe than alkali as it coagulates the surface protein, forms barrier for deep penetration.

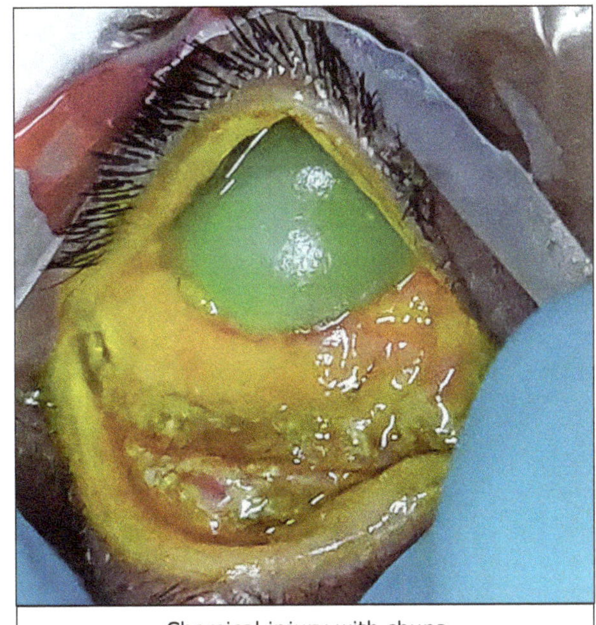

Chemical injury with chuna

i. Ammonia and sodium hydroxide are particularly harmful because of rapid penetration

j. **Signs and symptoms:**

1. Sudden onset of severe pain, epiphora and photophobia.
2. Acute periocular signs of injury include periorbital edema and erythema, deepithelialized skin, and loss of eyelashes and eyebrows.
3. Corneal epithelial damage
4. Limbal ischemia
5. Corneal cloudiness, sterile ulceration, edema, and occasionally perforation
6. Diminution of vision

k. **Grades of chemical injury: (Dua classification 2001)**

Grade of injury	Clock hours of Limbal involvement	Conjunctival involvement	Analog scale	Prognosis
I	0	0%	0/0 %	Very good
II	< or = 3	< 30 %	0.1 -3/1-29.9%	Good
III	> 3-6	> 30-50 %	3.1- 6/31-50%	Good
IV	>6-9	> 50-75%	6.1-9/51-75%	Good to guarded
V	> 9-< 12	75%- <100%	9.1-11.9/75.1-99.9%	Guarded to poor
VI	12	100%	12/100%	Very poor

Management:

a. **Emergency treatment**

1. **Copious irrigation of eye (Even before detailed eye examination):**
   a. A lid speculum is useful while irrigating the eye.
   b. Topical anesthetic should be instilled prior to irrigation, as it improves the comfort of the patient.
   c. Irrigation decrease duration of contact with the chemical and normalize the pH in the conjunctival sac as soon as possible
   d. A sterile neutral pH solution, such as balanced salt solution, Ringer lactate or normal saline should be used to irrigate the eye thoroughly.
   e. Commonly, ocular surface pH is checked using a litmus paper and irrigation is continued until pH normalizes.
   f. Tap water may be used if nothing else is available to avoid the longer duration of contact of the chemical with eye.
2. **Double-eversion of the upper eyelid (For thorough checking of fornices):** Used to identify and remove retained particulate matter in the fornices.
3. **Debridement of necrotic areas of corneal epithelium: Under the** slit lamp to promote re-epithelialization and remove associated chemical residue.
4. Admission of patients with severe injuries (Grade 4 onwards) in order to provide adequate eye care & effective monitoring.

b. **Management:**

1. **Medical management**: It is necessary to promote reepithelialization, decrease inflammation, prevent infection, avoid further epithelial and stromal break-down and minimize the sequelae.
2. **Topical corticosteroids**: Control acute inflammation after chemical injuries.

3. **Preservative free tear substitutes and lubricating ointment:** Reduce the risk of recurrent erosions, and accelerate visual rehabilitation
4. **Topical antibiotic drops**: Used for prophylaxis of bacterial infection (e.g. four times daily).
5. **Topical steroids and cycloplegics**: Used if necessary to reduce the pain and ciliary spasm.
6. **Ascorbic acid:** Used to reduce incidence of corneal thinning & ulceration.
7. **Oral tetracyclines/topical tetracycline preparation** are useful to avoid proteolytic melting of cornea.
8. **Autologous serum tears**: Contain many factors that promote healing and may be used to promote epithelialization
9. **Surgical management**: includes initial debridement of the necrotic material and amniotic membrane transplantation and tectonic grafting if necessary.
10. **Late surgical management:** Correcting eyelid abnormalities, management of glaucoma, limbal stem cell transplantation, and ultimately keratoplasty to restore visual function of the eye.

ACUTE ANGLE CLOSURE GLAUCOMA

1. Acute glaucoma is caused by sudden and rapid increase in intraocular pressure.
2. It results in damage to the optic nerve and causes vision loss.
3. An imbalance in the production and drainage of fluid in the eye leads to increase in intraocular pressure due to improperly functioning or blocked drainage channels.
4. If angle closes suddenly, symptoms are severe and dramatic.
5. So acute angle closure glaucoma is an emergency condition.
6. Immediate treatment needed to avoid the optic nerve damage and vision loss.

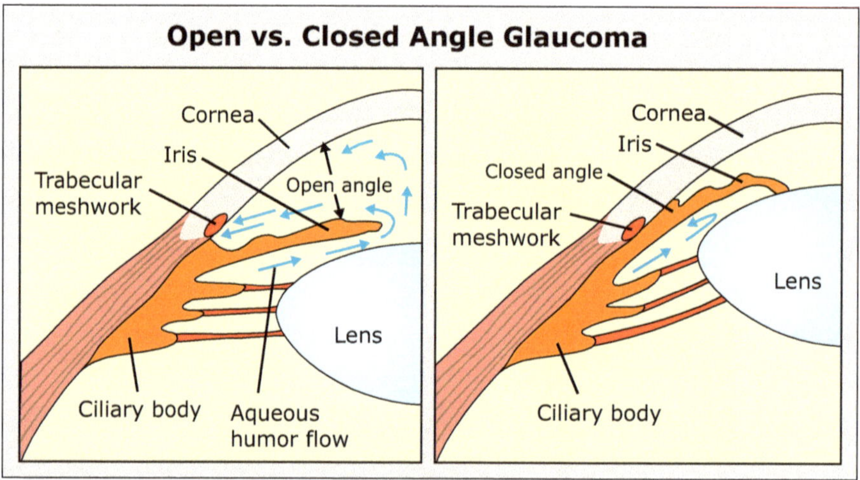

7. **Types of acute angle closure glaucoma**
   a. **Primary angle closure suspect (PACS)**
   b. **Primary angle closure (PAC)**
   c. **Primary angle closure glaucoma (PACG)**
8. **Signs and symptoms:**
   a. Severe headache
   b. Eye pain
   c. Diminution of vision
   d. Nausea /vomiting
   e. Colored halos
   f. Redness

9. **Signs in angle closure glaucoma:**
   a. Shallow anterior chamber
   b. Corneal edema
   c. Vertically oval mid-dilated fixed pupil
   d. Ciliary congestion
   e. Sphincter and iris atrophy
   f. Closed angles with raised IOP.
   g. Disc edema may be present.
10. **Management:**
    a. **Medical management (To reduce raised IOP)**
       1. **Antiglaucoma medications:** The use of **eyedrops, oral medications** (Osmotic agents such as glycerol or carbonic anhydrase inhibitors such as acetazolamide)
       2. **Intravenous medication** (Mannitol, an osmotic drug) are temporary measures used to bring the pressure down prior to surgical therapy.
    b. **Laser therapy:** Nd:YAG iridotomy procedure is performed to create hole in iris which facilitate flow of aqueous humor.
    c. **Trabeculectomy, if required.**
    d. A surgical iridotomy

VASCULAR DISORDERS OF RETINA

I] Central retinal artery occlusion (CRAO)

1. The arterial supply to the eye is provided by several branches from the ophthalmic artery, which is derived from the internal carotid artery
2. These branches include the central retinal artery, the short and long posterior ciliary arteries, and the anterior ciliary arteries.
3. When the flow of blood through the central retinal artery is blocked/occluded, it will cause sudden & complete retinal ischemia and ultimately tissue dies rapidly.

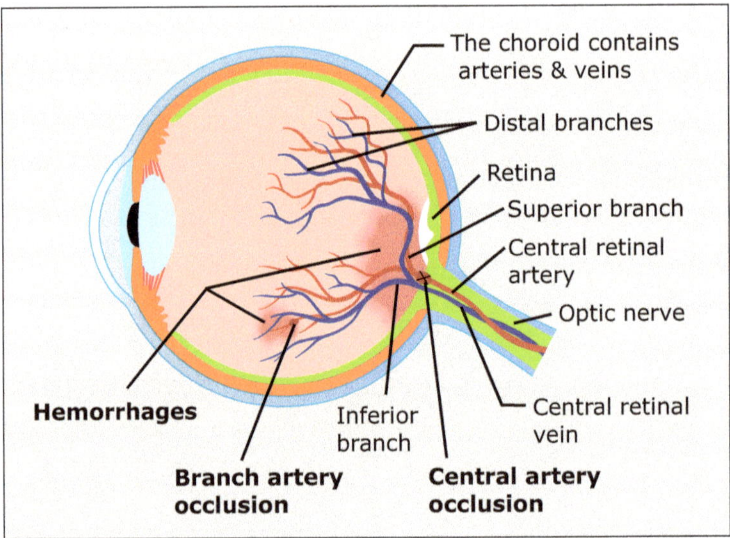

4. Most of the times obstruction of a retinal artery is due to an embolus and if it is associated with spasm often, it causes complete occlusion.
5. Central retinal artery occlusion (CRAO) is nearly always occur at the **lamina cribrosa,** where the vessels normally become slightly narrowed.
6. The eye suddenly may become blind due to complete occlusion.
7. In some cases a certain degree of central vision persists in spite of complete occlusion of the central artery. This is due to the presence of **cilioretinal artery**
8. In rare cases a cilioretinal artery alone becomes blocked.

9. History of smoking should be inquired.

Signs and symptoms	Investigations	Management
1. **Acute, Sudden and painless loss of vision in one eye** 2. **Cherry red spot with surrounding pale retina on fundoscopy** 3. **Relative afferent pupillary defect** 4. **Borcas segmentation of vessels.**	**Investigation for risk factors:** Routine blood investigation **Cardiovascular diseases evaluation:** ECG, auscultation, 2D echo, lipid profile. **Carotid doppler scanning:** look for carotid stenosis. **Thrombophilia screen:** **ESR or PCV, and CRP:** To identify Giant cell arteritis **CT scan /MRI brain:** Intracranial or orbital pathology **Plasma homocysteine level:** To exclude hyperhomocysteinemia. **Plasma protein electrophoresis**: Detect dysproteinemia such as multiple myeloma. **Autoantibodies:** Principally looking for vasculitis in younger patients.	1. **Supine posture:** Improve ocular perfusion 2. **Ocular massage:** (Apply direct Positive pressure over eyeball for 10–15 seconds followed by release & this is continued for 3–5 minutes): Useful to improve blood flow and dislodging thrombus or emboli. 3. **Topical and oral IOP lowering agent:** Topical timolol 0.5%, Tab acetazolamide, 4. **Breathing carbogen:** High oxygen (95%) and carbon dioxide (5%) mixture has dual effect, reduce of ischemia and vasodilatation. 5. **Sublingual isosorbide dinitrate**: Used to induce vasodilatation. 6. **Rebreathing' into a paper bag:** To elevate blood carbon dioxide and respiratory acidosis has been advocated, as this may promote vasodilation 7. **Mannitol or glycerol:** Causes reduction in intraocular pressure as well as increased intravascular volume 8. **Anterior chamber paracentesis** 9. **Transluminal Nd: YAG laser embolysis/embolectomy**

II] Retinal Venous thrombosis

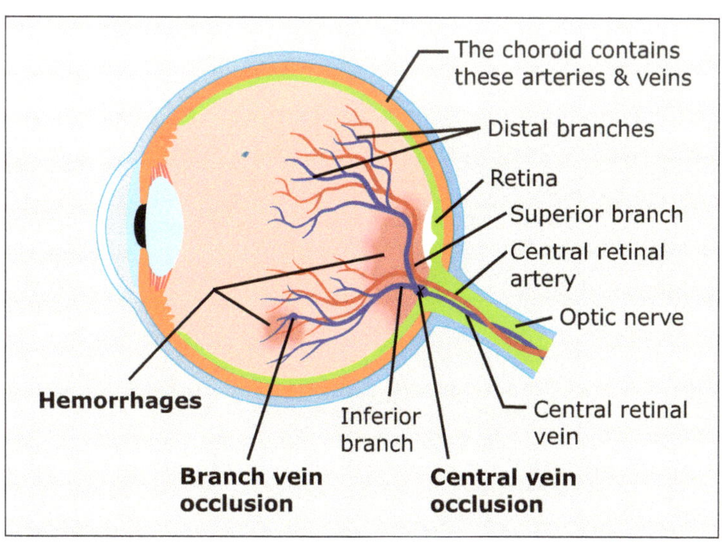

1. Central retinal vein drains into either superior ophthalmic vein or into the cavernous sinus directly.
2. Venous thrombosis usually occurs in elderly people with cardiovascular disease, diabetes mellitus, dyslipidemia, and chronic smokers.
3. In young people it may occur due to an infective periphlebitis
4. Venous thrombosis may also be due to local causes, such as a chronic glaucoma, orbital cellulitis or facial erysipelas.
5. Obstruction mostly occurs in the central vein just behind the lamina cribrosa.
6. After venous occlusion, venous and capillary pressure is increased which results into a stagnation of blood flow and retinal hypoxia.
7. Retinal hypoxia results in damage to the capillary endothelial cells, extravasation of blood constituents and release of mediators such as VEGF and inflammatory mediators.
8. Finally it results in a macular edema, vitreous hemorrhage and neovascular glaucoma.
9. Investigation and management of associated systemic diseases to reduce a chances of veno-occlusive (Ophthalmic or systemic) event in future.
10. **Types of central retinal venous occlusion:**
    a. **Non-ischemic CRVO**
    b. **Ischemic CRVO** (Poor prognosis).
11. **Two types of retinal venous occlusion:**
    a. **Central retinal venous occlusion:** Central retinal vein is occluded.
    b. **Branch retinal venous occlusion:** A single branch of the central vein is blocked

Signs and symptoms	Investigation	Treatment
Sudden unilateral blurring of vision **M**acular edema **V**itreous hemorrhage **N**eovascular glaucoma	**M**edical history **I**nvestigation related to risk factors like DM, HTN, dyslipidemia. **Diagnosis** 1. **Optical coherence tomography:** High definition image of the retina taken to determine the thickness of the retina. 2. **Ophthalmoscopy** 3. **Fundus fluorescein angiography:** Dye injected into a vein in the arm travels to the retinal blood vessels. Special photographs allow the physician to see the vessels.	1. **Macular edema:** **I**ntravitreal anti-VEGF agents **D**examethasone implant **L**aser photocoagulation 2. **Treatment of neovascularization:** a. **Panretinal photocoagulation (PRP)** should be performed without delay in eyes with NVI or angle neovascularization b. **Anti-VEGF agents** such as ranibizumab and bevacizumab have anti-angiogenic properties and may be used as adjuvant to pan-retinal photocoagulation.

RETINAL DETACHMENT

1. Retina is responsible for the absorption of the light and its conversion into electrical signals which are transferred to the brain via the optic nerve.
2. Retinal detachment is a separation of the neurosensory retina (NSR) from the retinal pigment epithelium (RPE).
3. Retinal detachment is due to accumulation of subretinal fluid.

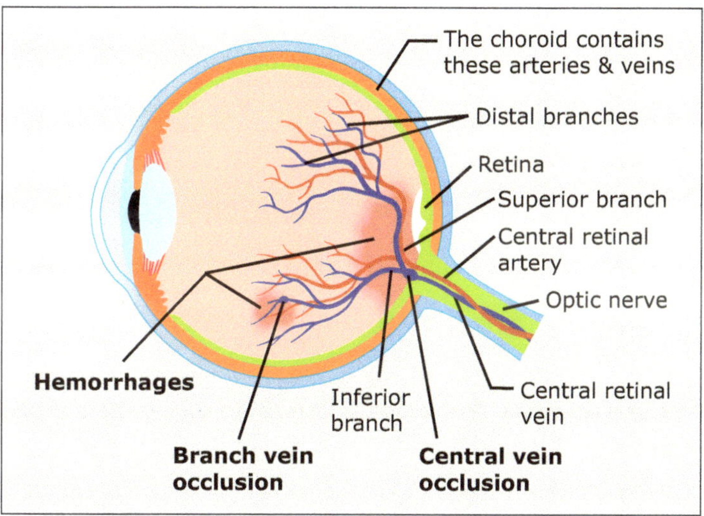

4. **Depending on the mechanism of subretinal fluid accumulation, retinal detachments traditionally have been classified into:**
   a. **Rhegmatogenous (Most common type):** In this type there is a hole or tear (Holes form due to retinal atrophy especially within an area of lattice degeneration and tears are due to vitreoretinal traction.) in the retina that allows fluid to pass through and collect underneath the retina, detaching it from its underlying blood supply.
   b. **Tractional:** Scar tissue caused by an injury, inflammation or neovascularization that grows on the surface of the retina and pulls the retina and thereby detaching it.
   c. **Exudative:** When fluid leaks out of blood vessels and accumulates under the retina (Occurs due to inflammation, injury or vascular abnormalities) In this type there are no holes, break in retina.
5. **Clinical features:**
   a. Sudden appearance of floaters (Mobile black spots)
   b. Very brief flashes of light in one or both eyes (Photopsia)

   c. Sudden diminution of vision usually painless
   d. A curtain- like dense shadow appears over field of vision

6. **Diagnosis:**
   a. **Ophthalmoscopy**
   b. **Fundus photography**
   c. **Ocular ultrasonography**

7. **Management:**
   a. **Three general principles used in the management of retinal detachment:**
      1. **Find all retinal breaks**
      2. **Seal all retinal breaks**
      3. **Relieve present and future vitreoretinal traction**
   b. **Cryopexy and laser photocoagulation:** To seal the retinal tears or holes
   c. **Scleral buckle surgery:** A silicone band is placed outside sclera to push it closer to retinal tear in order to close the tear.
   d. **Pneumatic retinopexy:** A gas (C3F8) bubble is injected into the eye over the retinal tear.
   e. **Vitrectomy:** To remove the vitreous humour from the eyeball and replace it with silicon oil or gas (tamponade).

CONJUNCTIVITIS

1. **Definition:** An inflammation of the conjunctiva.
2. Etiology of conjunctivitis is usually of infective or allergic origin.
   a. **Infectious:**
      1. **Bacterial:** (Staphylococcus aureus, Haemophilus aegyptius, H. influenzae, N. gonorrheae, N. meningitidis, Streptococcus pyogenes, Streptococcus pneumoniae, Moraxella lacunata, Proteus, Klebsiella, Escherichia coli, diphtheroids, etc.)
      2. **Viral:** Herpes simplex, adenoviruses, picornaviruses (coxsackie virus, enterovirus 70), myxovirus [measles], paramyxoviruses (mumps, Newcastle conjunctivitis), molluscum contagiosum, etc.
      3. **Chlamydial:** Adult or acute inclusion conjunctivitis, trachoma, lymphogranuloma venereum
      4. **Fungal:** Aspergillus, Candida, Nocardia, Leptothrix, Actinomyces, Rhinosporidium seeberi.
      5. **Parasitic**
   b. **Non-infectious:**
      1. **Allergic**
      2. **Irritants** (Physical, foreign bodies, contact lens use, radiation)
      3. **Endogenous or autoimmune**
      4. **Dry eye**
      5. **Toxic** (Chemical or drug-induced)
      6. **Factitious or self-inflicted, artefacta**
      7. **Idiopathic**
3. **Based on clinical presentation, the chief forms of infective conjunctivitis may be divided into two broad groups:**
   a. **Acute conjunctivitis**
   b. **Chronic conjunctivitis**
4. **Clinical features of conjunctival inflammation:**
   a. **Specific symptoms:**
      1. Red eye, swelling of the conjunctiva, and watering of the eyes are symptoms common to all forms of conjunctivitis.
      2. Congestion and increased secretion
      3. Congestion varies in degree and in distribution, and the secretion varies in nature and amount.

4. Itching is the hallmark of allergic disease, it may also occur to a lesser extent in blepharitis and dry eye.
5. Significant pain, photophobia or a marked foreign body sensation suggest corneal involvement.
6. **The nature of the secretion is of diagnostic importance:**

Discharge	Type of conjunctivitis
Watery discharge is composed of a serous exudate and tears	Acute viral or acute allergic conjunctivitis
Mucoid discharge	Chronic allergic conjunctivitis and dry eye
Mucopurulent	Chlamydial or acute bacterial infection
Moderately purulent discharge	Acute bacterial conjunctivitis.
Severe purulent discharge	Gonococcal infection.

b. **Non-specific symptoms:**

Lacrimation, grittiness, stinging and burning

5. **Diagnosis:**

a. If bacterial conjunctivitis is suspected, but no response to topical antibiotics is seen, swabs for bacterial culture should be taken and tested
b. A patch test is used to identify the causative allergen in allergic conjunctivitis
c. Conjunctival scrapes for cytology can be useful in detecting chlamydial and fungal infections.
d. Conjunctival incisional biopsy is occasionally done when granulomatous are suspected.

6. **Management:**

Bacterial	Viral	Allergic
A] Topical antibiotics: Usually four times daily for up to a week. **B] Systemic antibiotics:** required in the following circumstances **1. Gonococcal infection** **2. H. influenzae infection** **3. Meningococcal conjunctivitis**	**A] No specific treatment is typically unnecessary**: Spontaneous resolution of adenoviral infection usually occurs within 2–3 weeks. **B] Reduction of transmission risk** by strict hand hygiene, avoiding eye rubbing and towel sharing. **C] Topical steroids** May be required for severe membranous or pseudomembranous adenoviral conjunctivitis and in case of corneal involvement	**A] Artificial tears** for mild symptoms. **B] Mast cell stabilizers** (e.g. sodium cromoglycate, nedocromil sodium) **C] Antihistamines** (e.g. epinastine) **D] Dual action antihistamine and mast cell stabilizers** (e.g.olopatadine, alcaftadine) act rapidly and are often very effective for exacerbations

(Continued)

Bacterial	Viral	Allergic
C] Topical steroids: Use of topical steroid is unclear. **D] Irrigation:** Remove excessive discharge may be useful in severe purulent cases. **E] Contact lens wear:** Should be discontinued until resolution/ healing. **F] Reduce risk of transmission by regular hand washing and avoid sharing of towels.**	**D] Discontinuation of contact lens** wear until resolution of symptoms. **E] Artificial tears** four times daily may be useful for symptomatic relief. Preservative-free preparations may give best comfort. **F] Cold (or warm) compresses for symptomatic relief.** **G] Topical antihistamines and vasoconstrictors:** may be used for symptomatic relief. **J] Topical antibiotics** if secondary bacterial infection is suspected.	**E] Oral antihistamines** may be indicated for severe symptoms e.g. levocetirizine G] **Non-steroidal anti-inflammatory preparations** (e.g. ketorolac can provide symptomatic relief but are rarely used. **H] Topical steroids** are used in severe cases. **I] Eye drop cyclosporine** (Immunomodulator)

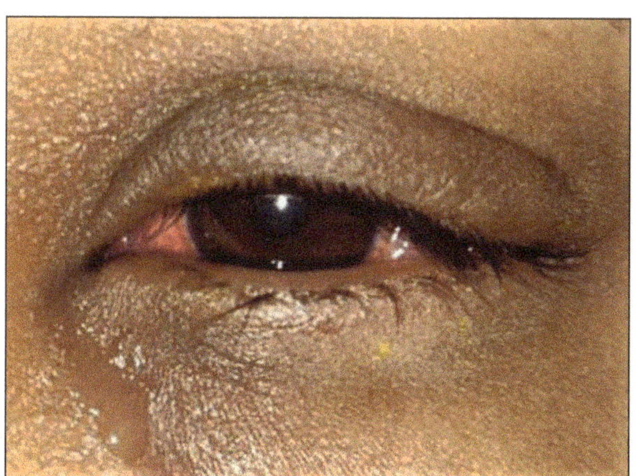
Lid edema with congestion in acute conjunctivitis

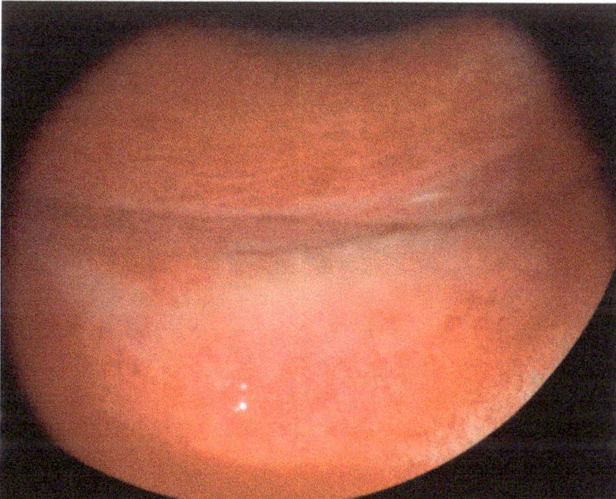
Pseudomembrane with petechial hemorrhage over tarsal conjunctiva in adenoviral conjunctivitis

INFECTIONS OF ORBITS

PRESEPTAL CELLULITIS

An infection of the subcutaneous tissues anterior to the orbital septum.

Causes:

1. Skin trauma
2. Insect bite
3. Spread from local ocular or periocular infection

Clinical features:

1. Swollen, tender red eyelids
2. Fever

Treatment

1. Oral antibiotics (amoxicillin + clavulanic acid)
2. Intravenous antibiotics in case of severe infection

BACTERIAL ORBITAL CELLULITIS

Serious infection of soft tissue behind the orbital septum.

Causes:

1. Infection originated from the paranasal sinuses especially from ethmoid sinus.
2. Infection can also spread from preseptal cellulitis, dacryocystitis, dental infections
3. Trauma
4. Ocular surgery
5. Blood borne spread

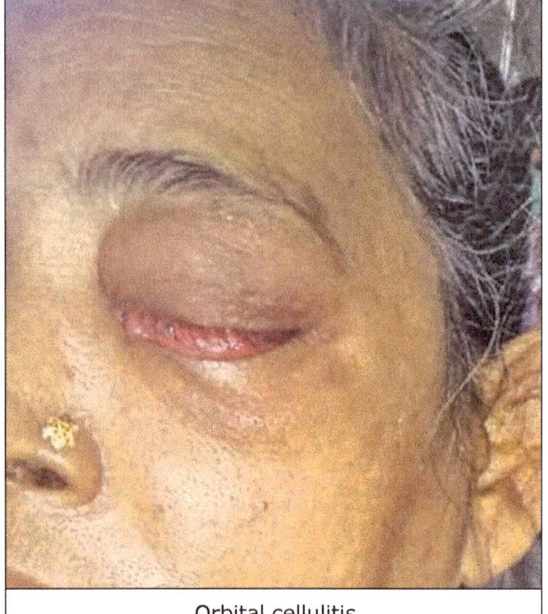

Orbital cellulitis

Clinical features:

Symptoms:

1. Swelling of eyelids
2. Pain on eye movement
3. Visual impairment
4. Double vision
5. Fever

Signs:

1. Tender, firm, erythematous, warm eyelids
2. Periocular edema
3. Conjunctival chemosis
4. Conjunctival injection and sometimes conjunctival hemorrhage
5. Proptosis and ophthalmoplegia (Loss of eye movement)
6. Visual acuity may be reduced and color vision impaired which raises the possibility of optic nerve involvement.

Investigations:

1. Complete blood count
2. Blood culture
3. Nasal discharge culture
4. High resolution CT scan of orbit, sinuses and brain or sometimes MRI scan is performed for diagnosis.
5. Lumbar puncture in patients with meningeal or cerebral signs.

Treatment:

1. Hospitalisation
2. Intravenous antibiotics
3. Antipyretics
4. Monitor optic nerve function and extent of erythema.
5. Drainage of abscess
6. Canthotomy or cantholysis in severe optic nerve compression

PHOTOKERATITIS OR ULTRAVIOLET KERATITIS

1. A painful eye condition caused by exposure of insufficiently protected eyes to the ultraviolet (UV) rays from either natural (e.g. Intense sunlight) or artificial (e.g. the electric arc during welding) sources.
2. Different terms used for photokeratitis are **Arc eye**, **Welder's flash.**
3. Any intense exposure to UV light can lead to photokeratitis.
4. Measures taken for eye protection to block most of the ultraviolet radiation, such as welding goggles with the proper filters, a welder's helmet, sunglasses rated for sufficient UV protection, or appropriate snow goggles.
5. **Symptoms of photokeratitis**:
    a. Pain
    b. Intense lacrimation
    c. Eyelid twitching
    d. Photophobia
    e. Foreign body sensation

Management

1. The pain may be temporarily reduced with anesthetic eye drops for the examination
2. Anesthetic drops are not used for continued treatment, as anesthesia of the eye interferes with corneal healing, and may lead to corneal ulceration
3. Cool compresses over the eyes and artificial tears may help symptomatically
4. Systemic (oral) pain medication is given if discomfort is severe.
5. Further injury should be avoided by isolation in a dark room, avoid rubbing the eyes, and wearing sunglasses until the symptoms improve.
6. Preservative free artificial tear drops are used
7. Topical steroids are to be used judiciously.

ENDOPHTHALMITIS AND PANOPHTHALMITIS

Endophthalmitis	Panophthalmitis
1. Inflammation of the vitreous and the inner coat of eye	**1. It is an intense purulent inflammation of the whole eyeball including the tenon's capsule.**
2. Mode of entry **a. Exogenous** 1. Infection introduced from the environment 2. Most commonly following surgery, trauma or keratitis. 3. Mainly bacterial **b. Endogenous** 1. Hematogenous spread of infection 2. Common predisposing factors are immunocompromised status, septicemia or IV drugs 3. Infection can occur from sinus 4. Mainly fungal **c. Secondary infection:** Orbital cellulitis, thrombophlebitis.	**2. Mode of entry** **a. Exogenous** 1. Infection introduced from the environment 2. Most commonly following surgery, trauma or keratitis. 3. Mainly bacterial **b. Endogenous** 1. Hematogenous spread of infection 2. Common predisposing factors are immunocompromised status, septicemia or IV drugs 3. Infection can occur from sinus 4. Mainly fungal **c. Secondary infection:** Orbital cellulitis, thrombophlebitis.
3. Etiological agents: **a. Bacterial** **E.g.** Staph epidermidis, Strepto Spp, S.aureus, haemophilus Influenzae, pseudomonas, pneumococcus. **b. Fungal** **E.g.:** Candida albicans, Aspergillus fumigatus, Cryptococcus neoformans **c. Viral** **d. Parasitic**	**3. Etiological agents:** **a. Bacterial** **E.g.** Staph epidermidis, Strepto Spp, S.aureus, haemophilus influenzae. **b. Fungal** **E.g.:** Candida albicans, Aspergillus fumigatus, Cryptococcus neoformans **c. Viral** **d. Parasitic**
4. Clinical features a. Ocular pain b. Blurring and diminished vision c. Headache d. Increased redness e. Discharge and watering f. Photophobia g. Blepharospasm	**4. Clinical features** a. Severe ocular pain b. Complete loss of vision c. Headache d. Marked redness e. Purulent discharge and profuse watering f. Photophobia g. Blepharospasm
5. Signs: a. Edema and hyperemia of lid b. Intense chemosis and conjunctival congestion c. Cloudy and edematous cornea d. Purulent discharge e. Corneal edema f. Hypopyon	**5. Signs:** a. Marked edema, hyperemia of lid. b. Ocular movements limited and painful c. Cloudy and edematous cornea d. Full pus in anterior chamber e. Marked chemosis and conjunctival congestion. f. Worsen g. Raised IOP h. Globe perforation i. Worsen hypopyon

(Continued)

Endophthalmitis	Panophthalmitis
6. Investigations a. Fundoscopic examination b. USG B-scan c. Vitreous biopsy d. Culture	**6. Investigation** a. Fundoscopic examination b. USG B-scan c. Vitreous biopsy d. Culture
7. Treatment a. Antimicrobial therapy b. Corticosteroid: Contraindicated in fungal infection c. Supportive therapy d. Vitreous aspirates e. Intravitreal antibiotic injections f. Vitrectomy	**7. Treatment** a. Antimicrobial therapy b. Anti-inflammatory and analgesics c. Evisceration (Its removal of the content eyeball leaving behind the sclera)

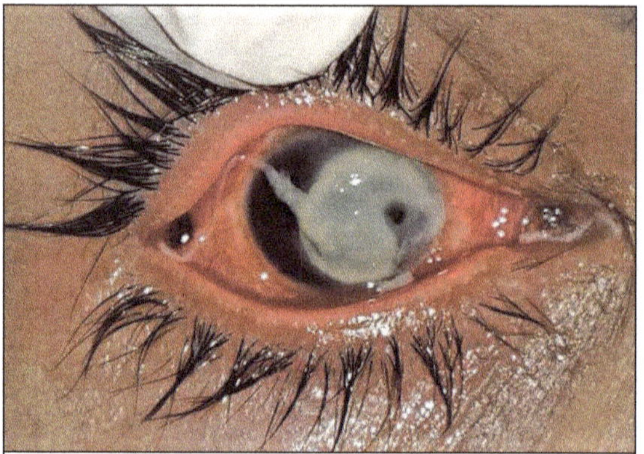

Corneal ulceration with perforation with endophthalmitis

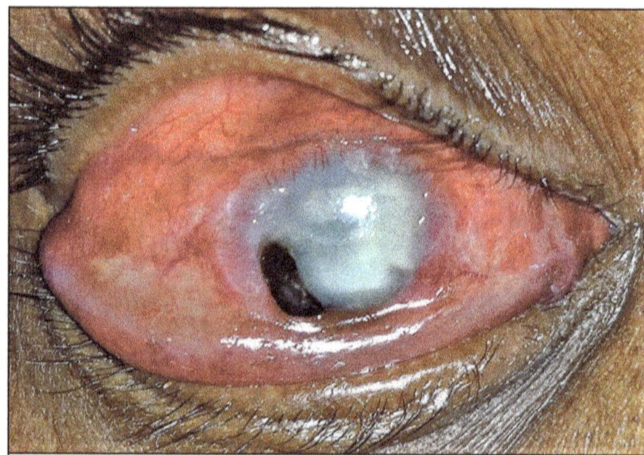

Panophthalmitis

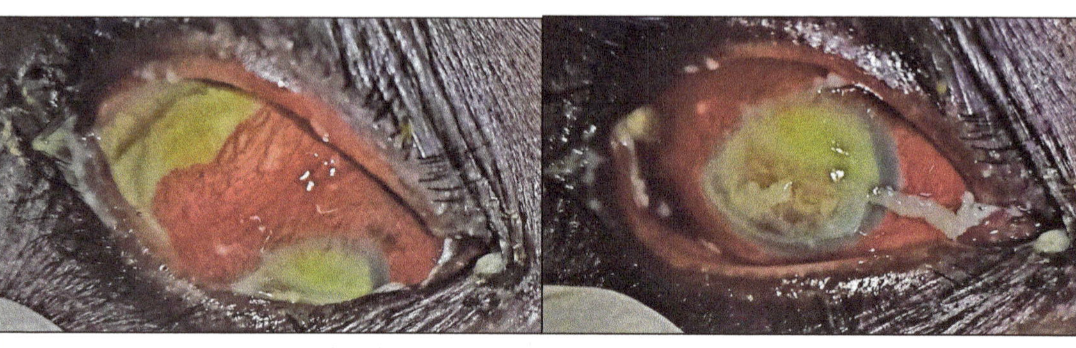

Panophthalmitis with superotemporal scleral abscess

EYE DONATION

1. Eye donation means donating the eyes of a person after death for transplantation with the family consent.
2. **Transplantation of Human Organ Act (THO), 1994** an Act to provide for the regulation of removal, storage and transplantation of human organs for therapeutic purposes and for prevention of commercial dealing in human organs and for matters connected therewith or incidental thereto.
3. **Importance of eye donation:**
   a. Eyes are considered more special than other organs as they have special power to visualize the world.
   b. However,due to some eye conditions ,many peoples lose their vision and the world becomes dark for them.
   c. Corneal impairment is a one of the common cause of blindness and which is curable in most of cases through eye donation.
   d. In such case, vision can be restored by corneal transplantation from donated eye.
4. **Who can donate?**
   a. Anyone irrespective of age, sex, blood group or religion can donate.
   b. Anyone with cataract or spectacles can donate eyes.
   c. Any patient suffering from hypertension, diabetes can also donate eyes.
   d. Eyes can be donated even if the deceased had not formally pledged (Signed consent form) for donating their eyes during their lifetime.
   e. Eye donation is consistent with beliefs and attitudes of all major religious and ethical traditions.
5. **Ophthalmic contraindications for procurement or use of cornea**
   a. Corneal pathology e.g. keratitis, opacities, dystrophies
   b. Malignant melanoma
   c. Retinoblastoma
   a. Previous intraocular surgery (Relative contraindication)
6. **Medical contraindications for procurement or use of cornea**
   a. Conditions potentially hazardous to eye bank personnel and fatal if transmitted
      1. Seropositivity, HIV or acquired immunodeficiency syndrome
      2. Active viral hepatitis
      3. Rabies
      4. Creutzfeldt-jakob disease

b. **Other contraindication**

1. Progressive multifocal leukoencephalopathy
2. Reye's syndrome
3. Congenital rubella
4. Active septicemia including endocarditis
5. Active meningitis
6. Active miliary tuberculosis
7. Death from unknown cause including unknown encephalitis
8. High risk groups individuals for HIV infection:

   Homosexuals, drug abusers, prostitutes, hemophiliacs.
9. Covid 19

7. **What should one do for eye donation?**

a. Dial 1919 (Toll free number, available 24 x 7) to contact the nearest eye bank within 6 hours of death.

b. Switch off the fans and keep the air conditioner on.

c. Raise the head with the help of a pillow by about 6 inches (To lessen bleeding during eye removal)

d. Place wet cotton on closed eyes

e. The eye bank team will reach at your home for collection

f. Procedure is simple, bloodless and Takes less than 15-20 minutes

g. After procedure, no disfigurement of the face of the donor.

h. For the other tests 10 ml of blood will be collected.

i. After removal, the eyes are analyzed, processed at the eye bank and then the cornea is transplanted.

Section

4

Orthopaedics Emergencies

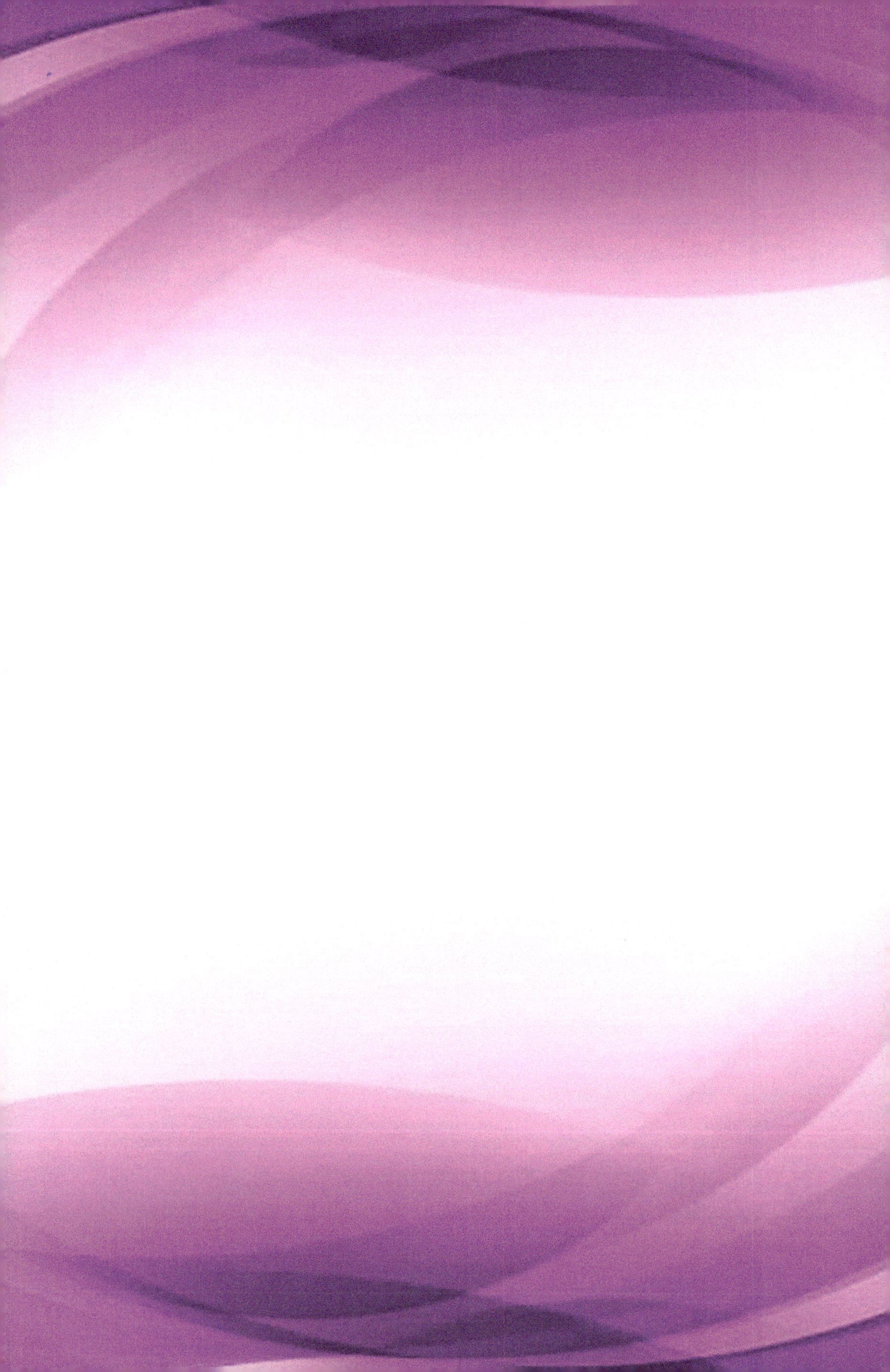

CHAPTER

4 Orthopedic Emergencies

EXTREMITY TRAUMA

1. Most extremity trauma occurs due to road traffic accidents, fall from height, machine operators.
2. Life threatening injuries should be identified first and treated as per ATLS guidelines.
    a. The ABCDE protocol is the standard management of trauma patients
    b. The aim of this system is to save "life before limb" i.e., to preserve heart, brain and lung functions.
    c. It requires continuous reassessment and adjustment in response to changing needs.
        1. **Airway:** Check that the airway is patent and protect it. Ensure that the cervical spine is protected especially in unconscious patients.
        2. **Breathing:** Check that there is adequate bilateral air entry and that there are no clinical signs of life-threatening chest conditions.
        3. **Circulation:** Detect shock and treat if present.

4. **Disability:** Briefly assess the neurological status using the AVPU mnemonic:

   Alert, verbal response, response to pain and unresponsive

5. **Exposure** Inspect the entire body along guidelines of secondary survey with a "log roll".

d. If there is an immediate life-threatening problem in A, you cannot proceed to B until the airway is secured and so on.

e. Proper stepwise management of extremity trauma is necessary so patients can regain optimal function.

3. The injured extremity is examined for soft tissue, bony and neuro-vascular injuries.

4. **History:**

   a. Mechanism of injury and amount of force in the incidence is important to understand the extent of trauma.

   b. The mnemonic AMPLE is a helpful tool in ascertaining history.

      1. **A: Allergies**
      2. **M: Medication**
      3. **P: Past medical and surgical history**
      4. **L: Last meal or drink**
      5. **E: Events of the injury**

5. **Examination:**

   a. Extremity injuries are evaluated when other life threatening injuries are managed and patient is stable

   b. Head to toe evaluation is done by a systematic approach

   c. **Stepwise examination in extremities injury as follows:**

      i. **Look:**

      Look at the whole limb i.e., back and front of limb for any localised swelling, bruising, wounds and any obvious deformity of the extremity.

      ii. **Feel:**

         1. Feel the limb for any bony tenderness, swelling and tenseness of the compartment.
         2. Check the pulses, assess the capillary refill, feel the temperature of the limb.
         3. Assess the function of nerves passing across the site of trauma.

iii. **Move:**

1. Movement of the extremity is done carefully without causing pain and discomfort.
2. Two types of movement are examined
   a. **Active:** Active movement is movement initiated and maintained by the patient
   b. **Passive:** Passive movement is when the examiner moves the limb.
3. Abnormal mobility at the site of fracture is noted.

d. **The injured extremity is then immobilized in a temporary splint or plaster slab to allow for transportation of the patient for radiological investigation, without risk of further neuro-vascular injuries.**

e. **Investigations:**

1. **Hematological investigation:** Complete blood count, renal function test, liver function test, blood grouping and cross matching.
2. **X-ray:** Routinely done in every cases of suspected extremity trauma ..

   Consider following points:

   a. 2 views in orthogonal planes to avoid missing a fracture
   b. Radiographs are required of the joint above and the joint below the fracture
   c. In pediatric patients it can be useful to consider a radiograph from the also from the opposite limb/uninjured side if doubt exists.
3. **CT scan:** Provides significant information about pattern of fracture.
4. **MRI Scan:** It provides useful information, particularly about the soft tissue injuries.
5. **Ultrasonography:** Ultrasound is very useful to define soft tissue injuries.

CLASSIFICATION OF FRACTURE AND ITS MANAGEMENT

1. Fracture is defined as a partial or complete break in the continuity of the bone.
2. Bony fracture is caused due to direct high force trauma, twisting injuries or stress.
3. Describing the bony injury depends on several characteristics and includes the:
   a. **Name of the bone**
   b. **Anatomical location**
   c. **Open/close fracture**
   d. **Pattern of fracture line:** Transverse, oblique, spiral, segmental or multifragmentary
   e. **Presence of displacement**: Un displaced or displaced
   f. **Type and degree of displacement**
      1. Angulation
      2. Translation
      3. Rotation
      4. Shortening
   g. **Associated joint pathology, dislocation or subluxation.**
   h. **Presence of pre-existing pathology**

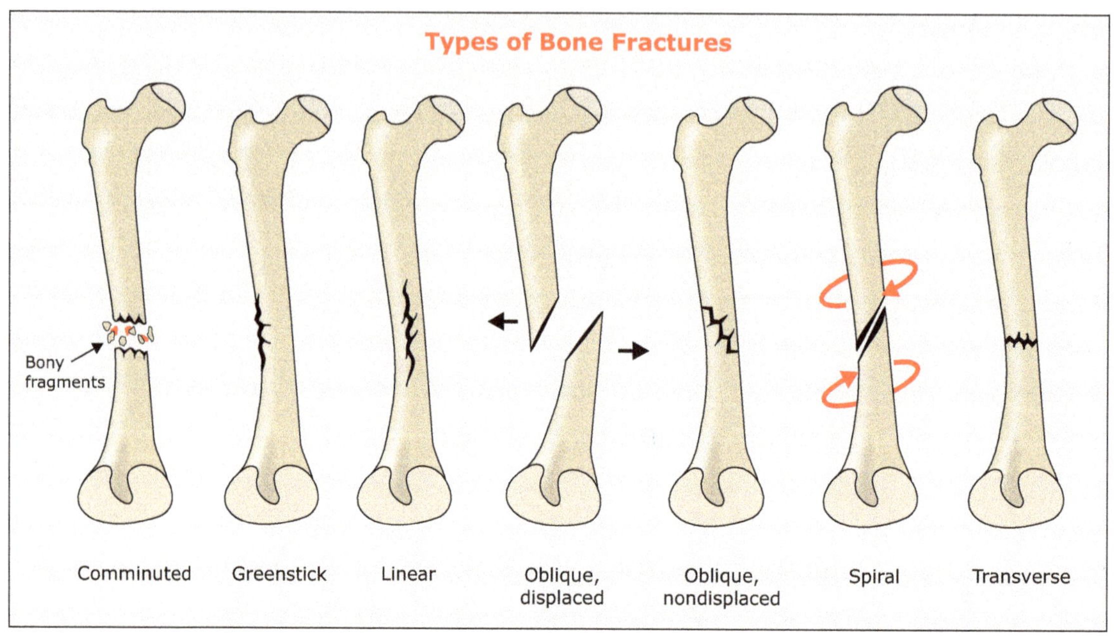

4. **Treatment:**
   a. The main principle of extremity fracture management includes reduction and stabilisation of the fracture
   b. The main objective of any treatment is to return the patient to normal function as early as possible
   c. **Treatment can be considered under the following headings:**
      1. **Reduce**
      2. **Hold**
      3. **Heal**
      4. **Rehabilitate**
   d. **Reduce:**
      1. Reduction means aligning the bone.
      2. The principle of reduction is to reverse the movement which created the fracture
      3. First know the degree of displacement of the fracture fragments.
      4. This process is extremely painful as a fracture itself without anesthesia.
      5. **In Fractures involving the articular joint surface:** we need to reduce displacement of fracture fragments perfectly to their normal anatomical position to avoid degenerative joint disease and to regain normal joint movement.
      6. **In Fractures that do not involve the joint surface:** Only needs mechanical alignment of fracture fragments and do not need to be reduced perfectly.
      7. **Fracture reduction can be done by following methods**
         a. Open reduction: If an acceptable closed reduction is not achieved or likely to succeed.
         b. Closed reduction: without exposing the bone and without tearing or further damaging the intact soft tissues and periosteum.
   e. **Hold**
      1. After reduction of fracture fragments in acceptable positions they then need to be held in that position until they heal.
      2. There are several methods of holding fracture fragments in place:

1. Plaster cast/splints
2. Traction
3. Kirschner (K-) wires
4. External fixation
5. Plates and screws
6. Intramedullary nails.

3. A combination of holding methods may be used for best results e.g., K-wires and a moulded cast

4. **Non operative and operative methods:**

Nonoperative	Operative
a. **Plaster immobilization** b. **Splint and traction** **Splint:** E.g. braun frame, thomas splint **Traction:** E.g. skeletal traction, skin traction	a. **Internal fixation:** Intramedullary nails, plates and screws. b. **External fixation:** Uniplanar or ring type. c. **Arthroplasty:** **Arthroplasty is indicated in:** Articular fractures that are not reconstructible, or injuries where the vascularity of the articular segment is compromised.

5. **Methods of holding fragments and their advantages and disadvantages:**

Methods of holding fracture fragments	Advantages	Disadvantages
Plaster cast **Plaster and splints** (Casts and splints are generally used to hold stable fractures or supplement the fixation of unstable fractures)	No surgery No interference with fracture site Affordable Adjustable No implants to remove	Limited access to the soft tissues Heavy to carry (particularly in the elderly) Interferes with function Poor mechanical stability Malunion Joint stiffness and muscle wasting. Compartment syndrome
Traction (Traction is defined as a stretching force on a limb to pull a fracture straight.)	No surgery No interference with fracture site Affordable Adjustable	Restricts mobility of patient Long hospital stay Skin pressure complications such as bed sores Pin site infection Thromboembolic complications due to chronic immobilisation
Kirschner (K) wires Used to hold small fragments in place. Used in a temporary fashion intraoperatively to hold fracture fragments in place until definitive fixation with plates and screws can be performed.	**Indication:** Used for temporary fixation or definitive fixation Less soft tissue damage Insertion is stress free. Tension band wiring e.g. fractures of the patella and olecranon Temporary immobilisation of a small joint	Pin tract infection Migration of pins Loss of reduction

(Continued)

Methods of holding fracture fragments	Advantages	Disadvantages
External fixation	**D**oes not interfere with fracture site **E**xternal adjustment is possible, if required **A**llow to access soft tissues for plastic surgey **R**apid stabilisation of fracture	**P**in tract infection **I**nterferes with plastic surgical procedures if pins not placed correctly **S**oft-tissue tethering **D**ifficult to carry for the patient
Plates and screw fixation	**U**sed when anatomical reduction is required **R**igid fixation **A**llows early mobilisation **C**an provide absolute or relative stability	**P**eriosteal/soft-tissue damage **N**ot allow early weight bearing **M**etalwork complications Possible need for plate removal
Intramedullary nails	**M**inimally invasive **E**arly weight-bearing **L**ess periosteal damage than open reduction **I**nternal fixation	**I**ncreased risk of fat emboli/chest complications **D**ifficult to treat infection **D**ifficult to remove if broken

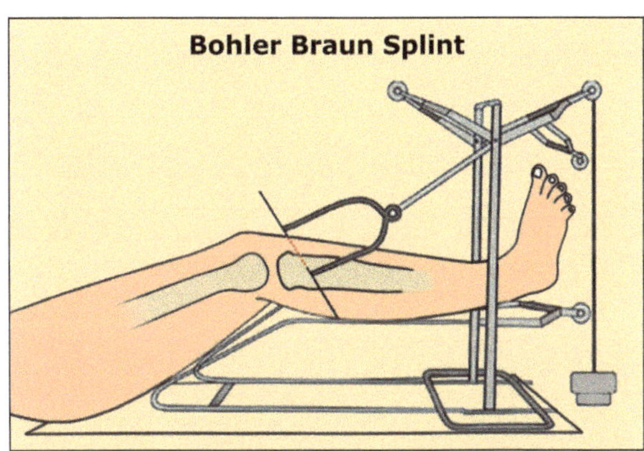

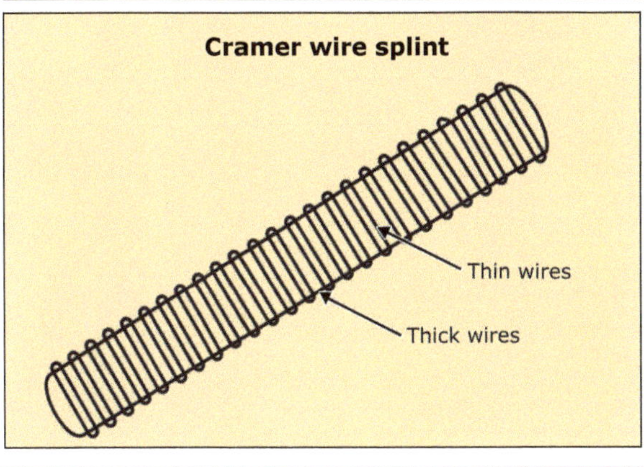

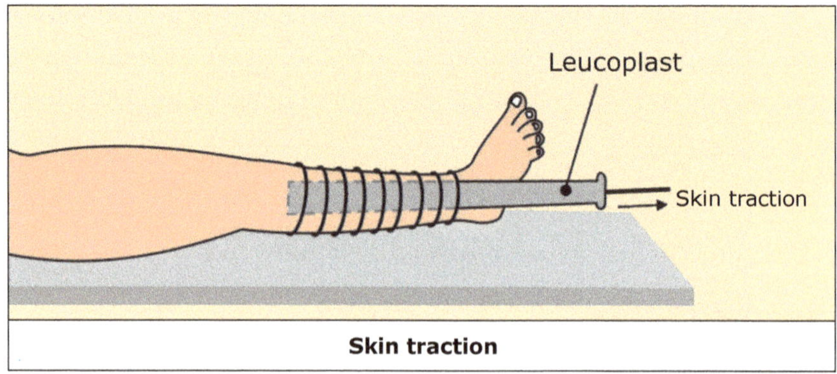

Skin traction

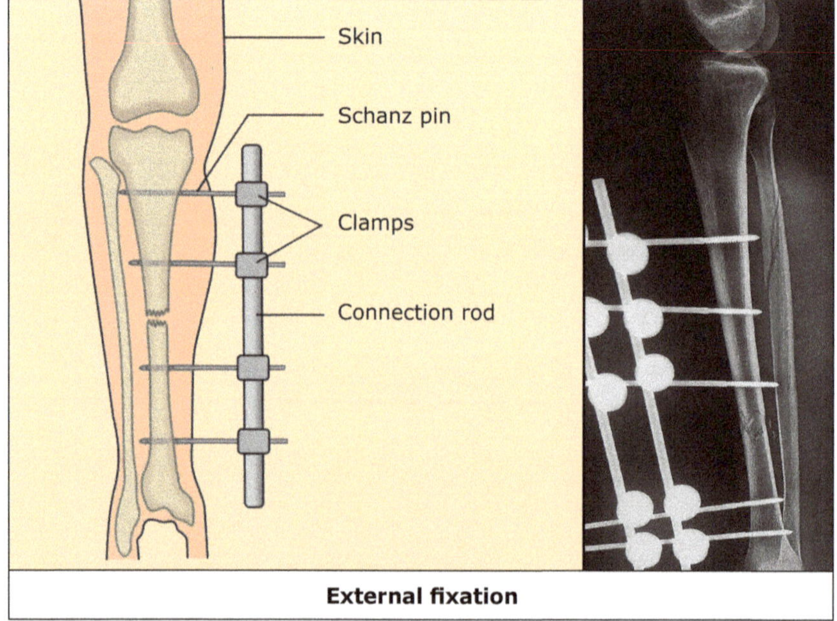

External fixation

Internal fixation

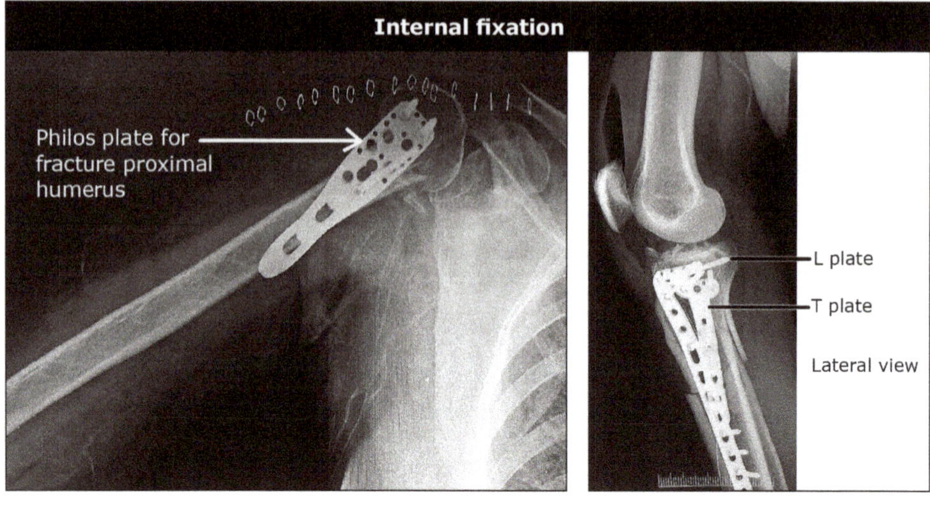

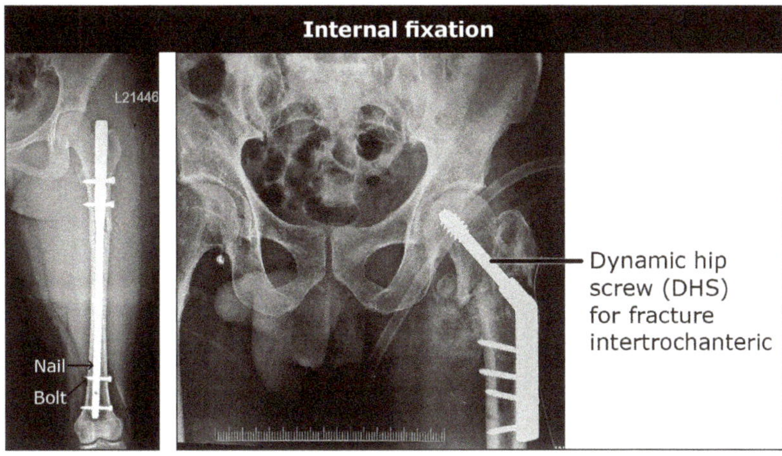

***The method of holding reduction is determined by:**

a. **Nature of the injury:** Open vs closed, simple vs comminuted fracture

b. **Location of the fracture:** Shaft vs periarticular.

c. **Age and functional requirement of the patient**

d. **Remodelling potential**

e. **General condition of the patient**

f. **Heal:**

   1. **Time for fracture healing depends on**

      a. **Patient's age**

      b. **Patient's comorbidities**

      c. **Bone involved**

      d. **Treatment used**

      e. **Nutrition**

   2. **Factors that slow down bone healing process:**

      a. **Diabetes mellitus**

      b. **Reduced blood supply**

      c. **Infection at fracture site**

g. **Rehabilitate:**

   1. Required to regain optimal function after fracture healing.

   2. Involves using specific exercises to regain/maintain mobility of joint and muscle strength.

   3. The aim is to restore the patient to a pre-trauma level of function

PELVIC FRACTURE

a. **History**

1. Pelvic fractures are serious & potentially life threatening injuries with little or no clinically obvious deformity.
2. These fractures are often associated with visceral injuries.
3. Most commonly due to motor vehicle accidents, fall and crush injury.
4. Typically, high energy blunt trauma is involved in fracture.

b. **Physical examination**

1. **Primary survey**
   a. Identify and begin treatment of life-threatening injuries immediately.
   b. In initial management we should follow the ATLS system, that is "ABCDE" of trauma care.
   c. Hemodynamic compromise from massive retroperitoneal hemorrhage must be looked out & in such cases immediate surgical exploration may be required.
2. **Secondary survey**
   a. The secondary is rapid but thorough head to toe examination assessment to identify all potential injuries.
   b. Pelvic compression/distraction test
   c. Examination of flanks, lower back, scrotum, labial hematoma, perineum, urethral injury, per-rectal and per-vaginal examination
   d. Reflexes
   e. Examination of extremities
   f. Associated Morel-Lavallee lesion (Internal degloving of skin)

c. **Investigation:**

1. **X-rays:** AP view, inlet view, outlet view
2. USG FAST, diagnostic peritoneal lavage to rule out associated abdominal trauma.
3. CT scan of bony pelvis and contrast enhanced CT of abdomen if associated visceral injury is suspected.
4. Other investigation: CBC, blood grouping and cross matching
5. Retrograde urethrogram in case of suspected urethral injury.

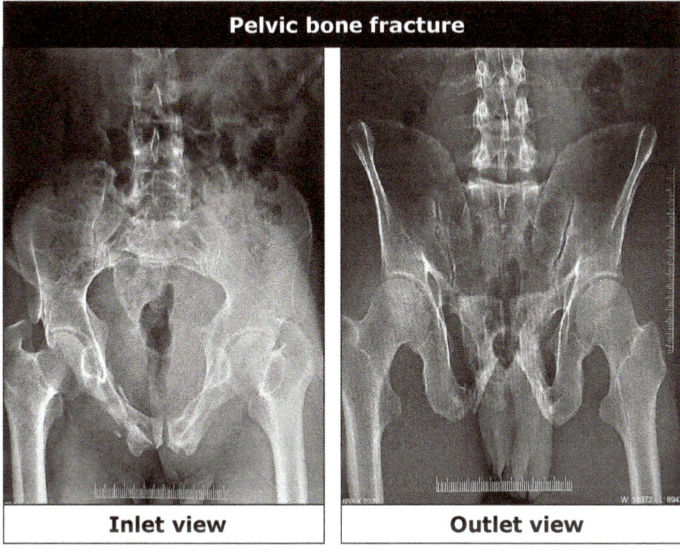

d. Management

1. The Pelvic should be stabilized by pelvic binder
2. Stabilization of the pelvic ring reduces blood loss from the pelvic vessels.
3. Embolization of vessels or surgical ligation may be needed in case of continued hemorrhage.
4. In case a complication like bladder or urethral injury is present, emergency urological reference must be sought.
5. Types of pelvic fracture and management

Young burgess classification

Type	Pattern	Stability
Lateral compression-1	Rami fracture and ipsilateral sacral ala compression fracture	Stable
Lateral compression-2	Iliac crescent fracture	Rotationally unstable
Lateral compression-3	Ipsilateral sacral ala compression and contralateral	Globally unstable
Antero-posterior compression 1	Pubic diastasis < 2.5 Cm	Stable
Antero-posterior compression 2	Pubic diastasis > and anterior sacroiliac diastasis	Rotationally unstable
Antero-posterior compression 3	Pubic diastasis > 5 cm and anterior-posterior sacroiliac diastasis	Globally unstable
Vertical shear	Vertical displacement of hemipelvis, fracture of pubis and sacro-iliac joint	Unstable
Combined	Complex fracture with combined elements	Variable

6. **Non operative treatment:**
    a. Most LC-1, APC-1 fractures.
    b. Pubic diastasis less than 2.5 cm.
7. **Absolute indication for operative treatment:**
    a. Open fractures or those with associated visceral injury requiring exploration.
    b. Open book fractures (APC-2) or vertically unstable fractures with associated hemodynamic instability.
8. **Operative techniques:**
    a. External fixation to aid in control of hemorrhage and stabilization of the patient.
    b. Internal fixation for definitive reconstruction of pelvic ring.
9. **Complications**
    a. Rupture of urethra
    b. Rupture of bladder
    c. Injuries to rectum or vagina
    d. Injuries to major blood vessels (common iliac artery or one of its branches may be damaged)
    e. Injuries to nerves (In marked vertical displacement of half of the pelvis, it is common for nerves of lumbosacral plexus to be injured)
    f. Ruptured of the pelvic diaphragm (In severely depressed pelvic fracture)

OPEN FRACTURE

1. An open fracture refers to a bone fracture in which the break in skin and underlying soft tissue directly communicates with the fracture and its hematoma.
2. Any fracture with an overlying wound should be considered an open fracture
3. The term previously used was a compound fracture.
4. Open fractures are caused due to high energy trauma with direct impact
5. Most commonly occurs in road traffic accidents, fall and firearm injury.

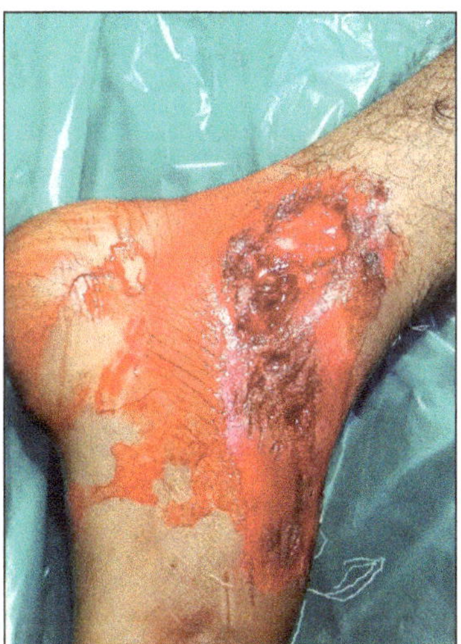

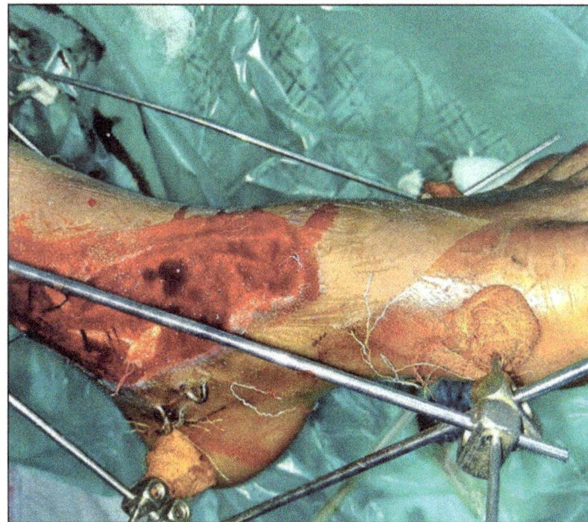

6. The **Gustilo and Anderson classification** of open fractures is the most frequently used for classification

I	**A**n open fracture with a wound less than 1 cm long and clean wound. **A**dequate soft tissue coverage **V**ascular intact **P**eriosteum intact Simple spiral or short oblique fracture
II	**A**n open fracture with a laceration more than 1 cm long without extensive soft tissue damage, flaps or avulsion. Minimal to moderate crushing component **A**dequate soft tissue coverage **V**ascular intact **P**eriosteum intact Simple transverse or short oblique fracture with minimal comminution.

III	Characterised by high energy injury (Firearm or farm injuries) Extensive damage to soft tissues and a high degree of contamination with severe crushing component Multifragmentary/Segmental and unstable fractures Periosteum stripping
A Subgroup of type III	Adequate soft tissue cover of a fractured bone after stabilisation despite extensive soft tissue damage. Vascular intact **Minimal Periosteal** stripping
B Subgroup of type III	Inadequate soft tissue cover of a fractured bone after stabilisation (i.e. flap coverage required) Vascular intact **Extensive Periosteal** stripping
C Subgroup of type III	Associated with an arterial injury requiring repair

7. The aim of open fracture management is to achieve bony union, reconstruction of limb and avoid infection.
8. The treatment of bone and joint infection is expensive, time-consuming for the professional as well as the patient.
9. **The treatment of open fractures:**

   A] Management in the emergency department

   B] The surgical phase

A] Management in the emergency department:

1. Stabilize patient as per ATLS protocol
2. Take a photograph for the documentation and to prevent the need of repeated opening of dressing to see by different doctors.
3. If the bone was out of the skin then quickly remove any macroscopic dirt by irrigation with saline and reduced the fracture/dislocation under the skin
4. Before and after reduction check the pulses and neurological status.
5. Once overall alignment is achieved, splint the affected limb.
6. Apply a moist saline dressing to the wound to avoid contamination.
7. Definitive debridement and washout of the wound should be done in the operation theatre at earliest.
8. Early administration of intravenous antibiotics is one of the most important steps in the management of open fractures.

9. A broad-spectrum antibiotic should be chosen covering gram-positive, gram-negative and if severe contamination, anaerobic organisms.
10. Look for compartment syndrome as it is possible even in open fractures.
11. A tetanus immunisation as per status.

B] The surgical phase

1. Severity of the injury must be graded as per a standardised scoring system like; mangled extremity severity score (MESS),

Skeletal/soft-tissue injury	
Low energy e.g. simple fracture, stab, small calibre gun shot wound	1
Medium energy e.g. open or multiple fracture, dislocation	2
High energy e.g. military shotgun injury, crush injury	3
Very high energy (as above with soft tissue avulsion)	4
Shock	
Stable (systolic BP > 90, RR maintained)	0
Transient hypotension (Respond to fluids)	1
Sustained hypotension	2
Limb ischemia (* doubled for limb ischemia > 6 hours)	
No ischemia (Pulse present)	0
Mild ischemia (Pulse reduced or absent but normal perfusion)	1*
Moderate ischemia (No dopplerable pulse, Reduced capillary refilling)	2*
Severe ischemia (Pulseless, no capillary refilling)	3*
Age	
< 30 yrs	0
30-50 yrs	1
> 50 yrs	2

If score is more than 7, limb salvage should be reconsidered in favour of amputation.

2. In salvageable limbs, stable fixation of the bony injury is very important to prevent damage of the soft tissues, allowing recovery and healing.
3. Thorough debridement of any contaminated or non-vital soft tissue is done. Wounds should be extended in line of the extremity to determine extent of injury.
4. Remove any loose or devitalised bone fragments.
5. Copious lavage of the wound is necessary.

6. Wound may be left open, closed over drain or vacuum dressing may be applied to aid in closure.
7. Repeated debridement may be necessary after 24-48 hours until there is no evidence of necrotic soft tissue or bone.
8. External fixator is used for immediate stabilization, to maintain alignment of the limb and allow for regular wound care.
9. Internal fixation after adequate soft tissue healing/plastic surgical coverage of the wound.

SPINE TRAUMA

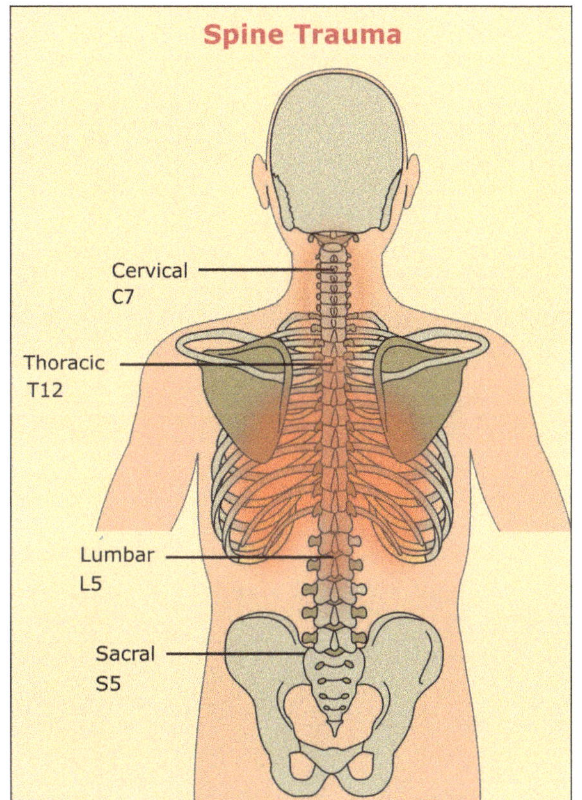

1. Injury to the spine occurs less frequently than fractures of the appendicular skeleton.
2. A **spinal cord injury** (**SCI**) is damage to the spinal cord that causes temporary or permanent changes in its function.
3. **Injury can occur at any level of the spinal cord and can be**
   a. **Complete injury:** A total loss of sensation and muscle function
   b. **Incomplete injury:** Some nervous signals are able to travel across the injured area of the cord.
4. Symptoms may include loss of motor function, sensation, or autonomic function in the parts of the body which supply nerves of the spinal cord below the level of the injury.
5. Damage results from physical trauma such as vehicle accidents, gunshots, falls, or sports injuries, but it can also be caused by nontraumatic causes such as infection, insufficient blood flow and tumors.
6. Motor vehicle accidents remain the leading cause of blunt spinal cord and vertebral column injuries.
7. Gunshot wounds causing the most penetrating spinal cord injuries and vertebral column injuries.
8. In blunt trauma patients, vertebral column fractures alone are more frequent than spinal cord injuries.
9. Spinal cord injuries result in severe long term effect and years of disability.
10. Blunt and penetrating mechanisms result in different types of spinal cord injuries.

Blunt trauma	1. Blunt trauma Cause cord injury through direct impact or indirect manipulation 2. Fractures and dislocations can collapse the spinal canal and directly compress cord tissue 3. May cause secondary injury through ischemia, bleeding or edema
Penetrating trauma	Either directly lacerate the spinal cord or cause indirect injuries through ischemia or vertebral fracture.

11. Mechanism of injuries

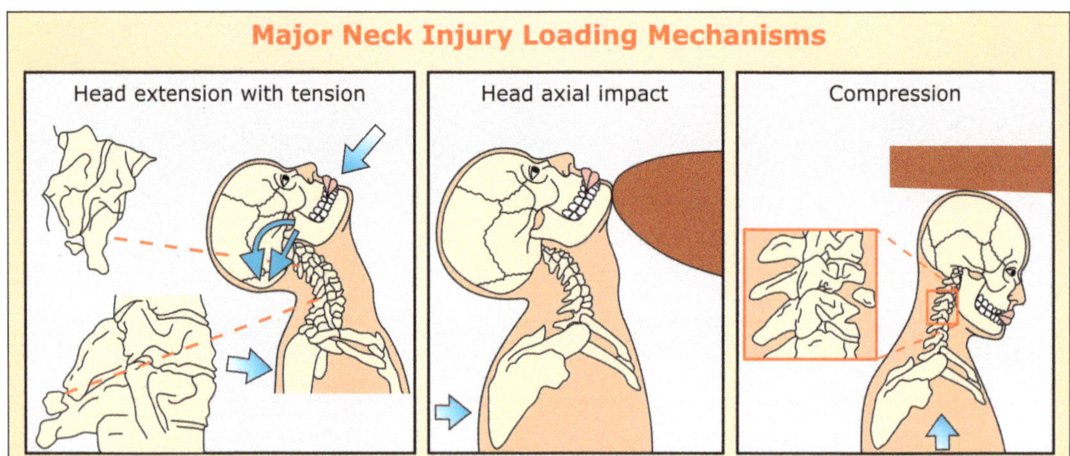

12. Mechanism of spinal injury:
   a. **Primary injury** – Physical tissue disruption caused by mechanical trauma.
   b. **Secondary injury** – Additional neural tissue damage as a result of the biological response to primary injury.

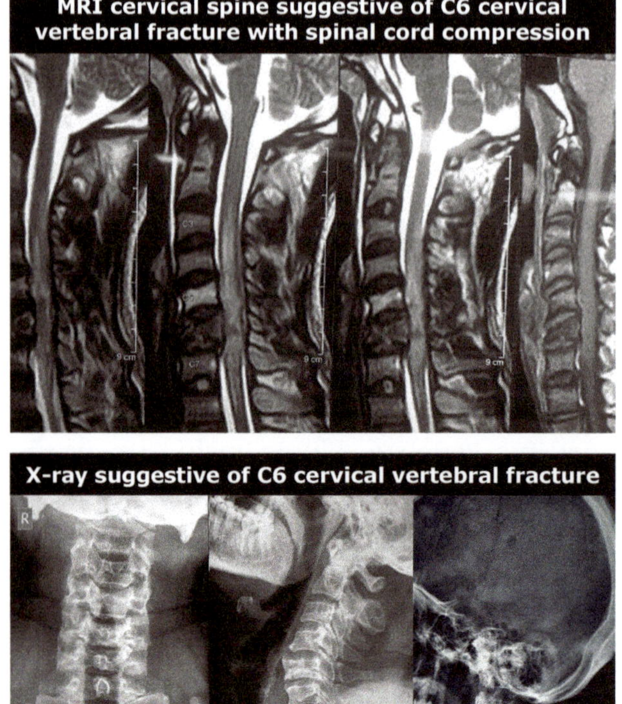

13. **Management:**

a. **Assessment:**

1. Assess the patient as per ATLS protocol and treat life threatening conditions first.
2. The spine must be protected at all times when dealing with suspected spinal trauma and multiple injured patients. This can be done manually, with cervical collars, with side head supports and strapping to a rigid spine board.

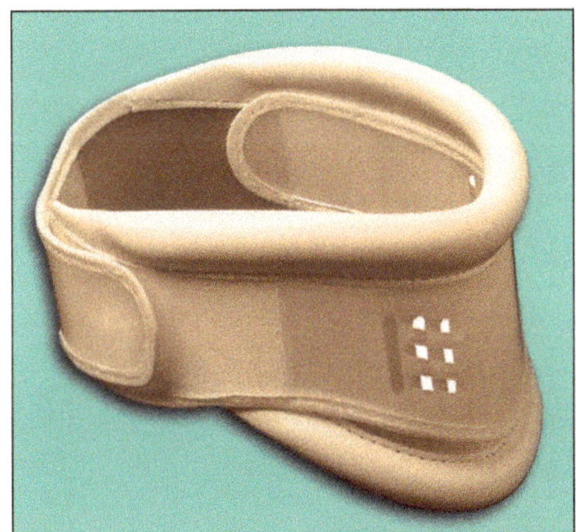

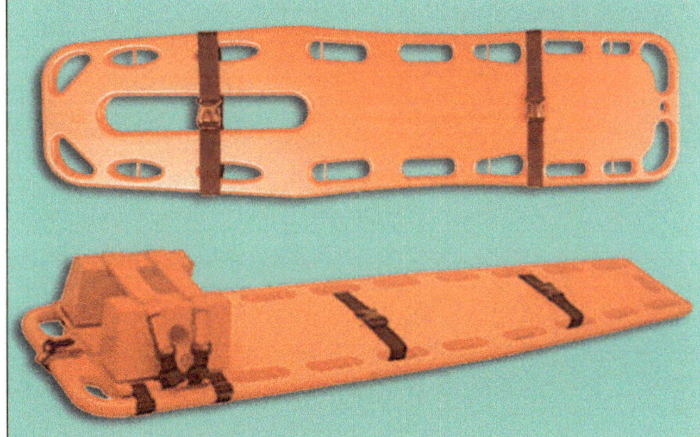

3. The spine should be immobilized in a neutral position on a firm surface.
4. Extreme care must be taken while log-rolling the patient as there is significant risk of injuring the spinal cord if there is vertebral instability.

b. **Spinal Shock:**

1. Physiological dysfunction of the spinal cord following trauma caused by sustained depolarization of neurons.
2. Characterised by flaccid paralysis, loss of reflexes and sensations.
3. Usually resolves in 24 hours with return of reflex arcs below the level of injury. Bulbocavernosus reflex is the first to return.

c. **Neurogenic shock:**

1. Hypotension is caused due to shut down of sympathetic stimulus from the spinal cord.
2. Characterised by associated bradycardia.
3. Managed with drugs to increase peripheral vascular resistance. Fluid overload must be avoided.

d. **Grading: (American Spinal Injury Association (ASIA) impairment scale is used)**

   1. **Complete –** No motor or sensory function in sacral segments.
   2. **Incomplete** – Sensory but no motor function is preserved below the level of injury.
   3. **Incomplete** – Sensory and motor function is preserved with muscle power less than 3/5.
   4. **Incomplete** – Sensory and motor function is preserved with muscle power more than 3/5.

e. **Treatment:**

   1. Immobilize the patient until the patient is cleared clinically and radiographically.
   2. I.V. methylprednisolone – the efficacy of steroid protocols is controversial.

      A loading dose of 30 mg/kg followed by a dose of 5.4 mg/kg over 24 hrs may be given as per institutional policy.
   3. Once the level of trauma is confirmed radiologically, the spinal cord is decompressed and vertebral column instrumentation is done to allow the cord to heal and to restore function of the vertebral column.

COMPARTMENT SYNDROME

1. Compartment syndrome is a raised pressure in an osteo-fascial compartment to a level that it compromises tissue perfusion below a critical value.
2. It may be associated with high and low energy injuries.
3. A compartment contains a group of muscles, blood vessels, nerves which are surrounded by very strong fascia.
4. Swelling inside the compartment leads to increase in pressure inside the compartment.
5. This increased pressure reduces or cuts blood flow to the compartment resulting in muscle ischemia and death of cells which further causes swelling & this vicious cycle continues.
6. We should be vigilant in traumatic patients with an altered level of consciousness for compartment syndrome.
7. Intracompartmental pressure may be measured using specialized catheters /device.
8. An absolute difference of 30 mm Hg between a patient's diastolic blood pressure and compartment pressure is taken as a cut-off.
9. **Causes of compartment syndrome:**
   a. Open /closed fractures (Most common)
   b. Soft tissue contusions
   c. Arterial injury
   d. Bleeding disorders including anticoagulation
   e. Burns (Particularly circumferential 3rd degree burns)
   f. Post-ischemic swelling (Reperfusion injury)
   g. Tight casts/dressings
   h. Injection injury, extravasation of intravenous infusion /drugs
10. **Types of compartment syndrome:**
    a. Acute
    b. Chronic
11. **Clinical diagnosis:**
    a. Pain out of proportion to the injury.
    b. Increasing pain
    c. Pain on passive stretch
    d. Paralysis, paraesthesia and pallor are late signs
    e. Pulselessness is an extremely late sign

12. Treatment:

a. Emergency treatment involves relieving pressure in the compartment to prevent ischemia and subsequent necrosis by early surgical decompression.

b. Remove the external compression if any i.e. cast, tourniquet.

c. Early preventive measures including limb elevation, active finger movement.

d. Monitor the vitals

e. Definitive treatment is adequate decompressive fasciotomy. This must be performed as an emergency procedure in operation theatre under general or local anesthesia.

JOINT INJURY

1. Traumatic Injury is commonest cause of dislocation and subluxations of joints
2. Dislocated joint is an emergency should be treated at the earliest
3. **Types of joint injury:**
   a. **Subluxation:** When the articular surface is displaced partially and there is some contact retained between them
   b. **Dislocation:** When the articular surface is displaced completely and there is no contact retained between them.

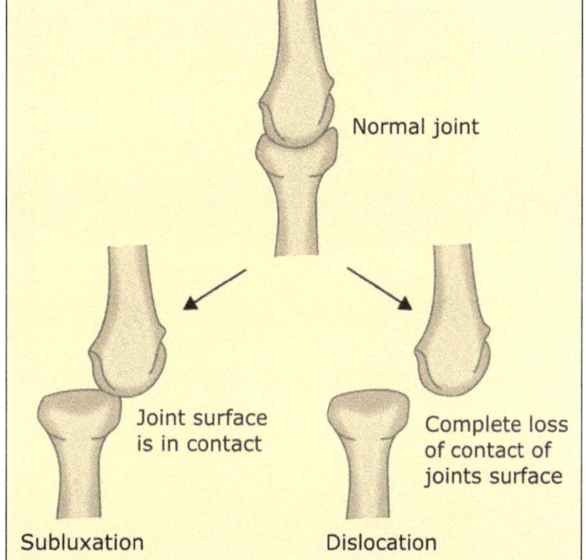

4. **There are two types of acquired dislocations :**
   a. **Traumatic:**
      1. Commonest cause of dislocations
      2. Different force is required to dislocated different joints
      3. Dislocation occurs due to damage to protective ligament or joint capsule.
      4. Traumatic dislocation having following different types

Type of dislocation	
Acute traumatic dislocation	Due to excessive force.
Recurrent dislocation	Due to weakness of the supportive structure of the joint which is as a result of improper healing in the first dislocation, so the joint dislocates repeatedly.
Fracture dislocation	In this type the dislocation of the joint there is a fracture of one or both or the articular bones.
Old unreduced dislocation	Non reduced traumatic fracture present as the old unreduced dislocation.

   b. **Pathological**:
      1. Articular surfaces destroyed by the infections, neoplastic lesion or the ligaments may be damaged due to some disease

5. **Clinical features**
   a. **Pain**
   b. **Swelling**

c. **Deformity of limb in joint dislocations:**

Joint dislocation	Associated deformity
Anterior shoulder dislocation	Abduction of upper limb
Anterior hip dislocation	Abducted and externally rotated lower limb
Posterior hip dislocation	Flexed, adducted and internally rotated lower limb
Posterior elbow dislocation	Flexion deformity of upper limb

d. **Loss of movement**

6. **Investigations**

a. **X-ray examination:**

1. Taken in two planes
2. X-ray of opposite joint (If doubt persist)

b. **CT scan:** If doubt persist after X-ray

c. **MRI scan:** Reveals Soft tissue injury

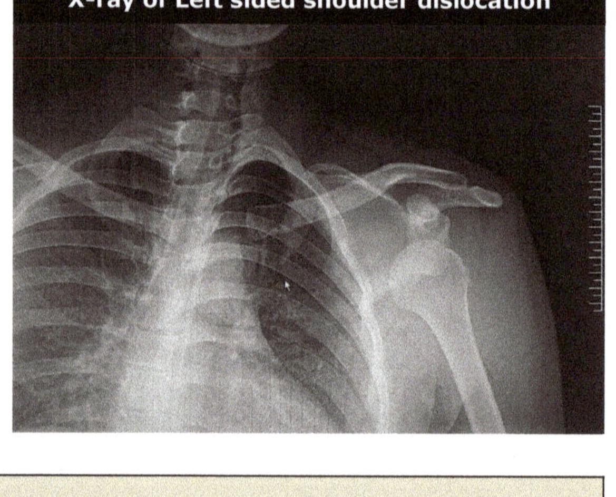
X-ray of Left sided shoulder dislocation

7. **Management**

Type of dislocation	Treatment option
Acute traumatic dislocation	**a. Conservative method** 1. Closed manipulative maneuvers 2. Prolonged traction **b. Operative method: Indicated if failure of closed reduction or dislocation is difficult to maintain by closed method**
Recurrent dislocation	**Operative method** Reconstructive procedure is required
Fracture dislocations	**Operative method**
Old unreduced dislocation	**Operative method:** In most cases requires operative intervention but in some cases if a dislocated joint is having good function no operative intervention requires.

8. **Complications**

a. Immediate

Neurovascular injury

b. Early

1. Recurrence
2. Persistent instability
3. Joint stiffness
4. Myositis ossificans

c. Late

1. Recurrence
2. Osteoarthritis
3. Avascular necrosis

VASCULAR INJURY

1. **Vascular injury requires urgent intervention to save the life or the limb of a patient.**
2. **Causes**
   a. **Penetrating injuries**

      Gunshot, stab injury

   b. **Blunt trauma**

      Bone fracture, joint dislocation, contusion

   c. **By invasive procedure**

      Arteriography, cardiac catheterization
3. **First priority in the vascular injury is to control the bleeding then do diagnostic work. Compressive dressing should be applied instead of a tourniquet or clamping vessels.**
4. **Signs of arterial injury**
   a. **Hard signs of arterial injury:**
      1. External arterial bleeding
      2. Rapidly expanding hematoma
      3. Palpable thrill, audible bruit
      4. Obvious arterial occlusion signs like pallor, pulseless, paresthesia, pain, paralysis, cold to touch

   b. **Soft signs of arterial injury:**
      1. History of arterial bleeding at the scene
      2. Diminished unilateral distal pulse
      3. Small non pulsatile hematoma
      4. Neurological deficit
      5. Abnormal velocity waveform on doppler study
      6. Penetrating injury or blunt trauma near major artery
5. **Diagnostic studies:**
   a. **Arterial Pressure Index (API):** Doppler-determined arterial systolic blood pressure in injured limb divided by systolic blood pressure in uninjured limb

   b. **Duplex doppler:** Widely used in peripheral vascular injury assessment

   c. **CT Angiography:** Gold standard for the evaluation of trauma-related vascular injuries

6. **Evaluation Algorithm:**

   a. **Hard Signs (> 90% risk of arterial injury)**

      Immediate arterial exploration is required in most of cases without further investigation

   b. **Soft Signs (30% risk of arterial injury)**

      1. Perform API → If < 0.9 then keep under observation for 24 hours & then perform serial API.
      2. **Consider:**
         a. Doppler ultrasound
         b. CT angiogram
         c. Evaluation of compartment pressure
         d. Ischemia time

7. **Management:**

   a. Admit the patient

   b. Assessment of blood loss by general condition ,pallor,pulse rate and blood pressure

   c. Analgesics for pain relief

   d. Broad spectrum antibiotics

   e. Large bore cannulas should be placed immediately .

   f. Administer warm IV crystalloids and control the site of bleeding by compressive dressing .

   g. Take blood for sampling for Complete blood count, blood grouping and cross match.

   h. Arterial blood gases: Lactate is useful to measure the degree of shock

   i. Administer the blood and blood products if unresponsive to the crystalloid fluid.

   j. Consult with vascular surgeon and shift the patient to operation theatre

   k. Fractured limb is reduced and stabilized with external fixator to maintain alignment before vascular intervention

   l. Vascular repair is achieved with the help of different procedures; e.g. End to end anastomosis, bypass, endovascular etc.

   m. Fasciotomy may be added if ischemia time is more than six hours.

MUSCLE AND TENDON INJURY

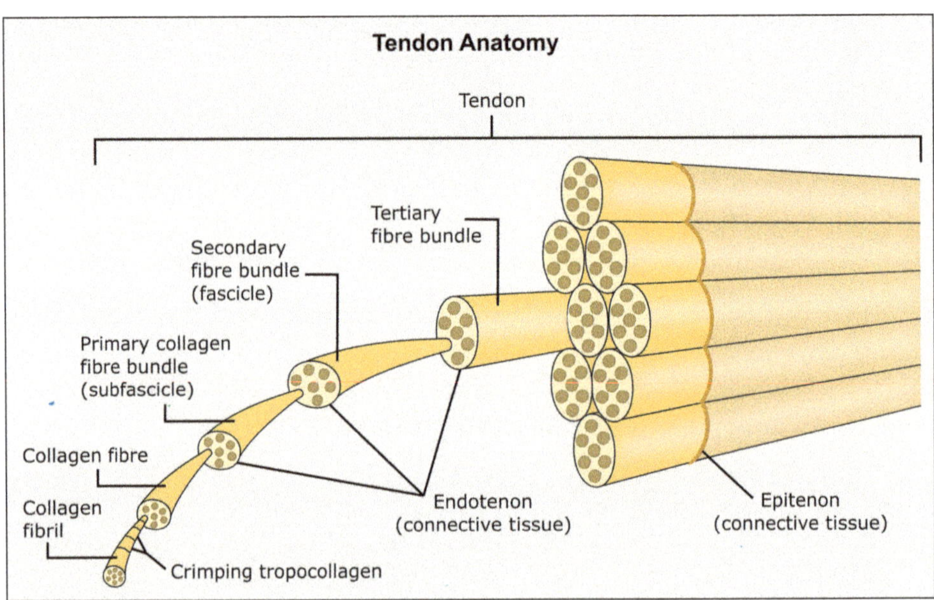

1. Muscles and tendons are parts of the musculoskeletal system and help in movement of body parts, weight bearing and other body functions .
2. Tendon is fibrous connective tissue that connects muscle to bone.
3. Most common cause of muscles or tendon rupture is sudden vigorous muscle contraction which occurs during sports & strenuous activities.
4. Penetrating trauma with a sharp object can also lead to muscle and tendon injury.
5. **Clinical features:**
    a. Limited limb movement
    b. Muscle weakness
    c. Restricted joint movement
    d. Inability to bear weight
    e. Pain and tenderness
    f. Redness and bruising
6. **Investigations**
    a. History and clinical examination of each muscle/tendon in isolation.
    b. Imaging
        1. Ultrasonography
        2. MRI scan

7. Management of tendon and muscle injury

Tendon injury	Muscles injury
1. In fresh rupture the best treatment is to regain continuity by end-to-end repair using various suturing techniques e.g. Kesselers stitch.	**Conservative** **a. Acute management (PRICE protocol)** 1. P = Protection (Protect from the excessive load) 2. R =Rest (Necessary to reduce the metabolic request over the injured site) 3. I =Ice application (Reduce the local temperature, the metabolic request and bleeding) 4. C =Compression (limit edema diffusion) 5. E =Elevation (Reduce edema)
2. When the gap is too much then Tendon graft is required. Palmaris longus, Plantaris are commonly used for grafting.	**b. NSAIDs** **c. Physiotherapy** **Surgical management** Surgical management involves suturing of the muscles with different suturing methods **Indication** 1. Complete rupture of muscle belly 2. Subtotal rupture associated with persistent pain and loss of strength

LIGAMENT INJURY /SPRAIN

1. Traumatic injuries to joints may result in ligament tears with associated joint subluxation or dislocation.
2. The history and physical examination is particularly important in the assessment of ligamentous injuries, along with radiological investigation for diagnosis
3. The anatomy and location of the joint have a major influence on susceptibility to injury:
   a. The hip joint is a stable ball and socket joint and hence major ligamentous injury and dislocation is therefore relatively uncommon.
   b. The knee joint is more commonly injured since it is a hinge joint with no bony stability and is more exposed to injury due to its location in the limb.
4. **Signs and symptoms:**
   a. Pain
   b. Swelling
   c. Bruising
   d. Decreased ability to move the limb
   e. If a ligament ruptures, one may hear a cracking sound
   f. Difficulty using the affected extremity
5. **Sprains are classified into three grades of severity, ranging from over-stretching to complete tearing of the ligament:**

Grades of injury	
Grade I (mild)	**S**light stretching of the ligament with some damage to fibers **M**inimal swelling and tenderness **M**inimal to no functional loss **N**o ligament laxity (Joint is stable)
Grade II (moderate)	**P**artial tear of ligament **M**oderate swelling, pain, or tenderness; **M**ild to moderate ligament laxity (Joint may be unstable)
Grade III (severe)	**C**omplete tear of ligament **S**ignificant swelling, bruising, and tenderness Positive for ligament laxity (joint instability) **R**ule out a fracture (In a severe sprain, the ligament may pull off a piece of the bone, resulting in an avulsion fracture)

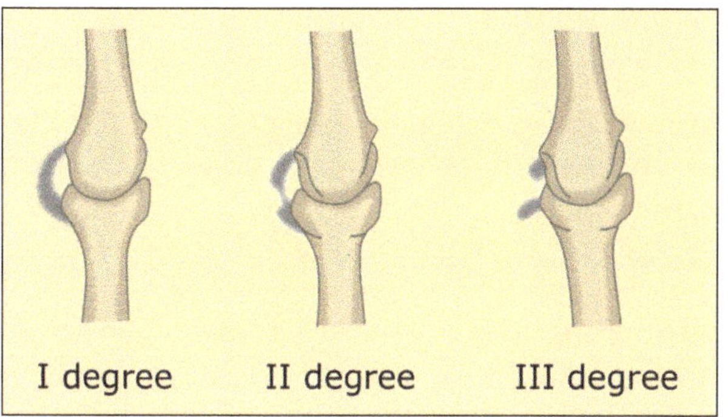

Diagnosis:

1. X-ray for fractures
2. **MRI:** Helpful to diagnose ligament injury

6. **Management: Follow the PRICE protocol as soon as possible after injury**

   a. **Protect:** Protect the injured site from repetitive injury.

   b. **Rest:** The sprain should be rested.

   c. **Ice application:**

      1. Ice should be applied immediately to the sprain to reduce swelling and pain.
      2. It can be applied for 10–15 minutes at a time, 3-4 times a day.
      3. Ice application to numb the pain.
      4. Used only for a short period of time (Not used more than twenty minutes): If used longer than 20 minutes can reduce the blood flow to the injured area and slows the healing process.

   d. **Compression:**

      1. Dressings, bandages should be used to immobilize the sprain and provide support.
      2. While wrapping the injured part, more pressure should be applied at the distal end of the injury and decrease pressure proximally i.e. towards heart.
      3. Compression should not be so tight to avoid reduction of blood supply

   e. **Elevation:** Keeping the sprained joint elevated (in relation to the rest of the body) will also help minimize swelling

   f. **Medications:** Non-steroidal anti-inflammatory drugs can relieve pain.

   Topical NSAIDs appear to be as good as those taken by mouth like diclofenac gel.

g. **Functional rehabilitation:** Rehabilitation exercises are used to prevent stiffness.

h. **Surgical treatment:** Surgical management is required in patient with ligament tear that does not heal adequately with conservative treatment and the joint shows persistent laxity.

   a. **Repair:**

      In an acute setting, the ruptured ligament may be repaired with sutures and allowed to heal.

   b. **Reconstruction:**

      In chronic injuries and for ligaments that do not have the ability to heal (e.g., ACL), reconstruction of the ligament using tendon grafts is the treatment of choice

NERVE INJURY

1. Nerve is the basic unit of the peripheral nervous system and functions of the limb depend on it.
2. Nerve injury may be caused by blunt, sharp or penetrating trauma .
3. It may result in a loss of sensations, paralysis, deformity and loss of functions.

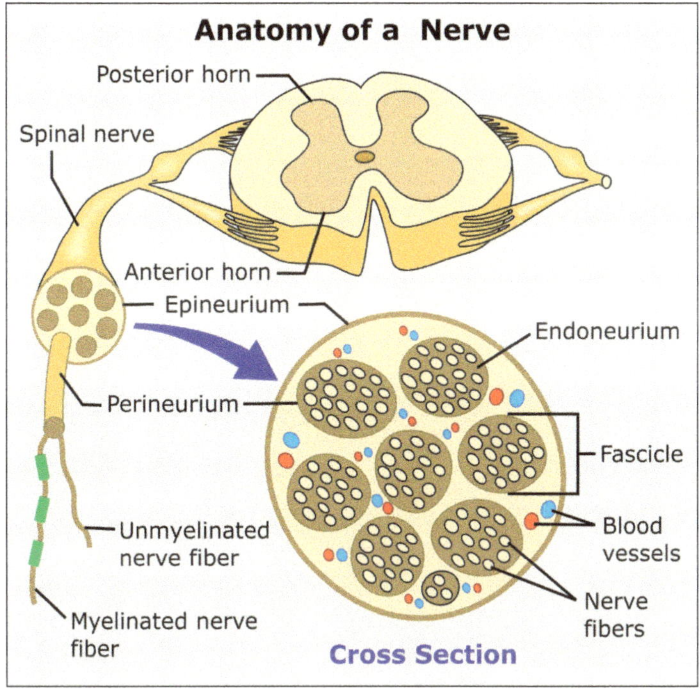

4. **Classification of nerve injuries:**

Seddon and sunderland classification

Seddon	Sunderland	Injury	Spontaneous recovery
Neuropraxis	Grade I	Focal segmental demyelination	Yes
Axonotmesis	Grade II	Damaged axon with intact endoneurium	Yes, but slower than neuropraxis
Axonotmesis	Grade III	Damaged axon and endoneurium with intact perineurium	Not very likely, surgical intervention is necessary
Axonotmesis	Grade IV	Damaged axon, endoneurium and perineurium with intact epineurium.	Highly unlikely, surgical intervention is necessary
Neurotmesis	Grade V	complete nerve transection	Not occurs, surgical intervention is necessary

5. **Signs and symptoms:**

   Functional loss is characterized as follows:

   1. **Loss of all sensations**
   2. **Paralysis of supplied muscles**

      Wasting is seen only as a late sign.
   3. **Sympathetic paralysis**

      Loss of sweating and vasomotor control is the most important early sign of degenerative lesions.
   4. **Loss of reflex arc.**

6. **Diagnosis:**
   1. History of trauma
   2. Symptoms
   3. Physical and neurological examination

7. **Investigations:**

   a. **Electromyography & Nerve conduction study (EMG-NCV):**

   Reduced muscle activity and altered nerve conduction velocity can be used to understand the exact level of injury in a peripheral nerve.

8. **Management:**

   a. It is important to recognize a nerve injury so that it can be repaired as soon as the condition becomes favorable.

   b. **Nerve repair in tidy open wound (Clean with minimal contamination)**
      1. Tidy wound mostly caused by glass or knife
      2. Primary repair by direct end to end suturing

   c. **Nerve repair in Untidy wound (Dirty and contaminated)**
      1. Careful excision of dead and contaminated tissue with adequate decompression is carried out and the skeletal is stabilized appropriately.
      2. Nerves are best identified, put in their normal anatomical position and tagged for later identification.
      3. Repair should be done after healthy skin cover has been achieved and sepsis ends.
      4. Nerve grafting may be needed in some cases to restore continuity in large gap/tense repair.

d. The course of spontaneous recovery

1. Neuropraxia recovers spontaneously in 6-8 weeks.
2. Axonotmesis/neurotmesis requires surgical intervention.
3. Nerve fibres regenerate at about the rate of 1 mm a day.
4. **Tinel sign is useful to know the evidence of recovery:**
    a. Tinel sign is performed by lightly tapping (percussing) over the nerve distribution to elicit a sensation of tingling or "pins and needles"
    b. A distally progressive Tinel's sign signifies nerve regeneration.
5. If there is no clinical or neurophysiological evidence of recovery at 3 months from fracture or dislocation and if tinel signs remain constant, then exploration and nerve repair required.

DISASTER MANAGEMENT

1. **Definition:** Any occurrence that causes damage, ecological disruption, loss of human life or deterioration of health and health services on a large scale which warrant an extraordinary response from outside the affected area.
2. There are many types of disasters such as floods, landslides, fires, earthquakes, snow storms, severe air pollution (smog), heat waves, epidemics, building collapse, toxicological accidents etc.
3. **Disaster management**
   a. Information regarding the disaster from disaster control
   b. Mobilise resources such as ambulances, essential drugs, manpower, instruments etc.
   c. Triage casualties
   d. Start emergency treatment
   e. Referral to other centres for definitive management
   f. Start definitive management
4. **Search and rescue:**
   a. Assessment of the damage and the number of casualties
   b. Most immediate help comes from the uninjured survivors.
   c. Search and rescue the injured survivors
5. **First aid:**

   Care for patients with minor injuries involves cleaning and dressing wounds, suturing lacerations and splinting simple fractures.
6. **Triage:**
   a. It is a cornerstone of the management of mass casualties.
   b. Aim of triage is to identify the patients who will benefit the most if treated earliest
   c. By sorting out the minor injuries, triage decreases the immediate burden on hospital.
   d. It helps to categorize patients in priority of treatment needed.
   e. Triaging of patient should be done by experienced senior doctor for proper management of patients.
   f. The principle first come, first treated is not followed in mass casualties.

g. Higher priority is granted to victims whose immediate or long-term prognosis can dramatically be affected by simple intensive care.

h. **The most common classification uses the internationally accepted four color code system**

1. **First (I):**

   Red (Immediate Critical) but likely to survive if treatment given early

   Examples: Severe facial trauma, tension pneumothorax, profuse external bleeding, hemothorax, flail chest, major intra-abdominal bleed, extradural hematomas

2. **Second (II):**

   Yellow (Urgent Critical), likely to survive if treatment given within hours

   Examples: Compound fractures, degloving injuries, ruptured abdominal viscus, pelvic fractures, spinal injuries

3. **Third (III):**

   Green (Non-urgent Stable) likely to survive even if treatment is delayed for hours to days **Examples:** Simple fractures, sprains, minor lacerations

4. **Last (0):**

   Black (Unsalvageable) Not breathing, pulseless, so severely injured that no medical care is likely to help

   Examples: Severe brain damage, very extensive burns, major disruption

7. **Essentials of casualty evacuation:**

   a. A quick re-triage is very useful in this situation.

   b. Decide which patients require referral to another institute.

   c. Select appropriate hospital for transfer for definitive management and care.

   d. Choose proper ambulance for transport.

   e. An adequate supply of essentials such as intravenous fluids, dressings, pain medication, oxygen must be arranged while transferring the patient in ambulance

8. **Once patients have been transported to health care facilities, they are managed using the ATLS protocol for emergency resuscitation and definitive treatment depends on individual needs of the patient.**

Section 5

Obstetrics and Gynecology Emergencies

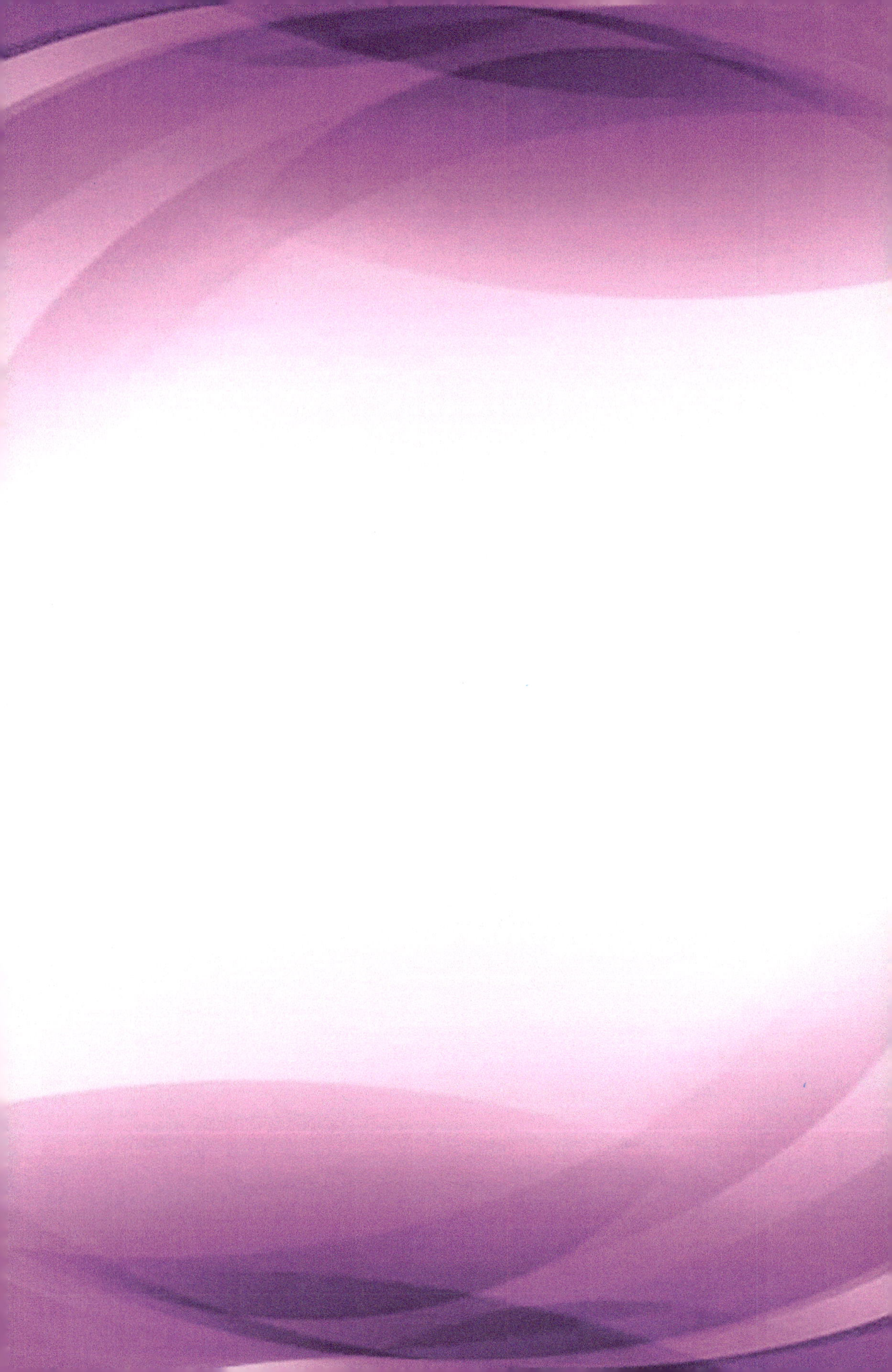

CHAPTER

5 Obstetric and Gynecology Emergencies

OBSTETRIC EXAMINATION

1. History

   a. **Current pregnancy basic details**: Name, age, occupation, marital status, consanguineous or non consanguineous marriage, ANC registration, gravidity, parity, EDD.

   b. **Menstrual history:** LMP, cycle length, irregular periods.

   c. **Current pregnancy history:** Trimester, method of confirmation of pregnancy, general health, vaginal bleeding, abdominal pain, vaccination, vaginal discharge, drug history, hyperemesis gravidarum, blood and sonography investigations, urinary problems.

   d. **Past obstetrics details:** Detail of previous pregnancy including MTP and Miscarriage, weeks of gestation, onset of labor, mode of delivery, date and place of delivery, birth weight and sex, neonatal and fetal life, complication and adverse outcomes.

   e. **Past gynecological history:** Contraception, menstrual history, cervical smear, coital problem.
   f. **Drug and allergy history:** Current medication, medication during pregnancy and details of adverse drug reactions.
   g. **Past medical and surgical history**: Diabetus, hypertension, endocrine problems, epilepsy, previous surgeries.
   h. **Family:** Chromosomal defect or hereditary illness, multiple pregnancy, consanguinity.
   i. **Social history:** No of family members, living status, earning members, domestic violence screening.
   j. **Personal history:** Diet, sleep, addiction, bowel and bladder habit.
2. **Gain verbal consent for examination**
3. **Inspection: shape, size, scar, linea nigra, striae, movement, color.**
4. **Palpate**
   a. **Fundal height in Cms**
   b. **Fetal parts**
   c. **Movement**
   d. **Number of fetus**
   e. **The lie (longitudinal/transverse/oblique)**
   f. **The presentation (cephalic/breech/other)**
   g. **The position (LOL/ROA/DOP etc.)**
   h. **Engagement of head**
5. **Auscultate: Fetal heart rate**

PRETERM LABOR

1. Preterm labor is defined as labor occurring before 37 completed weeks
2. It is one of the leading cause of perinatal morbidity and mortality.
3. **Etiology:** Most common cause of preterm labor is idiopathic followed by infection

High risk factors for preterm labor

History	Complication of current pregnancy	Iatrogenic	Idiopathic
1. Previous history of abortion or preterm delivery 2. Recurrent urinary tract infection 3. Smoking and alcohol habit 4. Low socio-economic status 5. Low nutritional status	1. Multiple pregnancy 2. Pre-eclampsia 3. Placenta previa 4. Abruptio placenta 5. Incompetent cervix 6. Malformation of uterus 7. Congenital malformation 8. Intrauterine death 9. Placental infarction 10. Polyhydramnios 11. Acute fever 12. Acute appendicitis 13. Toxoplasmosis 14. Abdominal operation	Indicated preterm delivery due to obstetric or medical complication	In Majority of cases

4. **Risk factor:**
   a. Short maternal height and weight
   b. Short cervical length
   c. Domestic violence
   d. Genital tract infections
5. **Sign/symptoms:**
   a. Backache
   b. Cramping in lower abdomen
   c. Pelvic pain/pressure
   d. Vaginal discharge or bleeding
   e. Regular uterine contraction with or without pain (at least one in every 10 min)

6. **Diagnosis (Based on history & physical examination)**
   a. Dilation (> 2 cm) and effacement 80% of cervix
   b. Length of cervix (measured by TVS) < 2.5 cm and funneling of internal os
   c. Vaginal discharge or bleeding
   d. Regular uterine contraction with or without pain (At least one in every 10 min)
7. **Investigation**
   a. Blood study (Complete blood count, serum electrolyte and blood glucose)
   b. Urine for routine analysis, culture and sensitivity
   c. Cervical culture
   d. Fetal fibronectin evaluation (Between 24 week and 34 week in cervicovaginal discharge is a predictor of PTL)
   e. Ultrasonography for fetal well being and placental localisation
   f. Transvaginal sonography for cervical length (Risk of PTL with length < 25 mm at 24 weeks gestation)
8. **Management:**
   a. If possible, try to prevent onset of labor
   b. Arrest preterm labor if not contraindicated
   c. Proper management of labor and appropriate care of neonate in neonatal intensive care unit (To prevent birth trauma, asphyxia and development of respiratory distress syndrome)

Pharmacological	Surgical treatment
a. Antibiotics: If infection is present **b. Steroids** (All preterm before 36 weeks) betamethasone or dexamethasone **c. Tocolytics (In early preterm):** To delay the delivery at least for 48 hours **e.g. Nifedipine, atosiban, progesterone, Magnesium sulfate.**	**a. Cervical cerclage** (Patients with prior preterm birth and having short cervix) **b. Cesarean section delivery** is not routinely recommended and is done only in obstetrics complication (Hypertension, abruption, malpresentation)

PREMATURE RUPTURE OF MEMBRANES (PROM)

1. **Definition**

   Spontaneous rupture of membrane any time beyond 28 weeks of pregnancy but before onset of labor.

   a. **Term PROM:** Beyond 37 weeks but before the onset of labor

   b. **Preterm PROM:** Before 37 weeks

2. **Causes**

   a. Membrane weakness (Decreased tensile strength and increased friability)

   b. Multiple pregnancy

   c. Polyhydramnios

   d. Infections (Proteolytic enzymes)

   e. Cervical incompetence

   f. Cervical length < 2.5 cm

3. **Signs and symptoms**

   Escape of watery discharge per vaginum either in the form of gush or slow leak.

4. **Diagnosis**

   a. **Speculum examination** (Liquor escaping out through the cervix)

   b. **Nitrazine paper/Litmus paper test for pH detection turn blue (Posterior fornix fluid)**

   c. **Ferning pattern under microscope (Posterior fornix fluid)**

   d. **Ultrasound:** To support diagnosis and also to know fetal wellbeing

   e. **Amnisure:** Rapid immunoassay test designed to detect high conc. of placental microglobulin (PAMG-1) which is present in amniotic fluid.

   f. **Nile blue test:** Centrifuged cells are stained with 0.1% nile blue sulfate showing orange blue colorization of the fat containing cells of fetus

5. **Investigations**

   a. Complete blood count

   b. Urine routine and culture

   c. High vaginal swab for culture

   d. Phosphatidyl glycerol estimation & lecithin /spingomyelin ratio

   e. Ultrasonography for fetal biophysical profile

   f. Cardiotocography for nonstress test

6. Management or premature rupture of membranes

Absence of chorioamnionitis, placental abruption, fetal distress and not in labor			**Presence of chorioamnionitis, placental abruption, fetal distress and in labor**
Management depends on gestational weeks			
<34 weeks	**≥ 34 weeks to <37 weeks**	**≥ 37 weeks**	
1. Prolong pregnancy for fetal maturity 2. Bed rest 3. Antibiotics, steroids 4. If possible consider delivery at 34 weeks 5. Neonatal care in intensive care unit	1. Wait for spontaneous onset of labor for 24 to 48 hours 2. If fails then induction with oxytocin 3. Cesarean section if non cephalic presentation 4. Neonatal care in intensive care unit	1. Wait for spontaneous onset of labor for 24 hours 2. If fails then induction with oxytocin 3. Cesarean section if obstetrics indication. 4. Neonatal care in intensive care unit (If required)	1. Expeditious delivery 2. Broad spectrum antibiotics 3. Neonatal care in intensive care unit

PROLONGED LABOR (FAILURE TO PROGRESS)

a. **Definition:** If the duration of 1st stage and 2nd stage of labor is more than the arbitrary time limit of 18 hours.

b. In nulliparous women the most common cause is inadequate uterine activity and in multiparous cephalopelvic disproportion.

c. Prolonged labor affects both the mother and fetus.

d. To understand the prolonged labor we have to know events of Labor, which are divided into three stages

1st stage	2nd stage	3rd stage
1. It starts from the onset of true labor pain and ends with full dilation of the cervix 2. Its average duration is 12 hours in primigravidae and 6 hours in multiparae 3. It includes latent phase and active phase 4. It is considered as a prolonged if duration is more than 12 hours	1. It starts with full dilation of cervix and ends with expulsion of fetus out of the cervix 2. Average time 2 hour in primi and 30 min in multiparae 3. It is considered as a prolonged if duration is more than 2 hours in primigravida and 1 hr in multiparae	1. It begins after expulsion of the fetus and ends with expulsion of placenta and membranes 2. Average time duration 15 min in both primigravidae and multiparae

e. **Causes**

	First stage	Second stage
Fault in power	1. Uterine inertia	1. Uterine inertia 2. Regional analgesia 3. Inability to bear down 4. Constriction ring
Fault in passage	1. Contracted pelvis 2. Full bladder 3. Cervical dystocia 4. Pelvic tumors	1. Cephalopelvic disproportion 2. Android pelvis 3. Contracted pelvis 4. Rigid perineum 5. Pelvic tumors
Fault in passenger	1. Malposition 2. Malpresentation 3. Anomalous baby	1. Malposition 2. Malpresentation 3. Big baby 4. Anomalous baby

f. **Diagnosis:**

1. Prolonged labor is not a diagnosis, but it occurs due to abnormality.
2. Actual cause of prolongation should be detected by proper abdominal and vaginal examination.

g. **Dangers to fetus and mother due to prolonged labor**

Fetal	Mother
Hypoxia	Distress
Intrauterine infection	Chorioamnionitis
Intracranial hemorrhage	Trauma to genital tract
Increased need of operative delivery	Puerperal sepsis
	Postpartum hemorrhage
	Increased need of operative delivery
	Subinvolution

h. **Management of prolonged labor it includes:**

1. **Prevention and early detection:** Antenatal or early intranatal detection of factors which may cause prolonged labor.
2. **Partograph** : Its use helps in early detection
3. **Emotional support**
4. **Change the position to increase the uterine contraction**
5. **Selective and judicious augmentation of labor with low rupture of membranes and followed by the oxytocin**
6. **Appropriate interventions**

First stage	Second stage
1. If suboptimal uterine contraction a. Amniotomy b. Oxytocin drip **2. Secondary arrest** a. Careful use of oxytocin b. In case of vaginal delivery is unsafe: Cesarean section	**1. Short period expectant management if FHS is reassuring and delivery near to happen** **2. If not then go for appropriate assisted delivery** a. Vaginal (Forceps or ventouse) b. Abdominal (Cesarean section)

CORD PROLAPSE

1. **Abnormal descent of the umbilical cord into the lower segment by the side of the presenting part or below the presenting part.**
2. Incomplete fitting of the presenting part in the maternal pelvis at time of rupture of membranes favors cord prolapse.
3. Cord prolapse may be spontaneous or iatrogenic.
4. This condition compromises blood flow to the baby.
5. Cord prolapse is one of the cause of fresh stillbirth.
6. Before declaration of fetal death, ultrasonography for cardiac movement of fetus or auscultation for fetal heart sound is to be done promptly.
7. Use of elective Cesarean section in noncephalic presentations will reduce a risk of cord prolapse.
8. **There are three clinical types:**

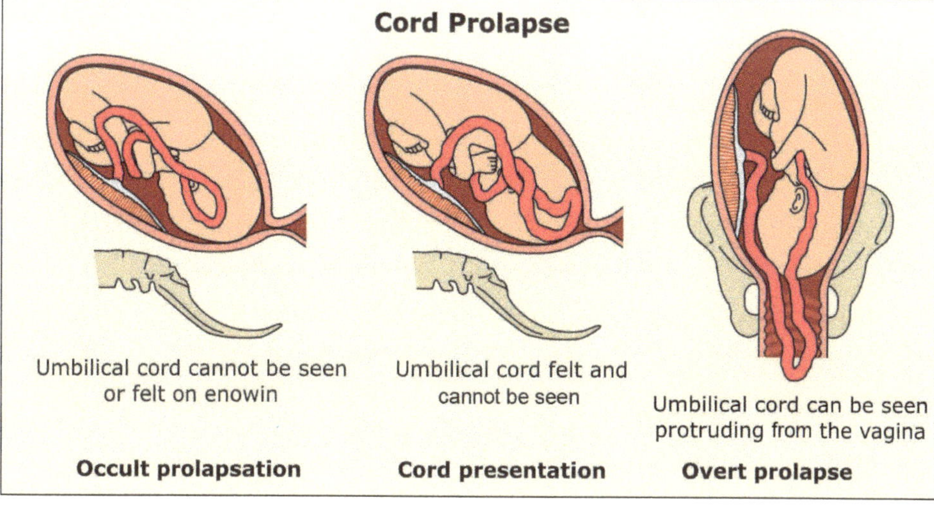

Clinical type of cord	Position of cord	Diagnosis
Occult prolapse	Present by the side of presenting of part	Difficult to diagnose Suspected in patients with continuous variable deceleration of fetal heart rate.
Cord presentation	Cord present below the presenting part. Intact bag of membranes	Pulsations of cord are felt on internal examination
Cord prolapse	Cord inside the vagina or outside the vulva Ruptured bag of membranes present	Cord can be palpated directly in vagina or outside.

9. **Etiological factors:**
   a. **For Spontaneous**
      1. **Malpresentation**
      2. **Polyhydramnios**
      3. **Low birth weight baby**
      4. **Prematurity**
      5. **Multiple pregnancy**
      6. **Abnormal lie**
      7. **Preterm labor**
   b. **For Iatrogenic**
      1. **Artificial rupture of membranes**
      2. **Manual rotation of the fetal head**
10. **Management:** Involves immediate delivery of viable babies by the quickest and safest route possible.
    a. **First aid**
       1. **Posture:** The exaggerated and elevated Sims position or Trendelenburg or knee chest position
       2. Bladder filing to lift the presenting part
    b. **The factors taken into consideration while taking decision**
       1. Baby is alive or dead
       2. Maturity of baby
       3. Cervical dilatation
       4. Presentation of fetus
    c. **If baby is alive:**
       1. Treatment of choice is cesarean section
       2. **If immediate vaginal delivery is possible:** In vertex presentation assisted delivery is conducted with forceps and ventouse and in breech presentation delivery is conducted by the expert hands only.
       3. **If immediate vaginal delivery is not possible:** Definitive management is cesarean section
    d. **If baby is dead:**
       1. Confirm with ultrasound
       2. Wait for spontaneous delivery
       3. If no spontaneous delivery occurs then go for destructive surgery.

MALPOSITION

1. Any position of the vertex other than flexed occipitoanterior one is called malposition.
2. Normal position of vertex is flexed occipitoanterior.
3. When an occiput is present directly over the sacrum or sacroiliac joint is called as occipitoposterior position.
4. Occipitoposterior position responsible for the prolonged labor.

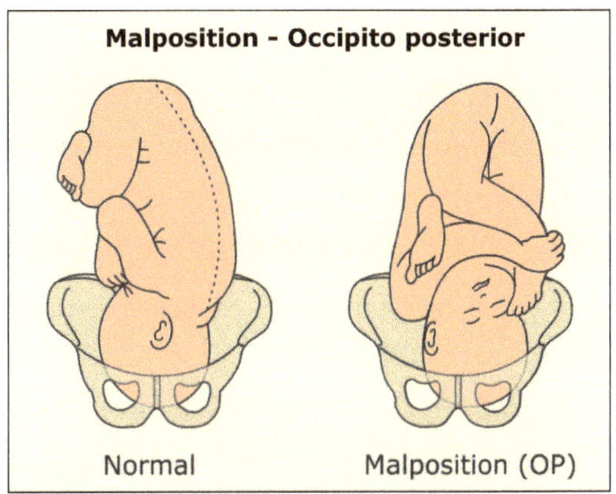

5. Three positions are described in occipitoposterior position right, left and direct.
6. In the right occiput lies on the right sacroiliac joint and in left occiput lies on the left sacroiliac joint.
7. In direct occipitoposterior position the occiput is lying in front of the sacrum.
8. **Etiological factor:**
   a. **Anthropoid/android pelvis:** Due to a wide posterior segment, the occiput lies comfortably.
   b. **Anterior attachment of placenta:** Causes deflexion of head.
   c. **High pelvic inclination:** Favors op position due to deflexion of head
   d. **Abnormal uterine contraction:** Leads to persistent deflexion of head.
9. **Diagnosis:**

Abdominal examination	Vaginal examination
1. Subumblical flattening due to absence of back 2. Limbs felt anteriorly 3. Non engaged head or high head in term. 4. Anterior shoulder lies away from the midline. 5. Heart sounds are well heard in flanks and frequently indistinct in the midline. 6. Sinciput did not feel prominent.	**1. In early labor** a. Early rupture of bag of membranes while examination. b. Due to deflexion of head anterior fontanel is well felt c. Posterior fontanel felt near the sacroiliac joint. **2. In late labor** a. Sutures and fontanels are not felt due to large caput formation

10. Management: (It is better to do cesarean section in the absence of skilled obstetrician)

a. In this position labor is prolonged so patient requires adequate IV fluid resuscitation and analgesia

b. If the mother and baby are in a good condition then spontaneous progress of labor occurs and no interference requires.

c. Partogram assessment is required to understand progress of labor.

d. Epidural analgesia is commonly used for pain relief.

e. In most patients the head rotates anteriorly and delivery occurs spontaneously.

f. In few patients the head rotate posteriorly and delivery may occur spontaneously or may require assistance.

g. In non-rotation or short anterior rotation spontaneous delivery is unlikely.

h. If progress of labor is unsatisfactory in expected spontaneous delivery, evaluate for the cephalopelvic disproportion and inadequate uterine contractions.

i. If cephalopelvic disproportion is not the cause of unsatisfactory progress of labor then start augmenting labor by oxytocin drip.

j. Cesarean section is indicated in the patient with cephalopelvic disproportion or non progress even after oxytocin.

MALPRESENTATION

1. **Breech presentation:** Buttocks in the lower pole of the uterus with longitudinal lie of fetus.
2. It is the most common malpresentation
3. **Types of breech presentation**

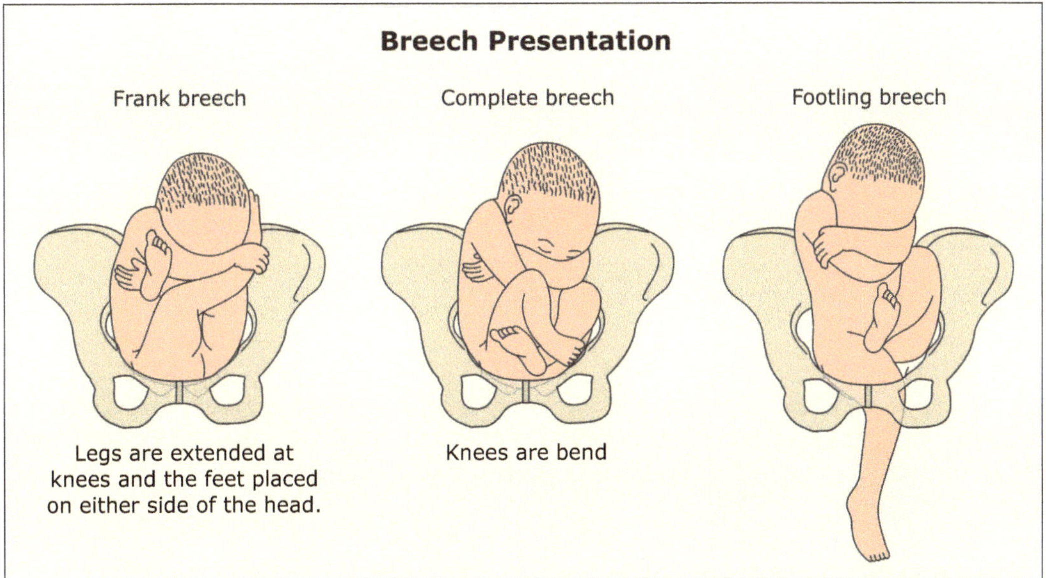

   a. **Complete:** In this presentation thighs are fixed at hip and legs are flexed at knees, presenting part includes buttocks, feet and external genitals. This is most commonly seen in multipara patients.

   b. **Incomplete**

      1. **Frank breech:** Thighs are flexed at hip joint but the legs are extended at knee joints, presenting part includes buttocks and external genitals. (Commonly seen in primigravida patients).

      2. **Footling presentation:** Both the thigh partially extend at hip and legs at knee joints, presenting part includes footling.

4. **Circumstances which favors breech presentation:**

   a. **Extended legs**

   b. **Preterm labor:** Common before 34 weeks of gestation

   c. **Multiple pregnancy:** Limits space for rotation

   d. **Polyhydramnios:** Distension of uterine cavity due to excessive amniotic fluids favors breech presentation.

e. **Hydrocephalus baby:** Head easily fits in fundus

f. **Septate or bicornuate uterus:** Favours adaption for breech.

g. **Contracted pelvis**

5. **Diagnosis:** Clinical and by sonography

Antenatal diagnosis	In labor
Patients complain of hard mass just below the ribs and causing difficulty in breathing especially at night. **Abdominal examination** **1. Complete breech** a. Hard and globular mass is felt on the fundal grip and head ballotable. b. Soft, broad and irregular mass felt on pelvic grip. c. Fetal back on one side and irregular parts to the other side on lateral grip. **2. Frank breech** a. Irregular small parts may be felt by the side of the head on the fundal grip. b. Irregular parts felt on one side and regular, hard on the other side on lateral grip. c. Small, hard and cone shaped mass is felt on the pelvic grip. **Vaginal examination** **a. In complete breech:** Soft and irregular parts are felt through fornix. **b. In frank breech:** Hard feel of the sacrum is felt, often mistaken for the head **Sonography**	**Abdominal examination** **1. Complete breech** a. Hard and globular mass is felt on the fundal grip and head ballotable. b. Soft, broad and irregular mass felt on pelvic grip. c. Fetal back on one side and irregular parts to the other side on lateral grip. **2. Frank breech** a. Irregular small parts may be felt by the side of the head on the fundal grip. b. Irregular parts felt on one side and regular, hard on the other side on lateral grip. c. Small, hard and cone shaped mass is felt on the pelvic grip. **Vaginal examination** **a. In complete breech:** Palpation of ischial tuberosities, sacrum and the feet by the sides of the buttocks **b. In frank breech:** Palpation of ischial tuberosities, anal opening and sacrum only **Sonography**

6. **Management**

a. Treating clinician have to make decision with proper communication with women with breech presentation about care and treatment (Informed decision)

b. **Management depends on**

1. Complicated factor associated with breech presentation
2. If external cephalic version fails or Contraindications for external cephalic version are present then two methods of delivery can be planned
   i. Elective cesarean section
   ii. Vaginal breech delivery

iii. External cephalic version

Contraindication for ECV	Suitable condition for ECV
1. Antepartum hemorrhage 2. Multiple pregnancy 3. Contracted pelvis 4. Congenital Malformed uterus 5. Fetal causes Dead fetus, IUGR, fetal abnormality, hyperextended head, large fetus > 3.5 kg 6. Ruptured membranes 7. Abnormal cardiotocography 8. Previous LSCS 9. Obstetrics complications like severe pre-eclampsia	1. To be done around 36 weeks or after 2. Well equipped labor room 3. Tocolytics if required 4. Fetal monitoring before and after ECV

iv. Criteria to allow the spontaneous vaginal breech delivery if ECV fails

1. Informed consent
2. Availability of an experienced obstetrician and neonatologist
3. Average fetal weight (In between 1.5 kg and 3.5 kg)
4. Frank or complete breech (Frank is preferred)
5. Flexed fetal head
6. Adequate pelvis

v. Indications for elective cesarean section

More than or equal to 38 weeks of gestation
Estimated baby weight > 3.5 kg
Hyperextended neck
Footling presentation
Pelvic inadequacy
Absence of expertise obstetricians
With medical or obstetrics complications

vi.

Antenatal management	In labor management
1. If external cephalic version successful **a. Delivery with vertex presentation** **2. If external cephalic version failed or not done** **a. Elective CS (If gestational age is more than equal to 38 weeks)** **b. Trial for vaginal delivery** **i. Satisfactory labor progress:** assisted delivery **ii. If fetal distress, arrest in progress, cord prolapse:** Go for cesarean section	**1. General management** **2. In first stage** a. Monitor the mother and fetus vitals. b. IV fluid infusion c. Epidural analgesia d. Pelvic assessment e. Oxytocin infusion for augmentation of labor. **3. In second stage** **a. Spontaneous labor** **b. Assisted labor** **c. Breech extraction** (Rarely done due to chances of trauma to mother and fetus) **4. In the third stage:** Occurs normally.

7. **Complications:**
   a. **Maternal**
      i. **Trauma to genital tract**
      ii. **Increased operative interference**
      iii. **Anesthesia related complication**
      iv. **Sepsis**
   b. **Fetal**
      i. **Head trauma: Intracranial hemorrhage**
      ii. **Birth injury**
         - **Fractures:** Fractures of femur, humerus
         - **Visceral organ injuries**
         - **Nerve injuries:** Erb's or Klumpke's palsy due to injury to cervical and brachial plexus.
         - **Vessels injury: Hematoma formation**
      iii. **Birth asphyxia**

MULTIPLE GESTATION: TWIN PREGNANCY

Multiple gestation: Twin pregnancy

1. When more than one fetus develops simultaneously in a mother's womb is called as multiple pregnancy
2. Twin pregnancy is the most common variety of multiple pregnancy.
3. Every multiple pregnancy is considered a high risk pregnancy.
4. **Types of twins**

   a. **Monozygotic/identical:** Single embryo divided into two (same sex, no of placenta depends on timing of division.

Time of division	**Morula stage** (cleavage within 1-3 days)	**Blastocyst** (cleavage within 4-8 days)	**Implanted blastocyst** (cleavage within 8-13 days)	**Formed embryonic disc** (cleavage within 13-14 days)
No of Amnion and chorion	Diamniotic and dichorionic	Mono chorionic and diamniotic	Monoamniotic and monochorionic	Conjoined twins

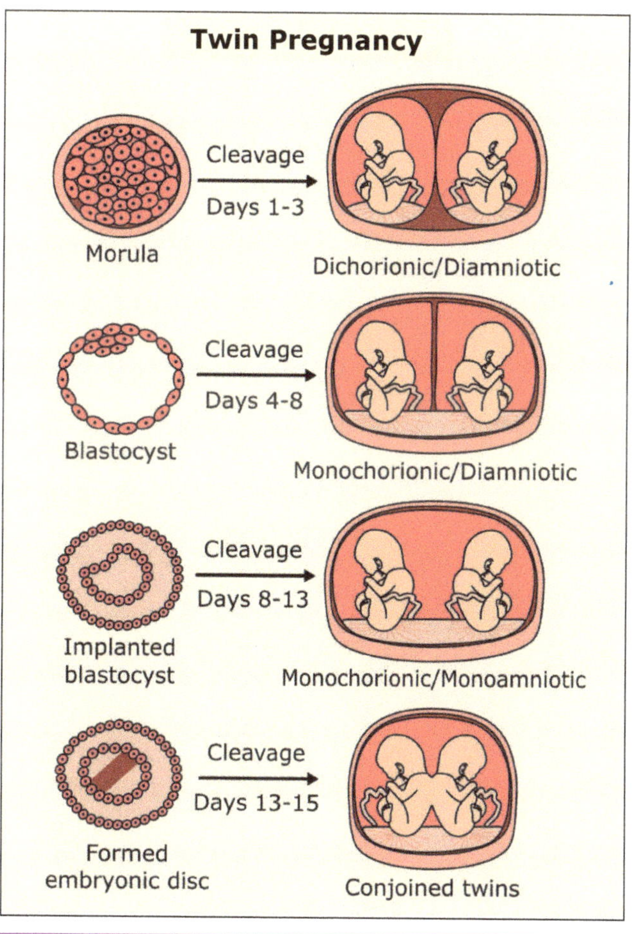

b. **Dizygotic/non identical:** In dizygotic sac each fetus is separated by separate amnion and chorion, two placenta which either completely separated or fused marginally appears single most commonly seen in IVF.

5. **Risk factors**
   a. **Heredity:** Mother's family history may be significant.
   b. **Fertility drugs and assisted reproductive techniques:** Gonadotropin used in fertility treatment and AFT increases the chances of multiple pregnancy
   c. **Maternal age and number of pregnancies:** Increases the frequency of twins.
6. **Diagnosis:**
   a. **Abdominal examination (Difficult to palpate or auscultate due to hydramnios)**
      i. Barrel shaped and unduly more elongated abdomen
      ii. Height of uterus more than the period of amenorrhea
      iii. Abdominal girth is more than normal at term
      iv. Finding of two fetal head
      v. Finding of too many fetal parts on palpation
      vi. Two different heart sounds are heard at two different spots by auscultation.
   b. **Sonography: Confirmation of diagnosis**
7. **Management:** This is a high risk pregnancy so it should be managed in a well equipped hospital in presence of skilled obstetricians and neonatologists.

Antenatal management	**In labor management** (Vaginal delivery is conducted if first presenting baby is in vertex presentation)
1. **Nutritional diet** 2. **Increased rest to avoid preterm labor after 24 weeks** 3. **Careful mother and fetal monitoring** 4. **Supplementation therapy:** Folic acid and iron supplementation	1. **Conduct the delivery of the first baby as like a normal delivery process.** 2. **Don't give methergine** 3. **Note down the lie of second baby** 4. **If the second baby in transverse lie then do the external version preferably in cephalic than podalic.** 5. **If fails then internal version under general anesthesia** 6. **If necessary do ARM or infusion oxytocin drip for augmentation of labor.** 7. **Watch for cord prolapse** 8. **Monitor the fetus intermittently** 9. **Deliver the second baby within 30 min of first delivery.** 10. **If second baby in longitudinal lie then with** a. **Vertex presentation** If vertex is low down then forceps delivery If vertex is high up ventouse or internal version b. **Breech presentation** Breech extraction

Pre-requesting for normal delivery	Indications for cesarean section
1. At least the first twin is with vertex presentation 2. Labor ward with sonography facility 3. Well equipped neonatal unit 4. Skilled obstetricians 5. Neonatologist 6. Blood units (at least one unit of cross matched) should be readily available.	1. Severe pre-eclampsia 2. Placenta previa 3. Contracted pelvis 4. Cord prolapse after delivery of first baby 5. Non cephalic presentation in both fetuses 6. IUGR or conjoined twins 7. Monoamniotic twins 8. Monochorionic twins with twin to twin transfusion syndrome.

8. Complications

Maternal	Fetal
1. Preterm labor **2. PIH and pre-eclampsia** **3. Hydramnios** **4. Antepartum hemorrhage** **5. Malpresentation** **6. Postpartum hemorrhage** **7. Increased operative interference** **8. Severe anemia** **9. Hyperemesis** **10. Gestational diabetes**	**1. Preterm birth** **2. Miscarriage** **3. Congenital malformation** **4. Cord prolapse** **5. Increased perinatal mortality** **6. Low birth weight (**Due to intrauterine growth retardation and preterm birth) **7. Monochorionic pregnancy complications** (Twin twin transfusion syndrome, twin anemia polycythemia sequence, selective fetal growth restriction)

ABORTION

1. **Definition:** Abortion is defined as the spontaneous or induced termination of pregnancy before fetal viability
2. Most the miscarriage/spontaneous abortion occurs within 20 weeks of gestation.
3. Cut off gestational age for abortion is 20 weeks
4. **Types of abortion**
   a. **Induced:** Classified as therapeutic (Done in response to a health condition of the woman or fetus) or elective (Chosen for other reasons).
   b. **Spontaneous abortion:** Miscarriage, also known as spontaneous abortion and pregnancy loss.
5. **Factors responsible for miscarriage**
   a. **Maternal factors**
      i. **Infections**
      ii. **Anatomical abnormalities:**
         a. Cervical incompetence and insufficiency
         b. Congenital malformation of uterus
         c. Uterine fibroid
      iii. **Medical disorders:** Risk factors associated with miscarriage are uncontrolled diabetes mellitus, thyroid disease, and systemic lupus erythematosus.
      iv. **Social and behavioral factors:**
         a. Alcohol consumption
         b. Regular and heavy smoking
      v. **Dietary:** Miscarriage risk less in women who consume a diet rich in fruits, vegetables, whole grains, vegetable oils, and fish
      vi. **Weight:** Obesity is also a risk factor
      vii. **Occupational and environmental factors:**
         a. **Occupational factors: Anesthetic agents, aniline, lead**
         b. **Environmental toxins** include dichlorodiphenyl trichloroethane (DDT), bisphenol A, phthalates etc.
      viii. **Surgical Procedures:** The risk of miscarriage caused by surgery is not well known but invasive prenatal genetic tests may increase risk of miscarriage.
      ix. **Unexplained**
   b. **Fetal factors**
      i. Chromosomal abnormality

ii. Numerical defect like trisomy, polyploidy monosomy

iii. Structural defect like translocation, deletion, inversion

iv. Multiple fetal pregnancy

v. Degeneration of villi

c. **Paternal factors:** Risk of abortion is increase with increase in paternal age but this association is not clear.

6. **Spontaneous Abortion Clinical Classification:**

a. **Threatened Abortion:** Condition in which the miscarriage has started but not progressed to state from which recovery is impossible (Recovery can be possible).

b. **Incomplete Abortion:** The miscarriage process already takes place, but entire product of conception are not expelled out and a some part of it is left inside the uterine cavity.

Bleeding follows partial or complete placental separation and dilation of the cervical os.

c. **Complete Abortion:** Complete expulsion of the entire products of conceptions and the cervical os subsequently closes

d. **Missed Abortion:** In this type dead products of conception that have been retained for days or weeks in the uterus with a closed cervical os.

e. **Inevitable Abortion:** In this type of abortion where the changes have progressed to a state from where continution of pregnancy is impossible

7. **Clinical types of abortion**

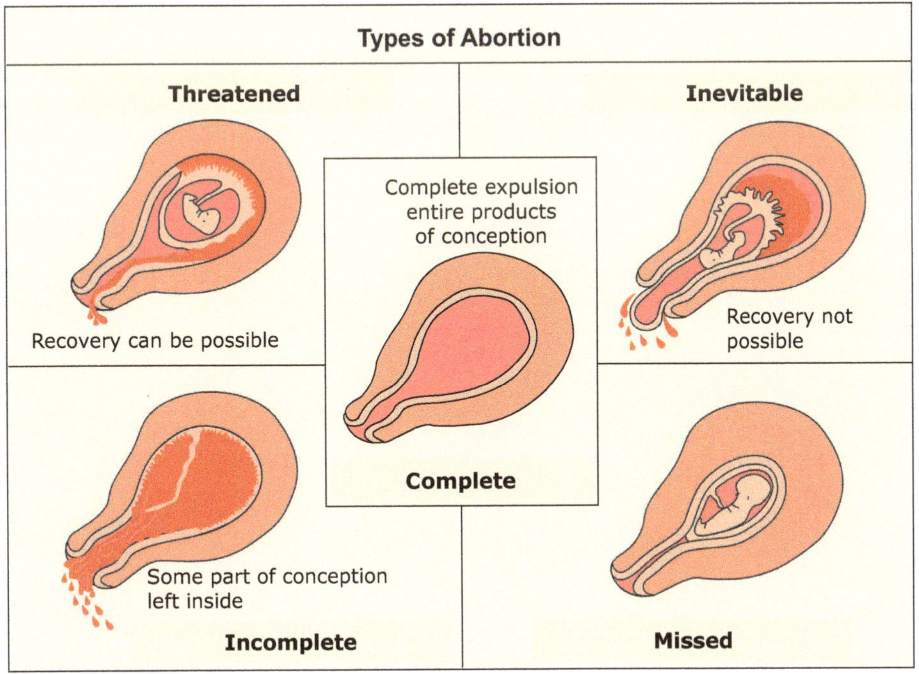

Clinical type of abortion	Clinical features	Management
Threatened abortion	**S**light PV bleeding, usually painless **M**ild backache or Dull aching pain in lower abdomen. **U**terus and cervix feels soft **I**nternal os (Orifice) is closed **U**ltrasound is diagnostic if USG is available then the pelvic examination is avoided.	**R**est **R**elief of pain **M**ost of pregnancy with threatened abortion go up to term **I**f pregnancy continues there may be chances of premature labor, placenta previa, IUGR.
Inevitable abortion	**P**V bleeding **C**olicky pain in lower abdomen **O**n digital examination: Internal os is open **O**n internal examination the product of conception can be felt.	**E**xcessive bleeding controlled by the Methergin 0.2 mg **I**V fluids and blood products for blood loss **I**f pregnancy is < 12 weeks, **suction and evacuation** is done **I**f pregnancy is > 12 weeks then expulsion by the **oxytocin infusion**
Incomplete abortion	**H**istory of Expulsion of fleshy mass out of vagina **C**ontinues pain in lower abdomen **P**ersistent vaginal bleeding **I**n internal examination: a. Uterus smaller than the period of amenorrhea b. Open internal os c. Per vaginal bleeding: Present with varying amount d. Expelled mass is incomplete	**T**ab Misoprostol 200 μg is used vaginally every 4 hourly **P**rophylactic Antibiotics is given **E**vacuation of retained products of conception. **E**arly abortion: **Dilation and evacuation** under general anesthesia or analgesia **L**ate abortion: Evacuation done under general anesthesia**, D&C** is done to remove the remnant of product of conceptus of tissue which are left inside the uterus.
Complete abortion	**H**istory of expulsion of fleshy mass out of vagina followed by **a. A**bdominal pain subsided **b. V**aginal bleeding becomes trace or absent **I**nternal examination reveals a. Uterus smaller than the period of amenorrhea b. Cervical os is **closed** c. Bleeding is trace d. Transvaginal sonography confirms the uterus is empty.	

(Continued)

Clinical type of abortion	Clinical features	Management
Missed abortion	The patient presents with features of threatened abortion followed by the following symptoms: **a.** Cervix feels firm and internal os closed **b.** Symptoms are disappeared **c.** Uterus becomes smaller in size **d.** Non-audibility of the fetal heart sound even with doppler ultrasound **e.** Immunological tests for pregnancy become negative	A] Uterus < 12 weeks: **1.** Prostaglandin E1 (Misoprostol) 800 mg is given vaginally and repeated after 24 hours if needed **2.** Expulsion occurs within 48 hours **3.** Suction evacuation done when medical method fails B] Uterus more than 12 weeks 1. 6 or 12 hourly Misoprostol tablets given vaginally 2. If this fails, then extra-amniotic instillation of solution of Ethacridine lactate is used 3. Antibiotics are given

8. **Various Regimens for Medical Termination of Pregnancy:**
   a. **First Trimester:**
      i. Mifepristone/Misoprostol
      ii. Misoprostol
      iii. Methotrexate/Misoprostol
   b. **Second Trimester**
      i. Mifepristone/Misoprostol
      ii. Misoprostol
      iii. Dinoprostone
      iv. Concentrated Oxytocin
9. **Septic abortion:**
   a. An infection of the placenta and fetus of a previable pregnancy.
   b. Septic abortion cases are now become rare.
   c. Infection is present in the placenta and there is a risk of spread to the uterus.
   d. Sepsis may develop in septic abortion which have serious complications .
   e. **Causative organism:**
      i. Most bacteria involved in septic abortion are part of the normal vaginal flora e.g. E. coli, klebseilla, anerobic streptococci, clostridium welchii etc.
      ii. Some infections are very serious and lead to severe necrotizing infections and toxic shock syndrome caused by group A streptococcus-S pyogenes.

f. **Signs and symptoms:**
   i. High grade fever
   ii. Chills
   iii. Severe abdominal pain
   iv. Prolonged or heavy vaginal bleeding
   v. Foul smelling discharge.
   vi. Hypotension
   vii. leukocytosis.

g. **Laboratory investigation**
   i. Complete blood count: Leukocytosis
   ii. Renal function test
   iii. Liver function test
   iv. Coagulation studies: PT, a PTT & fibrogen

h. **Radiological Investigation**
   i. Ultrasonography: To confirm specific location & origin of septic abortion
   ii. CT or MRI scan: To reveal findings of septic abortion

i. **Management:**
   i. Admit the patient
   ii. Start fluid resuscitation with intravenous fluids to maintain normal blood pressure .
   iii. Symptomatic treatment: Analgesic and antipyretics
   iv. Start broad spectrum antibiotics
   v. Suction and curettage: Performed to remove retained products of conception from the uterus .
   vi. Hysterectomy: If multiple abscesses are developed in the uterus, ovaries and fallopian tube.
   vii. Septic shock: Inotropic and respiratory support may be required.

j. **Complication:** If septic shock is not treated effectively and quickly then the patient may die.
   i. Septic shock
   ii. Acute respiratory distress syndrome
   iii. Renal failure
   iv. Disseminated intravascular coagulation
   v. Abscess formation

ECTOPIC PREGNANCY

Definition: Any pregnancy where the fertilized ovum gets implanted and develops outside the normal uterine cavity.

1. Normally, ovum and sperm meet in a fallopian tube and a fertilised egg implants into the uterus.
2. If implantation does not happen in the uterus then fertilised egg starts growing in the fallopian tube, rarely in ovary and very rarely in abdomen.
3. In nearly 95-97% of ectopic pregnancies fertilized egg are implanted in the various segments of the fallopian tube.
4. The remaining 5 percent of non-tubal ectopic pregnancies implant in the ovary, peritoneal cavity, cervix, or prior cesarean scar

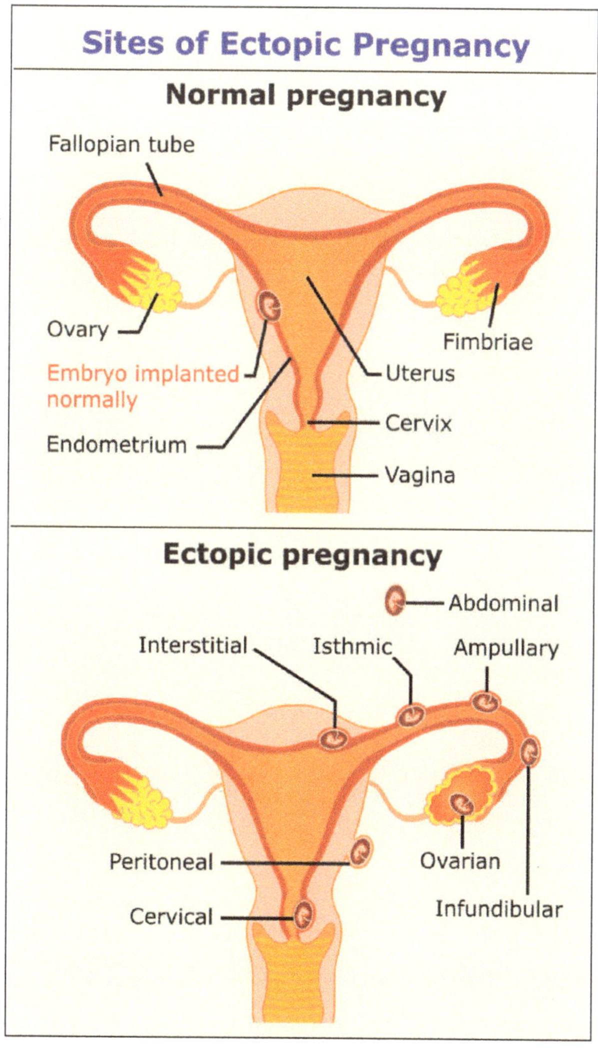

5. In a multifetal pregnancy one fertilised egg implanted in normal uterine cavity implantation and other implanted ectopically.
6. A ruptured ectopic tubal pregnancy is a surgical emergency.
7. **Etiology:**
   a. **Acquired:**
      i. Pelvic inflammatory disease (PID)
      ii. Scarring to the fallopian tubes (possibly from a ruptured appendix or previous pelvic surgery)
      iii. IUD use
      iv. Contraception failure
      v. Assisted reproductive technology (ART)
      vi. Endometriosis
      vii. A history of a sexually transmitted infection (STI)
      viii. A prior ectopic pregnancy
      ix. Genital tuberculosis
   b. **Congenital**
      i. **Tubal developmental defect:** Tubal hypoplasia, elongation, accessory ostia.
      ii. Tortuosity
      iii. Partial stenosis
      iv. Intramural polyps
   c. **Other risk factors:**
      i. Age 35-45 years
      ii. Cigarette smoking
8. **Clinical features:**
   a. The onset is acute
   b. Patient have **classic triad of symptoms** in tubal ectopic pregnancy
      i. **Lower abdominal pain**
      ii. **Amenorrhea (Positive pregnancy test)**
      iii. **Vaginal bleeding**
   c. With tubal rupture, lower abdominal and pelvic pain is usually becomes severe and frequently described as sharp, stabbing, or tearing type.
   d. Tenderness is present on abdominal palpation

e. If bleeding is mild then no symptoms and signs appear

f. If a patient has severe internal hemorrhage then the patient has clinical features of hypovolemic shock such as tachycardia, hypotension, pallor, cold and clammy extremities, dizziness.

g. In severe abdominal bleeding due to diaphragmatic irritation patient may have neck or shoulder pain specially on inspiration.

9. **Diagnosis:**

a. Diagnosis depends on history, detailed examination and investigation.

b. Take detailed history of obstetrics, contraception, previous surgery, addiction (e.g. smoking) and other relevant history

c. **To identify ectopic pregnancy, consider following important:**

i. **Physical findings**

ii. **Transvaginal sonography**

iii. **Serum beta hCG**

iv. **Diagnostic procedure (dilations and curettage, laparoscopy)**

v. **Laparotomy (occasionally): Useful in diagnosis (If doubtful)**

d. Rupture ectopic pregnancy undergo prompt surgical therapy

10. **Investigations**

a. **Routine investigations:** CBC, blood grouping and cross match, ESR

b. **Transvaginal sonography:** Performed to look for uterine or ectopic pregnancy.

c. **Serum beta hCG:** When the B-hCG value is greater than 1, 500 IU/L and sonography suggestive of empty uterine cavity, then mostly likely consider ectopic pregnancy.

d. **Laparoscopy:** Used for confirmation of diagnosis, removal of ectopic mass and can be used for direct injection of chemotherapeutic injection inside mass.

e. **Dilatation and curettage:** Performed once the pregnancy has been determined to be non-viable or in case its location cannot be verified on USG.

f. **Serum progesterone:** Level > 25 ng/ml indicate of viable intrauterine pregnancy and if < 5 ng/ml suggestive of an ectopic pregnancy.

g. **Laparotomy:** It is useful in doubtful condition as it gives direct visualisation.

11. **Management:**

a. **In unruptured ectopic pregnancy**

i. **Expectant:** Spontaneus resolution is possible if

- Initial serum hCG level less than 1000 IU/L

- Subsequent falling hCG level
- Ectopic mass diameter is < 4 cm.
- No evidence of bleeding or rupture on TVS.

ii. **Medical:**

- **Direct local:**
  1. **Methotrexate:** Under the guidance of sonography or laparoscopy.
  2. **Potassium chloride**
- **Systemic:**
  1. **Methotrexate: Single dose of methotrexate is given 1 mg/kg IM**
  2. **Actinomycin**

iii. **Surgical:**

- **Laparoscopy/Laparotomy**
  1. **Salpingostomy:** Made in fallopian tube and incision line kept open without sutures to heal it by secondary intention.
  2. **Salpingotomy:** Similar to salpingostomy but the incision line is closed by the sutures.
  3. **Salpingectomy:** Surgical removal of fallopian tube.

b. **In ruptured ectopic pregnancy**

i. In ruptured ectopic pregnancy there is internal hemorrhage patient may require blood transfusion depending on hematocrit level or hemoglobin

ii. Emergency treatment includes oxygen supply, fluid administration.

iii. In severe cases inotropic & mechanical ventilatory support may be required.

iv. Urgent surgery is indicated to stop ongoing blood loss and correction.

PLACENTAL ABRUPTION

1. **Definition:** The bleeding occurs due to premature separation (Partially or totally) of normally situated placenta i.e. implantation site.
2. It is a form of antepartum hemorrhage.
3. Abruption likely begins with rupture of a decidual spiral artery and then an expanding retroplacental hematoma develops which causes separation of placenta and compression of adjacent placenta.
4. Bleeding is almost always maternal.
5. Sometimes placental tears may cause fetal bleeding.
6. **Varieties of placenta abruptions:**

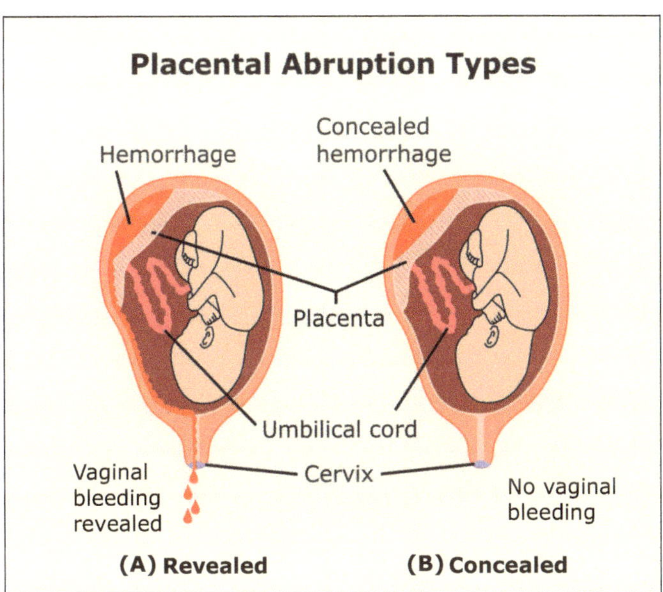

   a. **Concealed:**
      i. The blood collects behind the separated placenta
      ii. Blood does not become visible due to the presenting part.
   b. **Revealed:**
      i. The most common type
      ii. Blood becomes visible externally, coming out of the cervical canal.
   c. **Mixed:** In this type of abruption some parts collect inside and some become visible.

7. **Risk factors:**
   a. **Prior abruption:** Risk of recurrence for a woman with previous abruption
   b. Increased maternal age and parity
   c. Pre-eclampsia
   d. Chronic hypertension
   e. Chorioamnionitis
   f. Preterm ruptured membranes (PROM)
   g. Muti-fetal gestation
   h. Low birthweight
   i. Hydramnios
   j. Cigarette smoking (vasospasm)
   k. Single umbilical artery
   l. **Cocaine use:** Associated with increased risk of transient hypertension, vasospasm, placental abruption uterine leiomyoma.
8. **Clinical features:**
   a. In the early stages of placental abruption, there may be no symptoms
   b. Afterward the symptoms develop suddenly.
   c. Common symptoms include
      i. Sudden onset of abdominal pain or back pain
      ii. Uterine contractions that are continuous and do not stop
      iii. Vaginal bleeding (Bright red or dark)
      iv. Decreased fetal heart rate
      v. Decreased fetal movement
      vi. Enlargement of the uterus that is not appropriate to the gestational age.
   d. Clinical features of hypotensive shock: Hypotension, pallor, decreased urine output.
9. **Diagnosis:**
   a. **Mainly clinical findings**
   b. **Ultrasonography:** Even negative findings with USG examination do not rule out placental abruption.

c. **MRI may be helpful**

d. **Laboratory Tests:**

   i. **Complete blood count:** Low Hb

   ii. **Coagulation profile:** Clotting time increased, Fibrinogen level may be low, thrombocytopenia, Increased in partial thromboplastin time

   iii. **Urine for protein:** Proteins may present

10. **Management: maternal hospitalisation with continuous monitoring of fetus and maternal status.**

   a. **Assessment of the patient is done on following points:**

      i. Total amount of blood loss

      ii. Whether the patient is in labor or not (usually labor starts)

      iii. Maturity of fetus

      iv. Presence of any maternal complication along with type and grade of placental abruption.

   b. **Management in emergency**

      i. IV fluids like Ringer's solution drip is started

      ii. Arrange blood and blood products for transfusion if needed

      iii. Blood grouping

      iv. Blood investigations

      v. Close monitoring of maternal and fetal condition is done.

   c. **Definitive treatment: Immediate delivery**

      i. **If the patient is in labor:** Accelerate the labor by low rupture of the membranes and oxytocin drip if needed.

      ii. If patient is not in labor then

         - **Induction of labor**

            1. Done by low rupture of membranes.
            2. Oxytocin may be added.
            3. Inj. oxytocin 10 IU IV (slow) or IM or Inj. methergine 0.2 mg IV is given after delivery of baby to minimize postpartum blood loss.
            4. Oxytocics should be used to improve the uterine tone.

- **Cesarean section (Indication)**
    1. Fetal distress,
    2. Maternal hemodynamic instability.
    3. Severe abruption with live fetus

11. The major complications of placental abruption are:

   a. **Hemorrhagic shock**

   b. **DIC**

   c. **Renal failure**

   d. **Uterine atony and postpartum hemorrhage.**

PLACENTA PREVIA

1. In some women a placenta that is implanted in the lower uterine segment, either over or very near the internal cervical os.
2. In presence of placenta previa chances of bleeding are higher in second trimester.
3. It accounts 1/3 cases of antepartum hemorrhage
4. **The high risk factors for placenta previa are–**
   a. **Multiparity:** Elevates the risk for previa
   b. **Higher risk is associted with advanced maternal age (> 35 years)**
   c. **Smoking during pregnancy:** Carbon monoxide induced hypoxemia is responsible for placental hypertrophy
   d. **History of previous cesarean section**
   e. **Any other scar in the uterus** (Myomectomy or hysterectomy) or Prior dilation and curettage which have endometrial damage.
   f. **Women with large placental size:** (Big surface area of the placenta as in twins or erythroblastosis may lie in the lower segment).
   g. **Assisted reproductive technology (ART):** Used for conception elevates the risks for low lying placenta.
5. **Types of placenta previa:** It is divided into four types, depending upon degree of placenta covered internal opening of cervix.

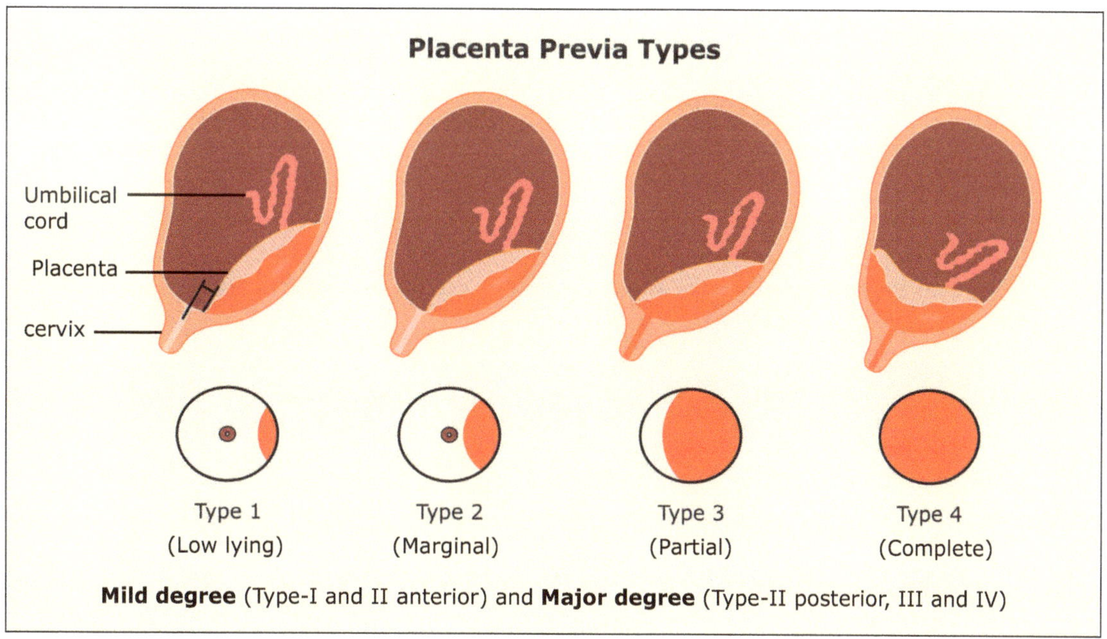

Mild degree (Type-I and II anterior) and **Major degree** (Type-II posterior, III and IV)

6. **For a clinical purpose, Types are graded into two:**
   a. **Mild degree (Type-I and II anterior)**
      i. **Type I (Low-lying):** Most part of the placenta lies on the upper segment and only the lower margin encroaches onto the lower segment but not up to the os.
      ii. **Type II anterior**
   b. **Major degree (Type-II posterior (Dangerous type), III and IV)**
      i. **Type II (Marginal):** In this the placenta reaches the margin of the internal os but does not cover it.
      ii. **Type III (Incomplete or partial central):** The placenta covers the internal os partially not completely.
      iii. **Type IV (Central or total):** The placenta completely covers the internal os even after it is fully dilated.
7. **Clinical features:**
   a. The only symptom of placenta previa is vaginal bleeding
   b. Bleeding is sudden in onset, painless (With pain if labor start simultaneously)
   c. Bleeding is bright red due to bleeding from uteroplacental sinuses.
   d. Bleeding is apparently causeless and recurrent.
   e. In the start the bleeding is mild as placental separation increases the bleeding increases.
   f. Bleeding usually start in a second trimester or later, but it can begin even before midpregnancy
8. **Diagnosis:** History may reveal the antepartum hemorrhage and sonography is confirmatory.
   a. **Localization of Placenta (Placentography)**
      i. **Sonography: Ultrasonography is the initial procedure either to confirm or to rule out the diagnosis.**
         - Transabdominal ultrasound (TAS)
         - Transvaginal ultrasound (TVS) (more superior than TAS)
         - Color doppler flow study
         - Transperineal ultrasound
      ii. **Magnetic resonance imaging (MRI):** For better diagnosis of placenta previa and placenta previa accreta

b. **Clinical examination:**

  i. If sonography is not readily available in the institute, diagnosis done by clinical examination.

  ii. A digital examination should not be done without planning to avoid severe hemorrhage.

  iii. A digital examination is done in an operating room and with preparations for immediate cesarean delivery (Double set technique).

9. **Management:** A placenta previa is managed based on fetal age and maturity, labor, and bleeding severity.

A] Immediate management:

1. Admit the patient
2. Assessment of blood loss by general condition, pallor, pulse rate and blood pressure.
3. Blood samples are collected for routine blood investigation along with blood grouping and cross match.
4. A large bore IV cannula inserted and Ringer lactate or normal saline infusion is started.
5. Abdominal examination for any uterine tenderness and auscultation to note the fetal heart rate.
6. Inspection of the vulva to note the presence of any active bleeding.
7. Confirmation of diagnosis is made from the history, physical examination and with sonographic examination.

B] Expectant management:

1. The expectant treatment is helpful to get more time for fetal maturity
2. But during this time period special care & observation to be done to avoid complications.
3. The expectant treatment is carried up to 37 weeks of pregnancy.
4. The baby becomes sufficiently mature up to 37 weeks.
5. **Expectant management is carried out in cases who have**
   a. Active vaginal bleeding is absent
   b. Mother is with Hemoglobin > 10 g % and hematocrit > 30% level
   c. Duration of pregnancy is less than 37 weeks
   d. Fetal well-being is assured (CTG and USG).

6. Preterm delivery may have to be done in conditions:
   a. Recurrence of severe hemorrhage and which is continuing
   b. The fetus is dead.

C] Definite management:

1. The definitive management is delivery.

a. Vaginal delivery is done when sonography suggestive of placental edge is clearly 2-3 cm away

b. Cesarean delivery is done when sonography suggestive of placental edge is within 2 cm from internal os.

POSTPARTUM HEMORRHAGE

1. Any amount of bleeding from genital tract of the mother after delivery of the child which compromises her reserve capacity, more than 500 ml for vaginal birth and above 1000 ml for LSCS
2. Early PPH within 24 hours
3. Secondary PPH after 24 upto 6 weeks
4. On the basis of amount bleeding PPH classified as follows:
   a. **Minor:** Blood loss greater than or equal to 500 ml within 24 hours after birth.
   b. **Severe:** Blood loss greater than or equal to 1000 ml within 24 hours after birth.
5. **Initial signs and symptoms of post partum hemorrhage**
   a. An increased heart rate
   b. Feeling faint upon standing
   c. Increased respiratory rate.
6. **Clinical features of hypovolemic shock will develop in patient with continuous heavy blood loss:** Cold extremities, low blood pressure and patient may become restless or unconscious.
7. **Postpartum hemorrhage (PPH) can be classified as**
   a. **Primary (early):** Primary PPH, the most common and severe, occurs within the first 24 hours after delivery
   b. **Secondary (late):** Secondary PPH occurs 24 hours to 12 weeks after delivery.
8. **Primary PPH is of two types:**
   a. **3rd stage hemorrhage:** Bleeding occurs before expulsion of placenta.
   b. **True postpartum hemorrhage:** Bleeding occurs following expulsion of placenta (Majority)
9. **Causes of primary PPH:**
   a. **Atonic uterus (80%):** (Failure of the uterus to contract properly after delivery)
   b. **Traumatic:** (Cervical, vaginal, or perineal lacerations)
   c. **Retained tissues:** Retained or adherent placental tissue
   d. **Coagulation disorder:** Due to formation of excessive fibrin
   e. **Inverted or ruptured uterus**

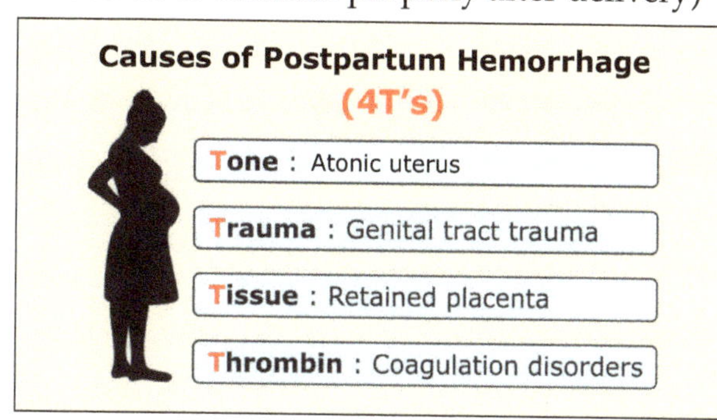

10. **Management of 3rd stage hemorrhage**

a. **Supportive management**

1. Keep the patient flat and warm.
2. Give oxygen by mask.
3. Insert two large bore (14 gauge) intravenous cannulas
4. Collect and send the blood for routine investigation and blood grouping and cross match.
5. Reserve 2 units (at least) of blood.
6. Start resuscitation with 1-2 liters of normal saline or ringer lactate.
7. Blood transfusion, if indicated.
8. Monitor vitals (pulse, blood pressure, oxygen saturation)

b. **Management of placental site bleeding**

1. Massage the uterus to make it hard.
2. If ongoing PV bleeding even after the uterus becomes hard then inspect genital tract for any injury.
3. Oxytocin 10 units IM or methergine 0.2 mg is given intravenously.
4. Start oxytocin drip solution (Normal saline or Ringer's solution) with oxytocin (1 L with 20 units) at 60 drops per minute.
5. Catheterize the bladder
6. If the placenta is separated remove it out by controlled cord traction method.
7. If the placenta is not separated remove it under general anesthesia

c. **Management of Traumatic bleeding**

Traumatic hemorrhage is managed by hemostatic suturing.

11. **Management of true PPH**

a. Feel the uterus by palpation

b. If uterus is atonic then

i. Massage the uterus to make it hard.

ii. Oxytocin 10 units IM/IV or Methergine 0.2 mg is given intravenously.

iii. Fluid resuscitation with intravenous fluids e.g. Normal saline or ringer lactate and Oxytocin is added in fluid.

iv. After placental expulsion look placenta and its membranes to understand any retention of product inside uterus.

v. Inspect genital tract of patient for any injury.

c. **If patient is still having atonic uterus**

i. Injection 15 methyl PGF2D 250 ug IM in the deltoid muscle every 15 minutes (Max upto 2 mg) **OR**

ii. Misoprostol (PGE1) 1000 Pg per rectum is effective **OR**

iii. Carbetocin 100

d. **Still uterus is atonic**

Then uterine tamponade is used

Any one method of following is used

i. **Tight intrauterine packing**

ii. **Balloon tamponade**

e. **If the above methods fail to control the PPH then surgical interventions required:**

i. Vascular ligation

ii. Uterine arterial embolization can be done using gel foam.

f. **Hysterectomy** is the final option when the uterus fails to contract and bleeding continues in spite of the above measures.

12. **Secondary PPH:**

a. Secondary PPH occurs 24 hours to 6 weeks after delivery.

b. Retained bits of cotyledon or membranes (most common) cause of secondary PPH.

c. **Causes:**

i. Retained bits of cotyledon or membranes.

ii. Uterine Infection

iii. Endometritis

iv. Hemorrhage from cesarean section wound.

d. **Internal examination:** Sepsis, subinvolution of the uterus and often an incompetence cervical os.

e. **Ultrasonography:** Useful in detecting the bits of placenta inside the uterine cavity.

f. **Blood investigation:** Anemia and sepsis

g. **Management:**

   i. IV antibiotics

   ii. **Retained bits of cotyledon or membranes:Immediately uterus is explored under general anesthesia**.

   iii. Suturing of sloughing wound.

   iv. If source of bleeding is cesarean section wound then laparotomy may be needed.

HYPERTENSIVE DISORDERS IN PREGNANCY

1. Hypertension that develops as a direct result of a gravid state is called pregnancy induced hypertension.
2. Gestational Hypertension is defined as having a blood pressure greater than 140/90 mm Hg on two separate occasions at least 6 hours apart.
3. If mother is having high BP during pregnancy then she will be at higher risk of developing complications.
4. Babies are also impacted with the high blood pressure.
5. Gestational hypertension can lead to a serious condition called pre-eclampsia.
6. In gestational Hypertension blood pressures reach 140/90 mm Hg or greater for the first time after mid-pregnancy, but in which proteinuria is not identified.
7. **Risk factors:**
   a. **Maternal causes**
      i. Obesity
      ii. First Pregnancy.
      iii. Mothers under 20 or over 40 years old
      iv. History of chronic Diabetes mellitus, hypertension (Particularly gestational hypertension) and renal disease
      v. Pre-existing hypertension, vascular disease
      vi. Thrombophilias
   b. **Pregnancy**
      i. Multiple pregnancy (Twins or triplets, etc.)
      ii. Placental abnormalities (Placental ischemia, hyperplacentosis)
   c. **Family history:** Family history of pre-eclampsia.
8. Four types of hypertensive diseases are described as follows
   a. **Pre-eclampsia and eclampsia syndrome**
   b. **Chronic hypertension of any etiology**
   c. **Pre-eclampsia superimposed on chronic hypertension**
   d. **Gestational hypertension** (Definitive evidence for the pre-eclampsia syndrome does not develop and hypertension resolve after 12 weeks postpartum)
9. Above classification differentiates the pre-eclampsia syndrome from other hypertensive disorders because it is potentially more ominous.

PRE-ECLAMPSIA

Definition:

a. Development of hypertension in pregnant women to the extent of 140/90 mm of Hg or more with proteinuria after 20 weeks of pregnancy in previously normotensive and non proteinuric women.

b. Pre-eclampsia is often silent, found unexpectedly in routine blood pressure and urine tests.

c. **Diagnosis of Pre-eclampsia [As per American College of Obstetricians and Gynecologists (ACOG)]:** Hypertension (BP > 140/90 mm Hg **after 20 weeks** in previously normotensive women) **plus**

   i. **Proteinuria** greater than or equal to 300 mg/24 h in urine **or**

   ii. **Urine dipstick:** 1 + persistent in random urine samples **or**

   iii. **Urine protein: creatinine:** Ratio greater than equal to 0.3

   Other diagnostic criteria (It is used in patients with new onset of hypertension but without proteinuria)

   1. **Thrombocytopenia:** Decreased platelet count
   2. **Renal insufficiency:** Creatinine level > 1.1 mg/dL or doubling of baseline
   3. **Liver involvement:** Serum transaminase levels twice normal
   4. **Cerebral and visual symptoms:** Headache, visual disturbances, convulsions.
   5. **Pulmonary edema (Fluid in lungs field): Crepitations heard in lung fields**

d. **Clinical features:**

Symptoms	Signs
Mild a. Slight swelling over the ankle b. Swelling may extend to the face, abdominal wall, vulva or over the whole body.	**Mild** a. Abnormal weight gain b. Raised blood pressure diastolic BP > 90 mm of Hg but < 110 mm of Hg
Alarming a. Headache b. Disturbed sleep c. Epigastric pain d. Diminished urine output e. Eye symptoms: blurring of vision, scotoma or at times a complete blindness. f. Cerebral symptoms: Headache, visual disturbances, convulsions.	**Alarming** a. Systolic BP 160 or higher or diastolic BP 110 or higher at two different occasions at least 4 hours apart. **b. Thrombocytopenia:** Platelet count < 1 lac./LL **c. Renal insufficiency:** Creatinine level > 1.1 mg/dL or doubling of baseline **d. Liver involvement:** Serum transaminase levels twice normal **e. Pulmonary edema: Auscultatory crepitations**

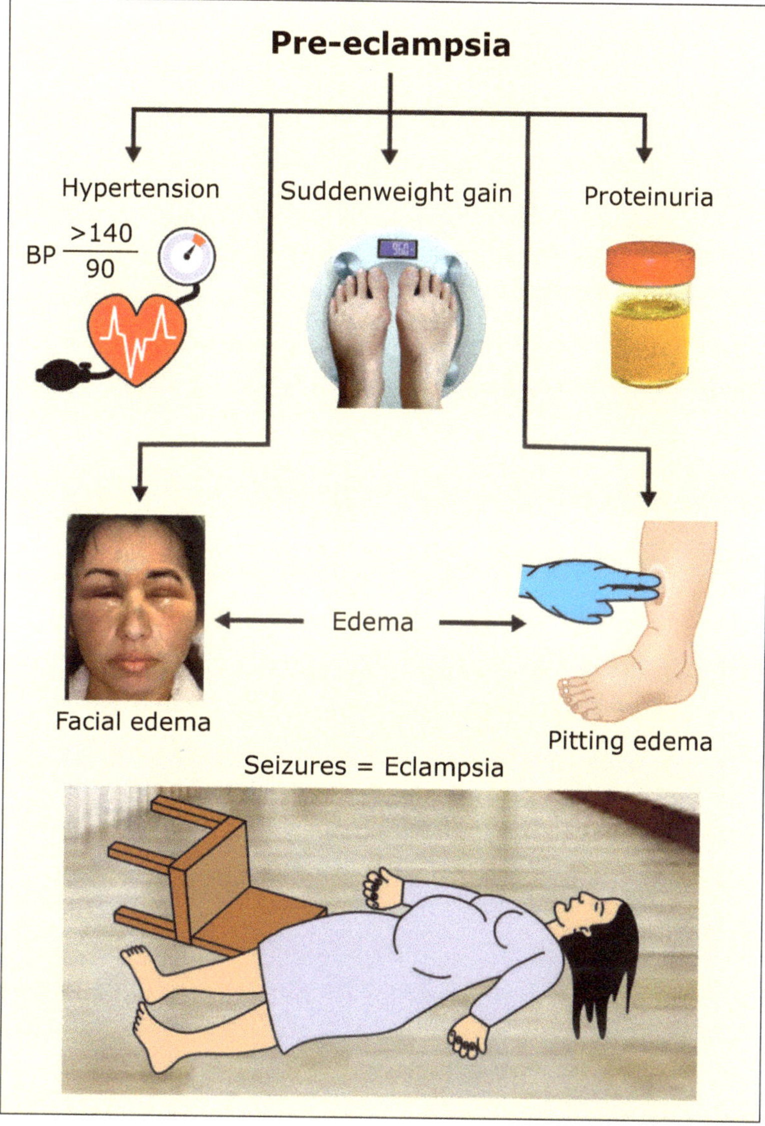

e. **Investigations:**

   i. **Blood investigations: CBC, serum creatinine, liver enzymes.**

   ii. **Urine examination: Urine protein in 24 hours collection.**

   iii. **Ophthalmic examination:** Ocular involvement is commonly seen in the majority of cases of pregnancy induced hypertension.

   iv. **Antenatal fetal monitoring:** Ultrasonographic evaluation for estimated fetal weight, amniotic fluid index, non stress test and biophysical profile if NST is negative.

f. **Management:**

i. The definitive treatment for pre-eclampsia is delivery of the baby and placenta.

ii. The timing of delivery depends on the maturity of the baby and risks for the mother.

iii. The severity of disease and the maturity of the baby are important factors which are considered in management

iv. Treatment can range from expectant management to delivery of baby by induction of labor or cesarean section

v. Antihypertensive agents

g. **General management:**

i. **Prophylactic measure:**

1. Mild-to moderate hypertension are managed at home
2. Outpatient management continues till the patient does not have worsening signs and symptoms and no harm to a fetus.
3. Calcium supplementation
4. Antioxidant vitamin E, C
5. Diet supplementation with fish oil, magnesium, zinc.
6. Low salt diet
7. Prophylactic low dose of aspirin (150 mg daily) is given for the prevention of pre-eclampsia in women at high risk and it is recommended to start before 20 weeks of pregnancy.

ii. **Observations:**

Maternal	Fetal
Blood pressure twice daily Urine volume and proteinuria daily Body weight twice daily Fundus examination once in week for ocular involvement Daily observation of edema Blood investigation at the time of admission.	Daily fetal movement count Serial USG doppler Non stress test and biophysical profile

iii. Medication to control blood pressure

1. Antihypertensives given for urgent control of hypertension:

Drug	Dose	Comment
Labetalol	IV 10-20 mg, then 20-80 mg every 20-30 min to a maximum dose of 300 mg Or Constant infusion 1-2 mg/min IV	Consider first line of drug Tachycardia and adverse effects are less. Contraindicated in the patient with asthma, congestive heart failure
Hydralazine	5 mg IV or IM then 5-10 mg IV every 20-40 min Or Constant infusion of 0.5 -10 mg/hour	Higher and frequent dosage are associated with hypotension, headaches, fetal distress may be more common than others.
Nifedipine	10-20 mg orally repeated in 30 min if needed then 10-20 mg every 2-6 hours	May observe reflex tachycardia and headache

2. Common oral antihypertensives in pregnancy:

Drug	Dosages	Comment
Labetalol	200-2400 mg/day orally in 2 or 3 divided dosage.	Well tolerated Avoided in asthma and congestive heart failure patients.
Nifedipine	30-120 mg/day orally in slowly release preparation	Do not sublingual form
Methyldopa	0.5-3 gm/day in 2-3 divided dosage	May not be useful in control of severe hypertension Childhood safety data upto 7 years of age

iv. Contraindications to conservative management:

1. Persistent symptoms or severe hypertension
2. Eclampsia, HELLP syndrome
3. Significant renal dysfunction
4. Pulmonary edema
5. Coagulopathy
6. Abruption
7. Previable fetus
8. Fetal compromise Present.

h. **Curative measures:**

i. The definitive treatment for pre-eclampsia is delivery of the baby and placenta.

ii. Conservative management for severe pre-eclampsia at < 34 weeks

1. Admit to labor ward
2. Maternal and fetal assessment
3. Consider $MgSO_4$
4. Treat dangerous hypertension
5. No contraindication should be present for conservative management

iii. If any contraindication for conservative management is present then conduct the delivery.

iv. If contraindications are not present then Initial 24-48 hour observation with

1. Daily maternal assessment
2. Daily fetal assessment
3. Corticosteroids for lung maturation of fetus
4. Daily serial lab evaluation for renal and HELLP syndrome
5. If contraindication does not develop then continue ongoing inpatient management
6. If contraindication develops then deliver the baby, If not then deliver at 34 weeks.

v. **Modes of delivery:**

1. **Vaginal delivery may be conducted in the vertex presentation by**
   - **If cervix is favorable:** Amniotomy with oxytocin
   - **If the cervix is not favorable:** Prostaglandin vaginal tablets (PGE2).
   - The 2nd stage of labor may be shortened by forceps delivery.
2. **Cesarean section indicated in following conditions**
   - Fetal distress
   - Failure of induction of labor
   - Malpresentation
   - Contracted pelvis
   - Late deceleration with oxytocin challenge test.

3. **Postpartum care:**
    - Methergine (Ergometrine) is better avoided as it may increase the blood pressure
    - Close observation of mother for 48 hours
    - Antihypertensives are continued for 48 hours with decreasing dose

i. **Complications**

i. **Maternal complications**

1. Eclampsia
2. Postpartum hemorrhage
3. Shock
4. Sepsis

ii. **Fetal complications**

1. Intrauterine death
2. Asphyxia
3. Prematurity, IUGR

ECLAMPSIA

1. **Definition: Pre-eclampsia when complicated with grand mal seizures or coma is called eclampsia in absence of known neurological disorder.**
2. In pre-eclampsia patients may have complications like GTCS convulsions which raises the risk to mother and fetus.
3. Onset of convulsions in pre-eclampsia is eclampsia.
   a. Eclampsia is most common in the last trimester
   b. The seizures of eclampsia typically present during pregnancy and prior to delivery (the antepartum period) but may also occur during labor, intrapartum delivery or postpartum delivery.
   c. **Clinical findings with eclampsia:**
      i. **Generalised tonic clonic seizures:** May be violent
      ii. **Postictal confusion occurs after seizures**
      iii. **Coma of variable duration can occur**
      iv. **Increased respiratory rate, lactic acidemia, hypoxia.**
4. **Laboratory investigations:**
   a. CBC
   b. LFT
   c. RFT
   d. Urine analysis
   e. Serum electrolyte
   f. PT INR
   g. Blood grouping and cross match
   h. **Angiotensin II test:** Angiotensin II is infused intravenously and blood pressure is monitored, if blood pressure raised by 20 mm after infusion then consider test positive and if not then consider negative.
5. **Management of eclampsia:**
   a. **Maintain airway, breathing and circulation**
   b. **Oxygen administration**
   c. **Ventilatory support if required.**
   d. **Prevention of injury to patient in convulsions**
   e. **Management of hypertension:**
      i. Most commonly labetalol, hydralazine.
      ii. **Nifedipine** can be used but used cautiously with $MGSO_4$ as both in combination cause hypotension.
      iii. **For refractory hypertension:** Nitroglycerine or Nitroprusside may be used.

f. **Intravascular fluid management:** Crystalloid fluid administered according to CVP, PCWP, and urine output and if administered without monitoring then it may elevate the risk of pulmonary and cerebral edema.

g. **Control and prevent convulsions:**

   i. Convulsions are prevented and treated using magnesium sulfate.

   ii. The dosages for severe pre-eclampsia are the same as for eclampsia.

   iii. In labor and delivery patients may have convulsions, so women with pre-eclampsia-eclampsia usually are given magnesium sulfate during labor and for 24 hours postpartum.

   iv. It may be given intravenously by continuous infusion or intramuscularly by intermittent injection

Continuous intravenous infusion (zuspan or sibai)	**Intermittent intramuscular infusion**
Give 4 to 6 gm loading dose of magnesium sulfate diluted in 100 mL of IV fluid administered over 15 to 20 min. Begin 1 gm/hr to 2 g/hr in 100 mL of IV maintenance infusion. **Monitor for magnesium toxicity:** **A**ssess deep tendon reflexes **R**espiratory depression (12 respirations) **U**rine output (<30 ml/hour) **Ch**est pain, block **M**agnesium sulfate is discontinued 24 hr after delivery	Give 4 g of magnesium sulfate as a 20% solution intravenously at a rate not to exceed 1 gm/min Followed by 10 gm of 50% magnesium sulfate solution, one half (5 g) injected deeply in the upper outer quadrant of each buttock. **Maintenance dose:** Give 5 g of a 50% solution of magnesium sulfate injected deeply in the upper outer quadrant of alternate buttocks 4 hourly, but only after ensuring that: **magnesium toxicity** Magnesium sulfate is discontinued 24 hr after delivery

h. Prevent complications and Deliver a viable fetus to resolve the pre-eclampsia

HELLP SYNDROME
(HE- Hemolysis EL- Elevated liver enzymes LP- Low platelets)

1. It is a variant of severe pre-eclampsia
2. Platelets less than 1 lac
3. LFT enzymes are twice the normal level
4. **Management:**
   a. Admit the patient
   b. Control the blood pressure
   c. Stabilize the patient
   d. Anti-seizures prophylaxis
   e. Correct coagulation profile
   f. Fetal condition assessment and monitoring

GYNECOLOGICAL CAUSES OF ACUTE ABDOMEN AND ITS MANAGEMENT

1. In female patient presenting with acute abdomen must always consider both surgical and gynecological causes
2. **Common gynecological causes of acute abdomen**
   a. **Pelvic inflammatory disease**
   b. **Endometriosis**
   c. **Tubo-ovarian abscess**
   d. **Ovarian cyst**
   e. **Fibroid**
3. **Clinical features, investigation and treatment of common gynecological causes:**

Causes	Signs and symptoms	Investigations	Treatment
Pelvic inflammatory disease Inflammatory condition of pelvic cavity that may involve the uterus, fallopian tube, pelvic peritoneum, or pelvic vessels. **Common pathogens:** **G**onorrhea **C**hlamydia **M**ycoplasma	**B/L L**ower abdominal pain **V**aginal discharge **B**urning pain on micturition **P**ain in sex **B**leeding after sex **I**rregular and excessive vaginal bleeding **G**eneral symptoms anorexia, fever, malaise, nausea and vomiting	**L**aparoscopy has been accepted as the gold standard for diagnosis **P**elvic examination (Tenderness on palpation or movement of uterus and cervix) **B**lood culture **S**onography **C**omplete blood count **C**-reactive protein **E**rythrocyte sedimentation rate **C**hlamydial test **G**ram stain of endocervix	**Bed rest** **Analgesics** **Antibiotic regimen** **I**ntravenous fluids **T**reatment of sexual partner **Outpatient (Reevaluate after 48 hours):** Inj. Ceftriaxone 250 mg IM once with doxycycline 100mg BD for 14 days with or without metro 400 mg BD for 14 days **Inpatient (according to CDC 2006):** Cefoxitin 6 h IV BD for 2-4 days plus doxycycline 100 mg BD orally or IV 12 hourly. **OR** Clindamycin 900 mg IV every 8 hours plus gentamicin 2 mg/kg IV loading dose followed by 1.5 mg/kg IV maintenance dose every 8 hours.

(Continued)

Causes	Signs and symptoms	Investigations	Treatment
Endometriosis Presence of endometrial glands and stroma outside the normal location	**Symptoms:** **D**ysmenorrhea **D**eep seated pelvic pain **D**yspareunia **H**ematuria **D**ysuria **I**nfertility **Signs:** **T**enderness in cul de sac **N**odularity in cul de sac **A**dnexal masses **A**dnexal tenderness	**Investigation** **Laparoscopy** (Gold standard) **T**ransabdominal ultrasound scan **C**A -125 **C**T/MRI scan **C**olor doppler flow **C**ystoscopy **S**igmoidoscopy **A**nti-endometrial antibodies **TNF**	**Asymptomatic and minimal endometriosis** **O**bserve for 6-8 hours **I**nvestigate for sterility **Symptomatic case** **Drug treatment** **C**ombined oral contraceptive pills **O**ral progestogens **D**anazol **A**romatase inhibitors **G**onadotropin releasing hormone RU-486 **Minimal invasive surgery** Destruction of endometrial implants in < 3 cm by Diathermy, cauterization or vaporization by CO_2 or ND: YAG laser **Surgery** Laparotomy Total hysterectomy with B/l oophorectomy
Tubo-ovarian abscess It is a consequence of pelvic inflammatory disease.	**A**bdominal pain and/Pelvic pain **N**ausea and vomiting **F**ever and general malaise	**H**istory of PID **L**ump in lower abdomen **T**enderness on pelvic examination **P**alpable adnexal mass **U**ltrasound **L**aparoscopy (confirms diagnosis)	**I**ntravenous fluid administration **A**ntipyretics **B**road spectrum antibiotics **G**uided drainage of TOA within 24-48 hours.
Ovarian cyst (Fluid filled sac in ovary or other tissue) **Types:** **Functional** **F**ollicular cysts **C**orpus luteum cyst **P**olycystic ovarian disease **Pathological** Dermoid Cystadenomas Endometriomas **Complications** **T**orsion **R**upture **H**emorrhage	**A**bdominal pain **P**ainful sexual intercourse **P**elvic pain before or during the menstrual cycle **In the abdomen**, patients may feel Fullness, heaviness, pressure, swelling, or bloating. **N**ausea and vomiting **C**hanges in bladder frequency and difficulty in bowel movements	**H**istory **P**hysical examination **U**ltrasonography **C**T scan **M**RI scan **Blood test** CA125 to rule out ovarian cancer **P**regnancy test: Positive in corpus luteum cyst **L**aparoscopy	**W**aitful Observation (usg after 1 month) **H**ormonal birth control pills **N**SAIDs **Surgical** **L**aparoscopy (Keyhole surgery) **L**aparotomy

(Continued)

Causes	Signs and symptoms	Investigations	Treatment
Fibroid **(The most common benign tumor of uterus)** **Complications** **T**orsion **D**egenerative (hyaline (most common), cystic, fatty, calcific, red	**Symptoms:** **A**symptomatic **M**enstrual abnormality **D**ysmenorrhea **P**ain during sexual intercourse **S**ubfertility **R**ecurrent pregnancy loss **L**ower abdominal or pelvic **A**bdominal enlargement	**History** **Pelvic examination** **Investigation:** **U**ltrasound and color doppler **S**aline infusion sonography **M**agnetic resonance imaging **L**aparoscopy **H**ysteroscopy **HSG** (Filling defect can be seen) **U**terine curettage	a. **Present on uterus body** **Medical (To minimize blood loss)** **Antiprogesterone:** Mifepristone **A**ntigonadotropins: Danazol, gestrinone etc. **G**nRH analogs: Gonadorelin, Buserelin, Goserelin etc. **C**ombined oral contraception **L**NG-IUS **P**rostaglandin synthetase inhibitors: Naproxen, Indomethacin, Aspirin etc. **S**elective progesterone receptor modulator: Mifepristone, Ulipristal, Asoprisnil etc. **Surgical** **M**yomectomy (Endoscopic or laparotomy) **H**ysterectomy **M**yolysis (Electrocautery, laser or cryo) **E**mbolotherapy b. **Present on cervix** **Supravaginal: Myomectomy or hysterectomy** **Vaginal:** Myomectomy or polypectomy

GYNECOLOGICAL CAUSES OF ABNORMAL UTERINE BLEEDING AND ITS MANAGEMENT

1. **Definition:** In absence of pregnancy, vaginal bleeding that occurs from the corpus that is abnormal in regularity, volume, frequency or duration.
2. Excessive blood loss negatively affects the person's quality of life.

Normal menstrual bleeding parameters	Abnormal uterine bleeding parameter
a. **Cycle interval:** 28 days (21-35)	1. **Cycle period** > 38 days or <24 days.
b. **Menstrual flow:** 4-5 days	2. **Menstrual flow:** > 7 days
c. **Menstrual blood loss:** 35 ml (20-80 ml)	3. **Blood loss:** > 80 ml.

3. Abnormal menstrual bleeding divided in two types
   a. **Acute:** In acute AUB urgent intervention requires.
   b. **Chronic:** Bleeding since the last 6 months but in chronic type acute bleeding may occur.
4. **PALM and COEIN classification of abnormal uterine bleeding**

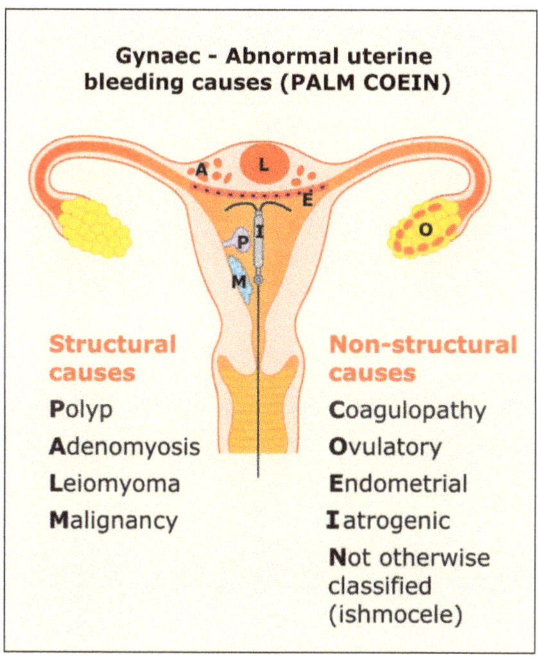

   a. **Structural cause (PALM)**
      i. Polyp
      ii. Adenomyosis

iii. Leiomyoma (Fibroids)

iv. Malignancy and hyperplasia

b. **Non structural cause (COEIN)**

i. Coagulopathy

ii. Ovulatory dysfunction

iii. Endometrial

iv. Iatrogenic

v. Not yet classified

5. **Assessment of patient with AUB:**

a. **Detailed history of current bleeding episode:** Length, duration, amount of loss, presence of clots and symptoms associated with hemorrhage.

b. **History**

i. **Menstrual history**

- Age at menarche
- Last menstruation period
- Menses frequency, regularity, duration and volume to know abnormality.

ii. **Sexual or reproductive history**

- Current contraception
- Obstetrics history
- PAP smear history
- History of sexually transmitted diseases

iii. **Family history:** Bleeding disorder in family.

iv. **Personal history:** Addiction of tobacco, alcohol or drug abuse

v. **Surgical history:** Recent or previous history of surgery

c. **Associated Signs and symptoms:**

i. Abdominal Pain, vomiting, nausea

ii. Discharge

iii. Fever

iv. Anorexia, Weight loss

v. Bowel/bladder symptoms

d. **Medical history and current Medications:** Warfarin, heparin, OC pills, NSAIDs.

e. **Physical examination**

i. **Signs and symptoms of acute blood loss**

- Giddiness
- Pallor
- Tachycardia
- Hypotension

ii. **To know etiology**

Disease	Symptoms and signs
PCOS	Obesity and hirsutism
Thyroid dysfunction	Thyroid enlargement, tenderness, Cold/heat intolerance, proptosis
Hyperandrogenism	Excessive or abnormal hair growth, clitoromegaly, acne.
Bleeding disorder	Petechiae, bruising
Cushing's	Moon facies, abnormal fat distribution, striae.
Hematological disorder	Splenomegaly

iii. **Confirmation of bleeding from the genital tract is present or not**

iv. **Abdominal examination:** For any masses, tenderness, organomegaly.

v. **Pelvic examination:** Speculum and bimanual

vi. **Laboratory investigation**

Acute AUB	Chronic AUB
a. Pregnancy test (Beta-hcg)	a. PAP smear/cervical cytology
b. Complete blood count	b. Hormonal assay
c. Kidney function test	c. Gonorrhea/chlamydia in high risk patients
d. Coagulation profile: PTT/INR	d. Endometrial biopsy in older patients.
e. Thyroid function test	e. Iron studies
f. Liver function test	
g. Iron studies	
h. Adrenal function	
i. If indicated then: VW factor assay, ristocetin cofactor assay, factor VIII.	

- **Imaging studies**
  1. Pelvic sonography
  2. Transvaginal ultrasonography

3. Hysteroscopy
4. Sonohysterography (Transvaginal ultrasound with intrauterine contrast)
5. MRI Scan

- **Cytopathology includes**
  1. PAP Smear
  2. Cervical biopsy
  3. Endometrial biopsy
- **Surgical:** D&C hysteroscopy

vii. **Management:** Treatment depends on multiple factors including fertility desire, etiology, medical condition of patient.

Etiology	**Management**
Polyps	**Surgical resection**
Adenomyosis	The definitive treatment is Hysterectomy or less commonly adenomyomectomy
Leiomyomas	**Medical management** a. Levonorgestrel releasing intrauterine device b. GnRH agonist c. Systemic progestins d. NSAIDs e. Tranexamic acid **Surgical management** a. Uterine artery embolization b. Endometrial ablation c. Hysterectomy
Malignancy	Surgical, adjuvant therapy or palliative therapy depending on stage
Coagulopathies	Tranexamic acid or Desmopressin
Ovulatory dysfunction	**Correction of endocrine disorders**
Endometrial disorder	**No specific treatment**
Iatrogenic	

Section 6

Medicine Emergencies

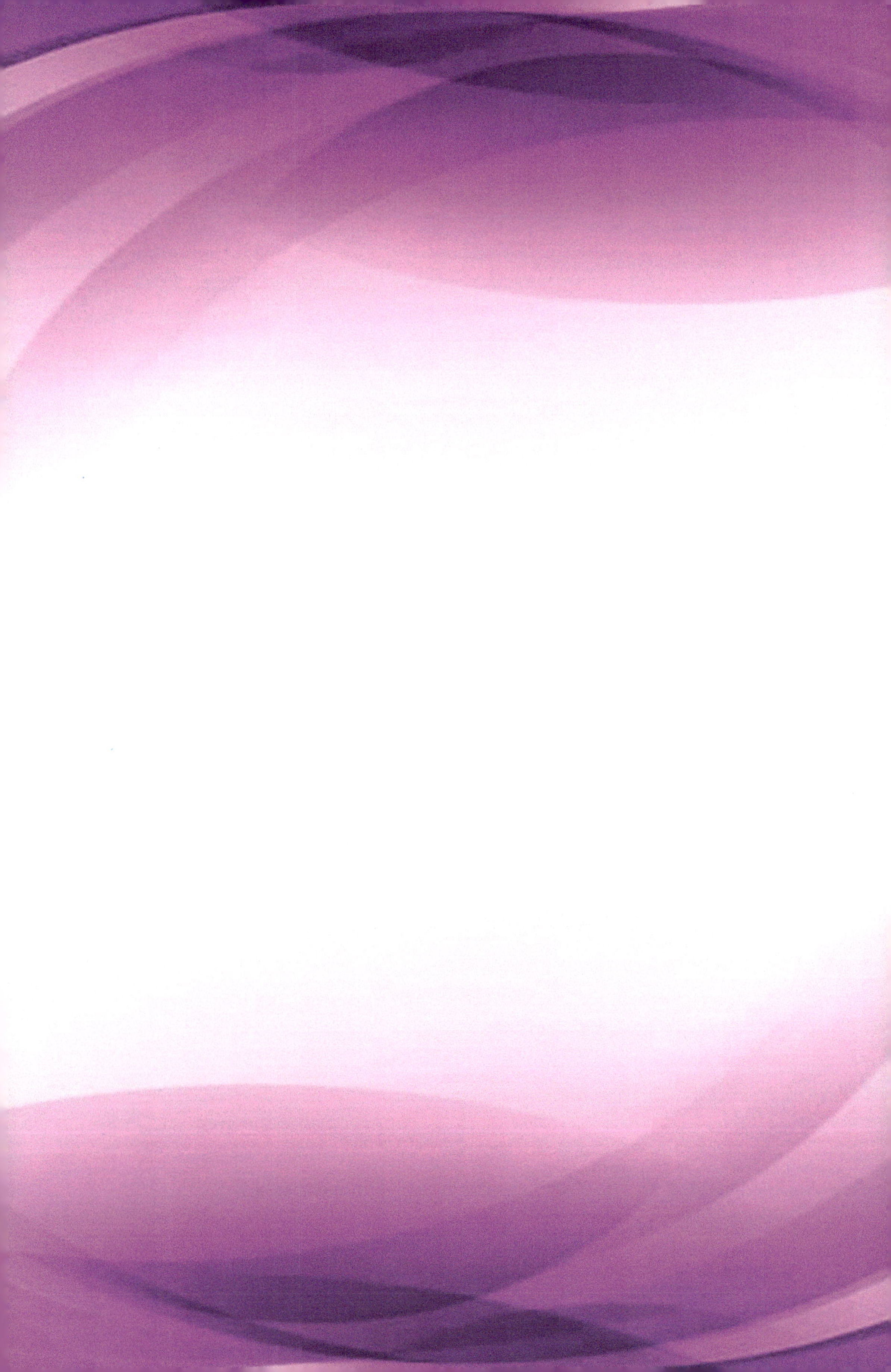

CHAPTER

6 Cardiovascular System

EXAMINATION OF THE CARDIOVASCULAR SYSTEM

Pulse	Rate, rhythm, volume, radio-radial delay, radio-femoral delay, other peripheral pulses, conditions of the arterial wall, any special character
Blood pressure	Hypotension or hypertension
Examination of neck veins	Neck veins Engorged or not If engorged then pressure (CVP), pulsation -present or not, hepatojugular reflux -present or not
Inspection	**1) Shape:** Presence any abnormality **2) Pulsation:** Apical pulsation; diffuse pulsation over precordium **3) Trachea:** Central/Deviated 4) Visible precordial bulge **5) Superficial veins on anterior chest wall:** Engorgement present or not **6) Polythelia (accessory nipple):** Which indicates underlying CHD, cardiomyopathy 7) Previous operative scar

(Continued)

Palpation	**a) Mitral area:** 1. Apex beat 2. Heart sound on palpation 3. Thrill **b) Pulmonary area:** 1. Pulsation 2. Heart sound on palpation 3. Thrill **c) Aortic area:** 1. Pulsation 2. Heart sound on palpation 3. Thrill **d) Tricuspid area:** 1. Left parasternal heave 2. Heart sound on palpation 3. Thrill **e) Pericardial rub** **f) Epigastric or suprasternal pulsation** **g) Palpate carotid artery for thrill**
Percussion	Not routinely performed
Auscultation	a) Heart rate b) Heart Rhythm c) Mitral area, pulmonary area, aortic area, tricuspid area for: 1. Heart sounds 2. Murmur 3. Abnormal sounds like opening snap, splitting heart sound, ejection click, S3 or S4 d) Auscultation over carotid arteries for bruit e) Pericardial rub

SYMPTOMS OF CARDIOVASCULAR DISORDER

1. Breathlessness
2. Chest pain
3. Palpitation (Arrhythmia)
4. Dizziness and syncope (Arrhythmia)
5. Swelling of feet (Peripheral edema), facial puffiness, or anasarca (Heart failure)
6. Hemoptysis (Mitral stenosis)
7. Cough with expectoration (Dry cough in LVF)
8. Visual disturbances (Retinal hemorrhage or embolism)
9. Digestive symptoms like anorexia, nausea, vomiting, pain in abdomen
10. Squatting or cyanotic spells
11. Cramping pain in the lower limb (Atherosclerosis)
12. Renal symptoms like oliguria (in CCF)
13. Generalised weakness or fatigue (Decreased cardiac output)
14. Fever, recent history of sore throat, mutiple joint pain & swelling, erythema marginatum, subcutaneous nodules
15. General symptoms like fever, anorexia, weight gain (Due to peripheral edema) or weight loss (Due to edema)

ISCHEMIC HEART DISEASE

1. Ischemia is a medical condition in which blood supply to body part is decreased or restricted.
2. In cardiac ischemia there is a decreased blood supply to the cardiac muscles.
3. This sudden deprivation of blood supply to the portion of heart resulting in heart attack.
4. Due to reduction of oxygen and nutrient supply to cardiac muscles, heart will not function properly.
5. Multiple factors are responsible for ischemic heart disease; most common are smoking, diabetes mellitus, increased cholesterol level.
6. **Patient with ischemic heart disease fall in two large groups**:
   a. **Acute coronary syndrome**
   b. **Chronic coronary artery disease**

(A) ACUTE CORONARY SYNDROME

Acute coronary syndrome (ACS) is a set of clinical signs & symptoms developed as result of reduction of blood supply to heart muscles through coronary arteries.

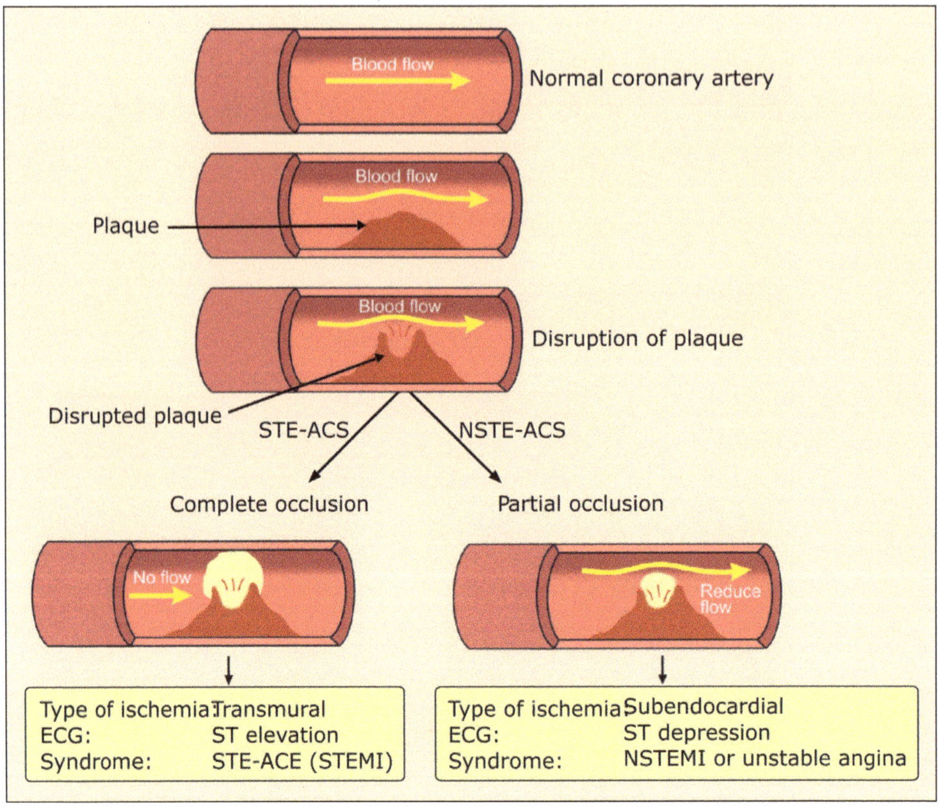

Acute coronary syndrome is commonly associated with three clinical manifestations: **ST elevation myocardial infarction (STEMI), non-ST elevation myocardial infarction (NSTEMI), or unstable angina.**

It includes:

1. **Non ST segment elevation myocardial infarction**: In NSTEMI there is evidence of myocardial necrosis present (Increase in cardiac markers)
2. **Unstable angina:** No evidence of myocardial necrosis.
3. **ST elevation myocardial infarction (STEMI)** Includes patients with acute myocardial infarction (Transmural) with ST elevation on their electrocardiogram

		NSTE-ACS		
	Stable Angina	**Unstable Angina**	**NSTEMI**	**STEMI**
Acute coronary syndrome due to decreased blood flow in coronary vessels	Angina pain develop when there is increased demand in the setting of a stable atherosclerotic plaque. The vessel is unable to dilate enough to allow adequate blood flow to meet the myocardial demand. Demand ischemia, no infarct	In unstable angina there is a partial occlusion of arterial lumen due to thrombosis formation on a disrupted atherothrombotic coronary plaque or on eroded coronary artery endothelium Partial occlusion Supply ischemia, no infarct	In this NSTE-ACS when there is a partial occlusion of arterial lumen due to thrombosis formation on a disrupted atherothrombotic coronary plaque or on eroded coronary artery endothelium Partial occlusion Subendocardial infarct	A STEMI is characterized by complete occlusion of the blood vessel lumen, resulting in transmural injury and infarct to the myocardium, which is reflected by ECG changes and a rise in troponins. Complete occlusion Transmural infarct
Troponins	Normal	Normal	Elevated	Elevated

(B) CHRONIC CORONARY ARTERY DISEASE

It includes patients with stable angina.

NON ST SEGMENT ACUTE CORONARY SYNDROME

In Non ST acute coronary syndrome the blood supply to heart muscles is partially reduced resulting in ischemia that only affects subendocardium.

Diagnosis of NSTE-ACS is done on the basis of the clinical presentation and cardiac biomarker

Pathophysiology:

1. Most commonly caused by an imbalance between oxygen supply and oxygen demand.
2. In Non ST segment acute coronary syndrome partial occlusion of arterial lumen occurs due to thrombus formation on a disrupted atherothrombotic coronary plaque or on eroded endothelium of coronary artery.
3. As, result of thrombus formation in coronary artery, blood supply to cardiac muscles reduced which results into a severe cardiac muscle ischemia or necrosis.
4. **Other causes of NSTE:**
   a. Coronary artery spasm, seen in the Prinzmetal variant angina.
   b. **Severe blood flow obstruction:** e.g. rapidly advancing coronary Atherosclerosis
   c. **Increased myocardial oxygen demand as compared to supply**: e.g. condition which are responsible for increased myocardial oxygen demand like high grade fever, hyperthyroidism, tachycardia which can precipitate acute coronary syndrome if there is fixed obstruction in coronary blood flow.

A. Unstable angina:

Typically chest discomfort is severe and has at least one out of three:

1. It occurs at rest (or with minimal exertion & lasting > 10 minutes)
2. Recent onset of chest discomfort (< 2 weeks)
3. It occurs with crescendo pattern (Distinctly more severe, prolonged, or frequent than previous episode)

B. Non ST elevation Myocardial infarction:

1. Diagnosis of NSTEMI is with above clinical feature and evidence of myocardial necrosis
2. Evidence of myocardial infarction seen as elevated level of biomarker of myocardial necrosis

Clinical features:

1. **Chest pain**
   a. Severe & usually lasting more than 10 minutes
   b. Occurs at rest or with minimal exertion

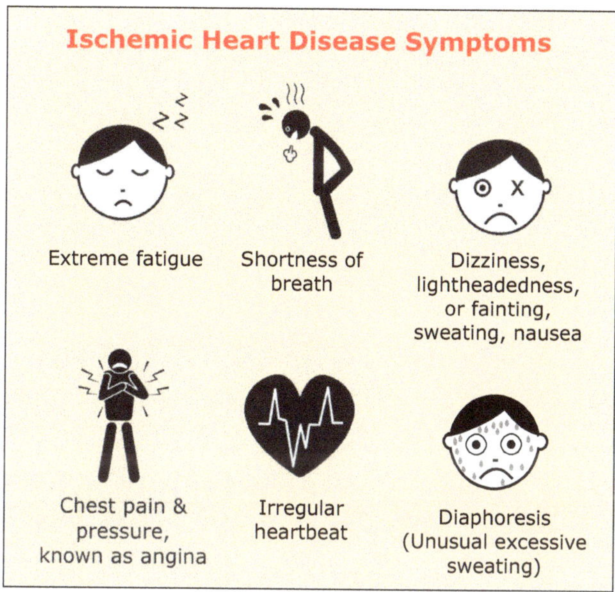

c. Typically located in substernal region or in the epigastric region

d. It may radiate to the left arm, left shoulder and/or neck

e. Pain may feel tight, crushing, squeezing or pressure type

2. Some symptoms are considered as equivalent to chest pain for evaluation of patient of myocardial infarction which includes following symptoms and seen more frequently in women, elderly and patients with diabetes mellitus.

   a. Breathlessness

   b. Epigastric pain, nausea

   c. Generalised weakness

3. **Physical findings in patient with large area of myocardial ischemia or a large NSTEMI:**

   a. Diaphoresis (Excessive sweating with no clear cause)

   b. Pale, cold skin

   c. Sinus tachycardia

   d. Basilar crepts due to cardiogenic pulmonary edema

   e. Sometimes, hypotension (Inferior wall involvement)

4. **Investigations:**

   a. **12 lead ECG:**

      1. Detect rest ischemia with serial ECG or continuous ECG i.e. ST segment depression and T wave inversion or flattening

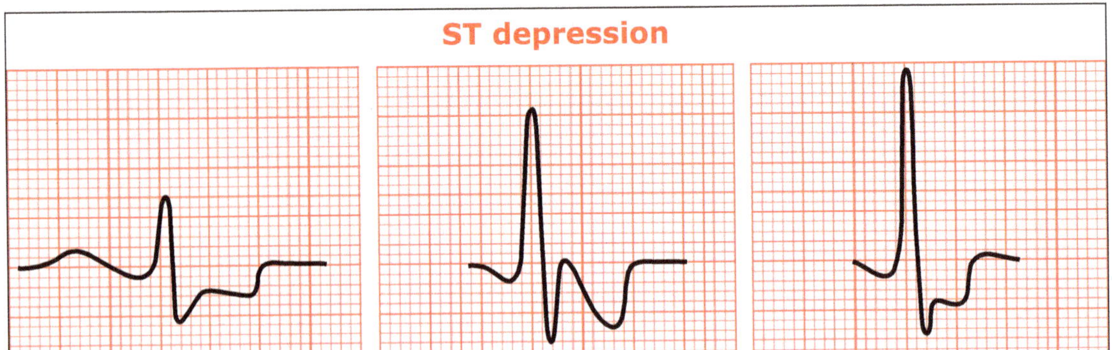

2. If no typical changes are seen, the term "non-ST segment elevation ACS" is applied.

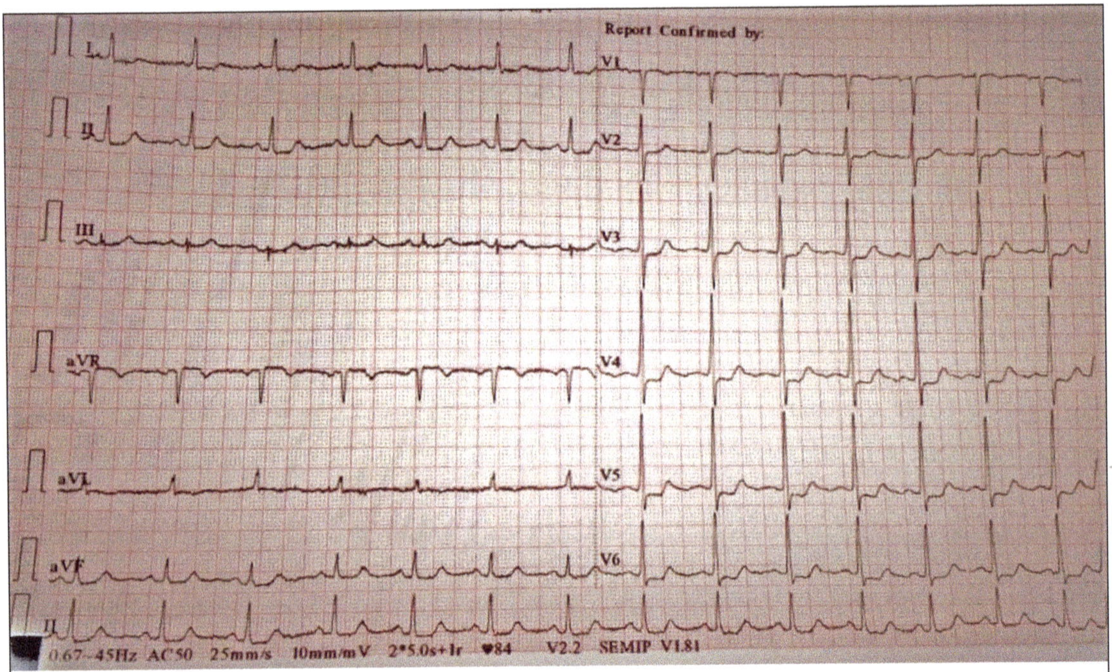

ECG showing ST depression in V3-V6 suggestive of sub-endocardial ischemia

b. **Cardiac marker**:
   1. Patients with NSTEMI have elevated biomarkers such as cardiac troponin I or T Which are specific and sensitive.
   2. CK-MB less sensitive biomarker as compare to troponin I & T.
   3. Cardiac markers help to distinguish patients with NSTEMI from those Unstable angina.

c. **Chest X-ray:** To rule out other causes of chest pain

d. **Blood test:** Routine blood investigation and lipid profile

e. **Cardiac imaging:** 2D echo used to detect abnormalities of heart walls motion and cardiac structures.

f. **Stress testing:** To see whether your heart is getting enough blood flow during exercise or not.

g. **Coronary computed tomography angiography (CCTA):** Imaging test that helps to know where plaque buildup in the coronary artery and how much coronary arteries are narrowed.

5. **Treatment**

a. **General measures**

1. Bed rest
2. Oxygen administration
3. Monitor vitals
4. Foley's catheterisation

b. **Medical treatment**

1. **Anti-ischemic treatment**

Anti-ischemic drugs	Uses in clinical condition	Contraindication
Nitrates (Sublingual or intravenous buccal spray) (5 min apart three doses (0.3-0.6 mg)) If pain persists after three oral doses then IV NTG is given (5-10 ug/min).	If patient experiencing ischemic pain Given till pain subsides or SBP<100 mm of Hg	Hypotension Use of sildenafil or phosphodiesterase 5 within 24-48 hours
B adrenergic blocker **(Metoprolol 5mg IV stat followed by every 5 min and used upto 15 mg)**	Started in the IV route in the severe ischemia Unstable angina	HR < 60/min, AV block, BP < 90 mm Hg, congestive cardiac failure
Calcium channel blocker (Amlodipine, nicardia, felodipine)	Variant angina Persistent symptoms and ECG suggestive of ischemia even after treatment with full dose of β blocker or nitrates (Recurrent ischemia) Contraindication to use β-blocker or nitrates	Pulmonary edema, Left sided failure

c. **Additional medical therapy:**

1. Angiotensin-converting enzyme inhibitors (ACE Inhibitors) or If not tolerated then angiotensin receptor blocker (ARB).
2. Early initiation of statins (Atorvastatin 80 mg/d) decreases recurrence of ACS and decreases complications related to PCI procedure.

d. **Anticoagulant:**

1. **Low molecular weight heparin**

2. **Bivalirudin**
3. **Enoxaparin**
4. **Fondaparinux**
5. **Unfractionated heparin**

e. **Thrombolytic:**

Antiplatelet drugs

1. **Aspirin:** Aspirin is a platelet cyclooxygenase inhibitors, should be initiated in starting.

   The typical loading dose is 300 mg/d, then start with lower doses 75 mg to 150 mg/day.

   Contraindication: Active bleeding, aspirin intolerance

2. **Clopidogrel:** Irreversible blockade of the P2Y12 receptor to inhibit platelet aggregation.

   Loading dose of 300 mg-600 mg followed by 75 mg.

3. The dual antiplatelet regimen should be continued for at least 1 year in patients with NSTE-ACS.

6. **Invasive therapy:** Coronary revascularization for restoring blood flow.

   It includes two procedures:

   a. **Percutaneous intervention:** Percutaneous coronary interventions, such as angioplasty alone or with a stent, can restore blood flow to the heart.

   b. **Coronary bypass grafting**

7. **Complications:**

   The acute complications of unstable angina and NSTEMI are similar to STEMI but occur at a lower rate.

   a. Acute myocardial infarction
   b. Bradyarrhythmias
   c. Cardiogenic shock
   d. Mitral regurgitation
   e. Ventricular septal rupture
   f. Rupture of left ventricular wall
   g. Dressler syndrome
   h. Life threatening arrhythmias e.g. ventricular tachycardia, ventricular fibrillation

ST SEGMENT ELEVATION MYOCARDIAL INFARCTION

1. It occurs due to complete artery occlusion results into the extensive myocardial ischemia called as transmural ischemia.

2. Retrosternal chest pain with profuse unexplained sweating for a period more than 30 minutes most likely suggestive of STEMI.

3. Mostly it presents in early morning hours but can present at any time.

4. Patients having unstable angina are at higher risk of precipitation of STEMI in situation with high oxygen demand.

5. Some situations precipitate STEMI e.g. Sudden emotional trauma, vigorous exercise (athlets)

6. **Clinical features:**

   Pain:

   1. Deep and visceral
   2. Usually pain is more severe, occurs even at rest and last for longer duration.
   3. Patient describes pain as tight, pressure, crushing or squeezing type.
   4. Typically pain at a central portion of the chest and/or epigastrium and it may radiate to the arms.
   5. Myocardial ischemic pain may radiate as high as the occipital area of skull and upto umbilicus.
   6. Painless STEMI occurs in the patient with diabetes mellitus due to autonomic neuropathy

7. **Other symptoms in STEMI:**

   1. **Weakness**
   2. **Profuse sweating**
   3. **Nausea, vomiting occurs due to stimulation of vomiting centre as result of severe pain.**
   4. **Anxiety and a sense of impending doom (Feeling of I will die)**
   5. **Sudden onset of breathlessness:** Commonly seen in elderly patients
   6. **Dry cough**
   7. **Hiccups (Inferior wall MI)**
   8. **Other less common findings:** Altered mental status, arrhythmias, peripheral embolism.

8. **Physical findings**

    1. In most of the cases patient is anxious and restless
    2. Pallor associated with sweating and cold, clammy extremities
    3. Patient with anterior wall infarct shows evidence of **sympathetic nervous hyperactivation**

       Tachycardia and/or hypertension
    4. Patient with inferior wall infarct shows evidence of **parasympathetic hyperactivity i.e. Bradycardia and/or hypotension**
    5. Mild pyrexia
    6. Features of complications (acute ventricular failure, pulmonary edema, arrhythmias)

9. **Investigations**

    a. **Electrocardiogram:**

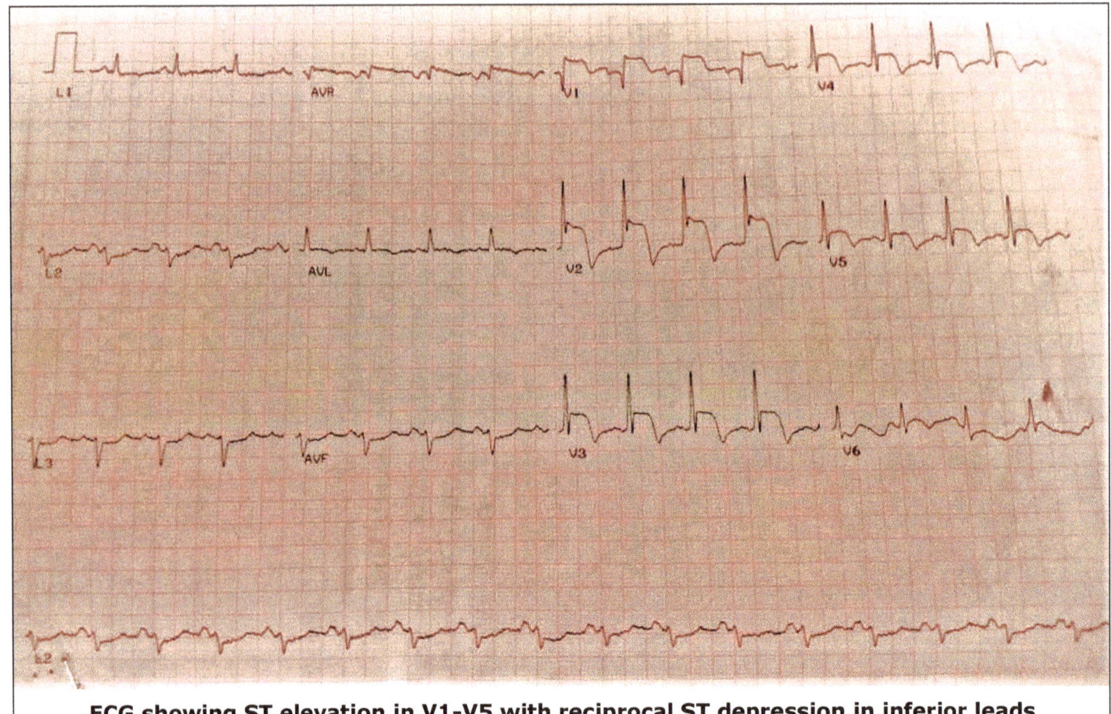

ECG showing ST elevation in V1-V5 with reciprocal ST depression in inferior leads suggestive of Anterior wall MI

1. New ST elevation at the J point in two contiguous leads of > 0.1 mV in all leads other than leads V2-V3

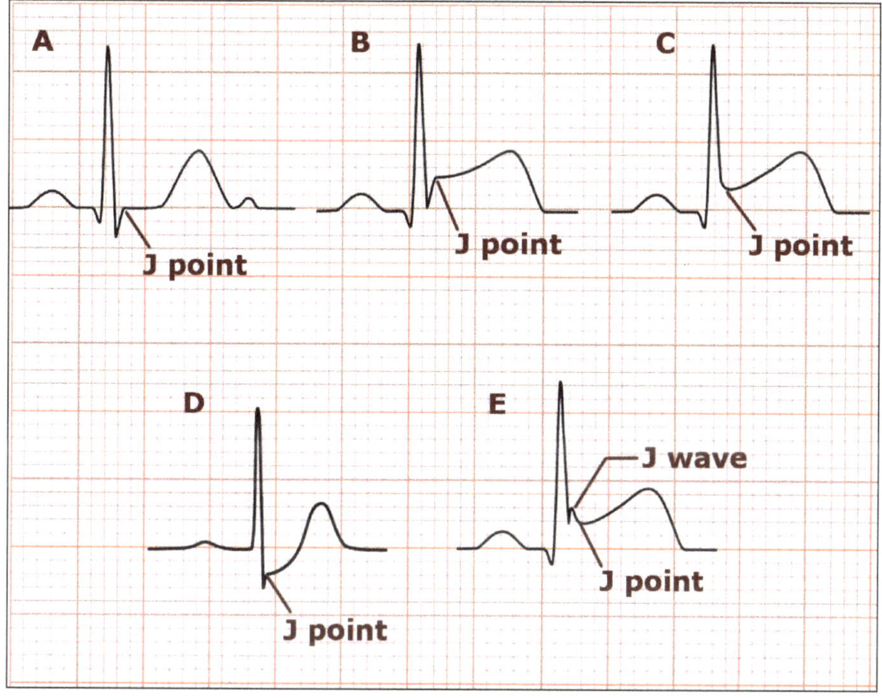

2. **For leads V2-V3 the following cut points apply:** ST elevation of ≥ 0.2 mV in men ≥ 40 years, ≥ 0.25 mV in men < 40 years, or ≥ 0.15 mV in women
3. **Other conditions which are treated as a STEMI:** New or presumed new LBBB, Isolated posterior MI
4. The presence of reciprocal ST depression helps to confirm the diagnosis
5. **Localization of Infarction:**

Septal wall: V1 and V2
Anterior wall: V2 to V5 (Classically changes seen in V3 -V4)
Lateral wall: V5 and V6
Extensive lateral wall: I, AVL, and V5 and V6.
Anteroseptal wall: V1-V4
Anterolateral wall: V3-V6, I, AVL
Extensive anterior wall: V1-V6
Inferior wall: II, III, aVF
High Lateral wall: I, aVL
Posterior wall: Tall R wave and ST depression in V1-V3 & V7, V8, V9

b. **Blood investigations**

1. **Serum cardiac markers**

a. **Troponin:** The most sensitive and specific test for myocardial damage. Troponin is a superior marker for detection of myocardial injury than CK-MB

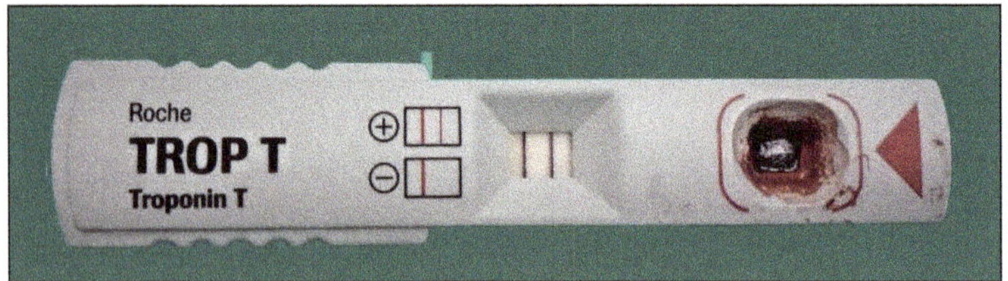

b. **Creatinine kinase:** It is relatively specific when skeletal muscle damage is not present.

c. **Lactate dehydrogenase:** LDH is not as specific as troponin.

d. **Myoglobin:** Low specificity for myocardial infarction

2. **ESR:** Raised in some cases
3. **Complete blood count:** Polymorphonuclear leucocytosis
4. **Renal function test:** Serum creatinine and blood urea level (Increased in AKI)
5. **Liver function test:** Liver enzymes are elevated in some patients
6. **Lipid profile:** To diagnose dislipidemia .
7. **B-type natriuretic peptide (BNP) or N-terminal pro-BNP:** Help to diagnose and understand severity of **heart failure**.
8. **D dimer:** If we are suspecting pulmonary embolism
9. **Chest X-ray:** Helpful to diagnose cardiomegaly and pulmonary edema

c. **Cardiac imaging:**

1. **2D echo:**

a. Detects abnormalities of wall motion, important in management decisions such as whether the patient should receive reperfusion therapy (e.g. fibrolysis, or PCI), left ventricular function which is a prognostic factor.

b. It can identify the right ventricular infarct, ventricular aneurysm, pericardial effusion, and LV thrombus

c. It is useful in detection and quantification of a ventral septal defect (VSD) and mitral regurgitation, two serious complications of STEMI

2. **Several nucleotide imaging techniques are used for myocardial perfusion imaging.**

3. **Cardiac MRI:** MI can accurately be detected with high resolution cardiac MRI technique referred to as late enhancement.

d. **Coronary Angiography:** To detect percentage of blockage and type of myocardial infarction

10. **Management:**

a. **Prehospital management:** Patients should recognise the symptoms of MI and should take medical attention immediately.

b. **In emergency department:**

1. Rapid identification of patient with STEMI and candidate for reperfusion therapy
2. Avoid inappropriate discharge of patients with STEMI.
3. The goal is to reduce the time in the contact and initiation of reperfusion therapy.

c. **Management in intensive care unit:**

1. Bed rest
2. Oxygen therapy
3. Nitrates may be given sublingually for pain relief by coronary vessels vasodilation
4. If pain persists even after giving of sublingual nitrates, IV infusion of nitroglycerine may be given, but blood pressure should be above 100 mm of Hg.
5. Aspirin is given orally in the dose ranging from 100-300 mg.
6. Transfer the patient to PCI capable hospital after fibrinolytic therapy (If not possible).
7. **Reperfusion therapy:**

i. **Candidate for reperfusion therapy:**

- When ST elevation of at least 2 mm in two contiguous precordial leads and 1 mm in two adjacent leads is present.
- Fibrinolysis is not helpful in Non-ST elevation myocardial infarction.
- Restoration of blood within golden period will limit infarct size of myocardium.
- Reperfusion done either by pharmacological drugs or by Percutaneous interventions (PCI).

ii. **Thrombolytic agents:**

- **Agents with fibrin specificity:**
  - Alteplase
  - Reteplase
  - Tenecteplase
- **Agents without fibrin specificity:**
  - **Streptokinase:** 1.5 million units IV infusion over 60 minutes
  - **Urokinase**

iii. **Cardiac catheterization and coronary angiography:**

- Failure of reperfusion (Persistence of chest pain and ST elevation > 90 min)
- Coronary artery reocclusion (Re-elevation of ST segments and/or recurrence of chest pain)
- Evidence of severe myocardial ischemia

HYPERTENSIVE CRISIS

1. In hypertensive crisis the blood pressure is severely elevated (SBP > or = 180 Or DBP 110)
2. Hypertensive crisis includes hypertensive emergencies and urgencies.
3. In hypertensive crisis, compensatory mechanism of our body does not get sufficient time to adapt and change accordingly.
4. Isolated systolic HTN is > or equal to 140 mm of Hg and diastolic < 90 mm of Hg
5. **Definitions:**
   a. **Hypertension urgency:** The situation in which the BP is marked elevated, without any clinical features of end organ damage (Brain, eyes, heart, kidney)

      In this condition, the control of the elevated BP can be done gradually.

   b. **Hypertension emergency:** The situation in which the BP is markedly elevated, but with clinical features of some end organ damage.

      In this condition, the elevated blood pressure is reduced on immediate basis with the help of IV antihpertensive drugs to reduce further end organ damge.

      1. **Accelerated hypertension:** Severely elevated HTN associated with evidence of vascular damage on fundoscopic examination, but without papilloedema. (SBP > 210 mm of Hg and DSP > 130 mm of Hg)
      2. **Malignant hypertension:** Severely elevated HTN (> 200/140 mm of Hg) associated with grade IV retinopathy (Papilledema) and renal dysfunction.
6. **Causes of hypertension:**
   a. **Primary hypertension:** High blood pressure which doesn't have a secondary cause.

      Multiple risk factors are responsible for primary hypertension

      1. Older age BP rises with age
      2. Diet (High fatty diet, salt rich diet, less dietary intake of fruits, green vegetables and fruits)
      3. Less physical activity
      4. Chronic alcoholic
      5. Family history
      6. Obesity (BMI > 30)

   b. **Secondary hypertension:**

      1. **Renal:** Renal parenchymal disorders, renovascular diseases

2. **Endocrine:** Pheochromocytoma, cushing's syndrome, Conn's syndrome, hyperthyroidism
3. **Miscellaneous:** Drugs (e.g. Beta 2 agonist, steroids, OC pills, coarction of aorta)

a. **Secondary HTN may be due to withdrawal of addictive material e.g. alcohol.**

b. **Rebound HTN due to discontinuing antihypertensive therapy, particularly beta adrenergic antagonists and central alpha 2 agonists**

7. **Initial evaluation:**

a. **History:**

1. Previous history of similar episode
2. Antihypertensive medication with dosing & frequency
3. Time since last intake of medicine
4. Use of other drugs or medications.

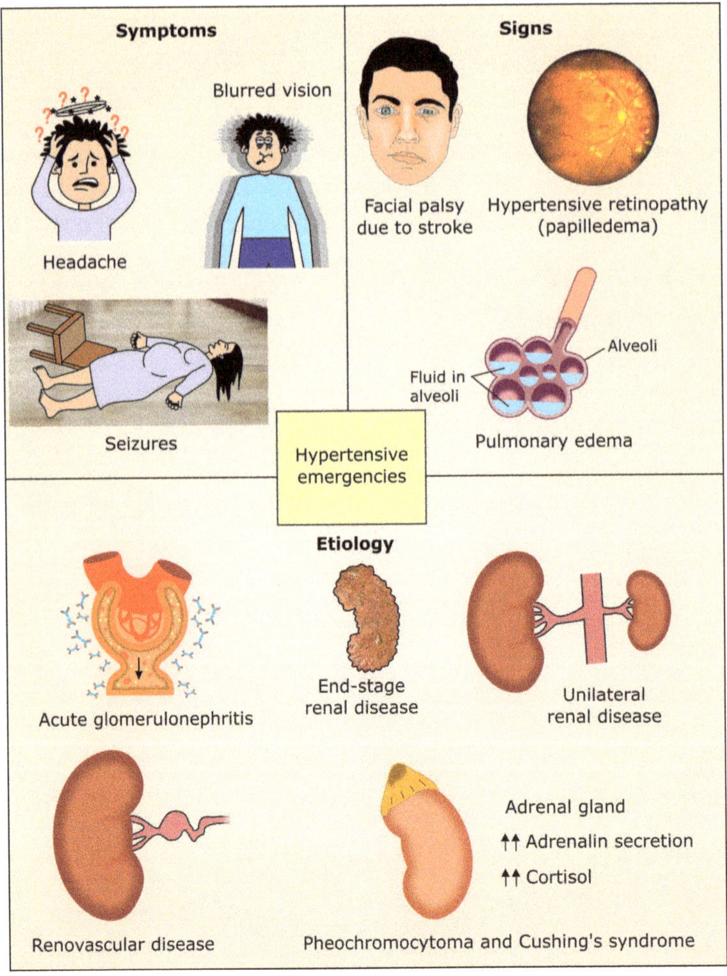

b. **Physical examination:** Identify the evidence of end organ damage or a secondary causes of hypertension

1. Altered sensorium (Hypertensive encephalopathy)
2. Elevated jugular venous pressure
3. Palpation of pulses in all extremities (For unequal pulses)
4. Evidence of left ventricular failure (Diastolic failure)
5. Auscultation for renal bruit or carotid bruit (artery stenosis)
6. Focused neurological deficit and fundoscopic examination
7. **Cushingoid features**: Weight gain, purple striae, fatty tissue deposition over neck, upper back and face.

c. **Investigations**

Routine investigations:

1. 12 lead ECG (LV hypertrophy, ischemia)
2. CT BRAIN (Scan if patient is unconscious and/or with convulsion) primarily to rule out IC bleed)
3. Complete blood count (Low Hb and high creatinine suggestive of chronic kidney disease)
4. Serum creatinine, BUN (Renal impairment)
5. Urinalysis for proteins and blood
6. Serum electrolyte
7. Plasma cholesterol
8. CXR (Cardiomegaly, heart failure)
9. **Investigations for secondary HTN:**
    a. Intravenous urogram if renal cause suspected
    b. Renal doppler (If renal disease is suspected)
    c. Radionuclide venography, renal arteriography (Renal arterial stenosis)
    d. 24 hours urine catecholamines, vanillyl mandelic acid (VMA)
    e. Plasma renin activity and aldosterone (If Conn's syndrome is suspected)
    f. Urinary cortisol, dexamethasone suppression test (Cushing's syndrome)
    g. Angiography/cardiac MRI (If coarctation of aorta is suspected)

8. **When to evaluate a patient for secondary hypertension:**
   a. Young age patient with significant hypertension
   b. Orthostatic hypotension
   c. Malignant hypertension
   d. Resistant or refractory HTN

9. **Treatment:**
   a. In hypertensive emergency:
      i. Rapid control of blood pressure is done with control of ongoing end organ damage.
      ii. BP control is done by rapidly acting parenteral antihypertensive agents as soon as possible to avoid permanent end organ damage and death.
      iii. Too rapid reduction of BP may cause cerebral damage, blindness, precipitate angina or renal hypoperfusion

   b. In hypertensive urgency:
      i. BP control is done more slowly than hypertensive emergency cases.
      ii. Targeted blood pressure is achieved more gradually than hypertensive emergency case.

   c. Parenteral drugs of choice in hypertensive emergencies:

Hypertensive encephalopathy and stroke	Nitroprusside, Nicardipine, labetalol
MI/Unstable angina	Nitroglycerine, Nicardipine
Acute LVF	Nitroglycerine, Loop diuretics
Adrenergic crisis	Phentolamine, Nitroprusside

   d. The intravenous drug doses of commonly used drugs in the management of hypertensive emergencies
      i. Labetalol: 2 mg/min upto a maximum dose of 300 mg IV or 20 mg over 2 min, then 40-80 mg at 10 min interval upto 300 mg total
      ii. Nitroglycerine: Initial 5 ug/min then titrated by 5 ug/min at 3-5 min interval; if no response is seen at 20 ug/min, Incremental increase of 10-20 ug/min may be used.

10. Complications

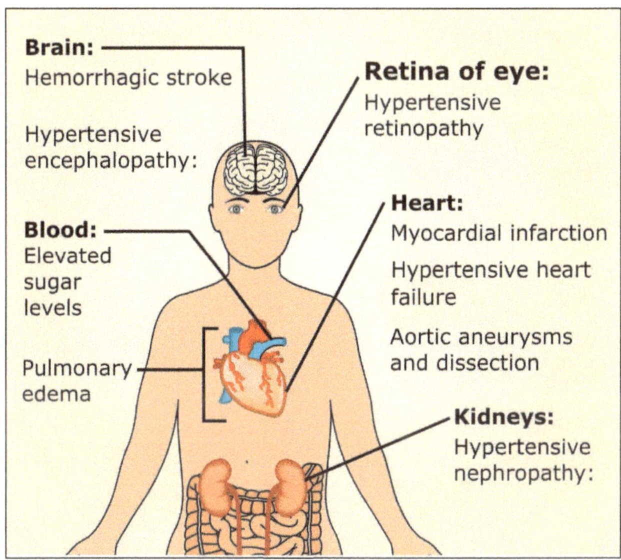

a. Changes in mental status, such as confusion

b. Bleeding into the brain (Stroke)

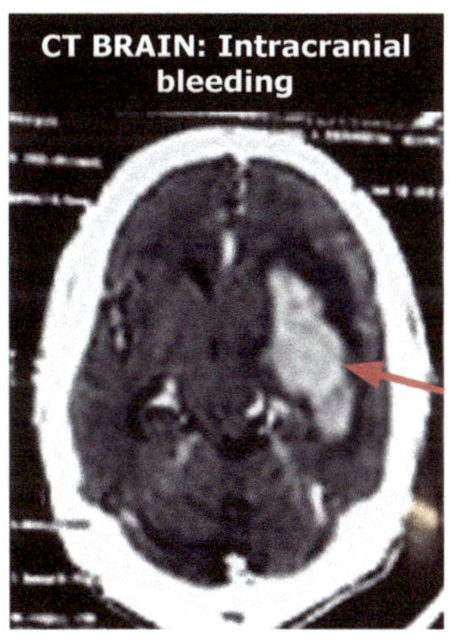

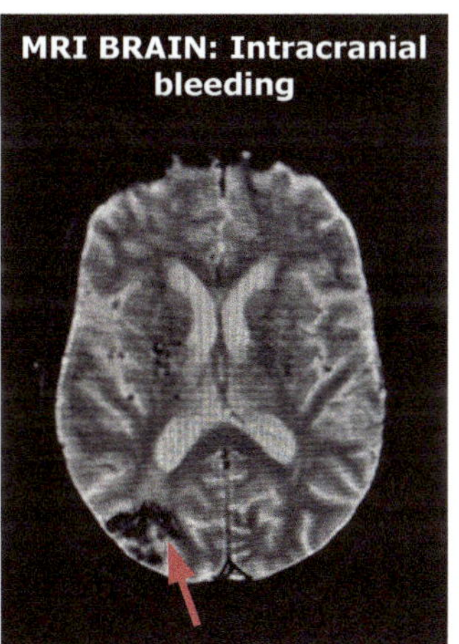

c. Heart failure

d. Chest pain (Unstable angina)

e. Fluid in the lungs (Pulmonary edema)

f. Heart attack

g. Aneurysm (Aortic dissection)

h. Eclampsia (Occurs during pregnancy)

SHOCK

1. **In shock there is intense and widespread reduction of blood supply to body tissues**
2. If delivery of oxygen and other nutrients to body tissues is not restored immediately then it may lead to irreversible cellular injury.
3. **Classification of shock**:
   a. **Hypovolemic**
   b. **Cardiogenic**
   c. **Septic**
   d. **Anaphylactic shock**
   e. **Neurogenic shock**

HYPOVOLEMIC SHOCK

1. Hypolemic shock occurs as result of significant loss of blood and body fluid.
2. Intravascular volume loss is at the level that the cardiovascular functions compromise and become unable to pump sufficient amounts of blood to meet body demand.
3. This is most common type of shock
4. It results from
   a. **Hemorrhage:** The loss of red blood cell mass and plasma
   b. **Fluid loss:** Significant fluid loss occurs in some conditions like continuous vomiting, loose motions, severe burn etc.

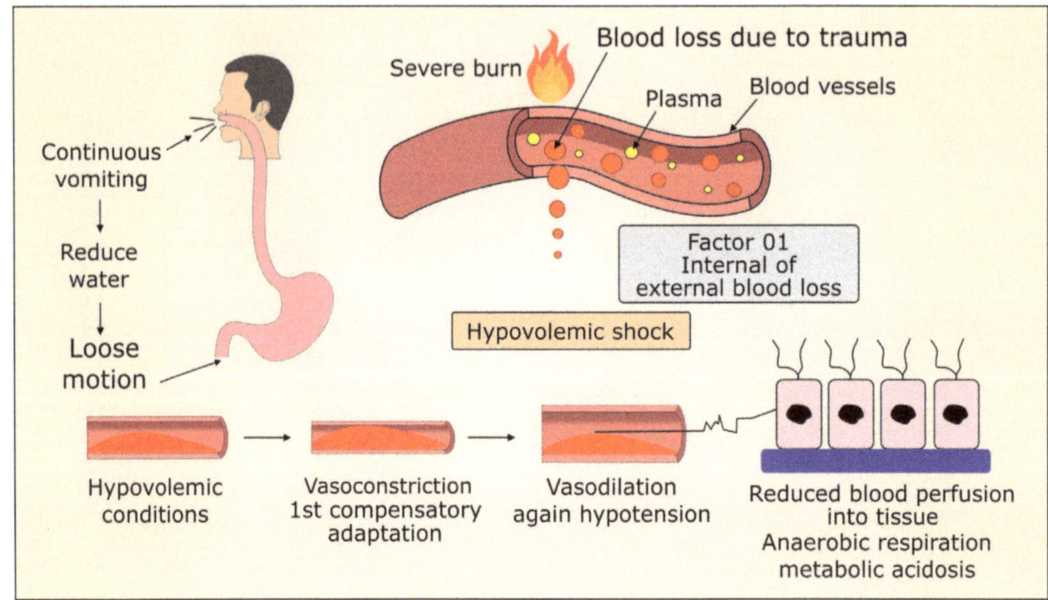

5. Traumatic hemorrhage is most common cause of hypovolemic shock
6. Signs and symptoms of the non-hemorrhagic and hemorrhagic hypovolemic shock are the same.
7. The normal physiological response to hypovolemic shock is to maintain perfusion of the brain and heart and for that reason blood is diverted from other organs.
8. Fluid and blood loss should be corrected as early as possible to avoid ischemic injury.
9. **Physiological response as follows:**
    a. Increased sympathetic activity (Increase in heart rate)
    b. Hyperventilation
    c. Increased blood flow from capacitance vessels to heart
    d. Release of stress hormone (Cortisol, adrenaline, norepinephrine)
    e. Reduction of urinary output (Oliguria), concentrated urine.
    f. Loss of intravascular volume compensated through the interstitial and intracellular fluid.

Mild (< 20% blood volume)	**Moderate (20-40% of blood volume)**	**Severe (> 40% of blood volume)**
A]	**B]**	**C]**
Cool extremities	**Signs and symptoms of [A] and**	**Signs and symptoms of [A+B] and**
Increased time of capillary refilling	Increased heart rate	Altered mental status
Diaphoresis	Increased respiratory rate	Low blood pressure
Collapsed vein	Low urine output	Hemodynamic instability
Anxiety	Postural changes	

10. **Investigation**
    a. **Complete blood count:** In hemorrhagic shock, hemoglobin and hematocrit level reduced.
    b. **Serum electrolyte:** Hypernatremia due to significant loss of water.
    c. **Renal function test:** Increased in BUN and serum creatinine due to prerenal failure
11. **Diagnosis:**
    a. Diagnosis is done by history, physical examination and clinical features.
    b. Readily diagnosed when there is:
        1. Signs of hypovolemia (Increased heart rate, tachypnea)

2. Source of volume loss is present (Acute gastroenteritis, vomiting, visible bleeding)

c. It is essential to differentiate between cardiogenic shock and hypovolemic shock as in both shock cardiac output is significantly reduced and most of clinical features are similar but definitive line of management is different.

d. Cardiogenic shock includes jugular venous distension, rales and S3 gallop that distinguish cardiogenic shock from hypovolemic shock.

12. Treatment:

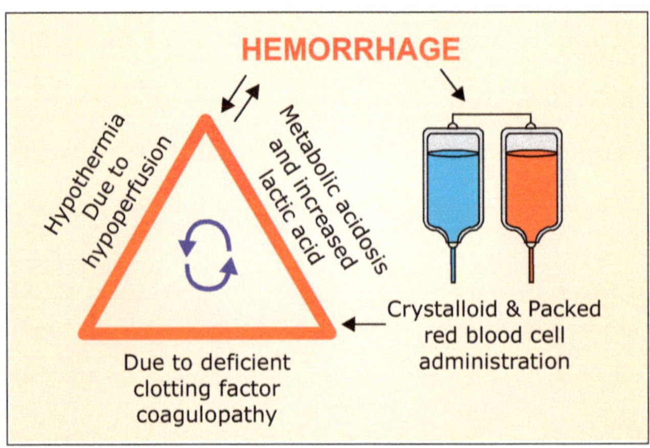

a. **Treatment includes**

1. **General measures:**
   - Oxygen supply
   - Foley's catheterisation (Monitor urine output)

2. **Respiratory support:** If a patient is not maintaining saturation mechanical ventilation may be required.

3. **Initial resuscitation**
   - **Fluid resuscitation:**
     i. Rapid re-expansion of circulating intravascular blood volume with IV fluids
     ii. It is initiated with rapid infusion of ringer lactate through a large bore intravenous line.
     iii. The infusion done to restore end organ perfusion.
   - **If continued hemodynamic instability:** after initial resuscitation clinical features of shock has not reversed then consider that there may be still significant blood loss is going on or volume loss is present and take necessary corrective steps.

- **Blood transfusion:** Indicated in patients with acute blood loss with Hb Conc. < 10 gm/dl.
- **Blood component transfusion:** Packed cell volume, fresh frozen plasma are administered early to avoid disseminated intravascular coagulation due to deficiet clotting factors.

4. **Intervention to control ongoing losses:**
   - Correct underlying condition responsible for the fluid loss.
   - In case of hemorrhage, control ongoing blood loss by rapid identification and control of source of bleeding.
   - Blood transfusion is indicated if Hb < 7 gm/dl
5. **After fluid resuscitation inotropic support:**
   - Inotropic support is given only after adequate fluid resuscitation to restore blood volume
   - Inotropic support with norepinephrine, vasopressin or dopamine.

CARDIOGENIC SHOCK

1. Cardiogenic shock is a medical emergency characterized by systemic inadequate blood flow due to cardiac dysfunction.
2. Heart cannot pump enough blood and oxygen to the brain, kidneys, and other vital organs.
3. Cardiogenic shock is due to dysfunction of ventricles.
4. LV failure accounts for most cases of cardiogenic shock which occurs due acute myocardial infarction.

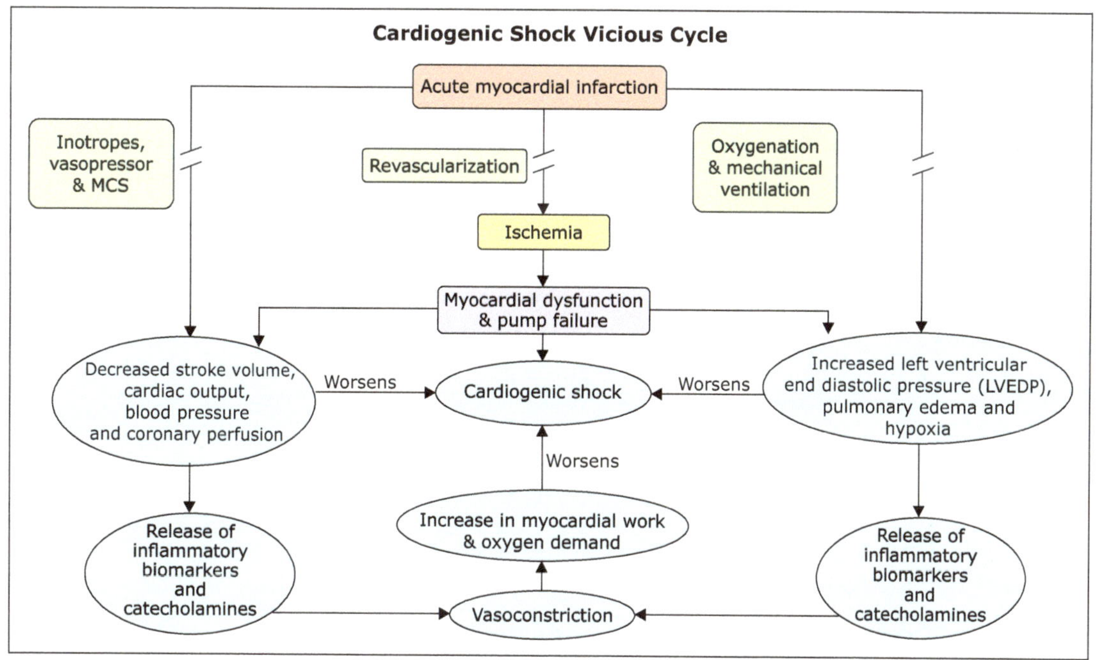

5. Most common causes of cardiogenic shock are cardiomyopathy, mechanical, arrhythmia.
6. In acute MI, shock is more common with ST elevation MI than with non -ST elevation MI.
7. **Etiology of cardiac shock:**

Cardiomyopathic	Mechanical	Abnormal heart rhythm
1. Acute myocardial infarction 2. Dilated cardiomyopathy 3. Myocardial depression in septic shock 4. Endocarditis, myocarditis	1. Mitral regurgitation 2. Ventricular septal defect due to acute myocardial infarction 3. Ventricular aneurysm 4. LV outflow obstruction	1. Tachyarrhythmias (SVT, VT, VF) 2. Bradyarrhythmia (Complete heart block) 3. Sick sinus syndrome

8. **Etiology of extracardiac obstructive shock:**
   a. Pericardial tamponade
   b. Constrictive pericarditis
   c. Acute cor. pulmonale
   d. Coarctation of the aorta
   e. Drug overdose or substance poisoning
9. **Clinical finding:**
   a. **Symptoms**
      1. Anxiety, restlessness, altered mental state due to decreased blood flow to the brain
      2. Breathing difficulty, tachypnea
      3. Cold clammy hands and feet
      4. Decreased urinary output
   b. **Signs:**
      1. Mental status altered (Due to less cerebral perfusion)
      2. Patient appears pale, diaphoretic
      3. Pulse is rapid & weak or slow due to high grade heart block
      4. Hypotension due to decrease in cardiac output.
      5. Increased jugular venous pressure.
      6. Tachypnea, cheyne-stokes respiration (sympathetic nervous stimulation, acidosis)
      7. Rales are present in most of patients with LV failure

10. **Laboratory findings:**
    a. **CBC:** WBC typically raised with left shift
    b. **RFT:** BUN and serum creatinine rise progressively (Renal hypoperfusion leads to AKI)
    c. **LFT:** Hepatic transaminases elevated due to liver hypoperfusion
    d. **ABG:** Metabolic acidosis, hypoxemia.
    e. **Cardiac markers:** Markedly elevated.
11. **Investigations:**
    a. **ECG:** Identify abnormal heart rhythms and myocardial infarction.
    b. **2D echo**: Useful to know motion wall deformity, valvular deformity, ventricular function, rupture of the interventricular septum or cardiomyopathy.
    c. **Left heart catheterization:** Diagnose and treatment of heart diseases
    d. **Pulmonary artery catheterization:** Excludes other causes of shock
    e. **Coronary Angiography for MI/ischemia**: Identify the obstruction in coronary blood vessels.
    f. **ABG:** Body acid base balance, body pH, arterial gases evaluation.
12. **Treatment:**
    a. Rest
    b. Correct hypoxia, acidosis with oxygen administration/ventilatory support if required.
    c. Intravenous fluids if hypovolemia
    d. **Vasopressors:**
        1. **Dopamine:** Drug of choice in cardiogenic shock with oliguric renal failure
        2. **Dobutamine:** It increases cardiac output with little effect on heart rate.
        3. **Noradrenaline:** It increases SBP and DBP with net decrease in heart rate. (It causes renal vasoconstriction and thus worsens renal failure)
    e. Antiarrhythmic drugs or insertion of pacemaker in case of arrhythmias.
    f. Thrombolytic therapy or CABG or PTCA to restore myocardial perfusion
    g. Correcting mechanical causes like mitral valve repair etc.
13. **Mechanical circulatory support:**
    1. Circulatory assisted devices can be used to support ventricles of heart.
    2. The most commonly used device is an intra-aortic balloon pump inserted in the aorta through the femoral vein. E.g. Intra-aortic balloon pump

SEPTIC SHOCK

1. **Definition:** Septic shock refers to sepsis with hypotension that cannot be corrected by the infusion of fluids.
2. Arterial blood pressure less than 90 mm Hg despite adequate fluid resuscitation.
3. It is a serious medical condition which leads to multiorgan failure and death.
4. **Sepsis:** The harmful body's response to infection which leads to damage to own tissue and organs.
5. Sepsis most commonly caused by the infection of bacteria but also by viruses, fungi or parasites.
6. Sepsis focus may present anywhere in the body.
7. **Clinical features:**

   A. Clinical features of septic shock

   a. Early stage sepsis

   1. Fever
   2. Malaise
   3. Shivering
   4. High respiratory rate
   5. Profound sweating
   6. Wide pulse pressure
   7. Normal blood pressure

   b. Later stage sepsis

   1. Altered mental status
   2. Cold clammy skin
   3. Patient appears pale
   4. Oliguria
   5. Hypotension
   6. Clinical features of multi organ failure

   B. Clinical features of septic focus

   1. **Urinary tract infection:** Lower abdominal pain, fever, dysuria
   2. **Abdominal organ infection:** Pain, tenderness, guarding, rigidity over abdomen, fever .
   3. **Large untidy wounds**

9. **Investigations:**

   a. Complete blood count: In early stage of sepsis leucopenia and later on leucocytosis is seen.

b. Septic work up: Blood culture, microscopy, culture and sensitivity of Urine, sputum, wound swab, endocervical swab is done .

c. Investigation to identify suspected source:

Chest X-ray, ultasonography (A+P)/Local, CT/MRI scan of body parts.

8. **Treatment**

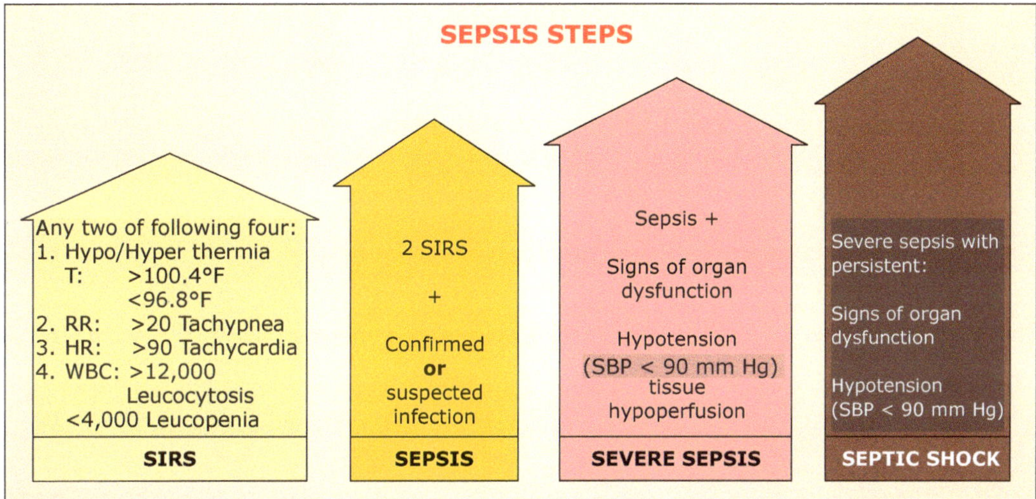

Management includes:

1. Management of systemic and local infection
2. Support airway, breathing and circulation
3. Symptomatic treatment

a. **Admit the patient to ICU**

b. **Secure IV line & collect blood samples for investigations**

c. **Start initial assessment of patient with resuscitation.**

d. **Circulatory support:**

1. **IV fluid administration:**

   a. Start with infusion of 1-2 litres of NS given within 1-2 hours

   b. Maintain CVP in between 8-12 cm of H_2O

   c. The urine output rate should be kept > 0.5 ml/kg per hour by continuing fluid administration

   d. Maintain the systolic pressure > 90 mm of Hg

   e. Monitor the circulatory adequacy by mental status, urine output and skin perfusion

2. **Vasopressor support nor-adrenaline, dopamine & dobutamine**

e. **Respiratory support:** Patient with progressive hypoxemia, hypercapnia, mental status deterioration or RS failure ventilatory support provided.

f. **Antimicrobial agents:** Initially broad spectrum antibiotics are initiated till availability of culture and sensitivity report and after getting report change antibiotics accordingly.

g. **Source of infection is treated:** Identify the source of infection and then control the source by surgical drainage of pus or both.

h. **Blood transfusion:** If Hb is ≤ 7 gm/dl with target Hb is 9 gm/dl.

i. **Critical illness related corticosteroid insufficiency (CIRCI):** Patients who develop hypotension that does not respond to fluid replacement therapy then suspect CIRCI.

If a patient is suspected of CIRCI then Hydrocortisone should be given.

ANAPHYLAXIS AND ANAPHYLACTIC SHOCK

1. **Definition:** It is a rapidly developing serious generalized immunological reaction occurring within minutes after combination of antigen with antibody bound to mast cells in individuals previously sensitized to the antigen.
2. Anaphylaxis is acute, potentially fatal, systemic type I hypersensitivity reaction mediated by IgE
3. It occurs due to exposure to specific antigens (Allergens)
4. Most exposures occur either by inhalation or ingestion of antigens.
5. **Common causes**
   a. Drugs and vaccines
   b. Bee/wasp stings
   c. Foods (Nuts, shellfish)
   d. Exposure to latex material: Surgical gloves, Foley's urinary catheter
6. **Clinical features:**
   a. **Respiratory system:**
      1. **Upper airway occlusion:** Swelling of lips, tongue, pharynx and epiglottitis.
      2. **Lower airway involvement:** Similar to acute severe asthma
   b. **Skin:** Pruritus, urticaria, erythema and angioedema
   c. **Cardiovascular system:** Hypotension and shock, arrhythmias, chest pain and ECG changes.

   d. **GI tract:** Nausea, vomiting, diarrhea, abdominal cramps.
   e. **CNS:** Headcahe, anxiety, confusion, coma
   f. **Eyes:** Itching and tears

7. **Management:**
   a. **Discontinue the allergen**
   b. **Give 100% oxygen**
   c. **Open and maintain airway:** Emergency endotracheal intubation and ventilatory support may be required
   d. **Give inhaled B2 agonist:** Salbutamol nebulization with oxygen for broncho-spasm.
   e. **Adrenaline is the drug of choice in the anaphylactic shock:** It is given as 0.5 ml of 1:1000 solution I.M (on lateral thigh)/S.C.

      Repeat after 5 min if there is no improvement
   f. **Antihistamine H1 blockers (Chlorpheniramine) and H2 blockers (Ranitidine)**
   g. **IV fluid administration (Rapid infusion 1-2 lit of saline)**
   h. **IV administration of hydrocortisone 100-200 mg slowly administered which reduces the severity/duration of symptoms.**
   i. **Admit/observe after initial treatment**

HEART FAILURE

1. **Definition: When the heart is unable to pump sufficiently to maintain blood flow to meet the body's needs**

   a. Heart failure occurs as a result of structural abnormality and functional impairment of ventricles of heart.

   b. Cardinal clinical symptoms of HF are dyspnea and fatigue and signs of HF are edema and rales.

   c. **In right sided heart failure:** There is a peripheral edema, raised jugular venous pressure, and hypotension

   But no evidence of pulmonary edema.

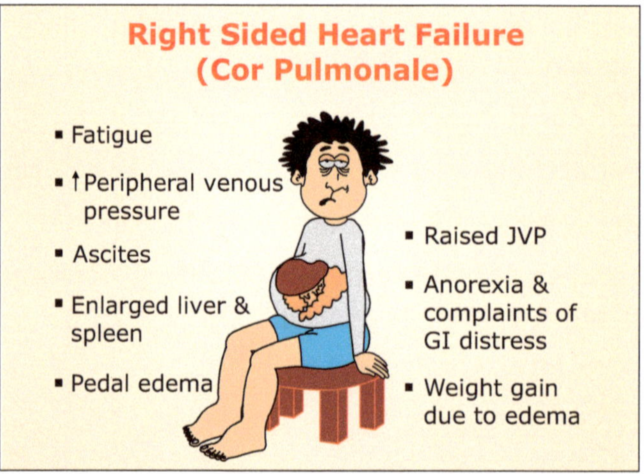

   d. **In left sided heart failure:** In most of the cases pulmonary edema is common involved. Other signs of left sided failure include cardiomegaly, third heart sound, tachycardia, tachypnea.

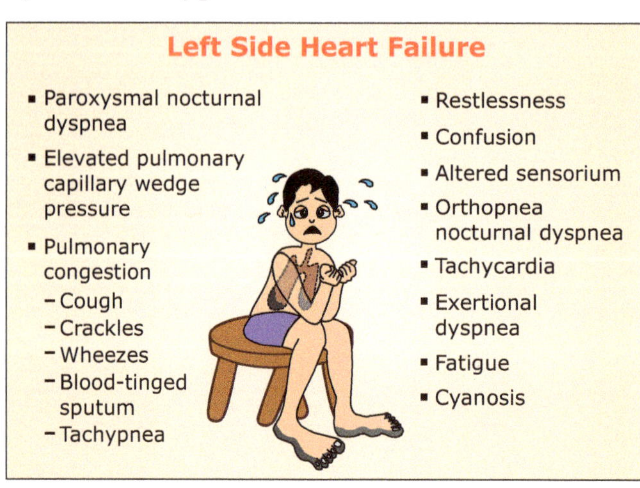

e. **Congestive cardiac failure:** Patients have signs and symptoms of both right and left sided heart failure.

2. **Functional classification (NYHA) of heart failure**

a. **Class I -** No symptoms and no limitation in ordinary physical activity, e.g. Shortness of breath while on walking or climbing staircase.

b. **Class II -** Mild symptoms (Mild shortness of breath) and slight limitation during ordinary activity.

c. **Class III -** Marked limitation in activity due to symptoms, even during less-than-ordinary activity, e.g. Shortness of breath on walking short distance and comfortable only at rest.

d. **Class IV -** Severe limitations in activity. (Patient have symptoms even at rest and mostly remain bed ridden).

e. No NYHA class listed or unable to determine

3. **Etiology:**

a. Coronary artery disease is most common cause of heart failure.

b. Clinical states which are involved in excessive blood flow requirement (systemic A-V shunting, chronic anemia) are responsible for development of heart failure.

Excessive blood flow requirement	1. Systemic A-V shunting 2. chronic anemia
Metabolic disorder	Thyrotoxicosis
Nutritional disorder	Beri-beri

c. **Causes of heart failure:**

Coronary artery disease	Myocardial infarction, myocardial ischemia
Chronic pressure overload	Hypertension, obstructive valvular disease
Chronic volume overload	Valvular regurgitation, congenital heart disease (shunts)
Chronic lung diseases	Cor pulmonale, pulmonary vascular disorder
Non ischemic dilated cardiomyopathy	Familial/genetic disorder, infiltrative disorder
Chronic arrhythmias	Chronic bradyarrhythmias, chronic tachyarrhythmias
Pathological hypertrophy	Primary (Hypertrophic cardiomyopathies) Secondary (Hypertension)
Restrictive cardiomyopathy	Amyloidosis Sarcoidosis

4. **Clinical manifestation:**

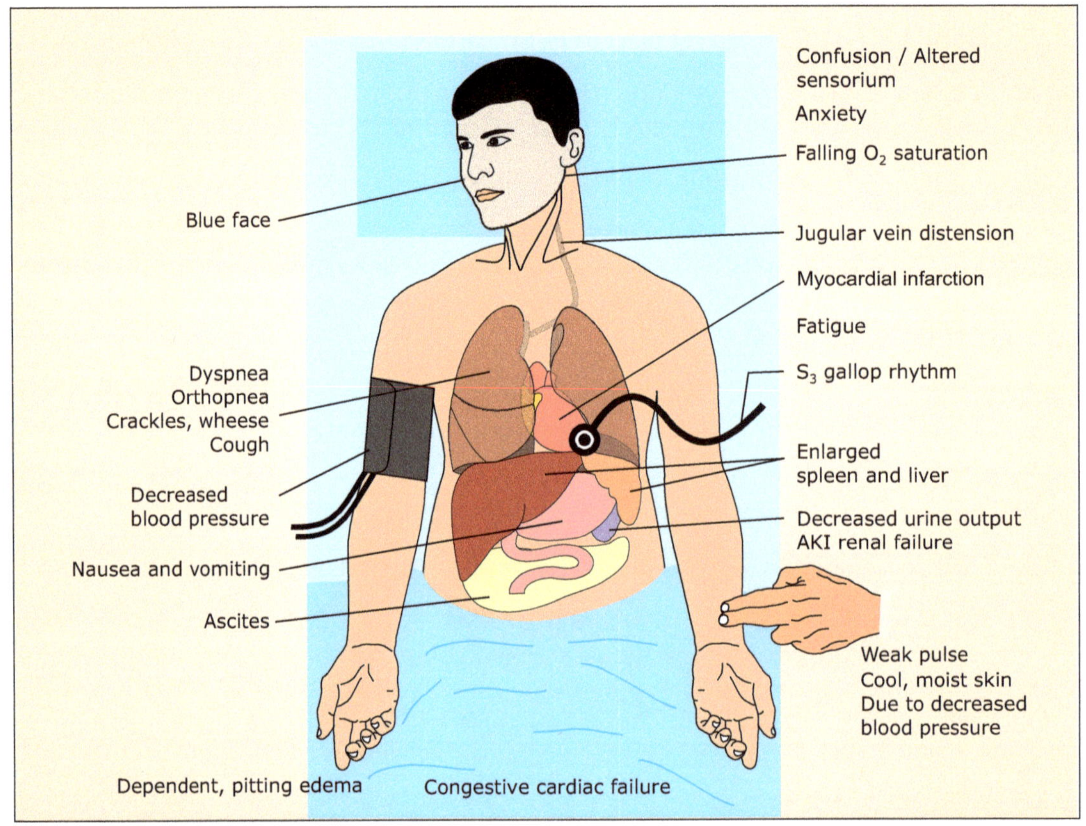

a. The cardinal symptoms of HF are fatigue and breathlessness.

b. **Fatigue**

c. **Dyspnea:**

1. In initial stages of heart failure dyspnea occurs during exertion but as disease progress it occurs with less strenuous activity and finally occurs even at rest.
2. There are multiple mechanism involved for development of shortness of breath such as pulmonary congestion due to left ventricular failure, respiratory fatigue, pulmonary compliance is reduced.
3. Rapid and shallow breathing is characteristic feature of cardiac dyspnea.
4. **Orthopnea:** Dyspnea occurs in supine position/recumbent position and this usually occurs in late stage of heart failure.

   Cause: Due to redistribution of fluid from splanchnic circulation and lower extremities into central circulation.

5. **Paroxysmal nocturnal dyspnea:**
   - Mostly occurs in night hours
   - In PND patients develop acute onset of dyspnea and coughing that awakens the patient from sleep.
   - Occurs after 1-3 hours of sleep
   - PND possibly because of two factors:
     1. **Raised pressure inside bronchial artery:** Airway compression
     2. **Interstitial edema:** Increased airway resistance .
6. **Cheyne-stokes respiration:** Apneic phase → arterial PO_2 falls and arterial PCO_2 rises → stimulate the respiratory centre → resulting in hyperventilation and hypocapnia, followed by recurrence of apnea.

d. Gastrointestinal symptoms:

1. Anorexia
2. Nausea
3. Abdominal pain
4. Abdominal fullness
5. Complain related to edema of bowel wall and/or a congested liver.
6. Right upper quadrant pain due to congestion of liver and stretching of liver capsule.

e. Cerebral symptoms: Altered mental status

5. **Physical examination:**

Help to determine the cause of HF as well as to assess severity of syndrome.

a. **In mild to moderate severe HF:** Patient becomes discomfortable after lying down for more than a few minutes.

b. **In more severe HF:** Patient need to sit upright for comfort, may have labored breathing, and unable to complete sentence because of shortness of breath.

c. Cold extremities due to vasoconstriction.

d. Cyanosis

e. Positive abdominojugular reflux

f. On auscultation crepitation are heard in lung fields due to accumultion of fluid in alveoli.

g. Pleural effusion most commonly seen in bilateral ventricular failure.

h. Hepato and splenomegaly
i. Ascites
j. Peripheral edema is a cardinal manifestation of HF.
k. Third heart S3 sounds gallop.

6. **Investigations:**
   a. **Routine lab investigations:**
      1. CBC
      2. Serum electrolyte
      3. Serum creatinine
      4. BUN
      5. LFT
      6. Lipid profile
      7. FBS and PPBS (in diabetes mellitus)
      8. Thyroid profile
   b. **Biomarker:** B-type natriuretic peptide (BNP) and N-terminal pro-BNP (NT-proBNP) which are released from the failing heart
   c. **Echocardiography:** A routine 12 lead ECG is done to access cardiac rhythm and determine the presence of LV hypertrophy or a prior MI.
   d. **Chest X-ray:** Features of pulmonary congestions with or without cardiomegaly

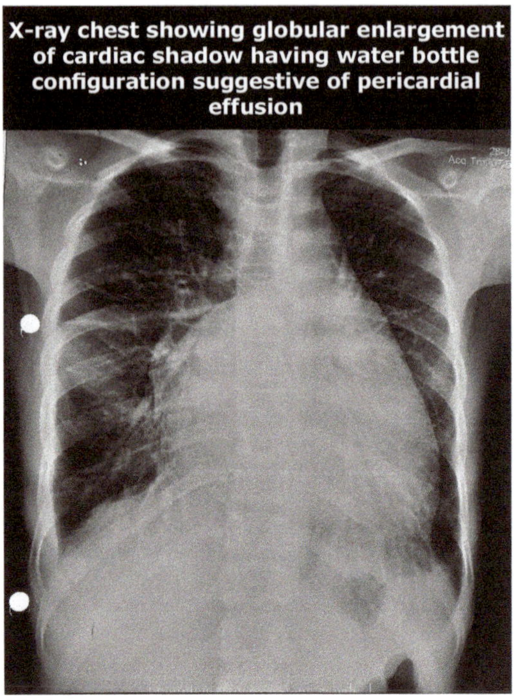
X-ray chest showing globular enlargement of cardiac shadow having water bottle configuration suggestive of pericardial effusion

e. **2D-echo:**

Provide information of LV size and ejection fraction as well as the presence or absence of valvular and/or motion wall abnormalities (Indicative of prior MI)

f. **Cardiac MRI:**

1. Useful to understand the cardiac functions and structural abnormalities.
2. Useful for determining the etiology of heart failure.

7. **FRAMINGHAM criteria for diagnosis of congestive cardiac failure:**

a. **MAJOR criteria:**

1. Paroxysmal nocturnal dyspnea
2. Neck vein distension
3. Crackles -lung field
4. Cardiomegaly on chest X-ray
5. Acute pulmonary edema
6. Third heart sound gallop
7. Increased venous pressure (> 16 cm of H_2O)
8. Positive hepatojugular reflux

b. **Minor criteria**

1. Extremity edema
2. Nocturnal cough
3. Dyspnea on ordinary exertion
4. Hepatomegaly
5. Pleural effusion
6. Tachycardia >120 bpm
7. Decreased vital capacity by 1/3

c. **For diagnosis: 1 major + 2 minor**

8. **Treatment:**

a. **In acute heart failure:**

1. Principles of management of acute decompensation is to identify the cause of precipitation and steps to correct it.
2. The immediate goal is to re-establish adequate perfusion and oxygen delivery to end organs. This entails ensuring that airway, breathing, and circulation are adequate.

Management:

1. **Hospitalization in intensive care unit:**

   Indications

   1. Patient with hypotension, decreased urine output with rising serum creatinine and BUN, or altered mental status in acute decompensated heart
   2. Patients who present with breathlessness, tachypnea, or hypoxemia (again, oxygen saturation of < 90%) at rest, or with significant arrhythmia.

2. **Respiratory support:** O_2 administration and non invasive respiratory support
3. **Drug therapy:**

Diuretics	Inotropic drugs	Vasodilators
In acute pulmonary edema removal of fluid is important to relieve the symptoms and to improve oxygenation	Increasing the contractibility	Act by reducing preload (venodilators), afterload (arteriolar dilators) or both (combined arteriolar and venodilators)
Diuretics of choice: Loop diuretics like furosemide and bumetanide To avoid the tolerance from the loop diuretics use thiazides or spironolactone in combination for chronic use	Dobutamine Dopamine **Cardiac glycosides** (Digoxin, digitoxin, strophanthin and ouabain) **Inodilators** (Inamrione, milrinone, enoximone and vesnarinone)	**Preload dilators:** nitrates **Afterload dilators:** Hydralazine, minoxidil and calcium channel blockers **(Not used in CHF)** **Agent reducing both preload and afterload:** ACE inhibitors, ARBs, Nitroprusside and alfa blockers.

Chronic heart failure management (Main aim is to decrease the work of heart by decreasing the preload and afterload and to prevent the mortality by reversing cardiac remodeling)

American heart association guidelines in treatment of chronic heart failure

Stage	Nature of heart disease	Treatment
A	No structural heart disease and no symptoms for HF Risk factors: DM, HTN, deranged lipid profile, familial cardiomyopathy	Lifestyle modification, stop smoking, salt restrictive diet, exercise, and treat the risk factor, ACE inhibitors are used to control BP
B	Structural heart disease with abnormal LV systolic function -MI, valvular disease but no clinical features of heart failure	Lifestyle modification, ACE inhibitors and β blockers
C	Structural heart disease and HF symptoms	Add diuretics and digoxin along with therapy as under stage A and B
D	Refractory HF symptoms to maximal medical Management	Therapy as listed under stage A, B, C mechanical assist devices, IV inotropic infusion, heart transplantation

b. **Cardiac assist device**

   1. Intra aortic balloon pump (IABP)
   2. Ventricular assist devices (VADs)
   3. Cardiac resynchronisation therapy/biventricular pacing

c. **Dialysis or ultrafiltration:** Indicated in patients with renal failure not responding to sodium, fluid restriction & diuretic therapy.

d. **Other Special considerations:**

   1. **Minimisations of medications that have deleterious effects in HF:**

      a. **Negative inotropes (e.g. verapamil, diltiazem)** should be avoided in the patient with impaired ventricular contractility.

      b. **NSAIDs:** Which antagonise the effect of ACE inhibitors and diuretics therapy, should be avoided, if possible

e. **Lifestyle modification:**

   1. Dietary restriction for sodium intake
   2. Stop smoking
   3. Stop alcohol consumption
   4. Weight reduction in obese patients
   5. Fluid and free water restrictions

BRADYARRHYTHMIAS

Definition: These are disorders of impulse formation or impulse conduction manifesting with slow ventricular rate < 60/min

1. These occur due to disorders of SA node or AV node.
2. SA node dysfunction and AV conduction block are the most common causes of pathologic bradycardia.

I. SA node dysfunction

1. The sinus node is a natural dominant pacemaker.
2. Sinus bradycardia refers to a heart rate of less than 60 bpm.
3. It may be pathological or physiological.
4. Causes of SA nodal dysfunction have been classified as intrinsic or extrinsic.
5. If Extrinsic dysfunction then it can be reversible
6. Intrinsic causes of sinus node dysfunction are degenerative (Due to pathological fibrous displacement).

Extrinsic causes	**Intrinsic causes**
Vasovagal stimulation Carotid sinus hypersensitivity	Age related degenerative fibrosis
	Coronary artery disease (Chronic and acute MI)
Drugs: 1. Beta blockers 2. Calcium channel blockers 3. Digoxin 4. Antiarrhythmics (Class I and III) 5. Ivabradine (HCN Channel blocker) 6. Clonidine (Other sympatholytics) 7. Lithium carbonate 8. Cimetidine 9. Amitriptyline 10. Phenothiazines 11. Narcotics (Methadone) 12. Pentamidine	**Inflammatory:** 1. Pericarditis 2. Myocarditis 3. Rheumatic fever 4. Chaga's disease 5. Lyme disease
Hypothyroidism	Senile amyloidosis, sarcoidosis, hemochromatosis

(Continued)

Extrinsic causes	**Intrinsic causes**
Sleep apnea	Congenital heart disease
Hypoxia	**Iatrogenic** 1. Radiation therapy 2. Postsurgical
Electrolyte abnormalities	Hyperkalemia, hypocalcemia
Hypothermia	Familial
Increased intracranial pressure (Cushing triad) Raised IOP	Myotonic dystrophy

7. **Clinical manifestations:**
    1. SA node dysfunction may be completely asymptomatic.
    2. Symptoms are due to both slow and fast heart rate.
        a. **Tachycardia:** Palpitations, angina and cardiac failure
        b. **Bradycardia:** Hypotension, syncope, fatigue and weakness
    3. In some patients SA node dysfunction may develop supraventricular tachycardia.
    4. In Sick sinus syndrome there is sinus node dysfunction and patient have combination of symptoms i.e. symptoms due to bradycardia and tachycardia .
8. **Diagnosis:** Based on the heart rate and electrocardiography
9. **Treatment:** Pacemaker implantation needed in irreversible SA node dysfunction.

II. Disorders of AV node

1. Main etiological causes of AV block are structural abnormality and functional impairment.
2. The functional causes like (Autonomic, metabolic/endocrine, and drug-related) tend to be reversible.
3. Most of causes produce permanent structural abnormalities along AV conduction segment such as fibrosis.
4. AV block is classified from first degree block to complete AV block based on severity.
5. Carotid sinus hypersensitivity, vasovagal syncope, may be associated with AV conduction block.

Causes of AV block:

1. **Metabolic/Endocrine:** Hyperkalemia, Hypothyroidism, Hypermagnesemia, Adrenaling insufficiency.
2. **Drug-Related:** Beta blockers, Calcium channel blockers, Antiarrhythmics (class I and III), Adenosine, Digitalis, Lithium.
3. **Infections:** Endocarditis, Diphtheria, Chagas' disease, Toxoplasmosis.
4. **Inflammatory:** SLE, Rheumatoid arthritis, Scleroderma.
5. **Infiltrative:** Amyloidosis, Hemochromatosis, Sarcoidosis.
6. **Neoplastic:** Lymphoma, Mesothelioma, Melanoma
7. **Traumatic:** Radiation, Catheter ablation.
8. **Coronary Artery Disease:** Acute MI.
9. **Congenital:** Congenital heart disease, Maternal SLE, Myotonic dystrophy.
10. **Autonomic nervous system activation:** Vasovagal stimulation

Types of AV block:

First degree AV block	As a result of delay in conduction of impulse through conduction system. One P wave for each QRS complex. PR interval prolonged (> 200 ms)
Mobitz type I block	It is a reversible block of the AV node. Progressive lengthening of PR interval Shortening of a RR interval Less chances of myocardial infarction
Mobitz type II block	In this AV block there is sudden failure of Purkinje and his cells for rapid conduction of impulse in conduction system. In this block there is a alternate conducted atrial beats and non conducted atrial beats. One P wave is not followed by a QRS complex. The degree of block can be expressed as 2:1 and 3:1 2:1 type of block meaning two P waves per QRS complex More chances of Myocardial infarction in this block
Third degree AV block	Complete failure of conduction from atrium to ventricle No association between the P waves and QRS complexes. Atrial contraction is normal but no beats are conducted to the ventricles In this ventricles are excited with depolarising focus within the ventricular muscles. QRS complexes are abnormally shaped, because of abnormal spread of depolarization from ventricular focus.

Signs and symptoms of second- and third-degree heart block include:

1. Fainting
2. Dizziness or light-headedness
3. Fatigue (Tiredness)
4. Shortness of breath
5. Chest pain

Diagnosis: Electrocardiographically.

Treatment:

1. Correction of electrolyte disturbance and ischemia.
2. Inhibit vasovagal stimulation.
3. Stop the drugs with AV nodal blocking properties .
4. IV atropine or isoproterenol given as it is useful in AV nodal block.
5. If patient have a second-degree heart block, a pacemaker is needed.
6. If patient have a third-degree heart block, pacemaker needed for the rest of life.
7. In third degree block, in an emergency, a temporary pacemaker might be used until you can get a long-term device.

TACHYARRHYTHMIAS

1. **Definition:** Heart rhythm with a rate >100 beats/min.
2. Tachyarrhythmias results from the disorders of impulse formation and disorders of impulse propagation.
3. Tachyarrhythmias due to impulse propagation is more common than impulse formation.
4. According to the origin of arrhythmias, tachyarrhythmias classified as supraventricular (origin above the bifurcation of bundle of His) and ventricular tachycardia.
5. When origin of impulse is not known then these arrhythmias can be classified morphologically into narrow complex tachycardia (Duration of QRS is < 120 msec) and broad complex tachycardia (Duration of QRS > 120 msec)
6. **Common causes of physiologic sinus tachycardia:**
   a. Exercise
   b. Acute illness with fever, infection, pain
   c. Hypovolemia, anemia
   d. Hyperthyroidism
   e. Pulmonary insufficiency
   f. Drugs: Theophylline, nifedipine, albuterol, hydralazine
   g. Pheochromocytoma
7. **Causes of tachyarrhythmias:**
   a. Damage to heart tissues from heart diseases
   b. Defective electrical pathway of heart since birth
   c. Disease or congenital abnormality of the heart

8. **Analysis of ECG in tachycardia:**

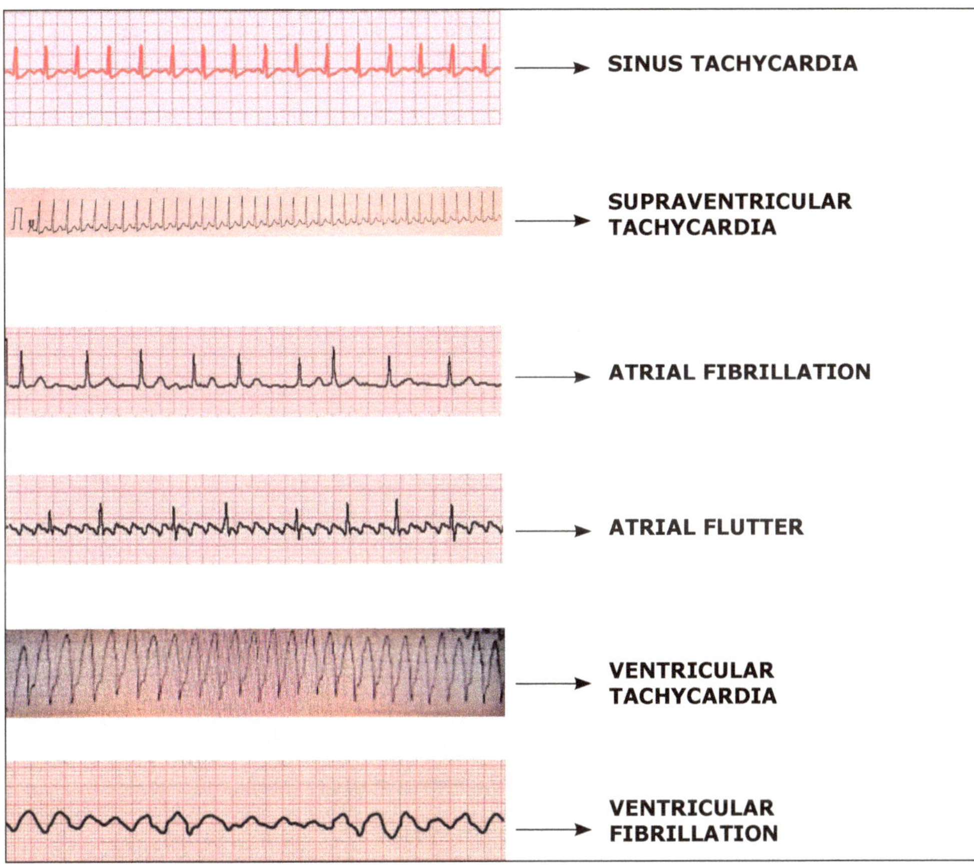

a. Rate, morphology and regularity of P wave

b. QRS morphology

c. Look for sinus P wave/fibrillation wave/flutter wave/ectopic P2 deflection

d. Response to carotid sinus massage/vagal maneuvers or not.

9. **Symptoms of tachyarrhythmias:**

a. **Symptoms**

1. Shortness of breath
2. Lightheadedness
3. Rapid pulse rate
   Heart palpitations
4. Chest pain
5. Fainting (syncope)

b. **Signs:**
   1. Rapid pulse rate
   2. Bounding pulse

10. **Management of tachyarrhythmias:**
   a. **Support airway, breathing and circulation**
      1. Give oxygen
      2. Insert IV cannula
      3. Monitor Blood pressure and SPO_2
      4. ECG (If possible record the 12 lead ECG)
      5. Identify and treat the reversible cause
   b. **Step I: Check whether patient is stable or unstable**
      1. **Signs of instability**
         a. Altered mental status
         b. Hypotension
         c. Chest pain
         d. Signs of heart failure
      2. **If unstable:**
         a. Synchronised DC shock (Upto 3 attempt)
         b. IV amiodarone can be given
   c. **Step II: If patient is stable then see QRS complex whether broad or narrow**
      1. **If QRS is narrow with**
         a. **Rhythm regular**
            1. **Empirically treat as AVNRT**
               a. Carotid massage
               b. Adenosine with or without calcium channel blocker
            2. **If patient not responding to above treatment then it may have atrial flutter**
               a. Drug therapy for rate control
               b. DC cardioversion
         b. **Rhythm Irregular**
            1. **Empirically treat as atrial fibrillation**
               a. **If onset > 48 hr**

1. Rate control with intravenous beta blocker or calcium channel blockers.
2. Digoxin may be added to rate controlling drugs.

b. **If onset < 48 hr**

Consider rhythm control (Intravenous loading dose of amiodarone or DC cardiovesion) or rate control

c. **Consider need of anticoagulation in patients with atrial fibrillation > 48 hours or associated with high risk factors.**

2. **If QRS is broad with rhythm**

a. **Regular**

1. **Empirically treat as ventricular tachycardia:**

   Loading dose of IV amiodarone or IV lidocaine and if unresponsive to drug therapy then use cardioversion

2. **If previously confirmed SVT with bundle branch block:** Adenosine

b. **Irregular**

1. **AF with BBB:** Treat as for narrow complex
2. **Polymorphic VT (Torsades de pointes):** Give intravenous magnesium along with or without DC cardioversion
3. **Pre-excited AF:** Amiodarone or DC cardioversion

CHAPTER

7

Respiratory System

EXAMINATION OF RESPIRATORY SYSTEM

I) **Primary assessment:**

1. **Altered mental status/not**
2. **Snoring, gurgling/stridor may indicate airway obstruction**
3. **Short history about the symptoms and cardiopulmonary disorders**
4. **Ask the full name:** If patient is unable to complete the sentence while speaking then it is mostly due to severe respiratory impairment and needs immediate respiratory support.
5. **Inspection:**
   a. Respiratory rate
   b. Use of accessory muscles
   c. Cyanosis
6. **Check blood pressure**
7. **SpO_2 saturation**
8. **Auscultation:** Auscultate the anterior and posterior chest wall, axilla (Infraaxillary)

Additional history:

1. Current or previous cigarette smoking (Packs per day)
2. Possible inhalational exposure
3. Travelling history
4. Duration, progress of symptoms and severity

II) Secondary assessment (Detailed examination):

Detailed history:

Symptoms

1. **Dyspnea:**
   a. Patients with obstructive lung diseases often complain of chest tightness or inability to get a deep breath.
   b. Onset and duration of dyspnea is helpful in determining the etiological factor
   c. Sudden onset is seen in laryngeal edema, bronchospasm, pulmonary embolism or pneumothorax
   d. Gradual progression of dyspnea on exertion seen in the COPD and idiopathic pulmonary fibrosis
   e. In asthmatics there is recurrent episodes of dyspnea due to specific allergens
   f. In congestive cardiac failure patient complains of a sense of air hunger.
2. **Cough:**
   a. Cough generally indicate disease of respiratory system
   b. Ask about duration of cough and whether associated with sputum production
   c. If cough associated with sputum producton ask about type and quantity e.g. Pink frothy (heart failure), blood in sputum (Pulmonary embolism).
   d. Chronic cough (> 8 weeks) commonly involved in obstructive lung diseases such as chronic bronchitis, chronic bronchiectasis.
3. **Hemoptysis:**
   a. Hemoptysis can be seen in many lung diseases, bronchogenic carcinoma and pulmonary embolism.

Physical examination:

1. **Inspection:**
    a) Shape, movement of chest
    b) Apical impulse (After standing on right side of patient and look tangentially over precordium)
    c) Look at patient for rate, rhythm, type, depth and breathing pattern
    d) Whether accessory muscles of respiration are working or not (Patients with respiratory distress often using accessory muscles of respiration to breathe)
    e) Wheezing or stridor
    f) Supraclavicular and infraclavicular fossae
    g) Intercostal suction
    h) Whether both the nipples are at the same level or not
    i) Venous prominence after coughing in standing or sitting position
    j) **Skin in front and back:** Pigmentation, sinus, ulcers, herpes zoster, any swelling, gynecomastia.
    k) Dilated veins and swelling in neck
    l) **Examination of Back:** Look for scoliosis, kyphosis, drooping of the shoulder, winging of the scapula, spinoscapular distance.

       Severe kyphoscoliosis can result in restrictive pathophysiology
    m) Fullness or depression: 1. Unilateral or bilateral
       2. Localised or generalised

2. **Palpation:**
    a) Surface temperature
    b) Tenderness (Rib tenderness in trauma, fracture or secondary metastasis, intercostal tenderness or punch tenderness in liver abscess)
    c) Position of trachea and the apex beat
    d) Movement of the chest
    e) Tactile vocal fremitus
    f) **Other palpatory findings:** Subcutaneous emphysema, friction fremitus, rhonchal fremitus, palpable pericardial rub.

3. **Percussion:**

Conventional percussion: Done on right and left
Shifting dullness: Done on right and left
Coin percussion: Done on right and left
Hepatic and cardiac dullness: Lost or not (both are lost in emphysema)

Percussion is used to distinguish between the pleural effusion and pneumothorax

4. **Auscultation:**

   1. Majority of the manifestations of respiratory diseases present as abnormalities of auscultation.

      a) Breath sounds

      b) Vocal resonance

      c) Adventitious sounds or added sounds

      - **Wheeze:**

        i. Wheeze is a continuous, high pitched whistling sound heard while breathing.

        ii. Wheeze are manifestation of airway obstruction and heard on expiration

        iii. Any condition which can cause narrowing of small bronchioles can result in wheeze.

        iv. Most common sign of asthma

        v. Congestive heart failure can also result in diffuse wheezes

      - **Crackles or rales:**

        i. Crackles are discontinuous, non-musical adventitious sounds normally heard in inspiration and sometimes on expiration.

        ii. Crackles are classified as fine and coarse crackles

        iii. Most common sign of alveolar disease

        iv. Alveoli filled with fluid results in crackles

        v. Pneumonia can cause focal crackles

        vi. Pulmonary edema is associated with crackles, generally prominent at the base

        vii. Egophony: Auscultation of sound AH instead of EEE when patient phonates EEE. It is helpful to distinguish between crackles associated with alveolar fluid and those associated with interstitial fibrosis **(Velcro crepts)**

- **Stridor:**

  Manifestation of upper airway obstruction (Mainly inspiratory)

- **Other systemic finding:**

  i. **Pedal edema:** Symmetrical then may be suggestive of cor pulmonale

  ii. **Jugular venous distension:** Sign of volume overload associated with right heart failure

  iii. **Pulsus paradoxus:** Ominous sign in the obstructive lung disease

  iv. **Clubbing:** Found in cystic fibrosis, Interstitial pulmonary fibrosis and lung cancer

  v. **Cyanosis:** Seen in the hypoxemic respiratory disorder that result in > 5 gm of deoxy Hb/dl. The majority of respiratory diseases falls in three major categories:

SYMPTOMS OF RESPIRATORY DISEASES

1. Sneezing and runny nose
2. Nasal congestion
3. Cough
4. Sore throat
5. Breathlessness
6. Chest pain
7. Sputum production
8. Hemoptysis
9. Fever
10. Weight loss

CLASSIFICATION OF RESPIRATORY DISEASES

The majority of respiratory diseases fall in three following major categories

1. Obstructive lung disease
2. Restrictive disorders
3. Abnormalities of the vasculature

Obstructive lung diseases	Asthma, COPD, Bronchiectasis, bronchiolitis, cystic fibrosis
Restrictive	
1. Chest wall/pleural disease	Kyphoscoliosis, ankylosing spondylitis, chronic pleural effusion
2. Parenchymal disease	Asbestosis, sarcoidosis, idiopathic pulmonary fibrosis, interstitial Pneumonitis.
3. Neuromuscular weakness	Guillain -barre syndrome, amyotrophic lateral sclerosis, Diaphramatic paralysis
Pulmonary vasculature diseases	Pulmonary embolism, pulmonary arterial hypertension (PAH)
Infection	Pneumonia, bronchitis, tracheitis
Malignancy	Bronchogenic carcinoma, metastatic diseases

ASTHMA

1. Asthma is a common long-term inflammatory disease of the airways of the lungs which is due to hyperresponsiveness of tracheobronchial tree to multiple intrinsic and extrinsic stimuli.
2. It is characterised by airflow obstruction and it varies markedly to both spontaneously and with therapy.
3. Inflammation of the airway causes thick, sticky secretion called mucus.
4. In asthma attacks, the bronchial smooth muscles constrict causing narrowing of airways causing airflow obstruction.

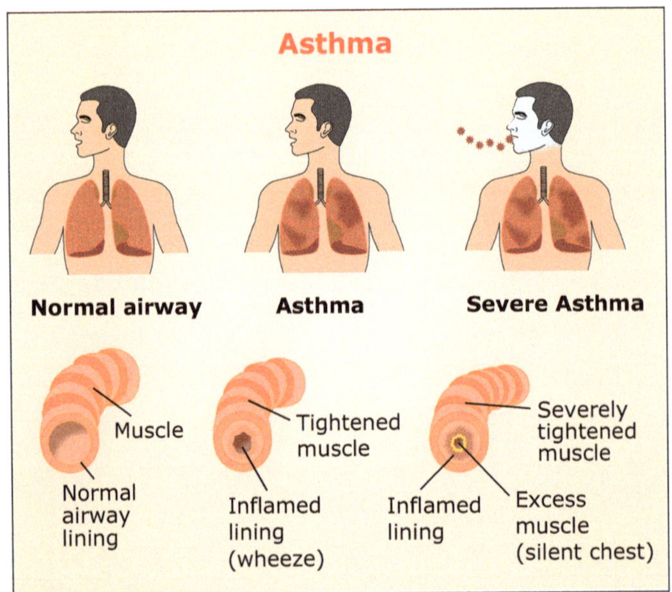

5. This swelling, mucus, and tight muscles can make your airways narrower than normal and it becomes very hard for patient to get air into and out of the lungs
6. **Asthma is caused by a combination of genetic and environmental factors:**

Endogenous factors	Environmental factors
Positive family history (genetic predisposition)	Indoor allergens
Atopy	Outdoor allergens
Airway hyperresponsiveness	Occupational exposure
High BMI	Respiratory infection e.g. viral infections
	Food additives: Tartazine, fish, nuts
	Passive smoker
	Acetaminophen

7. **Factor precipitating asthma:**
   a. Allergens
   b. Cold air
   c. Tobacco smoke
   d. Dust
   e. Emotional stress
   f. Upper respiratory viral infection
   g. Exercise and hyperventilation
   h. Sulfur dioxide and irritant gases
   i. Irritants (Household sprays, paint fumes)
8. **Clinical features**
   a. Breathlessness
   b. Cough
   c. Wheezing
   d. Symptoms are worse at night hours.
   e. Above symptoms are variable, both spontaneously and with therapy.
9. **Investigations:**
   a. **Pulmonary function tests:** Reduced FEV1, FEV1/FVC ratio.
   b. **Hematological tests:** Total serum IgE and specific IgE to inhaled allergens, may be measured in some patients
   c. **CT scan:** HRCT chest can detect structural abnormalities such as thickening of bronchial wall in asthma but non diagnostic for asthma.

      But useful in identification of associated condition or detect conditions which mimic asthma.
   d. **Skin test (Not routinely done):** Skin prick test for common allergens are positive in allergic asthma
   e. **Exhaled nitric oxide:** Test to see compliance with therapy
10. **Clinical classification of asthma**

	Symptoms	**Night time Symptoms**
Intermittent	$<$ 1 time a week asymptomatic and normal PEF between attacks	$\leq$ 2 times a month
Mild persistent	$\geq$ time a week but $<$ 1 time a day	$>$ 2 times a month
Moderate persistent	Daily use B2 agonist daily, attack affect activity	$>$ 1 time a week predicted
Severe persistent	Continuous limited physical activity	Frequent

11. **Diagnosis**

    Diagnostic steps for asthma:

    a. **Patient with respiratory symptoms (Are the symptoms typical of asthma)**

       If no typical symptoms of asthma then take further history and do tests for alternative diagnosis.

    b. **Detailed history/examination for asthma (Support diagnosis)**

    c. **Perform spirometry (Support diagnosis)**

    d. **The diagnosis should be confirmed and evidence documented for further reference and before starting controlled therapy.**

12. **Management of bronchial asthma**

    Asthma management includes:

    i. **Assess**
       a. Confirmation of diagnosis, if necessary
       b. Symptom control & modifiable risk factors
       c. Lung function
       d. Associated comorbidities
       e. Inhaler technique & adherence

    ii. **Adjust**
       a. Education & skills training
       b. Asthma medication
       c. Smoking cessation

    iii. **Review response**
       a. Symptoms
       b. Exacerbations
       c. Side-effects
       d. Lung function
       e. Patient satisfaction

    1. **Treatment of infection**

       Use of antibiotics should generally be reserved for patients with fever, purulent sputum and pneumonia.

    2. **Avoidance of allergens and other precipitating factor**

3. **Drugs:**

A. **Bronchodilator therapy:**

a. There are three classes of bronchodilators in current use: β2 -adrenergic agonists, anticholinergics, and methylxanthine.

i. **β2 adrenergic agonist:**

- **Short-acting β2 -agonists (SABAs):** Albuterol (salbutamol) and terbutaline are fast acting, short duration of action and used by inhalation route to abort an acute attack.
- **Long-acting β2-agonists (LABAs):** Salmeterol and formoterol, both of which have long duration of action and are given twice daily by inhalation route and useful in aborting acute attack as well as for prophylaxis.
- LABAs are used when the regular use of SABAs is needed to abort & control attack.
- LABAs should be given with ICS therapy because LABA alone do not control the underlying inflammation.

ii. **Anticholinergics:**

- Muscarinic receptor antagonists such as ipratropium bromide prevent bronchoconstriction and mucus secretion.
- Less effective than β2-agonists as they are slower acting bronchodilator

iii. **Methylxanthine:**

- Methylxanthines are given orally and having therapeutic effect of bronchodilation which is slow and sustained.
- It may be used as an additional bronchodilator in patients with severe asthma
- IV aminophylline was used for the treatment of severe asthma but due to side effects e.g. hypotension, tremors, convulsions, arrhythmias it is nowadays replaced with use of high dose inhaled SABA.

B. **Controlled therapies:**

a. **Inhaled Corticosteroids and Systemic Corticosteroids (Budesonide)**

b. **Cromones:** Cromolyn sodium and nedocromil sodium are used only to prevent acute attack of asthma by inhibition of degranulation of mast cells and sensory nerve activation.

c. **Anti-leukotrienes:**

   i. Cysteinyl-leukotrienes are potent bronchoconstrictors.

   ii. Useful as an additional therapy in some patients which are not controlled with low doses of ICS

d. **Anti-IgE**: Omalizumab inhibits IgE-mediated reactions to prevent the attack of bronchial asthma.

Clinical class of asthma	Treatment
Mild intermittent	1. Short acting β2 agonist
Mild persistent	1. Short acting β2 agonist 2. ICS low dose
Moderate persistent	1. ICS low dose 2. LABA
Severe persistent	1. ICS high dose 2. LABA
Very severe persistent	1. ICS high dose 2. LABA 3. OCS

Note: Short acting β2 agonist is required for symptomatic relief and steroids are mainstay because they decrease underlying inflammation.

ACUTE SEVERE ASTHMA (STATUS ASTHMATICUS)

1. **Acute severe asthma** is an acute exacerbation of asthma that does not respond to standard treatment of bronchodilators (inhalers) and corticosteroids
2. Status asthmaticus refers to severe bronchospasm that does not respond to aggressive therapies within 30 to 60 minutes.
3. It is a life-threatening episode of airway obstruction and is considered a medical emergency.
4. Complications include cardiac and/or respiratory arrest.
5. **Clinical features:**
   a. Patient is so breathless that they are unable to complete the sentences
   b. Patient may have cyanosis due to severe hypoxia
   c. Tachycardia (> 120 beats/min)
   d. Tachypnea (> 30 cycles/min)
   e. Sweating
   f. Pulsus paradoxus may be present
   g. Altered level of consciousness, confusion, exhaustion
   h. Silent chest
   i. Severe hypoxemia and PCO_2 is usually low due to hyperventilation
6. **Management:**
   a. High concentration oxygen therapy (Target saturation 90 to 95%)
   b. High dose of short acting β2 agonist by nebuliser (Repeat every 20 min)
   c. Systemic corticosteroids (Injection hydrocortisone 100-200 mg IV stat and further if necessary)
   d. If no response with above treatment then start ipratropium bromide by nebulisation or IV aminophylline (250 mg over 20 minutes)
   e. Monitor the treatment with oxygen concentration and PEF or FEV1
   f. In assisted ventilation, prefer non invasive ventilation before invasive.
7. **Indications for assisted ventilation:**
   a. Coma
   b. Respiratory arrest
   c. Exhaustion, confusion, drowsiness
   d. Deterioration of ABG tension despite therapy

CHRONIC OBSTRUCTIVE PULMONARY DISEASE

1. **Definition:** A pulmonary disease state in which there is airflow limitation that is not fully reversible caused by long term inhalation exposure to noxious substances such as tobacco smoke.
2. **Causes:**
   a. **Cigarette smoking:** COPD results from smoking-related inflammation and damage.
   b. **Occupational exposure:** Exposure to dust and fumes at workplace such as coal mining, gold mining and cotton textile.
   c. **Air pollution:** More COPD cases are seen in urban areas than rural area due to air pollution
   d. **Genetic consideration:** Severe alfa-1-antitrypsin deficiency is responsible for COPD.

Exogenous factors	**1. Greatest risk factor** a. Tobacco smoke **2. Important risk factor** a. Air pollution in urban areas b. Passive smoking c. Occupational exposure: Dust & fumes **3. Possible risk factor** a. Respiratory infections (viral, bacterial infections) b. Socioeconomic factors
Endogenous factors	1. **Greatest risk factor:** Severe alfa - anti trypsin deficiency 2. **Possible risk factor:** a. Aging b. Airway hypersensitivity c. Gene mutation d. Autoimmune response

3. **COPD includes:**
   a. **Emphysema:**
      1. In emphysema there is destruction and enlargement of the lung alveoli
      2. The walls of the air sacs (alveoli) of the lungs are damaged and lose their elasticity.
      3. As a result of damaged air sacs they break down easily leading to distension.
      4. Emphysema can also contribute to narrowing of the airways

b. **Chronic bronchitis:**

1. Clinically defined condition with chronic cough and phlegm (Thick tracheo-bronchial mucus product).
2. Chronic bronchitis is a condition in which chronic inflammation and swelling causes narrowing of airways than normal, so there is limitation to air flow.

4. **Clinical presentation:** Three most common symptoms of COPD are chronic cough, sputum production & dyspnea on exertion

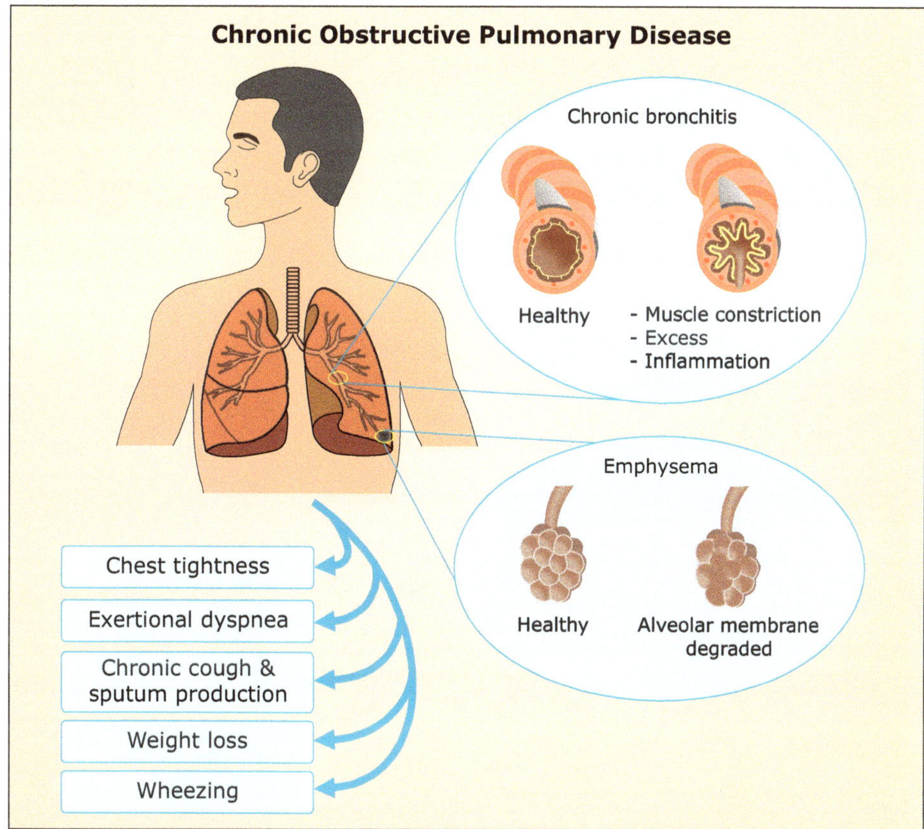

a. **Chronic cough:**

1. Chronic cough is often the first symptom to develop.
2. **Definition of chronic bronchitis:** When cough persists for more than three months each year for at least two years, in combination with sputum production and without another explanation.

b. **Sputum production:** In Some patients with COPD have increased amount of mucus production and secretion because of more no of mucus-producing cells (called goblet cells)

Sputum which can be clear, white, yellow or green in color.

c. **Exertional dyspnea**:

   i. It is a common symptom & often more distressing.

   ii. Shortness of breath of a prolonged duration, which worsens on exertion and worsens gradually over years.

5. **Physical findings:**

   a. Look for signs of active smoking including an odor of smoke or nicotine staining of fingernails.

   b. Barrel chest: It occur due to hyperinflation of lungs and enlarged lung volume.

   c. Hyper resonance note heard on percussion of chest.

   d. Patients with severe airflow obstruction often use accessory muscles (sternocleidomastoid, scalene group & pectoralis minor) of respiration.

   e. Patients may or may not develop cyanosis.

   f. In end stage of disease patient is cachexic with significant weight loss, bitemporal wasting and diffuse loss of subcutaneous fat.

   g. In some cases, signs of cor-pulmonale may be present.

   h. Clubbing is not a feature of COPD.

6. **GOLD criteria for severity of airflow obstruction in COPD:**

Gold staging	Severity	Spirometry findings (FEV1/FVC < 0.7) and
I	Mild	FEV1 > OR = 80% Predicted
II	Moderate	FEV1> or =50% but <80% predicted
III	Severe	FEV1 > or = 30% but <50% predicted
IV	Very severe	FEV1<30% predicted

7. **Investigation**

   a. **Chest X-ray:** Shows hyper translucency, low flat diaphragm or bullae, widened intercostal spaces and tubular heart are seen

   b. **Spirometry**

      i. Spirometry confirms the diagnosis

      ii. Post bronchodilator FEV1/FVC < 0.7

      iii. With increase in disease severity there is increase in total lung capacity, functional residual capacity, and residual volume

      iv. In emphysema patients there is a decrease in diffusion capacity of lungs.

X-ray with features of COPD

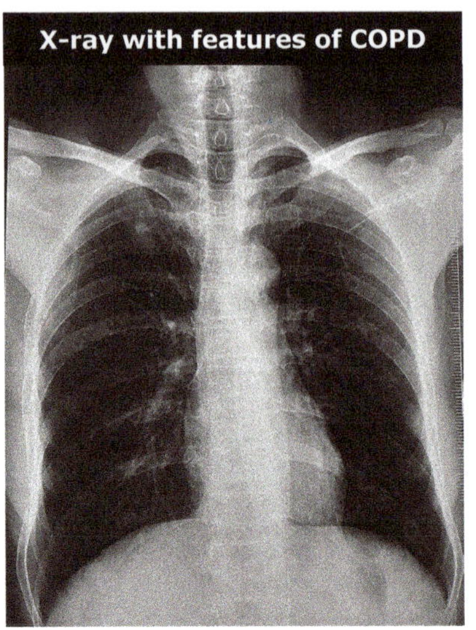

c. **Arterial blood gases:** It gives information regarding resting and exertional hypoxemia & acid base status.

d. **Screening for AAT deficiency**

e. **HRCT Chest:** It is useful to understand distribution of emphysema in the lung fields & to exclude other lung diseases .

f. **Routine blood investigations** : Complete blood count, particularly for hemoglobin and hematocrit levels.

8. **Management:** No cure for COPD is known, but the symptoms are treatable and its progression can be delayed

a. **Pharmacological**

i. Bronchodilators are used for symptomatic benefit in patients with COPD.

ii. **Inhaled anticholinergic Agents:** Ipratropium bromide is used for symptomatic relief & to reduce excerbation.

iii. **Inhaled beta Agonists:** Along with anticholinergic are given to provide more symptomatic benefits

iv. **Inhaled glucocorticoids:** When used in combination with a LABA, they have less rate of excerbation as compared to either ICSs or LABA alone.

In acute excerbation intravenous steroids are useful

v. **Theophylline:** Usually not recommended, but may be used as a second-line agent in those not controlled by other measures.

b. **Other pharmacological management**

i. **Macrolide antibiotics:** When there is respiratory infections

ii. **Alfa AT1 augmentation therapy** if serum level < 11um

iii. **N acetyl cysteine** can be used for its mucolytic and antioxidant properties.

iv. **Methylxanthine** can be added but constant blood level monitoring is required.

v. **O_2 therapy:** For patients with resting hypoxemia (Resting O_2 saturation $\leq 88\%$ or $< 90\%$ with signs of pulmonary hypertension or right heart failure), the use of O_2 reduces the mortality in these patients.

c. **Non pharmacological management**

i. **Vaccination:** COPD patients should receive the influenza vaccine annually & polyvalent pneumococcal vaccine is also advised to take to reduce serious illness and mortality.

ii. **Pulmonary rehabilitation:** To improve health-related quality of life, dyspnea, and exercise capacity.

iii. **Lung surgery:** Three forms of surgery may be considered for severe COPD:

- **Volume reduction surgery:** Used to remove damaged lung tissue (Has some mortality benefits).
- **Bullectomy:** Which is the removal of enlarged bullae from lungs .
- **Lung transplantation:** Recommended in very severe COPD cases.

PNEUMONIA

1. Pneumonia is a lung infection involving the lung alveoli (air sacs) and can be caused by microbes, including bacteria, viruses or fungi.

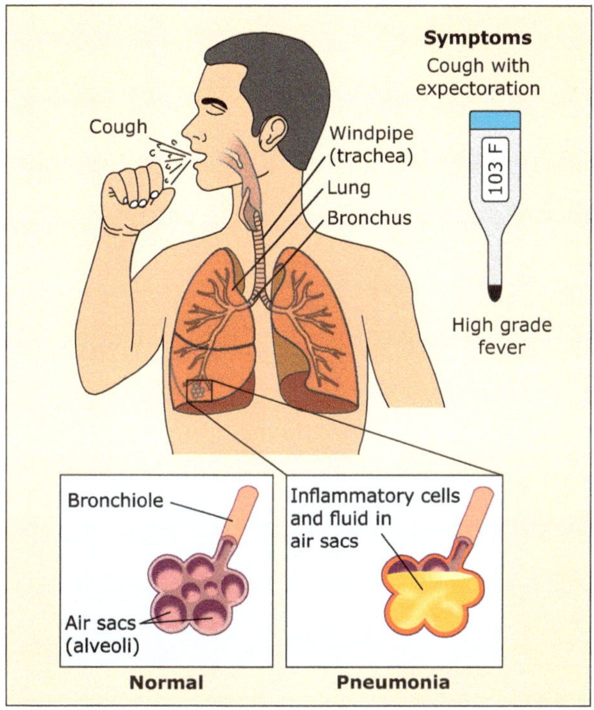

2. Pneumonia is usually caused by infection with viruses or bacteria and less commonly by other microorganisms.
3. In some patients who have a viral infection, such as influenza virus, will develop a secondary infection from bacteria such as Staphylococcus aureus while they are sick.
4. **Classification:**
   a. **Community acquired pneumonia**
   b. **Health care associated pneumonia**
      1. **Hospital acquired pneumonia**
      2. **Ventilator associated pneumonia**
5. **It may also be classified by the area of lung affected:**
   a. **Lobar pneumonia**
   b. **Bronchial pneumonia**
   c. **Acute interstitial pneumonia**

COMMUNITY ACQUIRED PNEUMONIA

6. **Etiology:**
   a. Potential agents in CAP includes bacteria, fungi, viruses and protozoa
   b. Most cases of CAP, However, are caused by relatively few pathogens
      1. Streptococcus pneumoniae
      2. H. influenza
      3. Respiratory viruses
      4. Mycoplasma pneumoniae
      5. Legionella spp.
      6. Respiratory viruses
      7. Chlamydia pneumoniae
7. **Risk factors:** Several risk factors place patients at risk for community-acquired pneumonia (CAP), Including comorbidities, lifestyle and patient characteristics
   a. **Patient characteristic**
      1. Extremes of ages
      2. Immunocompromised status
   b. **Comorbidities**
      1. Dementia, stroke, decreased level of consciousness
      2. COPD, asthma, bronchiectasis, cystic fibrosis
      3. Diabetes mellitus
      4. Heart diseases, failure
      5. HIV infection
      6. Renal failure
      7. Cancer
   c. **Life style**
      1. Alcohol or substance abuse
      2. A history of smoking
      3. Overcrowded living condition
8. **Clinical manifestation**
   a. Ask history regarding traveling, contact to birds, rabbits, underlying diseases & its treatment .
   b. Fever with tachycardia
   c. History of chills and/or sweat
   d. Cough with sputum (Mucoid, purulent, or blood tinged sputum)

   e. Hemoptysis (Gross hemoptysis is feature of CA-MRSA)
   f. Pleuritic chest pain if pleura is involved
   g. Gastrointestinal symptoms like nausea, vomiting and/or loose motions are seen in some patients.
   h. Other symptoms: Myalgia, headache, fatigue, arthralgia

9. **Physical examination**
   a. **Tachypnea:** Increased RR
   b. **Patient often uses accessory muscles of respiration**
   c. **Auscultation:** Crackles in lung fields, bronchial breath sounds and other signs of consolidation e.g. pleural friction rub.
   d. **Palpation:** Increased or decreased tactile vocal fremitus
   e. **Percussion**: Percussion note can vary from dull to flat

10. **Investigation:**
   a. Diagnosis of pneumonia is typically by clinical and radiographic methods
   b. Laboratory investigations aid in diagnosis.
   i. **Chest X-ray:** Shows evidence of consolidation & may show evidence of pleural effusion

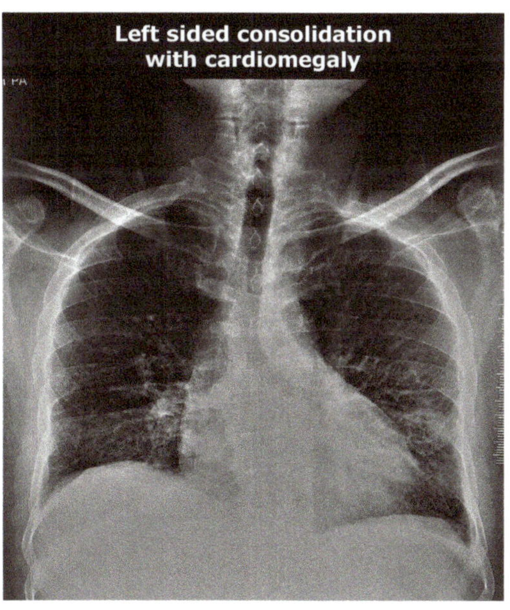

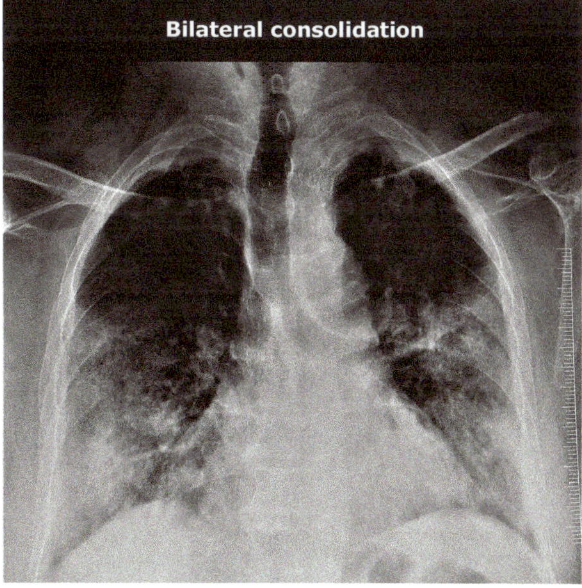

   ii. **Sputum examination (Gram's staining and culture)**
   iii. **Blood culture** (Blood sample should be collected before starting antibiotics therapy)

iv. **CRP**

v. **Urine antigen test** for legionella and pneumococcus

vi. **Polymerase chain reaction** for legionella, M. Pneumonias.

vii. **Reverse transcriptase polymerase chain reaction (RTPCR):** Covid-19 pneumonia

viii. **Serological tests:** Legionella, chlamydia

ix. **CBC with differential count**

x. **Oxygen saturation**

xi. **ABG**

xii. **Serum creatinine**

xiii. **FBS, PPBG AND LFT**

11. **Disease severity scoring:**

Useful to minimise unnecessary hospital admissions, to assess risk of adverse outcome, including severe illness and death.

a. **Pneumonia severity index (PSI)**

A prognostic model to identify patients at low risk of dieing.

1. To determine the **PSI score 20 variables** including age, coexisting illness, and abnormal physical and laboratory findings
2. Determination of the PSI is often impractical in busy emergency department setting because of multiple variables to be assessed.
3. Treat class 1 and 2 on outpatient basis
4. Class 3 as inpatient
5. Class 4 and 5 in ICU

b. **CURB 65 (age > 65 years):**

1. CURB 65 criteria is used to identify a severity of illness score
2. **It includes five variables**
   a. **Confusion (C)**
   b. **Urea > 7 mol/l (U)**
   c. **Respiratory rate > or equal to 30/min (R)**
   d. **Systolic blood pressure < or equal to 90 mm of Hg or diastolic < or equal to 60 mm of Hg**
   e. **Age > 65 years**
3. **Score 0 = Out patients**

4. **Score 2 = In-patient**
5. **Score 3 = Intensive care unit**

12. **Treatment:**
   a. Bed rest
   b. Hospitalisation, if required as per disease severity scoring system
   c. Oxygen therapy for hypoxemia
   d. Adequate hydration: IV fluids
   e. Analgesics and antipyretics
   f. Patients with severe CAP who remain hypotensive despite fluid resuscitation may have adrenal insufficiency and may respond to glucocorticoids.
   g. Assisted ventilation when necessary
   h. **Appropriate antimicrobial therapy (Depending on severity and pathogen responsible for CAP)**
      i. **A macrolide** (e.g. Clarithromycin 500 mg PO BD or azithromycin 500 mg once then 250 mg qd)
      ii. **A respiratory fluoroquinolones** (e.g. Moxifloxacin 400 mg PO or IV qd levoflox 750 mg PO)
      iii. β **lactam** (e.g. High dose amoxicillin 1 gm tid/amoxicillin 2 gm bid, ceftriaxone 1-2 gm IV qd, cefpodoxime 200 mg PO bid, Cefuroxime 500 mg PO bid plus macrolide).
      iv. **If pseudomonas is consideration:** An antipseudomonal β lactam e.g., piperacillin/tazobactam 4.5 gm IV q6h
      v. **If pneumococcal is a consideration:** The above β lactam plus aminoglycoside (amikacin 15 mg/kg qd) plus azithromycin
      vi. **If CA-MRSA is a consideration:** Add linezolid 600 mg IV q12 h or vancomycin 15 mg/kg q12h initially with adjusted doses.

HEMOPTYSIS

1. It is defined as expectoration of blood or bloody sputum
2. We have to distinguish hemoptysis from epistaxis (Bleeding from the nasopharynx) and hematemesis (Bleeding from the upper gastrointestinal tract).
3. **True hemoptysis:** Expectoration of blood from the lower respiratory tree, below glottis.
4. **Massive hemoptysis/life threatening**: Most commonly defined as > 600 ml of blood expectorated per 24 hours or 150 ml/hr.
5. Massive hemoptysis should be considered as a medical emergency & require rapid identification of cause and treatment.
6. **Etiology: (Based on anatomical location)**

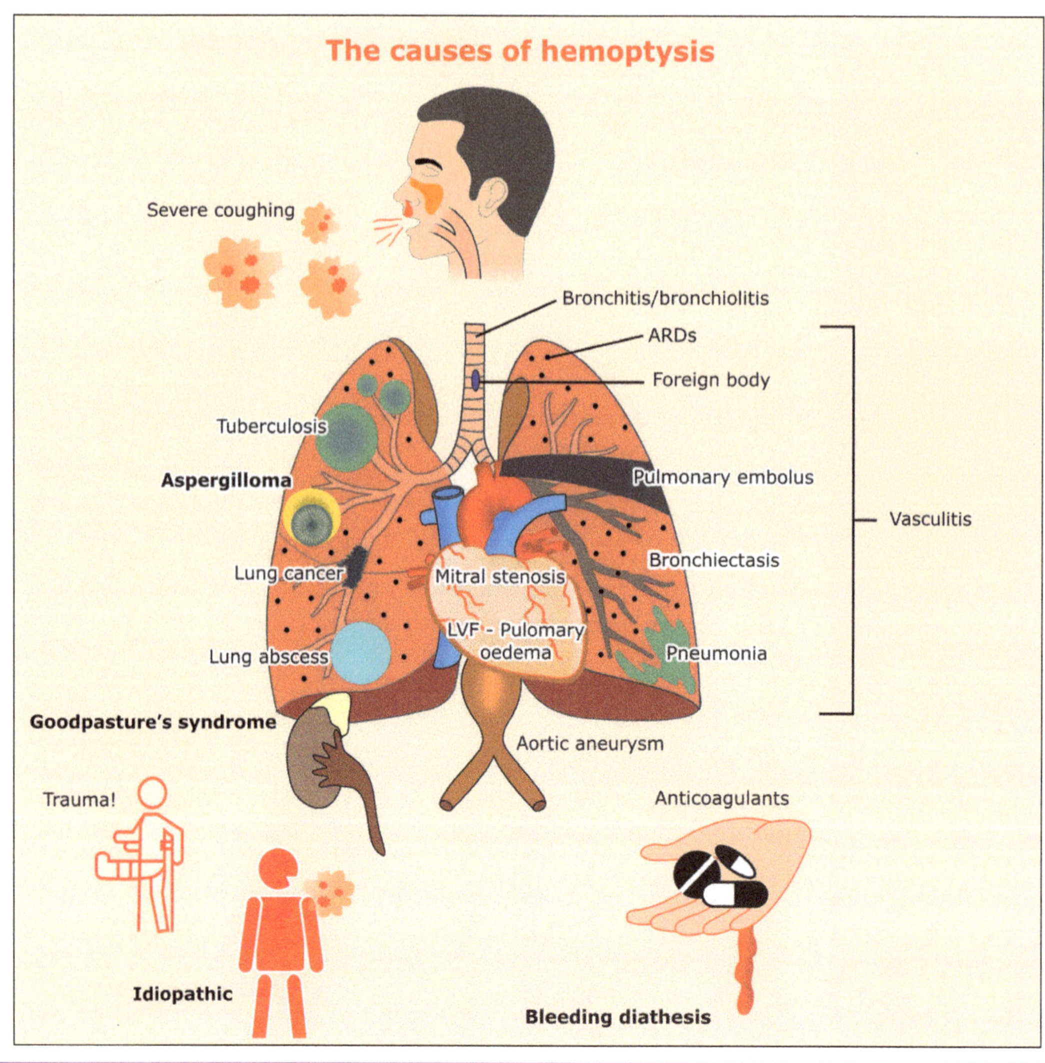

a. **Airway**: Bronchitis, Bronchiectasis, malignancy, foreign body, trauma, broncholithiasis.

b. **Parenchymal/alveoli:** Pneumonia, SLE, acute respiratory distress syndrome, rheumatologic vasculitides, goodpasture syndrome, ANCA positive, lung cancer.

c. **Vascular:** LV failure, mitral valve stenosis (Due to increase in pulmonary venous pressure), pulmonary embolism, arteriovenous malformation, varices/aneurysms.

d. **Etiologies involving multiple anatomical locations:**

   i. Cavitary lung disease (TB, lung abscess)

   ii. Thrombocytopenia (Leptospirosis, dengue, malaria)

   iii. Disseminated intravascular coagulation

   iv. Traumatic (Inhalation of toxic gases or acid aspiration)

   v. Diagnostic (Lung biopsy)

   vi. Therapeutic (Anticoagulants, antiplatelets)

   vii. Bronchovascular fistula.

e. **Idiopathic**

7. **Clinical presentation:**

   a. **Hemoptysis:**

      i. **Appearance:** Grossly bloody, blood tinged sputum, streaky, foamy

      ii. **Episodes:** Single or multiple

      iii. **Volume of blood:** Minimal/submassive/massive

      iv. **Prior episode of hemoptysis**

   b. **May be associated with other symptoms and signs related to underlying disorders.**

      i. **Fever, chills and dyspnea:** Respiratory tract infection

      ii. **Clubbing:** Bronchogenic carcinoma or bronchiectasis

8. **History and physical evaluation**

   a. **History:** Smoking, Prior/present respiratory disease, Malignancy, risk for coagulopathy, cardiopulmonary diseases, systemic inflammatory disease.

   b. **Physical examination**

      i. General appearance

      ii. Vitals (BP, PR, RR)

      iii. Oxygen saturation

      iv. Auscultation of chest: Crackles, wheeze.

9. **Diagnostic testing:**
   a. **Lab investigations**
      i. **Complete blood count:** To assess both the hematocrit and the platelets count
      ii. **Blood grouping and cross match**
      iii. **Liver function test**
      iv. **ABG: Hypoxemia**
      v. **Serum electrolyte**
      vi. **Coagulation profile**
      vii. **Renal function test and Urinalysis with microscopy**: To rule out possibility of pulmonary-renal syndromes presenting with hemoptysis
      viii. **Sputum studies:** Gram staining & culture, AFB, fungal & cytological studies
      ix. **BNP-** In chronic heart failure
10. **Immunological studies: ANA/ANCA screen**, anti-glomerular basement membrane antibodies, complement level, cryoglobulin.
   b. **Radiological Investigations**
      i. **Chest X-ray:** Standard chest X-ray done to find the cause of bleeding
      ii. **High resolution CT Chest:** Useful to understand cause of hemoptysis and if pulmonary embolism is suspected then CT chest angiography is needed.

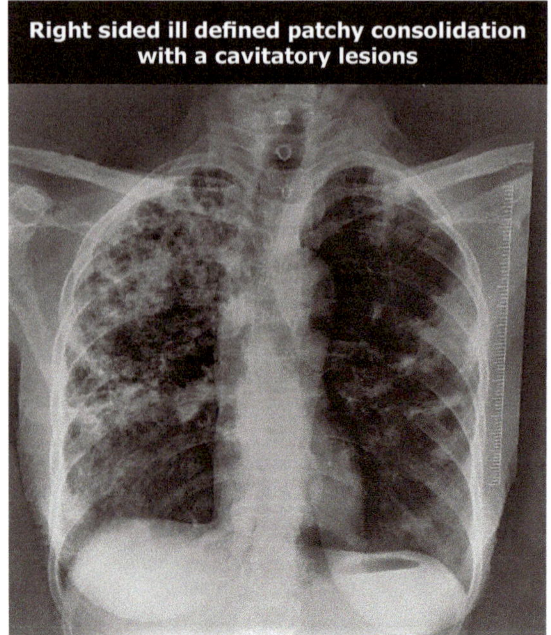
Right sided ill defined patchy consolidation with a cavitatory lesions

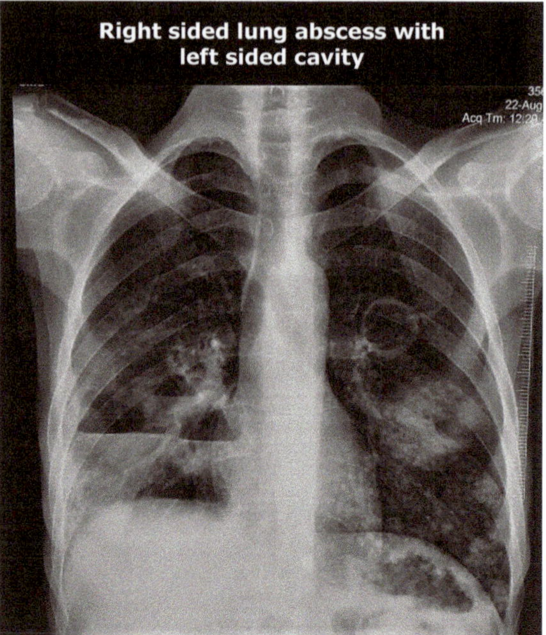
Right sided lung abscess with left sided cavity

c. **Diagnostic procedure: If all of the investigations are unable to diagnose, bronchoscopy should be considered.**

   i. **Fiber-optic bronchoscopy:** Generally useful to localize/lateralize bleeding source, identify potential site for embolization and to obtain brushing/biopsy.

   ii. **Bronchial and pulmonary arteriography:** Useful in persistent or recurring massive hemoptysis.

10. **Treatment:**

   a. **Non massive hemoptysis:**

      i. Antitussive and mild sedatives to control cough

      ii. Antibiotics for respiratory infections

      iii. Steroids for rheumatological conditions.

      iv. Treatment of heart failure

      v. Correct coagulopathy

      vi. Bronchoscopy if recurrent hemoptysis

   b. **Massive hemoptysis:**

      i. **Lateral decubitus position, affected lung down to minimize aspiration.**

      ii. **Initial stabilization:** Airway management with intubation, IV fluid

      iii. **Blood transfusion after blood grouping and cross matching**

      iv. **Bronchoscopy:** It is used for diagnostic and therapeutic management of hemoptysis.

      v. **Systemic procoagulants:** Factor VII, vasopressin

      vi. **Bronchial artery embolization**

      vii. **Argon beam coagulation**

      viii. **Endobronchial ballon temponade & electrocautery**

   c. **Surgical management:**

      Lobectomy/pneumonectomy: Surgical resection of the affected region of the lung is considered.

   d. **Referral**

      i. Interventional pulmonologists

      ii. Interventional radiologists

      iii. Thoracic surgeon

PULMONARY EDEMA

1. Pulmonary edema is fluid accumulation in the tissue and air spaces of the lungs
2. Fluid collection in the numerous air sacs in the lungs causes difficulty in breathing & may cause respiratory failure due to hypoxia.
3. Acute pulmonary edema is a medical emergency requiring immediate care.
4. In most of cases cardiac causes are commonly involved for development of pulmonary edema.
5. In non cardiogenic edema, fluid leaks into air sac from damaged capillary lining.
6. Cardiogenic pulmonary edema occurs when the capillary pressure exceeds the pressure of serum oncotic pressure and interstitial hydrostatic pressure.
7. This accumulated fluid causes hypoxia due to impairment of gas exchange.
8. **Types of pulmonary edema**
    a. **Cardiogenic**
    b. **Non cardiogenic**
9. **Causes of pulmonary edema:**

Cardiogenic	Non cardiogenic
1. Acute myocardial infarction or ischemia	1. Diffuse pulmonary infection
2. Left sided Heart failure	2. Inhalation of toxic smoke and irritant
3. Cardiomyopathy (Myocarditis)	3. Near drowning (aspiration of water)
4. Cardiac arrhythmias	4. Kerosine, insecticide poisoning
5. Heart valve problems (AS, AR, MS)	5. Aspiration of vomitus
6. Hypertensive crisis	6. Pulmonary embolism
	7. Severe sepsis, acute pancreatitis
	8. High altitude
	9. Intravenous narcotic or non narcotic drug overdose
	10. Head injury, major burn, chest trauma, multiple blood transfusion

10. Pneumonia (exudate) is not pulmonary edema (transudate)
11. **In cardiogenic edema**
    a. Engorgement of veins
    b. Increased central venous pressure
    c. Increased pulmonary capillary wedge pressure

12. In non cardiogenic edema

a. No engorged neck vessels

b. Normal capillary wedge pressure

c. Normal pulmonary capillary wedge pressure

d. Normal left sided atrial and ventricular pressure.

13. Clinical presentation:

a. Dyspnea (PND, orthopnea if cardiac cause)

b. Cough with expectoration of pink frothy fluid

c. Restlessness

d. Anxiety

14. Physical examination:

a. Use of accessory muscles

b. Hypoxemia

c. Cold extremities (Decreased peripheral perfusion)

d. Pulmonary congestion signs: Wheezing and crackles on auscultation

e. Tachypnea

f. Tachycardia

g. Signs of underlying heart disease (JVP raised, murmur, S3 gallop rhythm)

15. Diagnostic investigation:

a. Chest X-ray: Radiographic abnormalities include cardiomegaly, interstitial and perihilar vascular engorgement, Kerley's B lines, and pleural effusion.

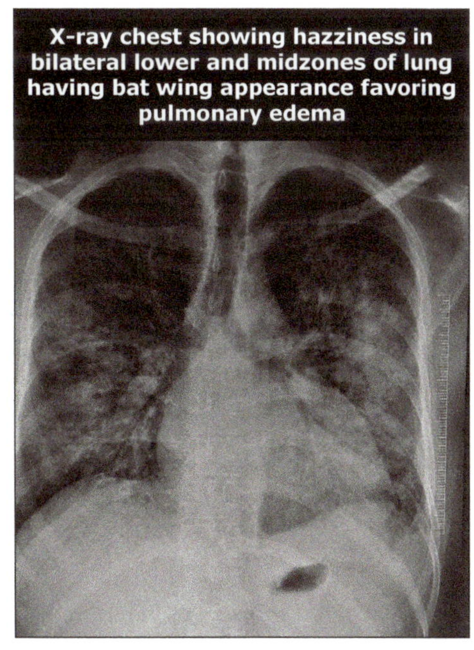

X-ray chest showing hazziness in bilateral lower and midzones of lung having bat wing appearance favoring pulmonary edema

b. ECG:

1. The electrocardiogram (ECG) may suggest acute tachydysrhythmia or bradydysrhythmias or acute myocardial ischemia or infarction as the cause of cardiogenic pulmonary edema.

2. LA enlargement and LV hypertrophy are sensitive, although nonspecific, indicators of chronic LV dysfunction

c. **Echocardiography: (Especially in the case of cardiogenic pulmonary edema)** Useful in diagnosis of impaired left ventricular function, high central venous pressures and high pulmonary artery pressures.

16. **Blood tests:**
    a. **A complete blood count**
    b. **Arterial blood gas analysis** (Amount of oxygen and carbon dioxide, blood pH)
    c. **Electrolytes (Sodium, potassium)**
    d. **Renal function (Creatinine, urea)**
    e. **Liver enzymes**
    f. **Inflammatory markers (C-reactive protein)**
    g. **Coagulation studies (PT, aPTT) are also typically requested.**
    h. **B-type natriuretic peptide (BNP):** Low levels of BNP (< 100 pg/ml) suggest a cardiac cause is unlikely.
    i. **Cardiac enzymes for myocardial infarction**

17. **Management:**
    a. Strict bed rest & relieve anxiety
    b. Placing the patient in a sitting position improves pulmonary function.
    c. Give oxygen to raise arterial oxygen saturation.
    d. If oxygenation is inadequate then use mechanical ventilation
    e. **Reduction of preload**
        1. **Diuretics:** Furosemide is a venodilator that decreases pulmonary congestion by profuse diuresis. An initial dose of 40-80 mg IV and can be repeated maximum dose of 200 mg.
        2. **Nitroglycerine (only if hypertensive cardiac failure):**
            a. Sublingual nitroglycerin (0.4 mg × 3 every 5 min) is first-line therapy for acute cardiogenic pulmonary edema.
            b. If pulmonary edema persists in the absence of hypotension, IV nitroglycerin can be given.
            c. A powerful vasodilator that potentiates the effect of furosemide.
            d. Contraindicated in right ventricular myocardial infarction
        3. **Nitroprusside:**
            a. It is useful in cardiogenic pulmonary edema due to valvular regurgitation or hypertension.

b. A potent venous and arterial vasodilator.

c. It is useful for patients with pulmonary edema and hypertension but is not given in patients with reduced coronary artery perfusion.

4. **ACE inhibitors:**

a. Reduces both afterload and preload

b. Recommended for hypertensive patients with acute LVF

c. In acute MI with heart failure, ACE inhibitors reduce short and long term mortality rates.

5. **Inotropic agents:** Such as dopamine, dobutamine may be helpful in patient CPE associated with hypotension or shock.

f. **Treatment of precipitating factors**

COR PULMONALE AND PULMONARY HYPERTENSION

1. **Definition:** Abnormal enlargement of the right side of the heart, as a result of disease of the lungs or pulmonary blood vessels.
2. Often referred to as pulmonary heart disease.
3. **Definition of PAH:** The sustained elevation of the mean pulmonary artery pressure (mPAP)
4. **Types:**
   a. **Acute cor pulmonale**
   b. **Chronic cor pulmonale**
5. **Causes:**

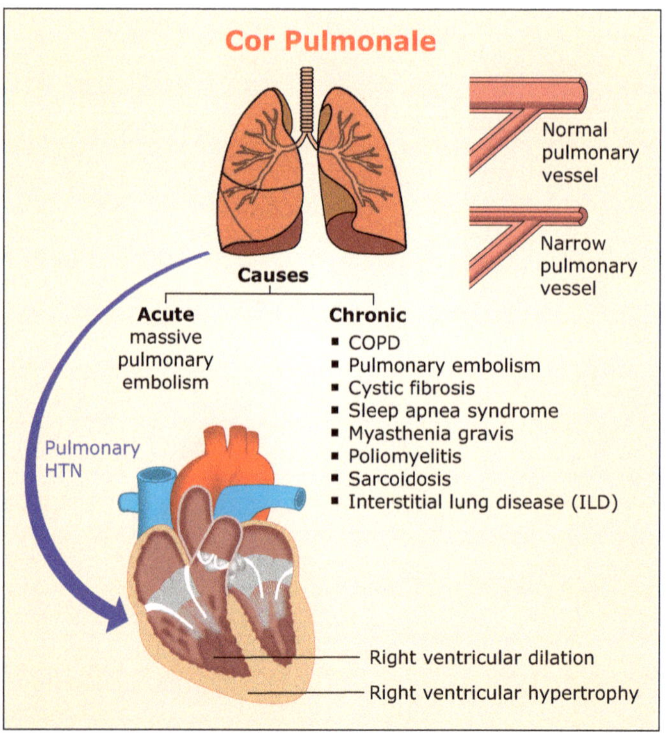

Acute	Massive pulmonary embolism
Chronic	1. **Pulmonary causes:** COPD, Pulmonary embolism, cystic fibrosis, Sarcoidosis, Bronchiectasis, ILD ARDS. 2. **Pulmonary circulation:** Recurrent pulmonary thromboembolism, primary pulmonary hypertension, chronic liver disease, pulmonary vasculitis. 3. **Thoracic cage abnormality:** Kyphosis, scoliosis 4. **Neuromuscular disorder:** Myasthenia gravis, poliomyelitis 5. **Hypoventilation:** Obstructive sleep apnea syndrome

6. **Acute cor pulmonale:**
   a. It results in right ventricular dilation and failure, but no hypertrophy.
   b. Acute cor pulmonale occurs following a massive pulmonary embolism with acute pulmonary hypertension.
7. **Chronic cor pulmonale:**
   a. In chronic cases there is hypertrophy and dilation of the right ventricle secondary to pulmonary hypertension.
   b. COPD is most commonly involved in chronic Cor pulmonale.
8. **Symptoms:**
   Features of both RV failure and Primary lung disease:
   a. Dyspnea (Not relieved by sitting up, due to pulmonary hypertension)
   b. Dry cough
   c. Chest discomfort: Due to dilatation of the root of pulmonary artery
   d. Swelling of feet or ankle
   e. Fatigue
   f. Palpitations
9. **Signs of right heart failure:**
   a. Elevated jugular venous pressure tachypnea
   b. Hepatomegaly
   c. Pulsatile liver
   d. Pedal edema
   e. Ascites
   f. Cyanosis (late finding)
10. **Investigations:**
   a. Chest X-ray: Shows prominent RA, RV and pulmonary artery
   b. ECG: Shows P. pulmonale, right axis deviation & right ventricular hypertrophy.
   c. Arterial blood gases
   d. 2D echocardiography: Useful for measurement of right ventricular thickness & heart chamber dimensions.
   e. Spirometry and lung volume
   To assess for obstructive or restrictive ventilatory abnormalities.

f. **Diffusing capacity for carbon monoxide (DLCO)**

It is usually reduced with parenchymal lung diseases, but isolated mild to moderate reduction is encountered in PAH.

g. **Chest CT:** Useful to identify underlying cause

h. **V/Q (Ventilation/perfusion ratio):** Useful in pulmonary embolism

i. **Pulmonary angiography:** Gold standard diagnostic test for pulmonary embolism

j. **Cardiac MRI:** For assessment of right ventricular structure and functions.

k. **Right heart catheterization**

Essential investigation if PAH is suspected and treatment is being considered.

11. **Treatment:**

a. **Treatment to decrease pulmonary HTN**

1. **Treatment of underlying lung disease**
2. **Long term oxygen therapy** is the only treatment shown to retard the progression of pulmonary HTN
3. **Vasodilatory/vaso-modulator therapy for PAH**

a. **Prostacyclin derivative:** Epoprostenol, Treprostinil, Iloprost

b. **Endothelin receptor antagonist:** Bosentan, ambrisentan

c. **PDE5 inhibitor:** Sildenafil, tadalafil

d. **Soluble guanylyl cyclase stimulator:** Riociguat

e. **Calcium channel blockers:** Nifedipine, amlodipine, diltiazem

b. **Treatment of right heart failure**

1. Optimize right ventricular preload and cardiac output
2. Right ventricular after load reduction
3. Inotrops for improving contractibility
4. Mechanical circulatory support devices e.g. ECMO

DROWNING

1. **Definition:** Drowning is a form of asphyxia due to aspiration of fluid into air passages, caused by submersion in water or other fluid

2. **Pathophysiology:**

   a. **In fresh water or brackish water:**

      1. After drowning water inhaled and absorbed in blood in few minutes
      2. Water absorbed in blood causes hypervolemia with hemodilution and increases workload of heart.
      3. Hemodilution occurs in fresh water drowning leads to hemolysis, hemoglobinaemia, and hemoglobinuria, marked hyponatremia and hyperkalemia.
      4. In lungs due to defective functioning of surfactant leads to pulmonary edema, hypoxia and secondary metabolic acidosis.
      5. Protein and hemoglobin are reduced.
      6. The serum becomes **hyperkalemic.**
      7. This increased fluid overload causes overburdening of the heart and produces the further increase in pulmonary edema.
      8. Cardiac arrhythmias leading to ventricular tachycardia and fibrillation occur, probably due to hypoxia and hemodilution.

   b. **Sea water drowning:**

      1. Due to high salinity of seawater, water is drawn from the blood into the lung tissue, and produces severe pulmonary edema and **hypernatremia.**
      2. It will cause hemoconcentration
      3. Bradycardia occurs probably due to raised plasma sodium level

3. **History:**

   a. **Immersion time**

   b. **Salt /Fresh water drowning**

   c. **Details of basic life support delivered and treatment given**

   d. **Find out any surgical ,medical and psychiatric cause which may responsible for drowning**

4. **Clinical features:**

   a. Altered mental state

b. Chest pain

c. Dyspnea

d. Tachypnea and tachycardia

e. Cyanosis

f. Coughing with expectoration of pink froth

g. Crepitation on auscultation

5. Investigation

a. Lab investigation

1. Complete blood count
2. Random blood glucose
3. Liver function test
4. Arterial blood gases
5. Serum electrolyte
6. Renal function test
7. PT, INR

b. Other investigation

1. Chest X-ray
2. CT brain or cervical spine, if suspected trauma
3. Abdominal, pelvic and extremity imaging, if clinically indicated.
4. Echocardiography

6. Management:

a. Patient should lie on back and hyperextend the neck and start primary assessment

b. Primary assessment: It includes airway, breathing, circulation, disability and exposure.

c. Mouth and nostril should be cleaned and air passage kept clear by repeated suction to avoid aspiration of content .

d. Initiate CPR at the earliest in person with respiratory distress or respiratory arrest to avoid cardiac arrest.

e. Respiratory support:

   1. Give 100% of oxygen
   2. Monitor oxygen saturation with the help of pulse oximetry and arterial blood gases analysis
   3. Consider intubation and mechanical ventilation in patients with altered mental state, severe respiratory distress, severe hypoxia and acidosis.

f. Stabilize body temperature

g. In the fresh water drowning an external defibrillator should be applied to the chest and electrolyte imbalance should be corrected.

h. In sea water hemoconcentration correction done by administration of hypotonic IV fluids.

ACUTE RESPIRATORY DISTRESS SYNDROME

1. **Definition:** A clinical syndrome of severe dyspnea of rapid onset of hypoxemia and diffuse pulmonary infiltrate leading to respiratory failure.
2. ARDS is caused by diffuse lung injury from many underlying medical and surgical disorders.
3. The risk of developing ARDS is increased in patients with more than one predisposing medical or surgical condition.
4. Lung injury may be direct or indirect.
5. ARDS is not a primary disorder, but is a consequence of a variety of infectious and noninfectious conditions
6. **Clinical disorders commonly associated with ARDS:**

Direct causes	Indirect causes
Aspiration of gastric contents	**Sepsis**
Near drowning	**Severe trauma:** multiple bone fracture, flail chest, head trauma, burns, lung contusions
Toxic inhalation injury e.g. NO, CO	**Pancreatitis**
Pneumonia	**Narcotics or non narcotic drug overdose**
Near drowning	**Multiple transfusion,** **Post cardiopulmonary bypass, DIC**

7. **Clinical features**
   a. Unexplained dyspnea
   b. Dry cough
   c. Cyanosis
   d. Labored breathing
   e. Crackles on both sided lung fields on auscultation

8. **Berlin diagnostic criteria**
   a. **Acute onset**
   b. **Bilateral infiltrates on frontal chest X-ray**
   c. **Severe hypoxemia ($PaO_2/FIO_2 \leq 300$ mm Hg+)**
   d. **No evidence of left heart failure or fluid overload**
   e. **The presence of a predisposing condition**

Portable chest X-ray showing fluffy shadows in bilateral lung fields, Right > Left

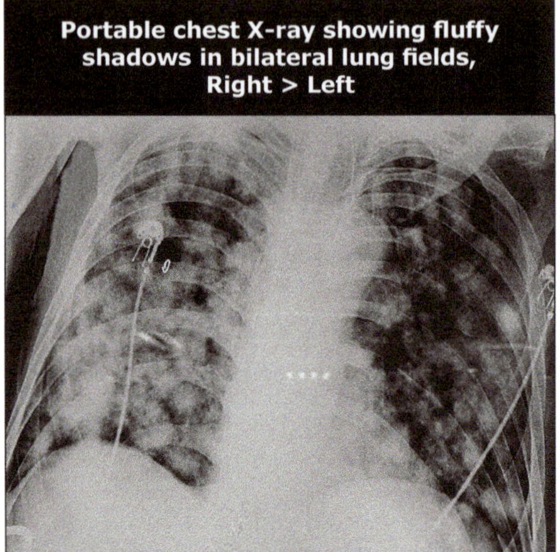

9. **Severity of ARDS (Berlin)**
   a. **Mild:** 200 mm of Hg PaO_2/FIO_2 < or equal to 300 mm of Hg
   b. **Moderate:** 100 mm of Hg PaO_2/FIO_2 < or equal to 200 mm of Hg
   c. **Severe:** PaO_2/FIO_2 < or = to 100 mm of Hg
10. **Pathophysiology:**
    a. **Exudative stage:** Diffuse alveolar damage in first week
    b. **Proliferative stage:** Resolution of pulmonary edema, Proliferation of type II pneumocytes along the alveolar basement membrane (7-21 days)
    c. **Fibrotic:** Fibrosis sets in with loss of elastic tissues & obliteration of vascular architecture.
11. **Treatment:**
    a. **Early recognition and treatment of underlying clinical disorder**
    b. **Prone position :** Improves oxygenation and reduces lung injury
    c. **Adequate nutrition with RT feeding**
    d. **Oxygen therapy:** Initially with face mask with high flow oxygen to achieve PaO_2 60 mm of Hg
    e. **Lung protective mechanical ventilation:**
       1. Lung protective ventilation is used that means low tidal volumes (6 mL/kg) to limit the risk of volume trauma and biotrauma
       2. Use positive end-expiratory pressure (PEEP) of at least 5 cm H_2O to prevent the collapse of small airways at the end of expiration to limit the risk of atelectrauma. **(Low tidal volume with high PEEP)**
    f. **Fluid management:**
       1. Fluid management is necessary to prevent excessive fluid accumulation in the lungs
       2. It s important to avoid fluid deficits and maintain intravascular volume
       3. Diuretics: It is used to remove excess fluid.
    g. **Neuromuscular blocking agents:** It is useful in early and severe ARDS with severe gas exchange abnormalities.
    h. **Glucocorticosteroids:** Steroid therapy is not recommended in ARDS, However,ARDS due to Covid 19, steroid use is recommended. ARDS due to leptospirosis steroid is contraversial.
    i. **Lung replacement with extracorporeal membrane oxygenation (ECMO):** It is useful in the neonatal respiratory distress syndrome.

CHAPTER

8

Gastrointestinal and Hepatobiliary System

GASTROINTESTINAL AND HEPATOBILIARY SYSTEM EXAMINATION

It includes examination of

1. Upper GI tract
2. Abdomen
3. Per rectal

A. Upper GI tract:

1. Breath (Halitosis or foul smell)
2. Teeth, lips, gum
3. Tongue (Deviation, color, texture)
4. Palate, tonsils, oropharynx
5. Cheek (Buccal mucosa)

B. Examination of abdomen:

a. Inspection:

1. Shape of abdomen
2. Flanks full or not

3. Vein dilation over abdomen may be seen in portal hypertension or vena cava obstruction
4. Bluish discoloration in flank or around umbilicus (Grey turner sign or Cullens) suggestive of hemorrhagic pancreatitis or retroperitoneal hemorrhage/intrabdominal hemorrhage
5. Any localised swelling, mass
6. Abdominal distension may be present due to intestinal obstruction, masses, tumors, heptomegaly or splenomegaly, pregnancy
7. Movement of abdomen with respiration (All quadrants moving or not)
8. Pulsations over abdomen
9. Peristaltic movement
10. **Condition of skin:** Striae, scar of previous surgery, pigmentation, ulcers, sinus, stoma, keloid, fistula in Crohn's disease
11. **Umbilicus:**
    a. Whether Inverted or Everted
    b. Whether situated in midway between the xiphisternum and symphysis pubis or not
    c. Venous prominence around the umbilicus (Caput medusae from portal hypertension)
    d. Umbilical hernia
12. **Hernial site examination:** Epigastric, inguinal, femoral, umbilical, incisional hernia)
13. **Secondary sexual character:** Groin, genitalia and hair

b. **Palpation: To evaluate internal organs and to examine for abdominal masses, for any tenderness, guarding.**

1. Superficial temperature
2. Tenderness or hyperaesthesia
3. Lump consistency, mobility
4. Check guarding or rigidity
5. Pulsation over abdomen
6. Fluid thrill
7. Girth of abdomen at the level of umbilicus
8. Cough impulse at Hernia sites
9. Palpate Liver, Spleen, Kidneys, Gallbladder, Colon

10. Rebound tenderness
11. Palpate at Mcburney's point, epigastric point, gall bladder point, renal angles for tenderness
12. Examination of hernial sites and its orifices
13. External genitalia, testis, groins (Inguinal lymph nodes, hernia, and femoral pulsation), urinary bladder
14. Palpate the both iliac fossa for colitis, pelvic colon for fecal mass

c. **Percussion: To determine size, density of abdominal organs and to detect air or fluid.**

1. Normally, on percussion abdomen is tympanic
2. Upper border of liver is dull
3. Shifting dullness and fluid thrill are used for detection of ascites

d. **Auscultation: To detect altered abdominal sounds, rubs or vascular bruits.**

1. Peristalsis
2. Hepatic/splenic rub
3. Venous hum
4. Bruit (Hepatic bruit, renal artery bruit, bruit of aneurysm of aorta)

C. **Per rectal examination (optional)**

1. It is important to examine anus.
2. It is important to diagnose rectal tumors and other forms of malignancy
3. To evaluate hemorrhoids
4. Digital rectal examination combined with fecal occult blood test which may be useful for diagnosing the cause of anemia or confirming GI bleeding in an emergency care setting.
5. In females, fullness in pouch of douglas is suggestive of ovarian cyst
6. In males, for the diagnosis of prostatic disorder

SYMPTOMS OF GASTROINTESTINAL AND HEPATOBILIARY DISEASES

1. Nausea, vomiting, hiccup
2. Heartburn, regurgitation
3. Water brash
4. Dysphagia, odynophagia, dyspepsia
5. Anorexia, indigestion
6. Flatulence (Belching or flatus)
7. Jaundice, yellow urine, pruritus (Obstructive jaundice)
8. Pain in abdomen
9. Fever (Amebicliver abscess, subphrenic abscess, spontaneous bacterial peritonitis, intestinal tuberculosis)
10. Distension of abdomen, swelling in abdomen
11. Mass in abdomen
12. Hematemesis, Melena, Hematochezia (Passage of fresh blood through anus), Bleeding per rectum.
13. Alteration in bowel habit
14. Diarrhea or constipation, mucus in stool, worms in stool
15. **Tenesmus:** Feeling of incomplete evacuation with constant desire for defecation (Bacillary dysentery, acute proctitis, CA rectum and impacted feces)
16. Difficulty in defecation with straining
17. **General symptoms:** Fatigue, generalised weakness
18. Loss of weight
19. Pedal edema in malnutrition, portal hypertension

Red Flag Sign of GI and Hepatobiliary System:

1. Persistent vomiting
2. GI bleeding
3. Progressive weight loss
4. Dysphagia
5. Protracted jaundice
6. Prolonged pyrexia
7. Chronic diarrhea
8. Anemia

ALCOHOLIC LIVER DISEASE

1. Liver is the largest internal organ important for keeping body function properly.
2. Alcoholic liver disease is one of the main causes of chronic liver disease.
3. The spectrum of alcoholic liver disease includes fatty liver, alcoholic hepatitis, and alcoholic cirrhosis.
4. Fatty liver is the most commonly observed abnormality in alcoholic spectrum.
5. Alcoholic liver cirrhosis is a common cause of end stage liver disease and hepatocellular carcinoma.
6. **Risk factors**
   a. **Sex:** Females are more susceptile to alcohol related injury than men.
   b. **Quantity of alcohol intake:** Quantity and duration of alcohol intake are responsible for the liver hepatitis and fibrosis.

      In men intake of > 60-80 gm/day for 10 years and in females > 20-40 gm/days for 10 years is responsible for liver hepatitis and fibrosis.
   c. **Hepatitis infection:** Hepatitis C infection accelerates the process of liver damage.
   d. **Diet:** Malnutrition worsen the alcohol induced liver damage by reducing regeneration of hepatocytes.
7. **Clinical features:**
   a. **Fatty liver:**
      1. In this condition excess fat build up in the liver.
      2. Patients are often asymptomatic.
      3. Patients usually present with upper right quadrant discomfort, nausea, and rarely jaundice.
   b. **Alcoholic hepatitis:**
      1. Inflammation of liver which contributes progression to fibrosis.
      2. Patient may develop symptoms like fever, spider nevi, jaundice, and abdominal pain.
      3. Portal hypertension, ascites, spider nevi or variceal bleed can occur even in the absence of cirrhosis depending upon the severity of disease.
   c. **Alcoholic liver cirrhosis:**
      1. In this stage normal healthy tissue is replaced by scar tissue.
      2. It requires months to years to develop.

3. **Clinical features of liver cirrhosis:**
    i. Fatigue, muscle wasting, asterixis
    ii. Anorexia
    iii. Abdominal pain, ascites, icterus
    iv. Weight loss
    v. Spider nevi develops on skin of face, neck-shoulders
    vi. Complications of cirrhosis e.g. GI bleeding, hepatic encephalopathy
    vii. In some patients complications may be the first sign of disease

8. **Laboratory features:**
    a. **In alcoholic fatty liver:** The typical lab findings in fatty liver are nonspecific
        1. **Liver function test:** Mild or normal elevation of aspartate aminotransferase (AST), alanine aminotransferase (ALT), and gamma-glutamyl transpeptidase (GGTP), and hyperbilirubinemia.
        2. Hypertriglyceridemia
        3. Hyperbilirubinemia
    b. **In alcoholic hepatitis:**
        1. AST and ALT are usually elevated two to seven fold and rarely > 400 IU.
        2. AST/ALT ratio is 2:1
        3. Hyperbilirubinemia
        4. Increase in the alkaline phosphatase level
        5. Raised PT/INR
        6. Ultrasonography shows fatty infiltration of the liver
        7. Ultrasonography examination is also useful to detect severity of disease.
    c. **Liver biopsy:** It may be helpful if alternate diagnosis being considered

9. **Treatment:**
    a. Immediate and total abstinence from alcohol
    b. Symptoms of alcohol withdrawal are managed by benzodiazepines and psychological therapy.
    c. Nutritional support should include vitamins (Folic acid, Thiamine, Vit E, Vit A) and minerals.
    d. The non-specific TNF inhibitor, pentoxifylline (A tumor necrosis factor inhibitor)

may be used in severe alcoholic hepatitis patients, hepatorenal syndrome but effect is unclear .

e. Patients with severe alcoholic hepatitis should be given prednisolone.

f. But, glucocorticoids are not given in patients with active gastrointestinal bleeding, renal failure or pancreatitis.

g. Early diagnosis and management of cirrhosis related complications.

10. **Liver transplantation:** Considered in cases with end stage cirrhosis.

LIVER CIRRHOSIS

1. **Definition:** Cirrhosis is a chronic condition characterized by diffuse replacement of healthy liver cells by fibrotic tissue due to liver damage.

    a. Cirrhosis is a condition that is defined on histopathological findings and has varieties of clinical manifestations and complications.

    a. It simply means nodule formation and scarring of liver .

    b. Clinical features of liver cirrhosis are the result of pathologic changes and reflect the severity of liver disease.

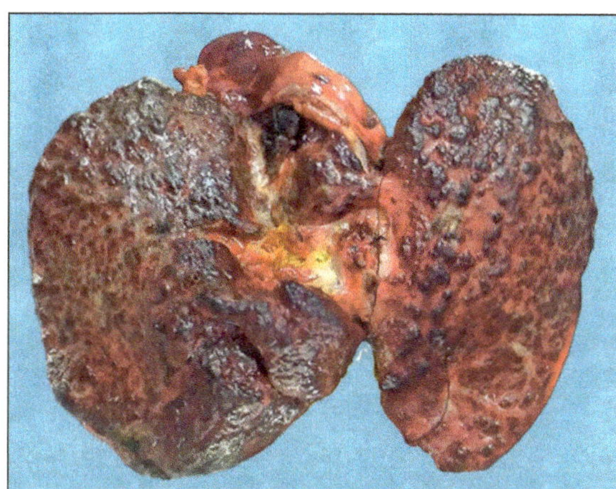

Cirrhotic liver with hepatocellular carcinoma. (Courtesy Dr. Prashant Rao from the book Clinics in Surgical Gastroenterology.)

    c. **Two different stages of liver cirrhosis**

        1. **Compensated:**

        In compensated liver cirrhosis there are sufficient healthy liver cells to do the job, so no symptoms or little.

        2. **Non compensated:**

        In decompensated liver cirrhosis healthy liver cells are overburdened for its functions and compensated liver progress to decompensated stage.

2. **Causes of cirrhosis:**

    a. **Chronic alcoholic**

    b. **Chronic viral hepatitis:** Hepatitis B, hepatitis C

    c. **Autoimmune hepatitis**

    d. **Non alcoholic steatohepatitis (NASH)**

    e. **Biliary cirrhosis:** Primary biliary cirrhosis, primary sclerosing cholangitis, autoimmune cholangiopathy due to bile duct obstruction

    f. **Cardiac cirrhosis:** Chronic heart failure with liver congestion

    g. **Inherited metabolic liver disease:** Hemochromatosis, Wilson's disease, alfa 1 antitrypsin deficiency, Fanconi syndrome.

h. **Toxins and drugs:** Methotrexate & amiodarone

i. **Cryptogenic cirrhosis:** Cause is not known

3. **Signs and symptoms:**

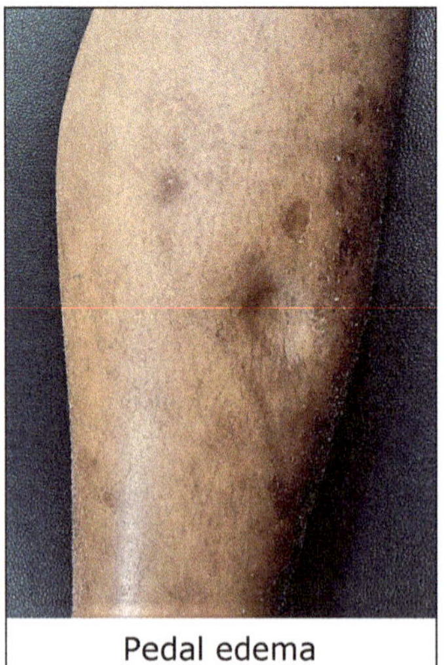

Pedal edema

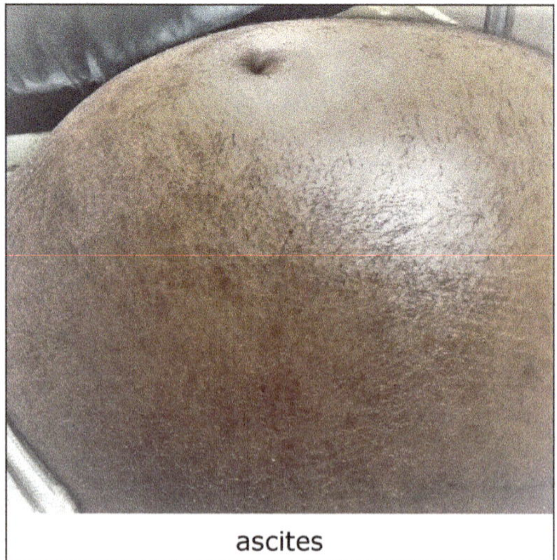

ascites

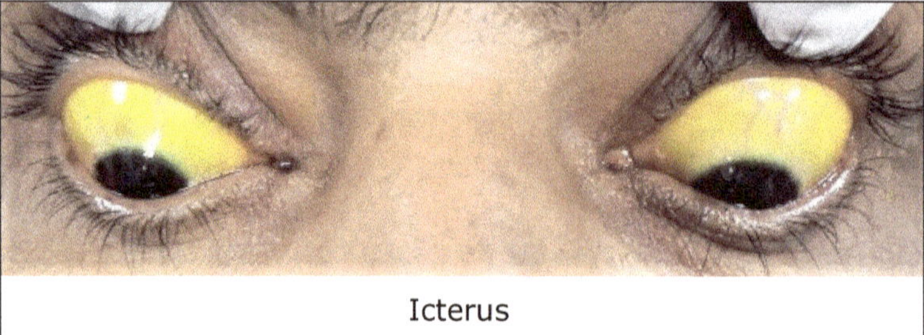

Icterus

a. **Palmar erythema:** Exaggeration of normal speckled mottling of palm due to altered sex hormone metabolism.

b. **Spider angiomas**

c. **Muscle wasting**

d. **Gynecomastia:** This is due to increased estradiol

e. **Parotid enlargement**

f. **Clubbing of fingers**

g. **Hypogonadism:** It manifest as infertility, loss of sexual drive and testicular atrophy in males and menstrual irregularities in females .

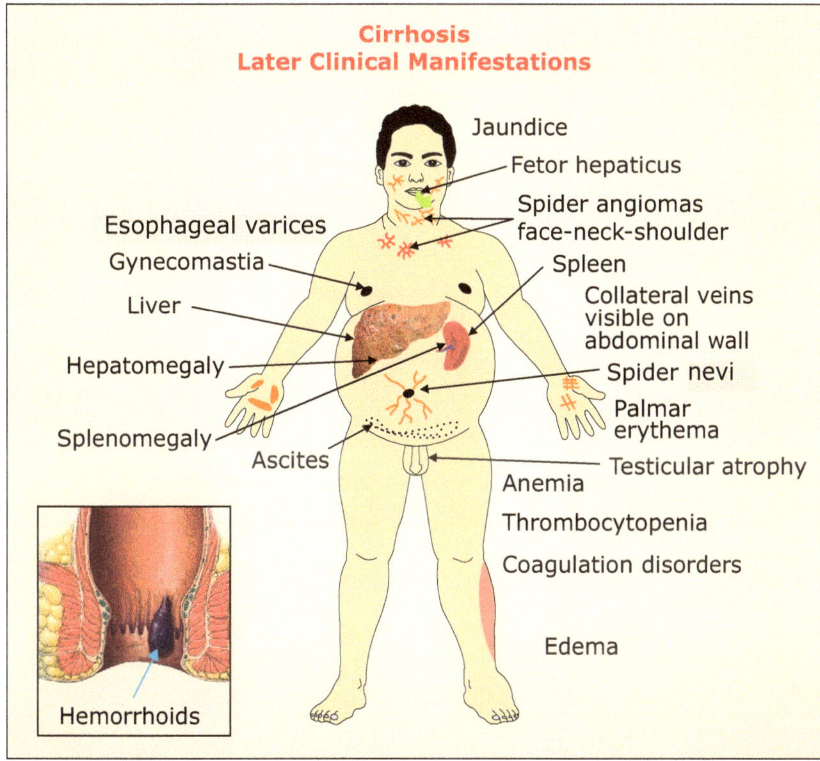

It occurs due to primary gonadal injury or suppression of hypothalamic or pituitary function

h. **Asterixis:** Bilateral asynchronous flapping of outstretched and dorsiflexed hands seen in hepatic encephalopathy

i. **Fetor hepaticus:** Musty odor of breath occur due to increased dimethyl sulfide

j. **Non specific symptoms include:**

1. Right upper quadrant abdominal pain
2. Fever
3. Generalized weakness
4. Nausea, and vomiting
5. Diarrhea
6. Anorexia, and malaise

P. Signs and symptoms of complications:

1. GI bleeding (Hematemesis or melena)
2. Ascites
3. Confused or exhibit a change in personality (Hepatic encephalopathy)

4. **Laboratory findings:**

    a. Laboratory tests may be completely normal in patients with early compensated alcoholic cirrhosis.

    b. In advanced liver disease, many abnormalities are usually present.

Complete blood count	**Anemia** (Due to chronic GI blood loss, nutritional deficiency, hypersplenism) **Thrombocytopenia:** Indicates presence of portal hypertension with hypersplenism. **Leukopenia** and **Neutropenia:** Due to splenomegaly with splenic migration
Liver function test	**S**erum bilirubin normal or mildly elevated **D**irect bilirubin is mildly elevated **S**erum alanine and aspartate aminotransferases are typically elevated (AST >ALT) & ratio is > 2 **Albumin:** Decreased due to impaired protein synthesis **Globulin:** Increased
PT INR	Prothrombin time often prolonged due to reduced synthesis of vitamin K dependent clotting factors.
Other laboratory studies performed in newly diagnosed cirrhosis patient	**Serology** for hepatitis viruses, autoantibodies **Ferritin and transferrin saturation** **Alfa 1- antitrypsin level**

5. **Diagnosis:**

    a. Diagnosis of alcoholic cirrhosis depends upon a history of alcohol intake, clinical features, physical findings, lab findings

    b. **Liver biopsy:** Helpful to confirm a diagnosis

    c. **Imaging:** Sonography, MRI scan, CT scan, helpful to diagnose liver cirrhosis & also to determine severity of disease

    d. **Gastroscopy:** To find the esophageal varices and to treat varices.

    e. **ERCP and MRCP:** Imaging of bile duct to diagnose a primary sclerosing cholangitis which can cause liver cirrhosis .

6. **Treatment of liver cirrhosis**

    a. **Prevent further damage**

    b. **Treatment of complication**

    c. **Liver transplantation**

7. Cause and treatment of liver cirrhosis

Hepatitis C	Interferon, antiviral medication (ribavirin), protease inhibitor
Hepatitis B	Antiviral medication (Tenofovir, lamivudine, entecavir, adefovir, telbivudine)
Chronic alcoholic	Abstinence
Biliary cirrhosis	**Primary:** Ursodeoxycholic acid **Secondary:** Regular biliary drainage
Autoimmune hepatitis	Prednisone, budesonide, azathioprine.
Inherited metabolic liver disease	**Hemochromatosis:** Phlebotomy **Wilson disease:** D-Penicillamine (Chelation therapy) **Alfa 1-antitrypsin deficiency:** Intravenous infusion of alfa 1-antitrypsin, liver transplantation.

8. Complications of cirrhosis

Portal hypertension	Gastroesophageal varices, portal hypertensive gastropathy, splenomegaly, hypersplenism, ascites, spontaneous bacterial peritonitis.
Hepatorenal syndrome	Type 1 and Type 2
Coagulopathy	Factor deficiency, fibrinolysis
Hematological abnormalities	Anemia, hemolysis, thrombocytopenia, neutropenia, leucopenia
Bone disease	Osteopenia, osteoporosis, osteomalacia
Hepatic encephalopathy	
Malnutrition	

PORTAL HYPERTENSION

1. **Definition:** Portal hypertension is defined as the elevation of hepatic venous pressure gradient (HVPG) to > 5 mm of Hg.
2. Portal hypertension occurs as a result of increased intrahepatic resistance to the blood flow through the liver due to regenerative nodules and cirrhosis.
3. Liver cirrhosis is the most common cause of portal hypertension.
4. **Classification of causes of portal hypertension:**

Prehepatic	Hepatic	Posthepatic
1. Portal vein thrombosis **2. Splenic vein thrombosis** **3. Massive splenomegaly**	**1. Presinusoidal** Schistosomiasis Metastatic carcinoma Congenital hepatic fibrosis **2. Sinusoidal** Liver cirrhosis Primary biliary disease Alcohol induced cirrhosis **3. Postsinusoidal** Hepatic sinusoidal obstruction Hepatic vein thrombosis	Budd-Chiari syndrome Inferior vena caval webs **Cardiac causes:** 1. Restrictive cardiomyopathy 2. Constrictive pericarditis 3. Severe congestive heart failure

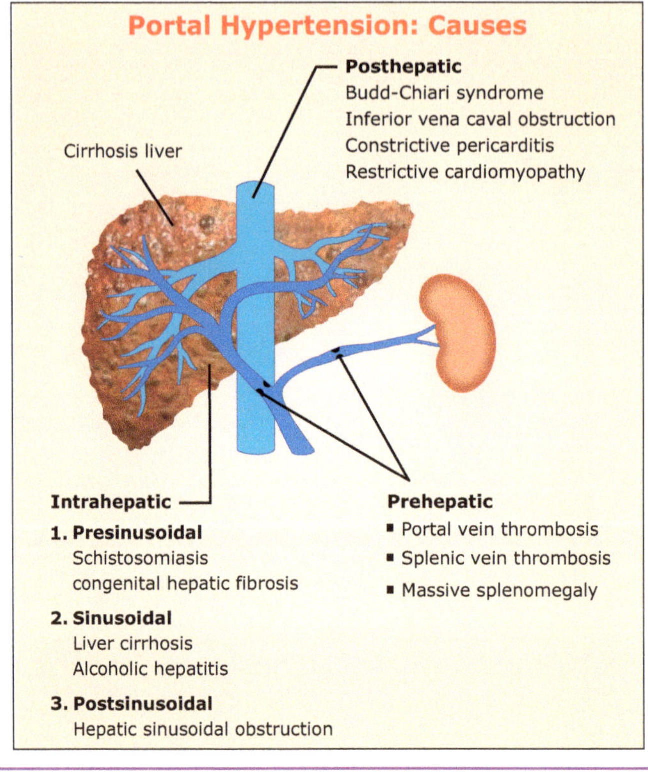

5. **The Primary Complications of portal hypertension:**

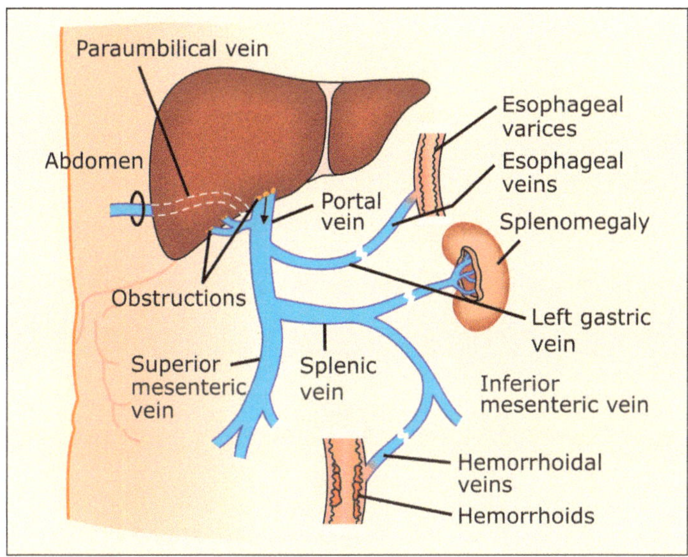

   a. **Gastroesophageal varices:** Patient may present with esophageal or gastric varices.

   b. **Ascites:** Development of ascites with peripheral edema.

   c. **Hypersplenism:** Associated with splenomegaly, reduction in platelets and white blood cells.

6. **Diagnosis:**

   a. **Diagnosis of portal hypertension is made on the basis of presence of**

      1. Thrombocytopenia and leucopenia
      2. Splenomegaly
      3. Ascites
      4. Hepatic encephalopathy
      5. Esophageal varices

   b. **Ultrasonography:** First line imaging for diagnosis of portal hypertension & also helps to diagnose portal vein thrombosis, splenomegaly.

   c. **Hepatic venous pressure gradient measurement:** A Gold standard for assessing the severity of portal hypertension. (Hepatic venous pressure gradient is defined as the difference between the wedged hepatic venous pressure and free hepatic venous pressure.)

   d. **Esophagogastroduodenoscopy** is the gold standard for the diagnosis of esophageal varices.

e. **CT scan or MRI abdomen:** Demonstrate nodular liver, ascites, splenomegaly and intra-abdominal venous collaterals.

f. **Interventional radiographic procedure:**

Help us to calculate the wedge to free gradient, which is equivalent to portal pressure.

g. **Portal venogram:** To detect portal venous obstruction.

7. **Treatment of portal hypertension:**

a. **Dietary and lifestyle modification**

i. Good nutrition which includes Folic acid, Thiamine, Vitamin E, Vitamin A and minerals

ii. Bed rest and Salt restriction

iii. Immediate and total abstinence of alcohol consumption

b. **Beta blockers:** Non selective beta-blockers are used to reduce portal and collateral blood flow to prevent variceal bleeding (e.g. Propranolol, nadolol, timolol)

c. **Management of complications:** Variceal bleeding, ascites

d. **TIPSS** (Transjugular intrahepatic portosystemic shunt): A stent is placed between portal and hepatic vein under radiological control for reduction of portal hypertension.

e. **Surgery:** Shunts (Distal splenorenal shunts), liver transplantation

f. **Endoscopic therapy**

i. **Endoscopic sclerotherapy:** Injection of sclerosant into varices

ii. **Band ligation**

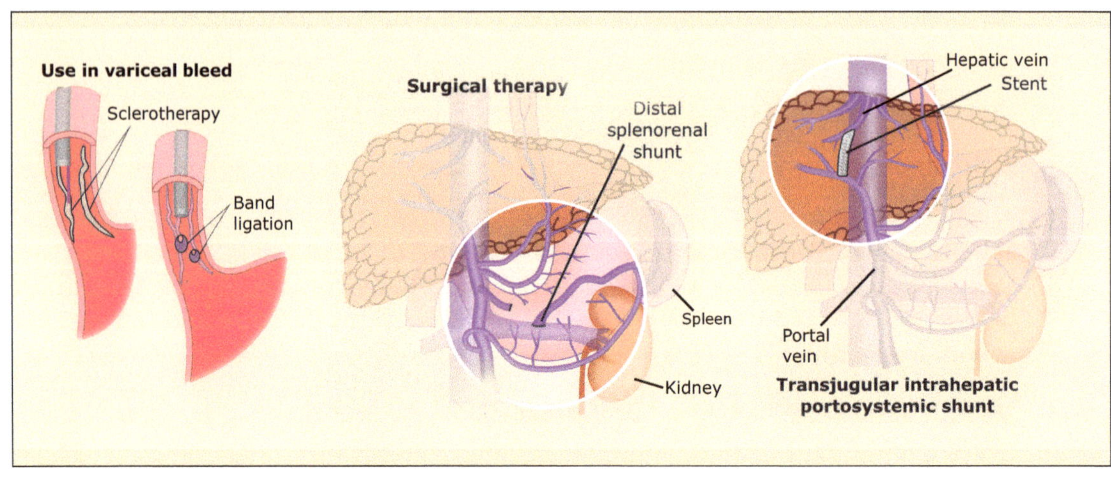

VARICEAL BLEEDING

1. Variceal bleeding is a consequence of portal hypertension.
2. Bleeding from varices is a major complication of portal hypertension and associated with high mortality rate .

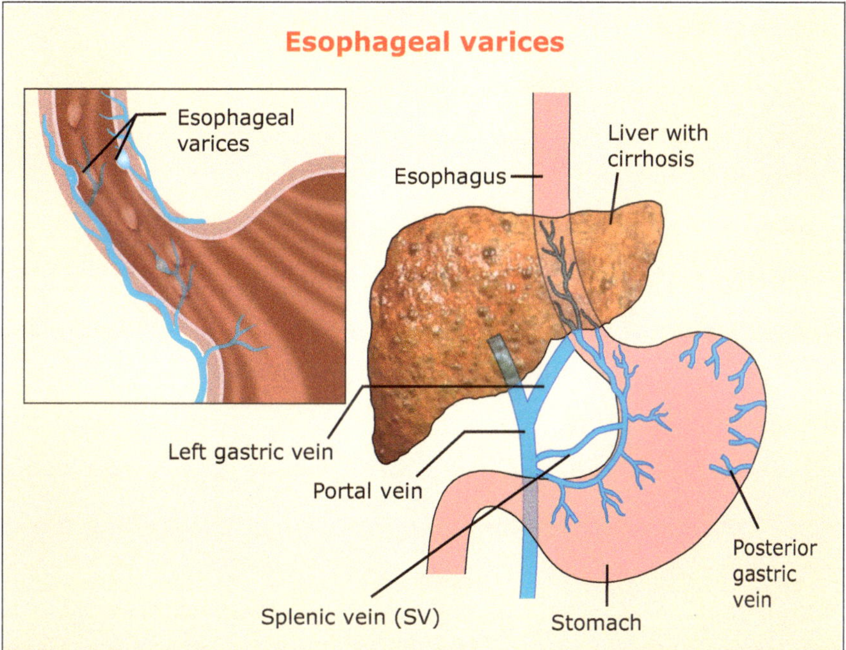

3. Esophagogastroduodenoscopy is the gold standard for the diagnosis of esophageal varices.
4. If not available then doppler ultrasonography is advised for detection of blood circulation in veins.
5. **Treatment:**
   a. **Primary prophylaxis**
   b. **Secondary prophylaxis:** Prevention of rebleeding.
6. **Primary prophylaxis:**
   a. Primary prophylaxis requires regular screening of cirrhotic patients for any high risk varices.
   b. Once high risk varices are identified by EGD scopy then treatment is given before bleeding either in the form of nonselective beta blockade (Propranolol, nadolol, carvedilol) or variceal band ligation/variceal sclerotherapy.
   c. Repeat EGD scopy is performed in patients with small varices.

7. **Management of acute bleed:**
   a. **Hospitalisation**
   b. **Resuscitation**
      1. Intravenous access and start fluid administration to correct hypovolemia
      2. Clear airway by suction
      3. High O_2 flow
      4. Insert Ryle's tube and give cold saline wash
      5. Blood samples are sent for routine blood investigations, blood grouping and cross match.
      6. Blood and blood product transfusion
   c. **Antiemetics and antacids are started.**
   d. **Prophylactic antibiotics:** Intravenous ciprofloxacin or ceftriaxone for 7 days are used to avoid bacterial infection such as spontaneous bacterial peritonitis.
   e. **Control active bleeding:**
      i. Use vasoconstricting agents like telmipressin, somatostatin or octreotide.
      ii. EGD scopy to be performed within 24 hours of bleeding (Once patient is stable)
      iii. Endoscopy is used as first line treatment to control bleeding acutely
      iv. In esophageal varices the variceal band ligation is done.
      v. In gastric varices the sclerotherapy with cyanoacrylate injection or variceal band ligation is used to control bleeding.
      vi. Balloon tamponade can be used in patients who cannot get the endoscopic therapy immediately.
      vii. If bleeding still continues then consider for transjugular intrahepatic portosystemic shunt (TIPS).
8. **Secondary prophylaxis (Prevention of recurrent bleeding):**
   a. Done by repeated variceal band ligation until varices are obliterated.
   b. Beta blockade used along with variceal band ligation has good results.

ASCITES

1. **Definition:**

   Ascites is the pathological accumulation of fluid within the peritoneal cavity.

   a. Healthy men may have little or no fluid in the peritoneal cavity but women normally may have up to 20 ml depending on the phase of menstrual cycle.

   b. Most common cause of ascites is portal hypertension due to cirrhosis.

   c. Ascites in the absence of cirrhosis generally results from peritoneal carcinomatosis, peritoneal infection or pancreatic diseases.

   d. Careful finding of cause is important for patient management.

2. **Causes of ascites based on the basis of serum ascites - albumin gradient**

   (The SAAG is useful for distinguishing ascites caused by portal hypertension from non portal hypertensive ascites.)

SAAG > 1.1 g/dl	SAAG < 1.1 g/dl
1. Liver Cirrhosis	1. Bacterial peritonitis
2. Alcoholic Hepatitis	2. Tuberculous peritonitis
3. Fulminant hepatic failure	3. Fungal peritonitis
4. Massive hepatic metastases	4. Malignant conditions: Massive hepatic metastases, Hepatocellular carcinoma, peritoneal carcinomatosis.
5. Cardiac ascites	5. Nephrotic syndrome
6. Constrictive pericarditis	6. Protein- losing enteropathy
7. Tricuspid insufficiency	7. Severe malnutrition with Anasarca
8. Budd-Chiari syndrome	8. Vasculitis
9. Veno-Occlusive syndrome	9. Granulomatous peritonitis
10. Portal venous occlusion	10. Eosinophilic peritonitis
11. Myxedema	11. Chylous ascites
12. Fatty liver of pregnancy	12. Pancreatic ascites
	13. Biliary ascites

3. **Pathogenesis:**

   a. **Pathogenesis of ascites in liver cirrhosis:**

Flowchart: Pathogenesis of ascites in liver cirrhosis

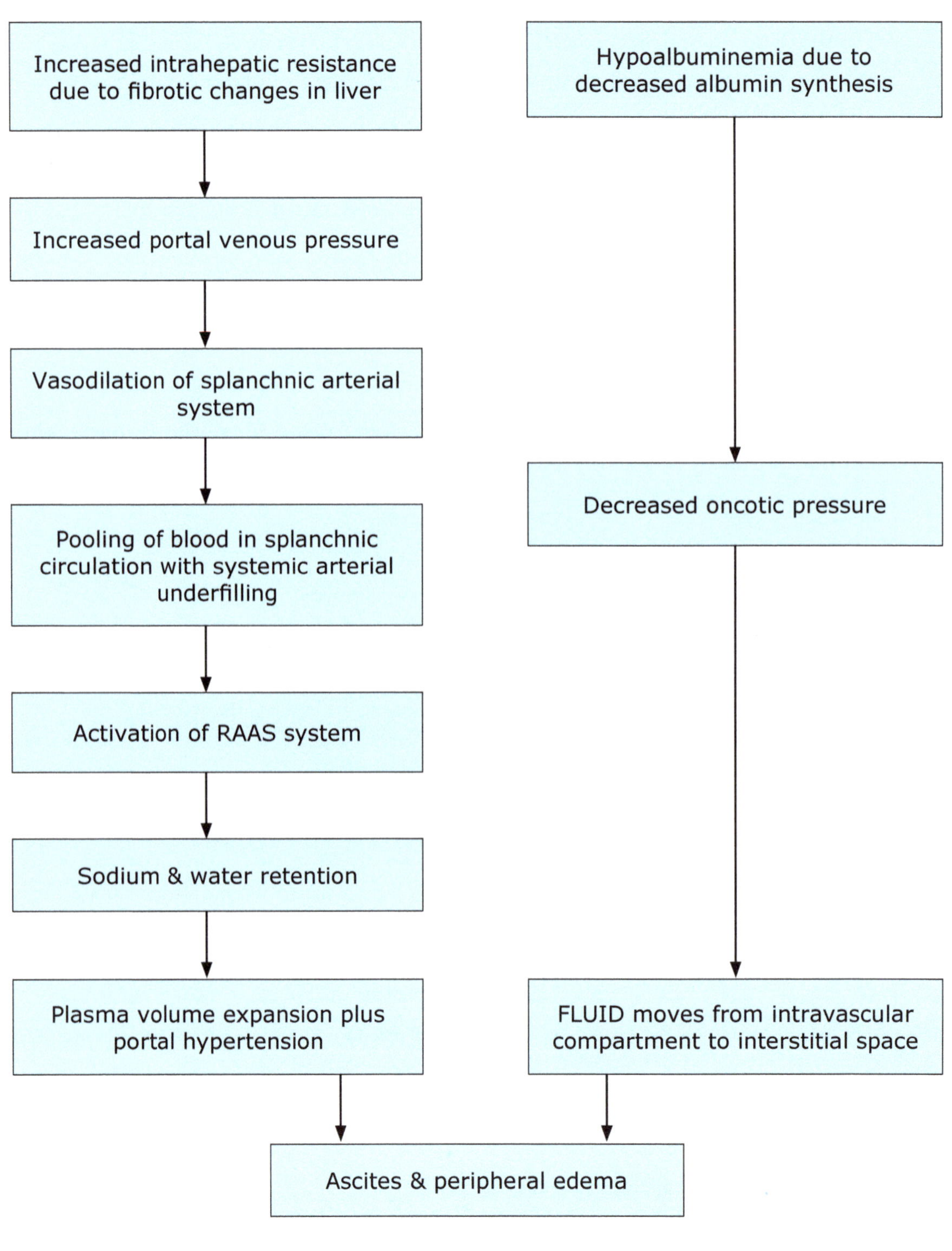

b. Pathogenesis of ascites in non-cirrohtic causes

Peritoneal carcinomatosis (Result from primary malignancies such as mesothelioma or sarcoma, secondary to abdominal malignancies such as gastric or colon adenocarcinoma, metastatic process from breast or lung carcinoma or melanoma)	Tumor cells lining the peritoneum produces a protein rich fluid that results into the development of ascites.
Tuberculous peritonitis	Tubercles deposited on the peritoneum produces a protein rich fluid
Pancreatic ascites	Leakage of pancreatic enzymes into the Peritoneum.

4. **History:**
   a. History related to risk factors for liver disease such as alcohol consumption, blood transfusion, tattoos (HIV, HBV infections).
   b. History of viral hepatitis, jaundice, tuberculosis .
   c. History related to cancer such as chronic fatigue, weight loss, GI bleeding (Hematemesis, melena), change in bowel and bladder habits.
   d. Medical history related to heart, renal, pancreatic, liver diseases.
5. **Clinical features:**
   a. Generalised swelling of abdomen with weight gain
   b. Umbilicus is everted or flushed with transverse slit
   c. Aching pain all over abdomen due to stretching due to fluid
   d. Shortness of breath due to massive ascitic fluid which disturbs the diaphragmatic function mechanically

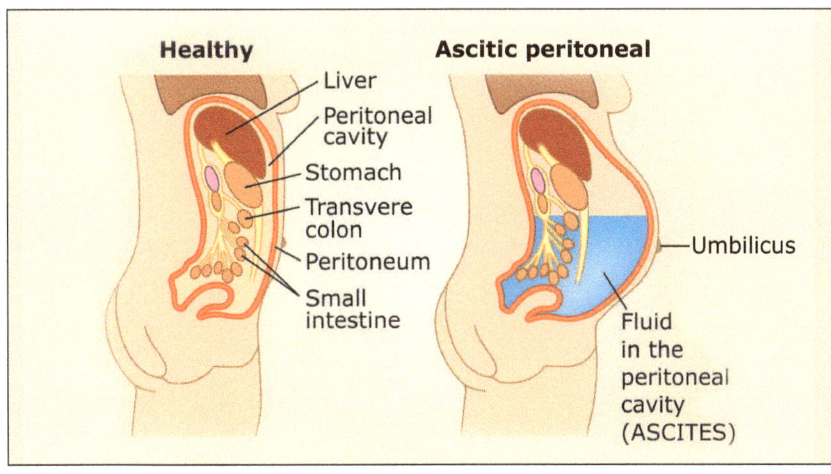

e. **Clinical features and etiological diagnosis :**

Clinical features associated with ascites	Etiological diagnosis
Bilateral pitting edema over lower limbs, Palmar erythema, Cutaneous spider angiomas, Gynecomastia, and muscle wasting	Chronic liver disease
Bilateral pitting edema over lower limbs, elevated JVP, dyspnea, PND or orthopnea	Congestive cardiac failure
Anasarca with hypoalbuminemia	Nephrotic syndrome
Weight loss, chronic fatigue, generalised weakness, left supraclavicular lymphadenopathy (Virchow's node), change in bowel habits	Abdominal malignancy
Fever, constipation, abdominal tenderness, constipation	Abdominal tuberculosis
Severe upper abdominal pain referring to back, guarding, rigidity and tenderness over upper abdomen/Generalised , fever, vomiting	Acute pancreatitis
Non pitting edema	Myxedema, Filariasis

g. **Palpation of abdomen:** Done for swelling or lump, tenderness, enlargement of liver spleen.

h. **Percussion of abdomen:** Fluid thrill and shifting dullness present

6. **Diagnosis:**

Diagnosis of ascites by physical examination, laboratory investigations and by abdominal imaging.

a. **Laboratory investigations:**

i. Complete blood count: Anemia, Infections

ii. **Liver function test :** Liver disease

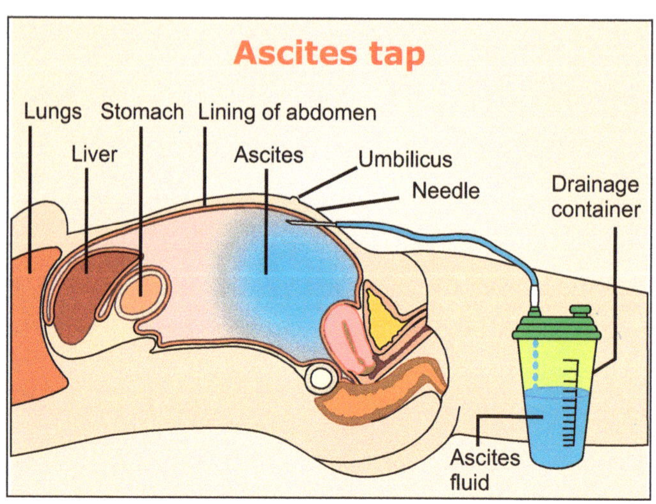

iii. **Renal function test:** Renal cause

iv. **PT INR:** High in liver cirrhosis

v. **Serum amylase or Lipase:** Acute pancreatitis

vi. **Serum cholesterol:** Increased in nephrotic syndrome and decreased in Liver cirrhosis

vii. **Plasma protein:** Low albumin level seen in Cirrhosis of liver, Nephrotic syndrome

viii. **Urine routine and microscopy:** Albumin in urine is seen in Nephrotic syndrome

ix. **Stool for occult blood:** Abdominal malignancy, Cirrhosis of liver

x. **B type natriuretic peptide (BNP):** Cardiac failure

b. **Ascitic fluid analysis:** When patients present with ascites for the first time diagnostic paracentesis is performed to characterize the fluid.

This should include the determination of total protein and albumin content, blood cell counts with differential, cultures, cytology and ADA.

Test performed of ascitic fluid

1. **Routine test**
   a. Cell count and differential count
   b. Total protein concentration
   c. Albumin concentration (SAAG)
   d. Culture in blood culture bottle
   e. Adenosine deaminase (ADA)
2. **Optional test**
   a. Glucose concentration
   b. LDH concentration (Intestinal perforation)
   c. Gram stain (Tuberculosis)
   d. Serum amylase (Pancreatitis)
3. **Unusual test**
   a. Cytology
   b. Tuberculous smear and culture

c. Triglyceride concentration

d. Bilirubin concentration

Appearance	Cell count	Total protein
Clear/straw colored Liver cirrhosis **Cloudy** Bacterial peritonitis, pancreatitis, **Bloody** Malignancy, hemorrhagic pancreatitis **Chylous** Lymphoma, tuberculosis, malignancy	**Red blood cells** None - normal > 100 ul - Malignancy > 1000000- Abdominal trauma **White blood cells** **< 300/microlitre:** normal **> 300/microlitre:** Ascitic fluid infection **≥ 25% of neutrophils:** bacterial peritonitis, cirrhosis **≥ 25% of lymphocytes:** TB, chylous ascites **Mesothelial cells:** Tuberculosis	**< 2.5 g/dl** Cirrhosis, late Budd Chiari syndrome, massive liver metastasis **≥ 2.5 g/dl** Congestive heart failure, constrictive pericarditis, IVC obstruction, early Budd Chiari syndrome, sinusoidal obstruction syndrome

SAAG	Cytology	Culture
> 1.1 g/dl Portal hypertension usually in setting of cirrhosis **< 1.1 g/dl** Infectious or malignant causes	For diagnosis of malignancy	In blood culture bottle

c. **Radiological investigations:**

i. **Chest X ray:** Pulmonary tuberculosis, cardiomegaly

ii. **Abdominal X ray erect:** Diffuse abdominal haziness may be seen due to ascites and to rule out intestinal obstruction in case of abdominal tuberculosis with constipation.

iii. **Ultrasonography of abdomen and pelvis:** To confirm ascites

iv. **CT abdomen and pelvis with contrast:** In suspected case of abdominal Tuberculosis, Acute pancreatitis, abdominal malignancy.

7. **Management**

a. **Bed rest:** It increases renal perfusion and hence diuresis

b. **Diet:** Salt restriction diet < 2 g of sodium per day

c. **Fluid restriction:** Restrict fluid intake to 1-1.5 lit/day

d. **Ascitic tapping:** Ascitic tapping is required in severe cases

   After ascitic tapping salt free albumin or dextran or hemaccel is infused to maintain the circulation.

e. **Diuretics:**

   i. Generally, spironolactone at 100-200 mg/day in divided dose is started

   ii. Furosemide may be added at 40-80 mg/day along with spironolactone particularly in patients with peripheral edema or no good response to spironolactone

   iii. **Other diuretics drugs:** Amiloride, bumetanide, torsemide may be used

f. **Treatment of etiological cause:** Tuberculosis, malignancy, CCF, nephrotic syndrome, Myxedema

g. **Refractory to medical treatment**

   i. **TIPSS**

   ii. **Shunts**

h. **Liver transplant:** In refractory cases with liver cirrhosis

HEPATIC ENCEPHALOPATHY

1. **Definition:**

   An alteration in mental status and cognitive function occurring in the presence of liver failure.

   a. Encephalopathy is commonly seen in patients with chronic liver disease

   b. It can also occur in fulminant liver failure.

   c. **It is developed due to following two factors:**

      1. **Raised level of ammonia in blood**

      2. **Inflammatory response to gut derived neurotoxins which is not removed by liver.**

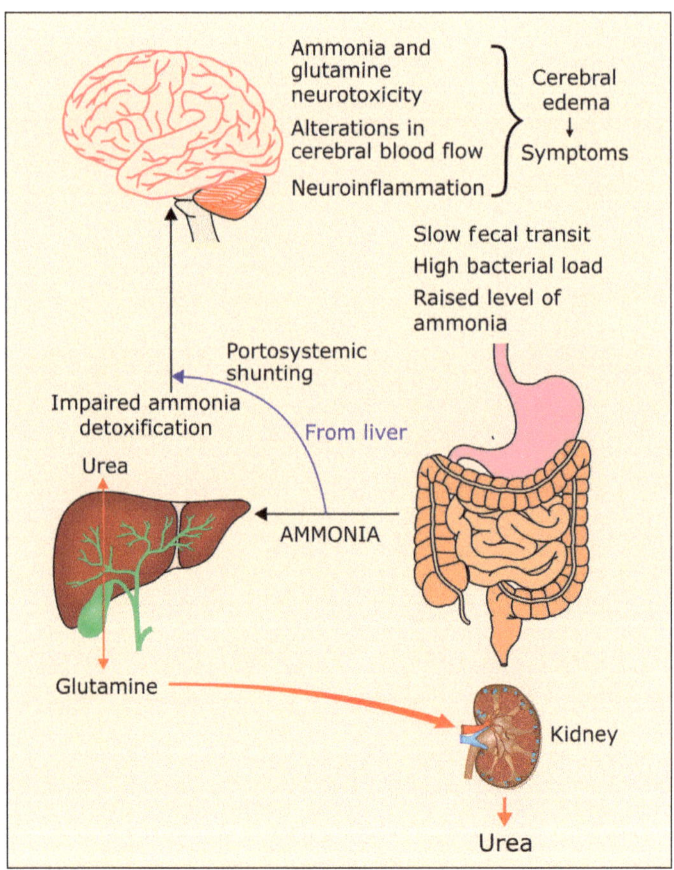

   d. Both above factors are responsible for cerebral edema and cerebral edema responsible for symptoms.

   e. Brain herniation is a complication of cerebral edema in acute liver failure which eventually leads to death.

2. **Causes:**

   Episodes can be precipatated by infections, GI bleed, constipation, electrolyte imbalance, or certain drugs & medication

   a. **Infection:** e.g. Pneumonia, urinary tract infection, spontaneous bacterial peritonitis, other infections.

   b. **Electrolyte imbalance:** Hyponatremia, hypokalemia, hypoxia, dehydration, alkalosis.

   c. **Excessive nitrogen load:** High intake of protein, GI bleed, kidney failure, constipation

   d. **Drugs and medications:** antipsychotics, alcohol intoxication, sedatives, narcotics

   e. **Others:** surgery, alcoholic hepatitis, GI bleed, TIPS.

3. **Clinical features**

   a. Onset may be gradual or sudden

   b. Patients may be confused or exhibit a change in personality.

   c. Poor concentration, judgment

   d. Loss of memory, slurred speech

   e. Reduced or loss of concentration

   f. Asterixis (Liver flap) is often present in encephalopathy patients.

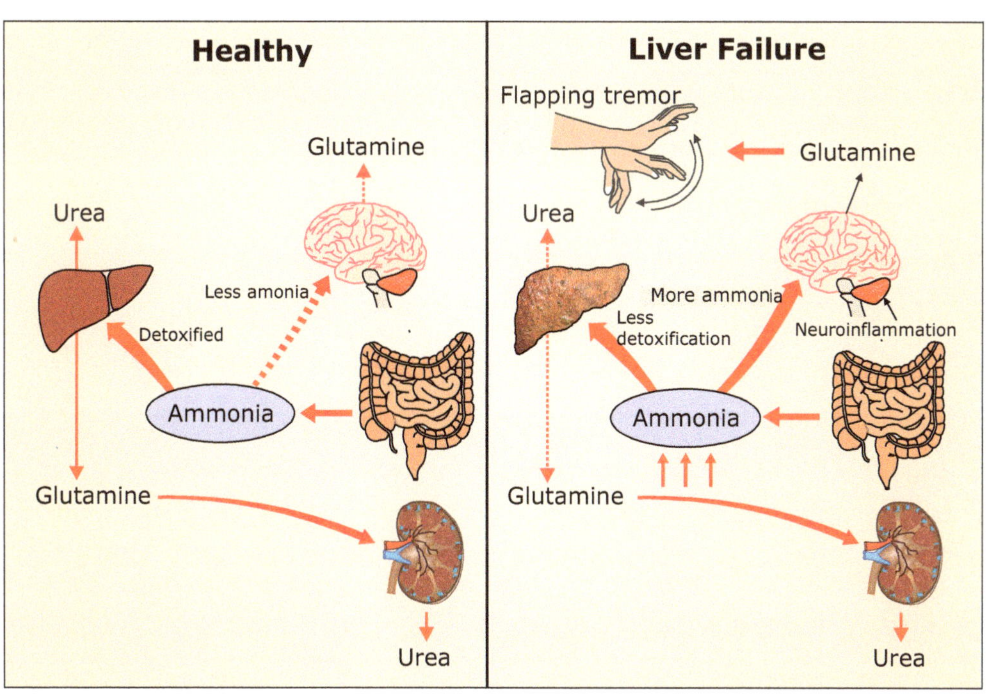

g. Encephalopathy often occurs together with other symptoms and signs of liver failure like generalised weakness, anorexia, abdominal pain, vomiting, nausea, ascites with pedal edema, jaundice and exaggerated tendon reflex.

4. **Diagnosis**

   a. Hepatic encephalopathy is diagnosed based on clinical findings and by excluding other causes of altered mental status.

   b. **Routine laboratory test**

      1. Liver function test
      2. Renal function
      3. Serum electrolytes
      4. Glucose level
      5. Cultures and Drug screening

   c. **A serum ammonia level:** Help to diagnose hepatic encephalopathy but it is not recommended.

   d. **Brain computed tomography (CT):** Helps to exclude other causes of altered mental status, such as intracerebral hemorrhage.

   e. **Brain magnetic resonance imaging (MRI):** Used to diagnose cerebral edema and other brain abnormalities associated with hepatic encephalopathy.

   f. **Electroencephalograph (EEG):** If seizure activity is suspected.

5. **Management based on the following strategy:**

   a. **Rule out other possible causes of encephalopathy**

   b. **Identify the precipitating cause in known case of chronic liver disease**

   c. **Empiric treatment**

6. **Management:**

   a. Hepatic encephalopathy is possibly reversible with treatment.

   b. Precipitating factors are diagnosed and treated / removed.

   c. Protect and maintain airway

   d. Monitor pulse, blood pressure, respiration and mental status

   e. Insert RT and Foley's catheter .

   f. Correct hypotension with IV fluids

   g. Correct electrolyte abnormalities

   h. **Cerebral edema:**

i. Head end elevation upto 30°
ii. Osmotic therapy with mannitol
iii. Judicious use of IV fluids
iv. Hyperventilation
v. Hypothermia

i. **Use of lactulose:**
   1. To avoid constipation
   1. A nonabsorbable disaccharide which results in colonic acidification.
   2. The goal of lactulose therapy is to promote 2-3 soft stools per day.

j. **Initiate empirical treatment (Bowel sterilisation)**
   1. Rifaximin at 550 mg twice daily has been very effective in treating encephalopathy.
   2. Neomycin 500 mg four times daily.
   3. Metronidazole 400 mg twice daily.

k. **Injection of Vitamin K**: 1 ampule of Vitamin K IM daily for 3 consecutive days for coagulopathy.

l. Avoid sedatives, narcotic drugs and restrict high protein diet.

m. Zinc supplementation is sometimes helpful in patients with encephalopathy and is relatively harmless.

n. Liver transplantation is the definitive management

FULMINANT HEPATIC FAILURE

1. Fulminant hepatic failure is a condition that develops rapid hepatocellular dysfunction specifically a coagulation abnormalities and associated with any degree of mental alteration in a patient without preexisting liver disease and with an illness of < 26 weeks duration.
2. **Divided in three types on the basis of length of illness**
   a. **Hyperacute (< 7 days)**
   b. **Acute (7-21 days)**
   c. **Sub acute (21 days to < 26 Weeks)**
3. **Causes:**
   a. **Infection:** Viral hepatitis A, B, C, D and E (Most common A, B and E)
   b. **Hepatotoxic drugs:** Acetaminophen, INH, alcohol
   c. **Vascular causes:** Budd Chiari syndrome, veno-occlusive disease
   d. **Pregnancy:** Acute fatty liver, eclampsia, HELLP syndrome.
   e. **Metabolic:** Wilson disease
   f. **Toxin exposure:** CCL 4 (mushroom poisoning)
   g. **Other:** Reye syndrome, primary biliary cirrhosis
4. **Clinical features**
   a. Generalised weakness
   b. Anorexia
   c. Abdominal pain, vomiting, nausea
   d. Jaundice and mental status changes (Mild to severe)
   e. Bleeding from orifices, melena
   f. Signs and symptoms of cerebral edema and cerebral herniation
   g. Patients may develop cardiovascular collapse, acute renal failure and sepsis.
5. **History:**
   a. **Alcohol abuse**
   b. **Medication history:** If patient is on any medications then detailed history of medications and doses
   c. **Onset and progression of mental status and jaundice**
   d. **Family history:** History of liver disease in family (Wilson disease)
   e. **History for risk factors for viral hepatitis:** travel, blood transfusion, sexual contact, body piercing.

6. **Physical examination**
    a. **Mental status:**
        1. **Grade I:** Mild confusion, irritability, tremors, asterixis, sleep reversal pattern
        2. **Grade II:** Lethargy, disorientation, inappropriate behavior, asterixis
        3. **Grade III:** Somnolence, severe confusion, aggressive behavior, asterixis
        4. **Grade VI:** Coma
    b. **Jaundice**
    c. **RUQ tenderness**
    d. **Hepatomegaly**
    e. **Ascites**
    f. **Raised ICP (Cushing triad):** Hypertension, Bradycardia, Irregular respiration
    g. **Decorticate posture**
7. **Initial investigation:**
    a. **Blood sugar:** May be low
    b. **Complete blood count:** Thrombocytopenia
    c. **Liver function test:** Elevated level of ALT, AST, ALP, bilirubin
    d. **Serum Electrolyte**
    e. **PT and INR:** INR > 1.5 that does not correct with the administration of vitamin K is a characteristic feature.
    f. **Arterial blood gas analysis**
    g. **USG with doppler:** For evaluation of obstruction of hepatic venous flow.
    h. **MRI scan brain:** Helpful to identify cerebral edema .
    i. **Liver biopsy:** Used to know etiology or prognosis
8. **Etiological:**
    a. **Viral hepatitis:** Anti-HAV IgM, HBSAg, anti HBc IgM, anti- HCV, hepatitis D virus IgM, Anti HEV, HSV IgM
    b. **Wilson disease:** Ceruloplasmin level, serum and urinary copper
    c. **Budd Chiari syndrome:** Hepatic doppler USG, abdominal CT and MRI
    d. **Toxicity:** Acetaminophen level
9. **Management:**
    a. **Admit the patient in intensive care unit**
    b. **Supportive therapy**

1. Bed elevation to 30 degrees
2. O_2 administration
3. Provide quiet dark environment
4. Insert RT and Foley's catheter

c. **Respiratory support with oxygen therapy, assisted ventilation (If required then intubate the patient)**

d. **Inotropic support: To maintain mean arterial pressure**

e. **Treat raised ICP:** Inj mannitol (0.5-1.20 gm/kg) of 20% Solution over 20-30 min.

f. **Identify and treat precipitating factors:** such as infections, GI bleeding

g. **Use of antibiotics** (Neomycin 500 mg, 4 times a day, metronidazole 400 mg, and rifaximin 550 mg BD)

h. **Correct electrolyte imbalance**

i. **Administration of Inj. Vit K:** At least one dose to be given.

j. **If bleeding present:** FFP (fresh frozen plasma) and activated factor VIIa or other blood products are needed.

k. **Serial monitoring:** Blood sugar, electrolytes, coagulation parameters, arterial blood gas analysis, blood pressure, fluid status and hydration.

l. **Lactulose syrup:** To produce 2-3 loose stools per day results in colonic acidification.

m. **Lactulose enema:** In patients who are unable to take orally

n. **Administration of N-acetylcysteine (NAC):** Given in case of acetaminophen induced hepatic failure or no relevant history present.

o. **Liver transplanatation** may be considered in patients with severe encephalopathy with poor prognostic factors

CHAPTER

9 Nervous System

EXAMINATION OF NERVOUS SYSTEM

A. Level of consciousness

B. Head and spine examination

C. Higher functions:

1. Level of consciousness
2. Orientation with time, place and person
3. Appearance and behavior
4. Speech and language
5. **Memory:** Immediate (seconds), Recent/short term (min/hr/days) and long/remote memory (past events)
6. **General Intelligence:** Judgment, calculation, attention and reasoning
7. Emotional state
8. Perception
9. Visuospatial function

D. Cranial nerve examination:

1.	**Olfactory**	Test the smell sensation with common objects like soap, toothpaste, coffee.
2.	**Optic**	Acuity of vision, field of vision, color vision, ophthalmoscopy or fundoscopy
3.	**Oculomotor (III), trochlear (IV), abducens (VI)**	**P**tosis, squint, enophthalmos or exophthalmos **P**ower of extraocular muscles **N**ystagmus **P**upil -size, shape, reflex (light, consensual, non- consensual and accommodation)
4.	**Trigeminal (V)**	**S**ensory function (Sensation over the face), motor function (masseter, pterygoids and temporalis), corneal reflex -rt and lt, jaw jerk, afferent
5.	**Facial (VII)**	1. Angle of mouth, nasolabial fold, ptosis, palpebral fissure. 2. Power of facial muscles 3. Upper half of face involved or not 4. Taste sensation of anterior ⅔ of the tongue 5. Dribbling of saliva, lacrimation 6. Corneal reflex, stapedial reflex, Efferent
6.	**Vestibulocochlear (VIII)**	**H**earing or auditory function -Watch test, Rinne test, Weber's test **V**estibular function -Positional nystagmus
7.	**Glossopharyngeal (IX) and vagus (X)**	**S**oft palate movement, gag reflex (Absent on side of lesion) **T**aste sensation on posterior ⅓ of the tongue **U**vula (Deviated to opposite)
8.	**Accessory (XII)**	**P**ower of sternomastoid, power of trapezius
9.	**Hypoglossal (XII)**	**P**ower of tongue muscles, atrophy (i.e. size, shape, wasting), fasciculation or any abnormal movements, deviation of tongue (Deviated to affected side)

E. Motor function

1. **Nutrition:** Attitude, atrophy, hypertrophy
2. **Tone:** Upper limb and lower limb (Check in both sides and both limbs)
   a. **Normally the tone of muscle is neither floppy or stiff**
   b. **In UML palsy:** Increased i.e spasticity (Pyramidal lesion) or rigidity (Extrapyramidal lesion)
   c. **In LMN palsy:** Decreased i.e Flaccidity

3. **Power:** Upper limb and lower limb (Check in both sides and limbs)

Grade	Meaning
o	Complete paralysis
1	Flicker of contraction possible
2	Movement possible if gravity is eliminated
3	Movement against gravity but resistance is not possible
4	Movement possible against some resistance
5	Normal power

4. **Coordination:** Upper limb -finger nose test and lower limb -heel shin test

F. Sensory function:

Superficial or exteroceptive	Deep or proprioceptive	Cortical
1. Pain 2. Touch 3. Temperature (hot and cold)	1. Vibration sense 2. Muscle sense 3. Pressure sense 4. Joint sense 5. Position sense	1. One point localisation 2. Two point discrimination 3. Stereognosis 4. Graphesthesia

G. Reflexes:

Superficial reflex	Deep reflex	Visceral reflex (sphincteric)	Other reflex
1. Abdominal: upper, middle, lower **2. Cremasteric** **3. Plantar response** Corneal and gag reflexes are superficial	1. Biceps 2. Triceps 3. Supinator 4. Knee 5. Ankle 6. Clonus (ankle and patellar)	1. **Swallowing:** Asked for dysphagia with liquid, solid, or both **2 Bladder:** Asked regarding retention of urine, incontinence of urine, urgency, or difficulty in controlling or initiating micturition and urethral sensations **3. Bowel** difficulty in defecation	**1. Glabellar tap** **2. Grasp reflex** **3. Palmomental reflex**

H. Cerebellar function:

1. Intention tremors
2. Hypotonia
3. Nystagmus (Jerky nystagmus)
4. Finger-nose test
5. Gait (Fall on the side of lesion)

6. Pendular knee jerk
7. Dysdiadochokinesia (Inability to perform rapid, alternating movements in a controlled, coordinated fashion)
8. Scanning speech

I. Autonomic nervous:

It includes sympathetic and parasympathetic nervous functions

1. Largely act unconsciously and regulate bodily function such as heart rate, digestion, respiratory rate, sexual arousal, urination, pupillary response, temperature regulation, sweating etc
2. Important function of sympathetic nervous system is tackling stress and emergency
3. Important function of the parasympathetic nervous system is assimilation of food and conservation of energy.
4. Autonomic nervous dysfunction leads to abnormal sweating, impotence, horner syndrome, nocturnal diarrhea

J. Peripheral nerves examination: Examined for the thickening, nodularity and tenderness. (e.g. In leprosy thickened peripheral nerves)

SYMPTOMS OF THE NERVOUS SYSTEM

A] **Higher functions:**

1. **Unconsciousness or alteration of consciousness:**
   a. **Level of consciousness**
      i. **Conscious:** Aware with self and environment
      ii. **Drowsy/lethargy:** Not fully awake/mildly depressed consciousness
      iii. **Stupor/semiconscious:** Arousal on vigorous external stimuli (Persistent & deep stimuli)
      iv. **Coma:** Patient doesn't respond to any external stimuli
   b. **Coma vigil:** Patient is comatose but patient's eyelids are open giving the appearance as of patient is awake
   c. **Akinetic mutism:** Partially awake patient who is immobile and silent seen in hydrocephalus, space occupying lesion around third ventricle.
   d. **Delirium:** Mental confusion and emotional disturbance
   e. **Catatonia:** Abnormality of movement and behavior arising from the disturbed mental state
2. **Appearance and behavioral abnormalities**
3. **Emotional state:** Mood, affect
4. **Orientation:** To time, place and person
5. **Handedness:** Left hemisphere is dominant in 90% of right handed and 50% of left handed persons
6. **General intelligence:** Dyscalculia, dysgraphia or agraphia, aphagia, astereognosis
7. **Memory:** Amnesia
8. **Perceptions:** Illusion, delusion or hallucination
9. **Visuospatial function:**
   a. **Apraxia:** Difficulty to perform skilled motor activities
   b. **Agnosia:** Failure to recognise known object with closed eyes
10. **Speech and language: Motor aphasia** (Can't talk but understand), **sensory aphasia** (Inability to understand spoken, written and tactile speech symbols) and **global aphasia** (Motor + sensory aphasia)

B] **Cranial nerves:**

1. Abnormal sensation of smell: Decreased or absent sensations

2. Visual disturbances, diplopia, squint, epiphora (watering from eyes), bells phenomenon (Unable to close eyelids)
3. Loss of taste sensation
4. Deviation of angle of mouth, facial asymmetry
5. Dysphagia
6. Hoarseness of voice
7. Difficulty in mastication
8. Loss of sensations over the face
9. Wasting of tongue, dysarthria
10. Vertigo, tinnitus, deafness or difficulty in hearing

C] **Motor system:**

1. Loss of power or weakness
2. Unsteady gait
3. Abnormal tone (hypertonia, hypotonia, atonia)
4. Abnormal movement
5. Fasciculations
6. Wasting of limbs (atrophy)
7. Limtation of functions
8. Pain in the muscles

D] **Abnormal reflexes**

E] **Sensory system**

1. Anesthesia
2. Paraesthesia
3. Tingling and numbness
4. Hyper or hypoesthesia
5. Sensation of walking on the cotton wool (Diabetes mellitus)
6. Analgesia

F] **Increased intracranial tension:** Headache, projectile vomiting, blurring of vision, hypertension, abnormal respiratory pattern, convulsions, coma.

G] **Cerebellar system:**

1. Unsteady of gait or H/O falling (Ataxia)

2. Weakness due to hypotonia
3. Incoordination of speech
4. Difficulty in while taking food, shaving (fine motor dysfunction)
5. Tremors of hand while reaching for object
6. Uncontrolled or repetitive eye movement

H] Autonomic nervous system:

1. Incontinence
2. Abnormal sweating
3. Impotence
4. Diarrhea or constipation
5. Precipitancy
6. Hesitancy
7. Retention of urine, feeling of sensation of bladder fullness

CEREBROVASCULAR ACCIDENT/STROKE

1. **Definition**:
   a. Acute focal neurological deficit that lasts more than 24 hours and occurs due to ischemic cerebral infarction (80%)or brain hemorrhage (20%).
   b. In ischemic stroke atherosclerosis is the most common pathology leading to occlusion of vascular territory.
   c. Neuroimaging shows evidence of abnormal vascular territory.
   d. **Transient ischemic attack**:
      i. Sudden focal neurological deficit resolves within 24 hours without evidence of brain infarction on brain imaging study.
      ii. Symptoms are transient.
      iii. Blood flow is quickly restored to brain tissue
      iv. Patient recovers fully within 24 hours .
   e. Types of stroke
      i. Progressive stroke: Focal neurological deficit which worsen with time.
      ii. Complete: Focal neurological deficit persists and do not worsen with time
2. **Causes of ischemic stroke:**

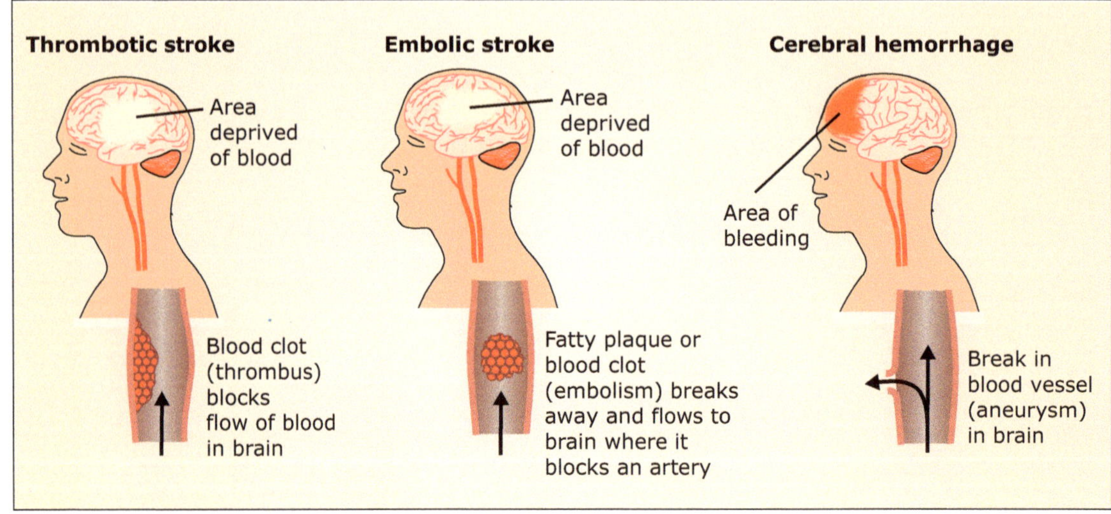

   a. Thrombotic stroke
      1. Large vessels ischemia
      Atherosclerosis, vasculitis, vascular spasm, non-inflammatory vasculopathy

2. **Small vessels ischemia (lacunar infarct)**

   Fibrinoid degeneration, microatheroma,

3. **Other causes of stroke**

   i. **Hypercoagulable disorder (inherited or acquired hypercoagulable states)**

      E.g. deficiency of protein C or S, antiphospholipid syndrome, oral contraceptive pills, pregnancy, Idiopathic thrombocytic purpura.

   ii. **Venous sinus thrombosis**

   iii. **Systemic lupus erythematosus**

   iv. **Moyamoya disease (**Narrowed internal carotid vessel)

   v. **Infections:** Meningitis, encephalitis, covid 19

   vi. **Fabri disease** (Certain type of fatty substance build up in cells and it narrows vessels)

b. **Embolic stroke**

   Atrial fibrillation, myocardial infarction, bacterial endocarditis, prosthetic valves, aortic arch, carotid bifurcation

3. **Causes of hemorrhagic stroke:**

   Intravascular malformation (aneurysm), uncontrolled hypertension, trauma, bleeding disorder.

4. **Clinical features:**

   a. **Facial weakness**

   b. **Limb weakness**

   c. **Slurred speech (**If dominant lobe is involved)

   d. **Headache:** severe headache in SAH, vomiting and altered mental state in ICH, Intermittent severe headache in aneurysm and head & neck pain in cerebellar stroke.

   e. **Vomiting:** Commonly seen in ICH, SAH

   f. **Seizures**: Acute hemorrhagic stroke

   g. **Altered mental status**: Hemorrhagic stroke

   h. **Fever:** Infective endocarditis.

5. **Risk factors:** Hypertension, atrial fibrillation, hyperlipidemia, diabetes, smoking, carotid stenosis

6. **Stroke mimics (D/D):**

   a. Complicated migraine

   b. Hypoglycemia

   c. Focal seizures
   d. Todd's palsy
   e. Encephalitis
   f. Meniere's disease
   g. Multiple sclerosis

7. **General physical examination:**
   a. Look for alertness/consciousness
   b. Look for Head and spinal injury
   c. Neurocutaneous markers e.g. shagreen patch, neurofibroma
   d. **Vital signs:** BP, SPO_2, peripheral pulses, carotid bruit
   e. **RS:** Rales, Crepts
   f. **Cvs:** Murmurs, gallop rhythm, cardiac arrhythmias

8. **Neurological examination:**
   a. Mental status and level of consciousness
   b. Cranial nerves
   c. Motor functions
   d. Reflexes
   e. Sensory function
   f. Cerebellar functions
   g. Meningeal irritation

9. **Investigations:**
   a. **Baseline investigation:**
      1. Complete blood count, ESR
      2. Blood glucose and urea
      3. Serum electrolyte and proteins
      4. ECG
      5. Chest X-ray
      6. PT INR, lipid profile
      7. Serological tests for syphilis
      8. Carotid doppler
   b. **CT brain:** Non contrast CT scan is performed to differentiate hemorrhagic stroke from ischemic stroke.

c. **MRI Brain:** It is a preferred investigation in patients with suspected posterior fossa infarcts and patients having transient ischemic attack.

d. **MRI angiography of the brain:** It is useful to evaluate blood vessels for stenosis, arterial dissection, aneurysm, occlusion or other abnormalities

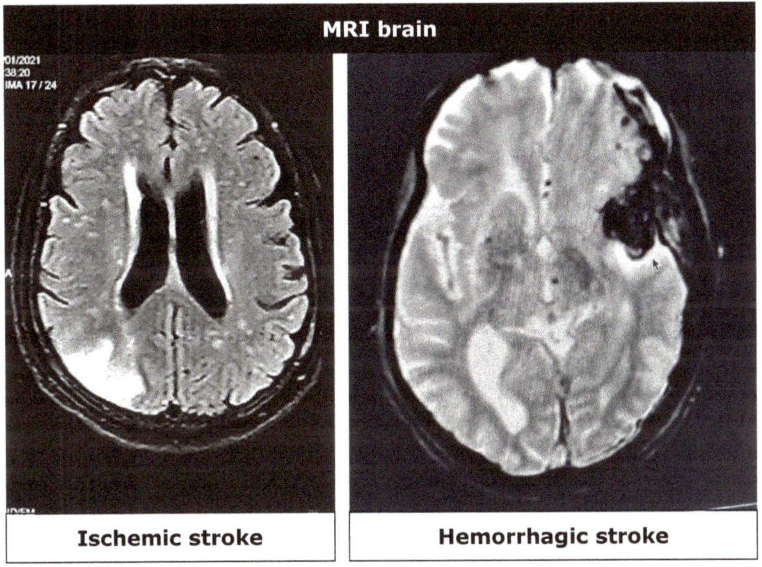

e. **Specific investigations: Specially in young patients**

1. **Antinuclear antibodies (ANA):** To detect systemic lupus erythematosus
2. **Rheumatoid arthritis (RA) factor**
3. **Antibodies to double stranded DNA (DsDNA):** To detect Systemic lupus erythematosus
4. **Anticardiolipin antibodies:** To detect systemic lupus erythematosus & anti-phospholipid syndrome.
5. **Lupus anticoagulant:** To detect systemic lupus erythematosus & antiphospholipid syndrome
6. **S. homocysteine:** Hyperhomocysteinemia
7. **Thrombophilia profile:** Protein C & S level

10. **Goals of line of management:**

a. Distinguishing stroke from stroke mimic such as seizures, encephalitis, migraine and metabolic encephalopathy.

b. Confirming stroke by clinical features, clinical examination and radiological investigations.

c. Confirm type of stroke ischemic or hemorrhagic.

d. Initiate treatment according to type of stroke.

e. Re evaluate the patient to understand the patient's condition to know whether the condition is improving or deteriorating.

11. **Management:**

Treatment goal is to reverse or lessen the amount of tissue infarction.

12. **Medical management:**

a. Maintain airways, breathing and circulation

b. **Check blood sugar:** Treat hypo or hyperglycemia if identified serum glucose kept at < 180 mg/dl

c. **Blood pressure:**

1. Routine lowering of blood pressure has been found to worsen outcome.
2. As collateral circulation of the ischemic brain is blood pressure dependent so blood pressure should not be lowered acutely and if lowered acutely then it may lead to hazardous complication.

   So, recent guidelines suggest that on the day first of ischemic stroke blood pressure is lowered by 15% (If BP > 220/120 mm of Hg)
3. Blood pressure should be lowered if there is malignant hypertension or associated with myocardial ischemia/infarction or if blood pressure is > 186/110 mm of Hg and thrombolytic therapy is replaced with necessary treatment.

d. **Management of cerebral edema:**

1. Head end elevation up to 30 degrees
2. Osmotic therapy with oral glycerol and mannitol.
3. If mannitol is contraindicated (Heart failure/renal failure) then use furosemide, it can be used as an alternative to mannitol
4. Inotropic support may be required to maintain adequate mean arterial pressure so as to maintain adequate central perfusion pressure
5. Hyperventilation is used to reduce raised ICP.
6. Hypothermia can be used to decrease metabolism of brain and also to reduce cerebral edema
7. Surgery (In refractory cases): Hemicraniectomy

In refractory cases of cerebral edema:

1. High dose barbiturate therapy
2. Hyperventilation

3. Hemicraniectomy
4. Hypothermia

e. **Intravenous thrombolysis in case of ischemic stroke:**

1. **Indication:**
   i. Diagnosis of acute ischemic stroke with neurological deficit
   ii. Onset of symptoms to time of drug administration < or equal to 4.5 h
2. **Contraindication:**
   i. Absolute
   - Raised BP > 180/110 mm of Hg despite treatment
   - Platelets 100000; HCT < 25%; Blood glucose < 50 or > 400 mg/dl
   - Rapidly improving symptoms
   - History of stroke or head injury within 3 months
   - History of intracranial bleed
   - Major surgery within previous 14 days
   - GI bleeding within the previous 21 days
   - Acute myocardial infarction
   - Coma or stupor

   ii. Relative
   - Use of heparin within 48 h, prolonged PTT, or elevated INR.
   - Minor stroke symptoms

f. **Administration of rtPA (Recombinant Tissue Plasminogen Activator):**

1. rTPA is a tissue plasminogen activator involved in the breakdown of clot e.g. alteplase, reteplase and tenecteplase.
2. Check the eligibility for rtPA (It is better to give within 4.5 hours but can be given upto 6 hours)
3. Administration of rtPA (Total dose of 0.9 mg/kg required out of that 10% given as bolus and remaining 90% given over 1 hour)
4. While administrating monitor BP regularly.
5. No other antithrombotic treatment within 24 hours
6. If neurologic status worsens or uncontrolled BP while monitoring, stop infusion, give cryoprecipitate, and brain reimaging done urgently.
7. Avoid urethral catheterization to avoid bleeding .

g. **Antithrombotic drugs:**

A. **COX Inhibitors:**

i. Aspirin is an antiplatelet agent effective in treatment of acute ischemic stroke .

ii. This is also useful in primary as well as secondary stroke prevention.

iii. Used to suppress the production of TXA2.

iv. It is given in dose range of 50 mg/day to 325 mg/day but most commonly used dose is 150 mg/day .

B. **Irreversible ADP Antagonist:**

1. **Ticlopidine:** Used in the patients who cannot tolerate aspirin and develops stroke even on aspirin.

   Dose: 250 mg PO BID

2. **Clopidogrel:** Dose 75 mg PO OD

C. **Glycoprotein IIa/IIIb inhibitors:** Abciximab given as an intravenous bolus of 0.25 mg/kg.

h. **Surgical management**

Carotid endarterectomy is useful in TIA patients with carotid stenosis (If > 50%).

i. **Rehabilitation:**

1. Rehabilitation includes early physical, occupational, and speech therapy.
2. The goal of rehabilitation is to maximise recovery in patients at the earliest by providing proper rehabilitation.

SEIZURES AND EPILEPSY

1. **Epilepsy: A condition characterized by recurrent and unprovoked seizures.**
2. **Seizure:** Each episode of neurological dysfunction occurring due to abnormal excessive synchronous neuronal activity in the brain is called seizure.
3. We can say a patient is having epilepsy if the patient has two unprovoked seizures that were not caused by some known and reversible medical cause such as low blood sugar.
4. Seizure may be convulsive or nonconvulsive.
5. Syncope symptoms mimics seizure, following are some clinical differentiating points:

	Seizures	**Syncope**
Preceding symptoms	None or aura (e.g. odd odor)	Nausea, diaphoresis, palpitation, tiredness
Posture at onset	Occurs at any position	Mainly in standing
Facial appearance	Cyanotic and frothing from mouth	Pallor
Unconsciousness	Occurs immediately and remain for minutes	Occurs gradually over seconds and remain for seconds
Disorientation and drowsiness after an event	Minutes to hours (Post ictal state)	Less than 5 minutes
Tongue biting	Often present	Rarely
Urinary incontinence	Sometimes	Sometimes
Stool incontinence	Rarely	Almost never

6. **Classification of seizures:**

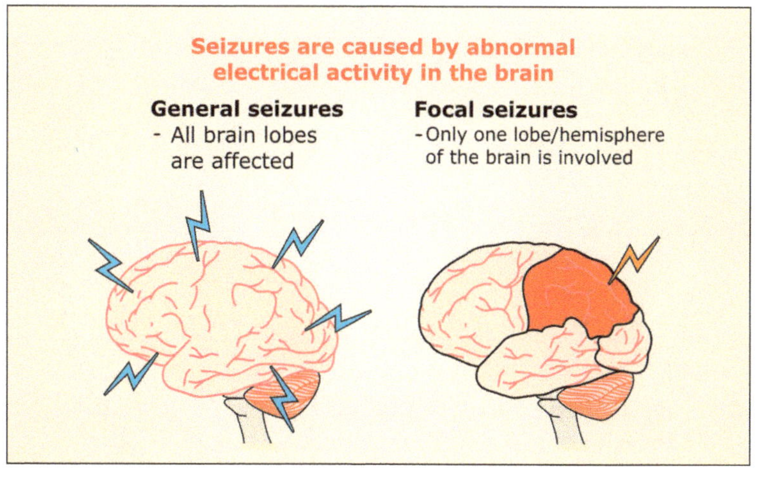

Based on the EEG and clinical features:

a. **Focal seizures: Seizure in which only one hemisphere or lobe of the brain is involved.**

b. **Generalised seizures**

 1. Absence -typical/atypical
 2. Tonic-clonic
 3. Tonic
 4. Clonic
 5. Atonic
 6. Myoclonic

c. **Epileptic spasm:** A sudden flexion, extension or mixed flexion-extension of proximal or truncal muscles lasting 1-2 seconds.

d. **Unclear seizures**

7. **Causes of seizures:**

 a. **Generalised seizures**

  1. **Primary** of genetic origin; there is a positive family history
  2. **Secondary:**

   i. **Infections:**

   Meningitis (Bacterial, tuberculosis), encephalitis, cerebral malaria, HIV, toxoplasmosis, syphilis, neurocysticercosis, toxoplasmosis

   ii. **Vascular pathology:**

   Malformation, aneurysm, infarction, hemorrhage

   iii. **Space occupying lesion:**

   Hematoma, arachanoid cyst, brain tumors, tuberculoma, abscess.

   iii. **Trauma:** Head trauma, birth injury

   iv. **Cerebral anoxia:** birth injury

   v. **Metabolic:** Hypoglycemia, hypocalcemia, hyponatremia, renal and hepatic failure.

   vi. **Drugs and Toxins:**

   - **Drug withdrawal:** Alcohol, barbiturates, benzodiazepines
   - **Antimicrobials/antivirals:** Acyclovir, isoniazid, quinolones, metronidazole
   - **Anesthetic and analgesics:** Tramadol, lignocaine, fentanyl, meperidine, sevoflurane, ketamine.

- **Psychotropics:** Antidepressants, Antipsychotics, lithium,
- **Antimalarials:** Chloroquine, Mefloquine
- **Alkylating agents:** Busulfan
- **Radiographic contrast:** Iodinised contrast agent
- **Drug abuse:** amphetamine, cocaine
- **Immunomodulatory drugs:** Cyclosporine, tacrolimus, interferon,

vii. **Collagen vascular disease:** SLE, sarcoidosis, storage disorder.

8. **History:**
   a. First goal is to know whether the seizure event truly occurred or not.
   b. In many cases the diagnosis of seizures is solely done on clinical grounds.
   c. History should focus on the symptoms before, during, and after the episode of seizure in order to differentiate a seizure from other differential of seizures
   d. History regarding
      1. Epileptogenic factors (Head trauma, meningitis, stroke)
      2. Previous seizure episodes, psychiatric illness.
      3. Alcohol consumption, last intake of alcohol
   e. If patient k/c/o epilepsy then medication, doses, last doses taken.
   f. Family history for genetic predisposition

9. **Clinical features:**

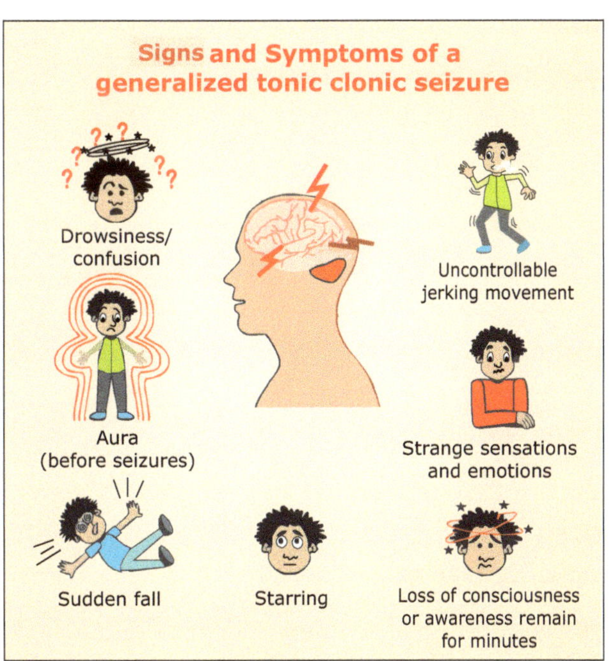

10. **Physical examination:**

    a. **Examination of patients for injuries:**

    E.g. Head injury, tongue bite, shoulder dislocation etc

    b. Check oxygen saturation and auscultate chest for findings of aspiration.

    c. Altered mental status is often seen after seizure.

    d. Check blood pressure (HTN), heart rate and rhythm, and other orthostatic changes for syncope.

    e. Fever for infection (Meningitis, cerebral malaria etc)

    f. **Mouth:** Tongue bite/laceration may be present

    g. **Neck:** - Neck rigidity (Meningitis), carotid (bruit)

    h. **Skin:** - Careful skin examination can reveal neurocutaneous disorders such as tuberous sclerosis or neurofibromatosis, or chronic liver or renal disease.

    i. **CVS**: Rhythm (syncope), murmur (emboli/stroke)

    j. **CNS:** Detail neurological examination to be done.

11. **Differential diagnosis**

    a. **Syncope**

    b. **Migraine**

    c. **Tics**

    d. **Narcolepsy**

    e. **Delirium tremens**

    f. **Psychotic: Panic attack, hyperventilation**

12. **Investigations:**

    a. **First seizure:**

        1. **Laboratory studies:** For metabolic or infectious disorders

        2. **Complete blood count with DLC:** Infectious disease (meningitis, encephalitis)

        3. **Blood for abnormal levels of serum electrolytes, calcium, magnesium, glucose.**

        4. **Liver and renal function test**

        5. **Urinalysis**

        6. **Toxicology screen**

        7. **Tests for syphilis & HIV**

        8. **Lumbar puncture:** Indicated in suspected cases of meningitis, or encephalitis.

9. **EEG studies:**
   i. Electrographic seizure activity during clinically evident seizure event clearly establishes diagnosis.
   ii. Absence of activity does not exclude a seizure disorder.
10. **Brain imaging:** All patients with new onset of seizures should be evaluated to know the underlying structural abnormality that is responsible for seizures.
11. MRI is superior to computed tomography (CT) for detection of cerebral lesion associated with epilepsy.

b. **Breakthrough seizures:** Seizure that occurs despite the use of anticonvulsants therapy that have otherwise successfully prevented seizures in the patient.
   1. All above laboratory investigations
   2. Anticonvulsant drug level.
   3. MRI brain
   4. EEG: If patient does not return to normal level.

13. **Management in active seizure episode:**
   a. Keep the patient away from dangers like electricity, fire, machine, water
   b. Turn the patient to semi prone position and avoid aspiration of secretion.
   c. Avoid head trauma by providing support to head or by providing cushion under the head.
   d. Avoid tongue bite by using a padded gag or rolled handkerchief between the teeth.
   e. Intravenous benzodiazepine (Lorazepam 0.1 mg/kg or midazolam 0.2 mg/kg, clonazepam 0.0015 mg/kg) is considered as the first line of therapy.
   f. **General measures:**
      1. Use railed cot
      2. Secure Intravenous line
      3. Clear the airway and oxygen therapy, if necessary
      4. Monitor pulse, blood pressure, respiration and mental status
      5. Ryle's tube and Foley's catheter insertion
      6. Check patient for head injury and other injuries
   g. **Identify and treat the underlying causes** such as metabolic disturbance, tumors, fever, hypoglycemia
   h. **Select and start appropriate drug for each seizure type**

1. **GTCS:**
   i. **First line:** Valproic acid (DOC), lamotrigine
   ii. **Alternative:** Phenytoin, carbamazepine, topiramate, oxcarbazepine, barbiturates
2. **Focal:**
   i. **First line:** Carbamazepine (DOC), lamotrigine, phenytoin, levetiracetam
   ii. **Alternatives:** All other except ethosuximide and benzodiazepines.
3. **Typical absence:**
   i. **First line:** Valproic acid (DOC), ethosuximide
   ii. **Alternative:** lamotrigine, clonazepam
4. **Atypical absence/myoclonic/atonic:**
   i. **First line:** Valproic acid (DOC), lamotrigine, topiramate
   ii. **Alternative:** Clonazepam, clobazam, felbamate, rufinamide

i. **Start the anticonvulsant therapy** with a single drug in a small dose and increase the dose gradually over a period of 4 to 6 weeks

j. **Drug therapy has to be monitored.**

k. **Avoid precipitating factors**

STATUS EPILEPTICUS

1. **Definition:**

    1. It is defined as a series of seizures without fully recovering consciousness between these seizures.
    2. Duration of seizure activity more than 5 minutes.
    3. It is a medical emergency & should be treated immediately.

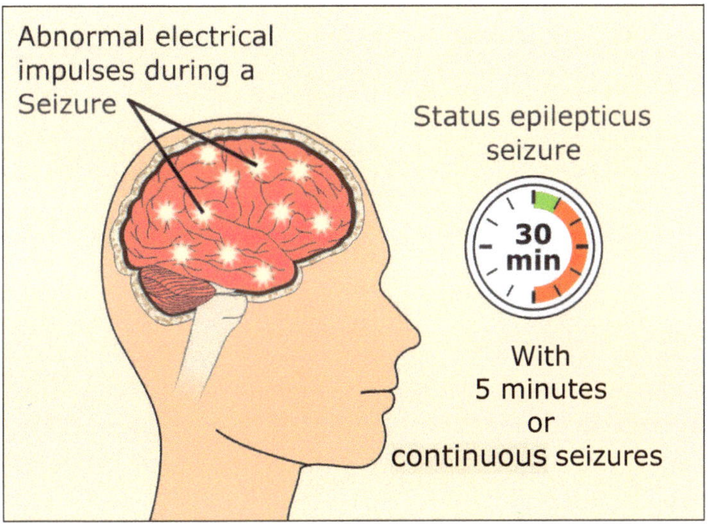

2. **Classification:**

    a. Convulsive:

    1. Generalised tonic clonic status
    2. Partial (epilepsia partialis continua)

    b. Nonconvulsive:

    1. Complex partial seizure
    2. Absence seizure

3. **Etiology:**

    a. **Sudden withdrawal/insufficient dosage antiepileptic drugs** in a known epileptic patient

    b. **Cerebrovascular disease** due to venous thrombosis

    c. **Infections:** Meningitis, encephalitis

    d. **Metabolic disturbance**

   e. **Alcohol withdrawal**
   f. **Hypertensive encephalopathy**
   g. **Brain tumors**
   h. **Anoxic brain injury**

4. **Management:**
   a. General measures:
      i. Use railed cot
      ii. Secure Intravenous line
      iii. Clear the airway and oxygen therapy, if necessary
      iv. Monitor pulse, blood pressure, respiration and mental status
      v. Ryle's tube and Foley's catheter insertion
      vi. Check patient for head injury and other injuries
   b. Intravenous benzodiazepine (Lorazepam 0.1 mg/kg or midazolam 0.2 mg/kg, clonazepam 0.0015 mg/kg) is considered as the first line of therapy.
   c. Then add IV antiepileptic drugs (Administration of long acting anticonvulsant like phenytoin or fosphenytoin 20 mg/kg, valproic acid 20-30 mg/dl or levetiracetam 20-30 mg/kg loading dose with maintenance dose of 5 to 10 mg/kg via glucose free IV fluid).
   d. If established and early refractory SE (30 min-48 hours) then

      Inj phenobarbitone 5 mg/kg → 15 mg/kg.
   e. In some patients continuous benzodiazepine infusion may be required

      (IV midazolam 0.2 mg/kg → 0.2-0.6 mg/kg/h), IV infusion done with respiratory support.
   f. If seizures still persist then general anesthesia with neuromuscular blockade is required (IV midazolam, pentobarbital)
   g. After controlling the seizures successfully, identify the causative factors and manage or remove it.
   h. Anticonvulsants drug dosage are maintained. (Phenytoin 4 to 7 mg/kg/day, phenobarbitone 1-5 mg/kg/day IV or oral BD)

5. **Complication:**
   a. Hyperthermia
   b. Metabolic acidosis

c. Hypoglycemia
d. Cardiac arrhythmias
e. Pulmonary edema
f. Rhabdomyolysis
g. Myoglobinuria
h. Aspiration pneumonia
i. Hypotensive shock
j. Chronic encephalopathy

ACUTE MENINGITIS

Definition: Meningitis is an inflammation of the meninges in a response to infection of leptomeninges (pia-arachnoid mater).

Acute meningitis may be

a. **Bacterial (Septic or Pyogenic and Tubular)**

b. **Viral**

c. **Fungal**

Acute Bacterial Meningitis

1. **Definition: Inflammation of the meninges caused by the bacteria.**
   a. It is a medical emergency and should be treated promptly
   b. If not treated promptly, patient may lead to death or permanent disability.
   c. The classical clinical triad of acute bacterial meningitis include is headache, neck stiffness and fever.
2. **Pathogens for acute pyogenic meningitis:**

Common (More than 80% of cases)	Less common
Streptococcus pneumoniae (50%)	**Listeria monocytogenes** Important cause of meningitis in neonates (<1 month of age), pregnant women, individuals >60 years, and immunocompromised individuals of all ages
Neisseria meningitidis (25%)	**Aerobic gram - negative bacteria** E.g. E. coli, klebsiella, pseudomonas aeruginosa, b. proteus
Haemophilus influenzae H. influenzae causes meningitis in unvaccinated children and older adults	

3. In India, meningococcal meningitis is the most common cause of bacterial meningitis.
4. Listeria is more common pathogen in neonates, pregnant women and older people (> 60 years)
5. **Clinical features:**

   Clinical features may progress rapidly within few hours or slowly worsen over several days.

   a. **Symptoms and signs of infection**
      1. High grade fever

2. Malaise
3. Headache, bodyache
4. Vomiting
5. Seizures: Focal or generalised
6. Septic shock
7. Photophobia
8. Tachycardia, tachypnea
9. **Meningococcal meningitis:** Purpuric/petechial skin rash, ecchymoses
10. **In pneumococcal meningitis:** Associated lung, ear, sinus infection
11. **In H.influenzae meningitis:** Upper respiratory and ear infection in children associated with meningitis.

b. **Symptoms and signs of meningeal irritation**:
   1. Pain in the neck, stiffness of neck (Increased tone of neck muscles)
   2. Kernig's and Brudzinski's signs are positive.

c. **Symptoms and signs due to raised intracranial tension:**
   1. Headache, projectile vomiting, blurring of vision
   2. **Signs of increased ICP include:**
      i. Altered mental status/decreased awareness
      ii. Decreased pupillary reaction
      iii. Papilledema
      iv. Decerebrate posturing
      v. Cushing triad (Bradycardia, hypertension and irregular respirations).
   3. The most serious complication of an increased ICP is cerebral herniation.

d. **Focal neurological deficit:**
   1. Unilateral cranial nerve palsies
   2. Visual field defect
   3. Hemiparesis
   4. Monoplegia

6. **Diagnosis:** It is made on the basis of clinical features, examination of CSF & neuroimaging findings.

7. **Investigation**

a. **Total or differential leukocyte count:** Polymorphonuclear leucocytosis

b. **Blood culture:** Positive in some cases

c. **Normal CSF picture**

Appearance	Cells	Glucose	Proteins	Organism
Clear	**Lymphocytes <4/mm**	**40 mg/dl/2/3 of serum glucose**	**20-40 mg%**	**nil**

d. **Cerebrospinal Fluid (CSF) Abnormalities in Bacterial Meningitis**

White blood cells	100 µL to 10,000 µL
Glucose	< 40 mg/dl (Low)
CSF/serum glucose	<0.4 (**Marked low)**
Protein	> 0.45 mg/dl **(Elevated)**
Gram's stain of CSF sediment	Positive (in > 60%)
CSF Culture	Positive (in > 80%)

e. **Fundus examination:** Should be done before lumbar puncture to exclude papilledema

f. **X-ray chest:** It may show a patch of consolidation in pneumococcal pneumonia

g. **CT brain (P+C) or MRI brain:**

1. CT scan is useful to diagnose complication of meningitis such as brain abscess, hydrocephalus.
2. MRI show areas of cerebral edema & ischemia.

H. **Lumbar puncture:**

1. Commonly done after CT scan/MRI scan
2. Contraindicated in gross papilledema

8. **Management:**

a. **Antibiotic therapy: as per etiological agent**

b. **Steroid therapy:**

i. Adjunctive dexamethasone therapy (10 mg intravenously) is administered 15–20 min before the first dose of an antibiotic.

ii. **It is given within 6 hourly for 3 days**

c. **Supportive therapy**

1. Antipyretics for fever
2. Analgesia for headache and bodyache
3. IV fluids to maintain hydration
4. Antibiotic should be initiated within one hour of arrival

   e.g. Ceftriaxone 4 gm/day + Vancomycin 45-60 mg/kg/day for 10-14 days

   Add rifampicin chemoprophylaxis 600 mg BD for 2 days in N. meningitidis
5. Monitor electrolytes disturbances and corrected appropriately.
6. If patient is having photophobia then nursing care is provided in the dark room
7. **In signs of raised ICP:**

   i. Head end elevation up to 30 degrees

   ii. Osmotic therapy with oral glycerol and mannitol.

   iii. If mannitol is contraindicated (Heart failure/renal failure) then use furosemide, can be used as an alternative to mannitol

   viii. Placement of ventricular shunt to measure ICP

   iv. Hyperventilation is used to reduce raised ICP.

   v. Hypothermia can be used to decrease metabolism of brain and also to reduce cerebral edema.

9. **Complications:**

   a. Cerebritis

   b. Cerebral infarct

   c. Venous sinus thrombosis

   d. Vasculopathy

   e. Subdural empyema/effusion

   f. Hydrocephalus

   g. Brain abscess

VIRAL MENINGITIS

1. Viral meningitis is more common than bacterial meningitis.
2. It is self limiting illness recover without any sequelae or residual deficit.
3. Virus is a common cause of aseptic meningitis i.e in which bacteria cannot be isolated from CSF.

4. It is usually acute in onset.
5. **Causative viruses:** Enteroviruses, Epstein-Barr virus, herpes simplex viruses I & II, mumps, HIV, cytomegalovirus
6. **Clinical features:**
   a. Fever
   b. Malaise
   c. Myalgia
   d. Anorexia, nausea and vomiting
   e. Abdominal pain, and/or diarrhea.
   f. Headache is almost always present and is frequently associated with photophobia
   g. Neck rigidity
   h. Mild lethargy/drowsiness.
   i. The disease is self-limiting and symptoms resolve within a period of 10 days.
7. **Investigation:**
   a. **CSF Examination:**

Total CSF cell count	25–500/μL
Protein concentration	Normal or slightly elevated 20-80 mg/dl
Glucose concentration	Normal
CSF/serum glucose ratio	> 0.6
Gram's stain of CSF	Organisms are not seen
CSF culture	May be negative

   b. **Polymerase chain reaction** Used for diagnosing CNS viral infections.
   c. **Serological tests:** Serologic studies remain important diagnostic tools.
   d. **Neuroimaging (CT/MRI scan):**Performed only in patients with profound alteration in consciousness, seizures, focal neurologic signs or symptoms, atypical CSF profile, or in immunocompromised patients .
   e. **Other tests:**
      1. Complete blood count and differential leukocyte count
      2. Erythrocyte sedimentation rate (ESR)
      3. C-reactive protein
      4. LFT and RFT
      5. **Blood biochemistry:** Serum electrolytes, glucose, creatine kinase, amylase, and lipase.

8. **Management mainly includes supportive treatment:**

   a. **Hospitalization:**

   In patients who are immunocompromised, profound alteration in consciousness, seizures, or the presence of focal signs and symptoms of encephalitis or parenchymal brain involvement.

   b. **General measures**

      1. Secure intravenous line
      2. Ryle's tube and Foley's catheter insertion
      3. Monitor pulse, blood pressure, respiration, mental status

   c. **Symptomatic and supportive care**

   Use of analgesics, antipyretics, antiemetics, maintain hydration with intravenous fluids

   d. **Fluid and electrolyte:** If imbalance then should be corrected

   e. **Antiviral therapy:**

      1. Antiviral therapy includes acyclovir, famciclovir or valacyclovir
      2. Acute HIV meningitis may respond to combined antiretroviral therapy with zidovudine
      3. Avoid use of steroids in immunocompromised patients
      4. Vaccination is best preventive method against poliovirus, MMR or varicella associated meningitis

TUBERCULOUS MENINGITIS

1. Tuberculous meningitis is caused by mycobacterium tuberculosis infection of the meninges and results from hematogenous spread of tubercular bacilli from primary source.
2. It is commonly a subacute or chronic in onset, but occasionally may present as an acute form.
3. TBM is commonly seen in patients with HIV.
4. **Clinical features:**
   a. Fever, headache are cardinal features
   b. Anorexia, nausea, vomiting, abdominal pain
   c. Night sweat, weight loss
   d. Seizures
   e. Kernig's sign and Brudzinki signs may be positive.
   f. Focal neurological deficits include hemiparesis, cranial nerve palsies and involuntary movements.
   g. In advanced disease:
      1. **Profound alteration in level of consciousness such as stupor or coma**
      2. **Signs of brain dysfunction:** Decorticate or decerebrate rigidity, fixed dilated pupils, bradycardia or cheyne-stokes type of breathing.
5. **Diagnosis:**
   a. CSF examination :

   Findings in TBM are as follows:

Color of CSF	Clear or straw colored
Acid fast culture	M. tuberculosis positive
proteins	Raised (100-500 mg/dl)
Sugar	Slightly low (Less than 40 mg/dl or 50% of blood sugar)
Leukocytes	Raised number of leukocytes

   b. Test for diagnosis of TBM:
      1. **Routine tests:**
         a. Complete blood count and differential leukocyte count
         b. Erythrocyte sedimentation rate (ESR)
         c. C-reactive protein

d. Liver function test and renal function test

e. **Blood biochemistry:** Serum electrolytes, glucose, creatine kinase, amylase and lipase.

2. **Indirect tests method:** Host specific immune response to the M. tuberculosis bacteria

a. Adenosine deaminase level in CSF (i.e more than 10 U/L)

b. Bromide partition

c. Antibody to AFB in CSF

3. **Direct tests method:** Detection of mycobacteria or its antigenic products

a. Microscopy: Z-N stained CSF smear examination

b. Gene X pert of CSF (CBNAAT)

c. M.tuberculosis antigen in CSF (ELISA)

d. M.tuberculosis DNA (PCR)

e. CSF tuberculostearic acid by gas chromatography or mass spectroscopy

3. **CT/MRI scan:** Hydrocephalus, brisk meningeal enhancement and/or intracranial tuberculosis.

6. **Management:**

a. **Symptomatic & supportive care:** Bed rest, analgesics, antipyretic, antiemetics, maintain hydration.

a. **Antitubercular drugs:** Start antitubercular therapy according to TB guidelines

b. **Corticosteroid therapy:** Reduces inflammation of the surface of the brain and associated blood vessels.

Steroid dose: Dexamethasone 12-16 mg/day for 3 weeks then taper over 3 weeks

c. **Surgery:**

Surgical drainage is required in patients with deteriorating level of consciousness with enlarging obstructive hydrocephalus.

COMA

1. **Definition:** It is a deep state of unconsciousness in which the patient cannot be awakened and does not respond to any type of external stimuli or inner need.
2. A deep sleep-like state from which the patient cannot be aroused.
3. **The causes of coma divided into three broad categories:**
   a. Metabolic causes without neurological signs
   b. Meningitis syndrome (Bacterial, viral, tuberculous meningitis)
   c. Disease associated with prominent focal neurological signs (hemorrhagic/ ischemic stroke)

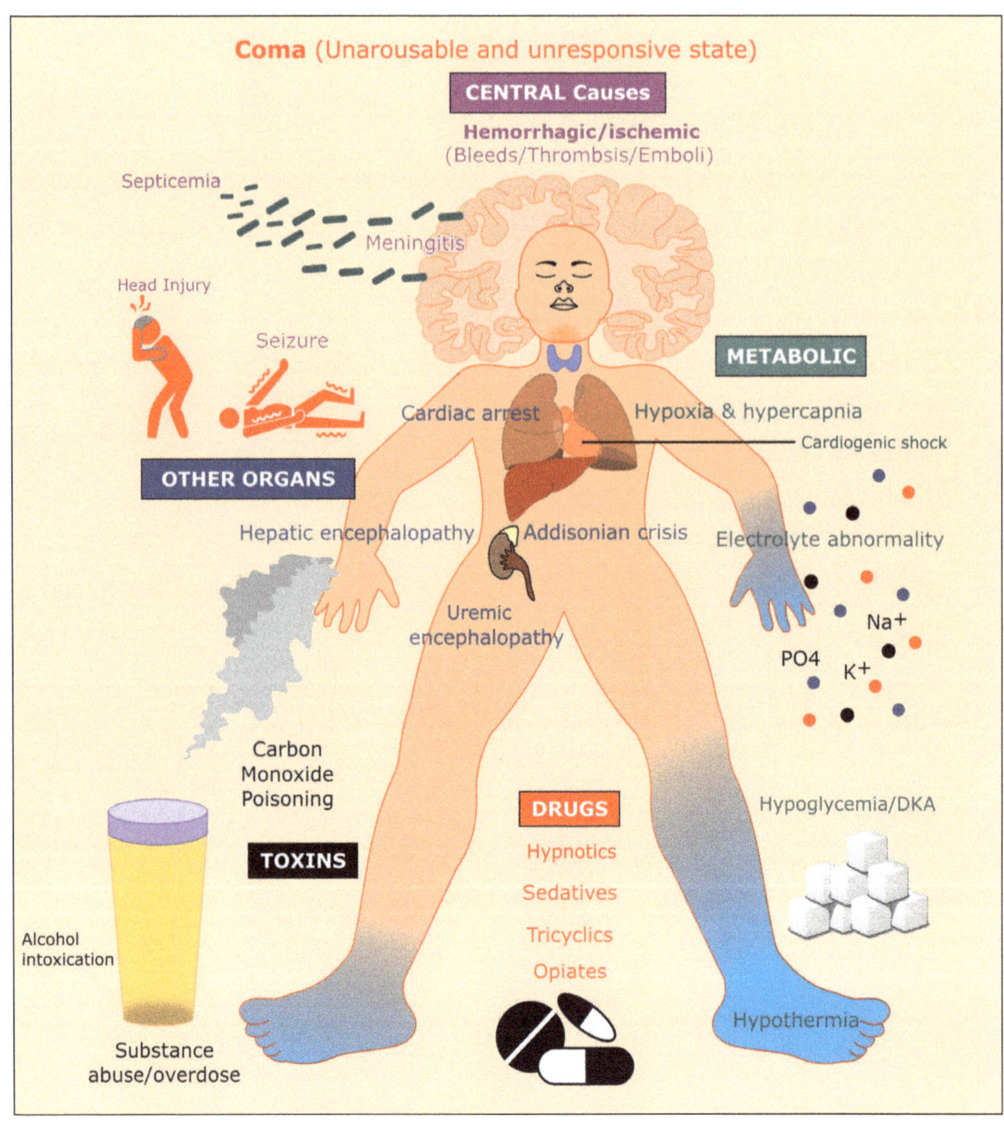

4. **Causes of coma:**
   a. **Severe Systemic Infections:** Pneumonia, malaria, typhoid fever, septicemia, meningitis, encephalitis
   b. **Metabolic:** Hypoglycemia, Diabetic ketoacidosis, Hepatic coma, Uremia, Hyponatremia, Hypercalcemia, Anoxia, Nonketotic Hyperosmolar hyperglycemia, hypo and hyperthyroid states.
   c. **Trauma:** Head injury (Epidural and Subdural hemorrhage, brain contusion, widespread traumatic head injury)
   d. **Ischemic:** Brainstem infarction due to basilar artery thrombosis or embolism, Cerebellar and pontine infarction, brain anoxia
   e. **Hemorrhagic:** Subarachnoid hemorrhage from ruptured aneurysm, AV malformation, Cerebellar and pontine hemorrhage.
   f. **Intoxication:** Alcohol, sedative drugs, opiates
   g. **Epileptic:** Post seizure status, status epilepticus, nonconvulsive status epilepticus.
   h. **Neoplastic:** Brain tumor with surrounding edema
   i. **Hypertensive:** Hypertensive encephalopathy, eclampsia
   j. **Other:** Shock, Severe hyperthermia, hypothermia, brain abscess, thrombotic thrombocytopenic purpura, cerebral vasculitis, gliomatosis cerebri, pituitary apoplexy, intravascular lymphoma.
5. **Principle causes of coma:**
   a. **Lesions that damage the RAS**
   b. **Destruction of large portions of both cerebral hemispheres**
   c. **Suppression of reticulo-cerebral function:** Drugs, toxins, or metabolic derangements such as hypoglycemia, anoxia, uremia and hepatic failure.
6. **History:**
   a. **Neurological symptoms:** Confusion, seizures, vomiting, weakness, double vision, headache, fever.
   b. **Onset of symptoms:** How rapidly the neurological symptoms develop
   c. **Medical diseases:** Chronic liver, kidney, lung, heart or other medical diseases
   d. **Use of medications and drugs**
   e. **Addiction of alcohol, narcotic drugs**
7. **General physical examination:**
   a. **Fever:** Systemic infection, bacterial meningitis, encephalitis, heat stroke, neuroleptic malignant syndrome.

b. **Temperature:**

1. **Malignant hyperthermia:** Anesthetics, or Anticholinergic drug intoxication
2. **Slight rise in temperature:** Status epilepticus
3. **Hypothermia:** Hypoglycemia, Hypovolemic shock, extreme hypothyroidism (Myxedema), intoxication of barbiturates, sedatives.

c. **Respiratory system**

1. **Tachypnea:** Systemic acidosis or pneumonia
2. **Pattern of respiration**
   a. **Cheyne stokes:** Cerebral hemisphere is affected
   b. **Central neurogenic hyperventilation:** Midbrain is affected
   c. **Apneustic:** Lower pontine is affected.

d. **Blood pressure**

1. **Marked hypertension:** Hypertensive encephalopathy, Raised ICP (Head trauma or intracranial hemorrhage)
2. **Hypotension:** Coma from alcohol, or barbiturate intoxication, Hypovolemic shock, myocardial infarction (inferior wall), septic shock, profound hypothyroidism, or addisonian crisis

8. **Neurological examination:**

a. **General**

1. Head, neck and ear for trauma
2. Fundoscopy (Papilledema)
3. Signs of meningeal inflammation

b. **Level of consciousness: GCS scale**

c. **Brain stem function**

1. Eye movement
2. Corneal response
3. Respiratory pattern

d. **Posturing:**

1. **Decorticate posturing** (Flexion of elbows and wrists and supination of the arm, shoulder adduction and lower extremities extension) Results from damage to one or both corticospinal tract.
2. **Decerebrate posturing** (Extension of the elbows and wrist with pronation,

adduction and internal rotation of shoulder with extension of lower extremities): Results from damage to the upper brain stem.

e. **Motor function**

1. **Motor response**
2. **Deep tendon reflexes**
3. **Muscles tone**
4. **Plantar reflex**

	Brainstem coma	**Hemispheric coma**
Type of unresponsiveness	Looks asleep	Looks awake (eyes open)
Bodily position	Looks unnatural	Looks natural (appears to be a comfortable posture)
Respiration	Apneustic or ataxic	Normal or Cheyne Stokes
Spontaneous reflexes	Yawning or sneezing not seen (Coughing, Swallowing, or Hiccuping does not rule out brainstem coma)	Yawning, sneezing may be seen
Pupillary functions	Abnormal response	Normal response
Eye movement	Caloric testing shows normal response	Caloric testing reveals slow phase without fast phase spontaneous roving conjugate movement indicate brain stem disinhibition due to hemispheric coma

9. **Investigation:**
   a. **Complete blood count**
   b. **Arterial blood gases**
   c. **Liver function test**
   d. **Renal function test**
   e. **Serum electrolyte**
   f. **CSF examination**
   g. **Brain imaging: CT Scan or MRI scan for diagnosis of cerebral causes of coma**
   h. **Urine toxicology scan**
10. **Management of coma:**
   a. Use railed cot and give Semi-prone position to the patient
   b. Assess pulse, blood pressure, breathing and mental status

c. Maintain clear airway
d. Oxygen therapy (If hypoxemia)
e. Check head injury/spinal injury
f. Secure intravenous access and correct dehydration with intravenous fluids
g. Insert RT and Foley's catheter
h. Check random blood sugar and correct hypoglycemia/hyperglycemia
i. Correct electrolyte abnormalities
j. **Administration:**
    1. Intravenous dextrose if hypoglycemia
    2. Injection thiamine 100 mg in 100 ml NS, if alcoholic
    3. Naloxone (If opiate overdose)
    4. Flumazenil (If diazepam overdose)
    5. If cerebral herniation/Raised IOP present:
        i. Head end elevation up to 30 degrees
        ii. Osmotic therapy with oral glycerol and mannitol.
        iii. If mannitol is contraindicated (Heart failure/renal failure) then use furosemide, can be used as an alternative to mannitol
        ix. Placement of ventricular shunt to measure ICP
        iv. Hyperventilation is used to reduce raised ICP.
        v. Hypothermia can be used to decrease metabolism of brain and also to reduce cerebral edema.
    6. **Operable cause:** Refer to neurosurgery
    7. **Non operable cause:** Manage conservatively as per cause

CHAPTER

10

Acute Febrile Illness

MALARIA

1. Malaria is a protozoan disease.
2. It is transmitted by the bite of infected female Anopheles mosquitoes.
3. Six species of the genus Plasmodium cause nearly all malarial infections in humans.
4. These are P. falciparum, P. vivax, P. ovale, P. malariae, and the monkey malaria parasite P. knowlesi.
5. Two of these species P. falciparum and P. vivax possess the greatest threat of complication.
6. P. vivax is the second most significant species after P. falciparum.
7. Most deaths are caused by P. falciparum malarial parasites.
8. P. vivax, P. ovale and P. malariae generally cause a milder form of malaria.
9. Cerebral malaria is the most severe form of P. falciparum malaria associated with a high level of parasitemia.
10. In P falciparum exo-erythrocytic stage is absent so no relapse occurs.

Symptoms

1. Fever: A fever episode usually starts with shivering and chills, followed by a high grade fever, followed by sweating and after some time body temperature return to normal.
2. Malaise & fatigue
3. Headache may be severe in malaria

4. Abdominal discomfort
5. Nausea and vomiting
6. Convulsions
7. Coma

Signs

1. Tachycardia
2. Mild jaundice is common among adults; usually resolves over 1–3 weeks.

Management

1. **Acute uncomplicated malaria due to P.vivax, malariae and ovale infection:**
   a. Oral chloroquine 4 tablets stat (600 mg) followed by 2 tablets 6 hours later (300 mg) and 2 tablets on the 2nd day and 3rd day morning.
   b. Radical cure is essential since chloroquine is ineffective against hepatic forms
   c. Oral primaquine 7.5 mg BD for 14 days is required to prevent relapses in vivax and ovale infections.

   According to NBVDCP (National vector borne disease control programme):

Malarial parasite	Male and females (non pregnant)	1st trimester pregnancy	2nd or 3rd trimester pregnancy
P. vivax or P. ovale	Chloroquine +primaquine (14 days)	Chloroquine	Chloroquine
P. falciparum or P. malariae	Artemisinin based combination therapy + primaquine (Single dose 45 mg)	Quinine	Artemisinin based combination therapy
Mixed	Artemisinin based combination therapy + primaquine (Single dose)	Quinine	Artemisinin based combination therapy

   Primaquine is contraindicated in pregnancy, infants and G6-PD deficiency

2. **WHO recommended Artemisinin based combination therapy**

   1. **Artemether-lumefantrine (North-eastern state)**
   2. **Artesunate-mefloquine**
   3. **Artesunate-sulfadoxine-pyrimethamine (Rest of india)**
   4. **Artesunate-amodiaquine**
   5. **Dihydroartemisinin-piperaquine**

Severe falciparum malaria including cerebral malaria:

1. Severe falciparum malaria is a medical emergency requiring intensive care and careful management

2. In severe malaria, parenteral antimalarial treatment should be started immediately.
3. Artesunate is a drug of choice given by either IV or IM injection
4. Artesunate should be given as a loading dose of 2.4 mg/kg IV every 12 hourly for one day then daily (i.e. 0, 12, 24, 48 hours).
5. No dose adjustments are required in liver dysfunction or renal failure.
6. It can be used in pregnant women with severe malaria.
7. If artesunate and artemether is unavailable, then quinine or quinidine is used.
8. Both quinine and quinidine will cause dangerous hypotension if injected IV rapidly; they must be administered carefully.
9. Intravenous quinine is given in 10% dextrose given as an infusion of 20 mg/kg over a period of 4 hours as a loading dose, followed by 10 mg/kg after every 8 hours till patients regain consciousness and start taking orally.
10. Once a patient starts orally then starts oral therapy 10 mg/kg after every 8 hours to be given for 10 days including the parenteral therapy duration.
11. If the patient remains seriously ill or in acute renal failure, maintenance doses of quinine or quinidine should be reduced to prevent toxicity.

Manifestations of Severe Falciparum Malaria Manifestations and their Management

1. Unarousable/cerebral malaria

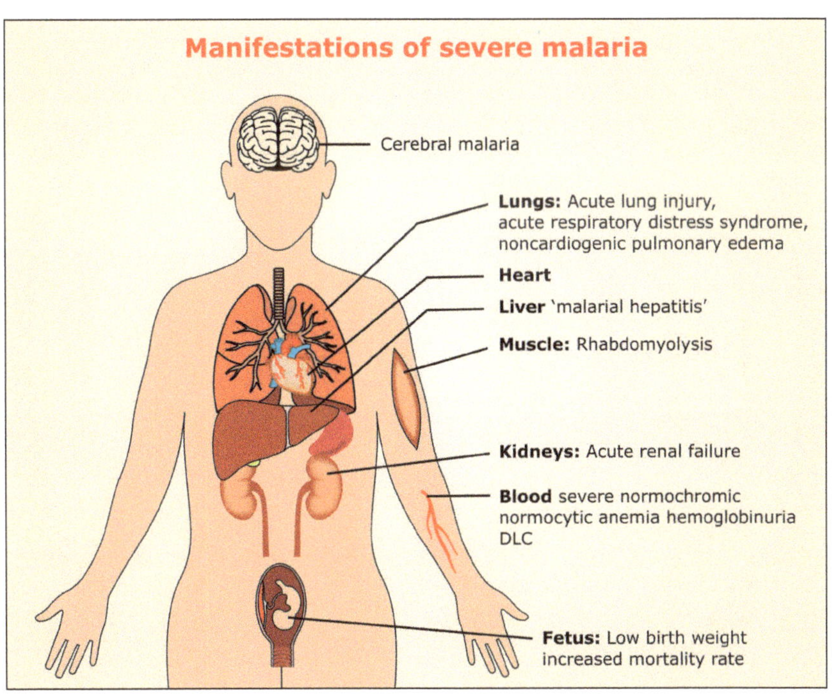

2. Acidemia/acidosis
3. Acute renal failure
4. Pulmonary edema/Acute respiratory distress syndrome
5. Hypoglycemia
6. Hypotension/shock
7. Bleeding/disseminated intravascular coagulation
8. Repeated generalised Convulsions
9. Severe normochromic, normocytic anemia
10. Other manifestations: Hemoglobinuria, jaundice, extreme weakness

DENGUE

1. Dengue is a mosquito-borne viral infection which belongs to genus flavivirus, family flaviviridae.
2. The disease is also called 'break-bone' fever and it affects infants, children and adults alike.
3. The incubation period is 4 to 7 days
4. **Dengue fever has following three clinical manifestation:**
   a. **Classic dengue (Febrile illness)**
   b. **Dengue hemorrhagic fever (Bleeding)**
   c. **Dengue shock syndrome (Severe hypotension)**
5. The infected Aedes aegypti mosquito is the main vector that transmits the viruses to humans.
6. The viruses are passed to humans through the bite of an infected mosquito, which mainly acquires the virus while feeding on the blood of an infected person.
7. The full life cycle of dengue fever virus includes mosquito as a vector and humans as the main victim and source of infection.
8. The dengue virus (DEN) comprises four distinct serotypes DEN-1, DEN-2, DEN-3 and DEN-4
9. Genotypes of DEN-2 and DEN-3 are frequently associated with severe dengue disease.
10. Secondary dengue infections are more severe due to circulating antibodies and may lead to DSS and DHF in hyperendemic areas.

Clinical Manifestations

A person infected by the dengue virus develops severe flu-like symptoms.

A] Classic dengue fever:

1. In persons suspected to have dengue presents with a **high grade fever (40°C/104°F)** and accompanied by following symptoms:
   a. **Severe headache**
   b. **Pain behind the eyes & on movement**
   c. **Anorexia, nausea, Vomiting**
   d. **Swollen glands**

e. **Muscle and joint pains**: Severe back pain with severe myalgia for which common term **break bone fever** is used.

f. **Rash:** Macular erythematous rash which blanches on pressure may be seen on the trunk within 24 hours of fever, there may be flushed face with redness of eyes and rash which fades over a few days.

2. **Signs:**

a. Scleral congestion

b. Abdominal tenderness

c. Lymphadenopathy

d. Pharyngeal congestion

e. Positive tourniquet test for capillary fragility i.e. more than 10 petechiae over 2.5 cm^2 area.

f. Flushed face

B] Dengue hemorrhagic fever:

Dengue hemorrhagic fever is characterized by clinical features of classic dengue fever and

a. Thrombocytopenia (< 1 Lac/cmm)

b. Increased vascular permeability results of leakage of intravascular fluid to interstitial space so hemoconcentration occurs.

c. Plasma leakage evidenced by rise in hematocrit level.

d. Hemorrhage may be seen in the form of petechiae, purpura, ecchymoses, bleeding per mucosa, GIT bleed, cerebrovascular bleed, a positive tourniquet test.

e. Pleural effusion, ascites and hypoalbuminemia may develop.

C] Dengue shock syndrome:

It is a complication of dengue hemorrhagic fever with clinical features of circulatory shock

a. **Tachycardia**

b. **Hypotension < 90 mm Hg for adults**

c. **Narrow pulse pressure < 20 mm Hg**

d. **Cold extremities**

e. **Restlessness, irritability, altered mental status**

Diagnosis

1. **Laboratory findings:** Leukopenia, thrombocytopenia < 1 lac, elevated hematocrit and liver enzymes and hypoalbuminemia.
2. **Dengue NS-1 virus antigen:**
   a. NS1 tests detect the non-structural protein NS1 of dengue virus. This protein is secreted into the blood during dengue infection.
   b. NS1 is detectable during the acute phase of dengue virus infections.
   c. NS1 tests can be sensitive during the first 0-7 days of onset of symptoms.
   d. After day 7, NS1 tests are not recommended.
3. **Antibodies test:**
   a. These tests are primarily used to help diagnose a current or recent infection.
   b. This test detects two different classes of antibodies produced by the body in response to a dengue fever infection i.e. IgG and IgM.
4. Diagnosis may require a combination of these tests because the body's immune system produces varying levels of antibodies over the course of the illness.
5. **Molecular test (Polymerase chain reaction): Isolation of dengue virus.**

Management: Treatment is symptomatic and supportive

1. Tepid sponge baths.
2. Analgesics such as acetaminophen (Paracetamol)
3. Advise a patient to remain stay well hydrated by taking fruit juices, plenty of water.
4. Avoid prescribing aspirin (Acetylsalicylic acid), aspirin-containing drugs due to antiplatelets property which may precipitate bleeding.
5. No specific antiviral therapy available for dengue.
6. **IV fluid administration (in indoor patients):**
   a. Mild circulatory hypotension requires fluid replacement by mouth but close monitoring of patient's vital is required.
   b. Patients presenting with hypovolemic shock with thrombocytopenia require hospitalisation for fluid replacement.
   c. Fluid administration is continued till patient recover from shock
   d. Fluids which are used for resuscitation in dengue are dextrose containing fluid, Ringer lactate or plasma expanders

7. **Oxygen therapy: In severe hypoxemia patient with respiratory distress**
8. **Inotropic support:** Inotropic support with fluid therapy to maintain BP above 90 mm of Hg to resuscitate hypovolemic shock in severe dengue cases.
9. **Blood transfusion:** In patients with massive hemorrhage
10. **Thrombocytopenia or Coagulopathy:** Cryoprecipitate or platelet transfusion is given to avoid coagulopathy.

LEPTOSPIROSIS

1. The spirochetal disease which is caused by leptospira species
2. It is transmitted by both wild and domestic animals.
3. The most common animals that spread the disease are rodents, especially rats, which are the most important reservoir.
4. It is often transmitted by animal urine or by water or soil containing animal urine coming into contact with breaks in skin, eyes, mouth, or nose.
5. In mild form, leptospirosis may present with nonspecific symptoms such as fever, headache, and myalgia.
6. Severe leptospirosis, characterized by jaundice, renal dysfunction, and hemorrhagic diathesis, is often referred to as **Weil's syndrome**
7. The incubation period is usually 1–2 weeks
8. **Clinical features:**

   a. **Mild Leptospirosis:**

      I. **Flu-like symptoms**

         i. Sudden in onset

         ii. Fever with chills

         iii. Headache (Intense, localized to the frontal or retro-orbital region)

         iv. Myalgia (Intense and especially affects the calves, back and abdomen.)

         v. Nausea and vomiting

         vi. Abdominal pain

         vii. Conjunctival suffusion (Redness without exudate) and myalgia

      II. **Physical findings include:**

         i. Mild jaundice may be present

         ii. Conjunctival congestion/pharyngeal congestion

         iii. Lymphadenopathy

         iv. Hepatomegaly, and splenomegaly

         v. Macular, maculopapular rash is often seen & which; may be erythematous, or hemorrhagic (petechial or ecchymotic)

         vi. Lung auscultation may reveal crackles due to pulmonary edema.

b. **Severe leptospirosis:**

   I. Onset of severe leptospirosis is similar to mild leptospirosis.

   II. Patient comes with complain of cough, chest pain, breathlessness, and hemoptysis.

   III. The classic presentation of severe leptospirosis, often referred to as **Weil's syndrome,** which includes classical triad of hemorrhage, jaundice, and acute kidney injury.

   IV. Severe bleeding that most commonly involve the lungs (pulmonary hemorrhage), gastrointestinal tract (Melena, hemoptysis), hematuria, and skin (petechiae, ecchymosis) and bleeding from venepuncture sites.

   V. Pulmonary hemorrhage is seen in ET tube when a patient is intubated.

   VI. Other complications associated Necrotizing pancreatitis, Cholecystitis, rhabdomyolysis, and aseptic meningitis.

   VII. Patient may die of septic shock with multiorgan failure

9. **Investigations:**

   a. **Complete blood count:** Leukocytosis and thrombocytopenia

   b. **Liver function test:** Serum bilirubin, AST, ALT may be elevated

   c. **Renal function test:** Urea & creatinine may be elevated.

   d. **Serum electrolyte:** Hypokalemia and hyponatremia due to increased excretion of potassium by kidneys.

   e. **Chest X-ray:** It may demonstrate diffuse alveolar opacities.

   f. **Urine analysis:** May reveal proteinuria, presence of white blood cells (pyuria), and microscopic hematuria.

   g. **Diagnostic test for leptospirosis:** Diagnostic tests for detection of leptospirosis include dark field microscopy, IgM Elisa, microscopic agglutination test, polymerase chain reaction

10. **Treatment and Chemoprophylaxis of Leptospirosis:**

   a. **Mild leptospirosis (for 5 to 7 days):**

      i. Doxycycline (100 mg PO bid) (Not to be given in pregnant female) or

      ii. Amoxicillin (500 mg PO tid) or

      iii. Ampicillin (500 mg PO tid)

   b. **Moderate/severe leptospirosis (for 7 days):**

      i. Crystalline Penicillin (1.5 million units IV or IM q6h) or

ii. Ceftriaxone (2 g/d IV) or

iii. Cefotaxime (1 g IV q6h)

c. **Chemoprophylaxis:**

i. Doxycycline (200 mg PO once a week)

d. **Supportive care for severe leptospirosis:**

i. Hospitalisation

ii. Symptomatic treatment: Antipyretics, analgesic, antiemetics

iii. Antibiotics for chemoprophylaxis

iv. Administration of IV fluids to maintain hydration

v. In severe hypotension inotropic support may be required

vi. Blood transfusion in severe hemorrhage

vii. **Thrombocytopenia or Coagulopathy:** Cryoprecipitate or platelet transfusion is done

viii. Electrolyte abnormality such as hypokalemia and hyponatremia if present should be corrected

ix. Peritoneal dialysis or hemodialysis may be needed in patients with renal failure

x. Rapid initiation of hemodialysis has been shown to reduce mortality risk and typically it is necessary only for short periods

xi. Patients with pulmonary hemorrhage may benefit from mechanical ventilation with low tidal volumes to avoid barotrauma

ENTERIC FEVER

1. Enteric fever includes typhoid and paratyphoid.
2. It is a febrile illness caused by Salmonella typhi and salmonella paratyphi A, B, C.
3. Transmission occurs through contaminated water and food.
4. Salmonella paratyphi, a bacterium that usually causes a less severe illness.
5. The bacteria are deposited in water or food by a human carrier and are then spread to other people in the area
6. The reservoir of infection includes patients suffering or convalescing from typhoid or chronic carriers of typhoid (Food handler).
7. The untreated patients may develop complications during the 2nd and 3rd week due to toxaemia and septicaemia.
8. In untreated cases, sometimes it may be fatal.
9. **Clinical features**

   Incubation period of typhoid fever is 5-14 days

   Onset is insidious

   a. **During first week**
      - i. Remittent fever
      - ii. Headache
      - iii. Bodyache
      - iv. Malaise
      - v. Constipation
      - vi. Leucopenia
      - vii. Relative bradycardia

   b. **Between first and second week**
      - i. Fever: (Step ladder pattern)
      - ii. Abdominal pain
      - iii. Abdominal distension
      - iv. Loose motions
      - v. Splenomegaly
      - **vi. Rose spots:** These are the pink papules appers over the trunk and abdomen

c. **Beyond third week**

   A number of complications can occur in this week

   i. Intestinal hemorrhage due to bleeding in congested Peyer's patches can occur.
   ii. Intestinal perforation in the distal ileum
   iii. Hepatitis, Hepatic abscess, Necrotising cholecystitis
   iv. Typhoid encephalopathy
   v. Bronchitis, Pneumonia
   vi. Nephritis, Hemolytic uremic syndrome
   vii. Thrombocytopenia with risk of bleeding

d. **Diagnosis**

   i. The diagnosis is suggested by the clinical features
   ii. The definitive diagnosis of typhoid fever depends on the isolation of S. typhi organisms from the blood or bone marrow or stool culture.
   iii. Blood is the preferred in first week of infection when bacterial load is highest.
   iv. Stool culture may be used for the detection of chronic carriers.
   v. The Widal test, a serologic assay for detecting antibodies to the O and H antigens of Salmonella

10. **Management**

   a. Antipyretics for fever
   b. Analgesia for headache and bodyache
   c. IV fluids to maintain hydration
   d. Dehydration is less common in typhoid but may be seen in complication
   e. **Antimicrobial therapy (Anyone of the following):** 3rd generation cephalosporins becomes antibiotics of choice as chloramphenicol resistant cases are increased nowdays.

      i. Ceftriaxone
      ii. Ciprofloxacin
      iii. Ofloxacin
      iv. Azithromycin 1 gm/day
      v. Amoxicillin 1 gm TID orally

f. **Intravenous therapy**

i. Ceftriaxone and cefoperazone are equally effective in dosage of 1 gm twice a day I.V or 50 mg/kg for 7 to 10 days

ii. In pregnancy, the third generation cephalosporin is preferred over fluoroquinolone.

iii. Electrolyte imbalance to be treated accordingly

g. **Treatment of Carriers**

Carrier state in absence of gallstones treated as follows

i. Ciprofloxacin 750 mg BD x 4 weeks to sterile the gallbladder

ii. Cholecystectomy if lithiasis is present

COVID 19

1. The covid-19 pandemic has led to a dramatic loss of human life worldwide.
2. Coronavirus disease is an infectious disease caused by a newly discovered coronavirus.
3. Most people who fall sick with COVID-19 develop mild to moderate illness and recover without hospitalization, only needing isolation along with supportive therapy.
4. In some cases, mostly in patients with co-morbidity needs hospitalization and prompt management
5. It is mainly transmitted through droplets generated when an infected person coughs, exhales or sneezes.
6. You can get infection in following ways
   a. Inhalation of infected droplets of saliva or discharge from nose when an infected person coughs, exhales or sneezes.
   b. Viruses can enter through eyes, nose or mouth after having contact with contaminated surfaces of Covid 19.
7. **Clinical features:**
   a. Fever
   b. Cough
   c. Myalgia
   d. Fatigue
   e. Shortness of breath
   f. Runny nose
   g. Sore throat
   h. Diarrhea
   i. Loss of smell/taste
8. **Investigations**
   a. Diagnostic investigation
      1. Rapid antigen test
      2. RTPCR (Confirmatory test)
   b. Routine blood investigation
      1. Complete blood count
      2. Random blood sugar

3. Liver function test
4. Renal function test

c. **Inflammatory markers**

1. C-reactive protein
2. D-dimer
3. Interleukin 6
4. Procalcitonin
5. Ferritin
6. Erythrocyte sedimentation rate

d. **Radiological investigation (To help in diagnosis & progression of disease)**

1. Chest X-ray
2. CT scan

9. **Management**

Mild (Upper respiratory tract symptoms without shortness of breath/hypoxia)	Moderate (Increased rate of respiration >24 cycles/min, shortness of breath, SPO_2 90% to 93% on room air)	Severe (Increased rate of respiration >v30 cycles/ min, shortness of breath, SPO_2 < 90% on room air)
1. **Home isolation (if pre-requesting facilities are available)** 2. **Contact and droplet precautions** 3. **Supportive and symptomatic management** a. Maintain hydration b. Antipyretics c. Antitussive d. Gargles e. Vitamins and minerals supplementation f. Tab ivermectin and cap. Doxycycline (as per weight & if not contraindicated)	1. **Supportive measures:** Maintain hydration, antipyretics 2. **Oxygen support with non-rebreathing face mask** 3. **Encourage awake proning in all patient** 4. **Anti-inflammatory therapy/ Immunomodulatory therapy** **e.g.** Injection methylprednis-olone (0.5 mg to 1 mg/kg into two divided doses per day) or dexamethasone 5. **Anticoagulant therapy (Prophylactic) If no contraindication:** **e.g. LMWH (Enoxaparin 0.5 mg/kg per day SC), unfractionated heparin**	1. **Supportive measures:** Maintain hydration, antipyretics, antibiotics therapy 2. **Respiratory support** a. High flow nasal cannula b. Non invasive ventilation c. Ventilatory support 3. **Encourage awake proning in all patient** 4. **Anti-inflammatory therapy/ immunomodulatory therapy** **e.g.** Injection methylpred-nisolone (0.5 mg to 1 mg/ kg into two divided doses per day) Or dexamethasone

(Continued)

Mild (Upper respiratory tract symptoms without shortness of breath/hypoxia)	Moderate (Increased rate of respiration >24 cycles/min, shortness of breath, SPO_2 90% to 93% on room air)	Severe (Increased rate of respiration >v30 cycles/ min, shortness of breath, SPO_2 < 90% on room air)
4. Seek immediate help a. High grade fever SPO_2 < 94% b. Severe cough particularly for 3 to 5 days of onset of symptoms c. Worsening symptoms with high risk groups (e.g. Diabetes, hypertension, IHD, CKD)	**6. Monitoring** **a. Respiratory rate** **b. Work of breathing** **c. Oxygen requirement** **d. Radiological investigation** **(If worsening):** 1. Serial CXR 2. HRCT chest **e. Blood investigations** **1. Routine investigation:** CBC, LFT, RFT every 24 to 48 hourly. **2. Inflammatory markers:** CRP, ESR, D-dimer, Interleukin -6 every 48 to 72 hourly.	**5. Anticoagulant therapy (Prophylactic) If no contraindication:** **e.g.** LMWH (Enoxaparin 0.5 mg/kg per day SC), unfractionated heparin **6. Monitoring** **a. Respiratory rate** **b. Work of breathing** **c. Oxygen requirement** **d. Radiological investigation** **(If worsening):** 1. Serial CXR 2. HRCT chest **e. Blood Investigations** **1. Routine investigation:** CBC, LFT, RFT every 24 to 48 hourly. **2. Inflammatory markers:** CRP, ESR, D-dimer, Interleukin- 6 every 48 to 72 hourly

10. **Injection ramdesivir and Injection tocilizumab are used in specific circumstances (Emergency utilization authentication/off label use)**

*** Kindly refer frequently updated management of covid 19 as per Ministry of Health and Family Welfare (MoHFW)**

CHAPTER

11

Endocrinology and Metabolism

HYPEROSMOLAR HYPERGLYCEMIC STATE

1. It is characterised by the extreme hyperglycemia (Blood sugar > 600 mg/dl) and hyperosmolarity (> 320 mOsm/kg) with dehydration without significant ketoacidosis. 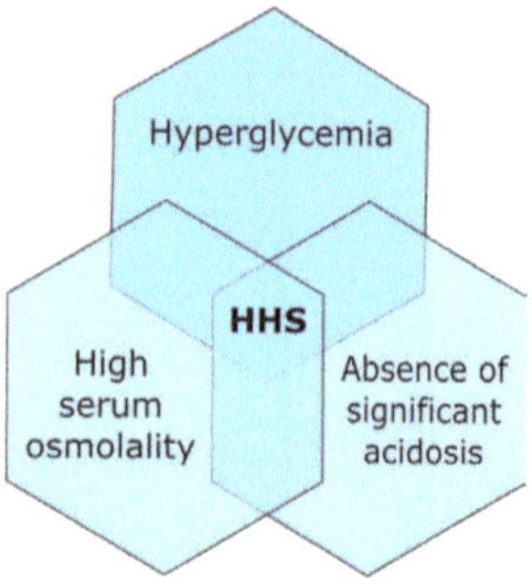
2. This condition most commonly occurs in type 2 diabetic patients and may occur in type 1 diabetes mellitus also.
3. Insulin deficiency and dehydration are the underlying causes.
4. Hyperglycemia leads to intravascular volume depletion due to osmotic diuresis.

5. **Etiology:**
   a. The main risk factor is a history of type 2 diabetes mellitus
   b. Older age (50–70 years)
   c. Medical conditions (Cerebral vascular injury, pneumonia, stroke, myocardial infarction, sepsis)
   d. Inadequate water intake/dehydration
   e. Lack of sufficient insulin, non compliance with antidiabetic medication
   f. Deranged renal function
   g. Certain medications (Glucocorticoids, beta-blockers, thiazide diuretics, calcium channel blockers, and phenytoin) can induce hyperglycemia
   h. Stress, infection, stroke, alcohol, cocaine abuse.
6. **Clinical features:**
   a. Altered mental status (Drowsiness, coma, lethargy)
   b. Symptoms of Hyperglycemia: Polydipsia, Polyuria, polyphagia

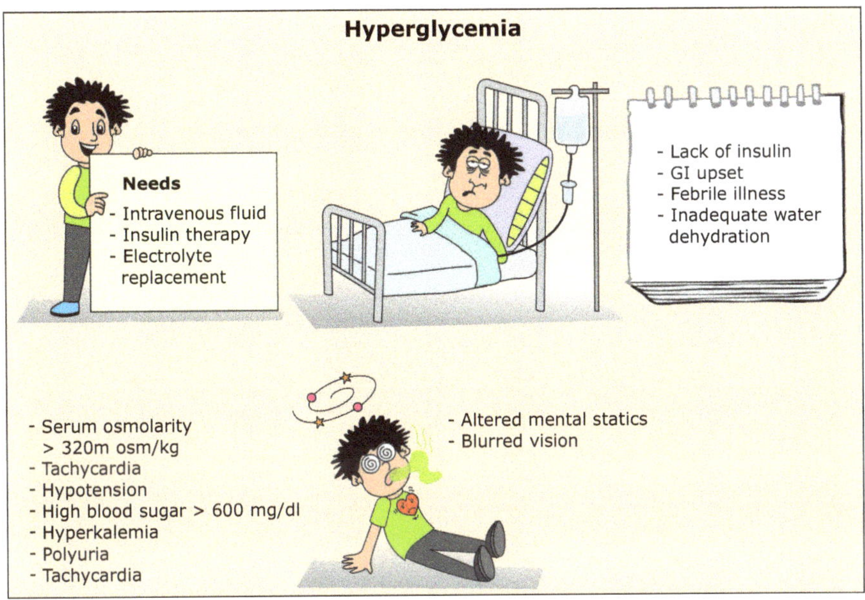

c. **Dehydration:** Dry mouth, dry skin, increased thirst.

d. **Weight loss**

e. **Generalised Weakness**

f. **Hyperviscosity and increased risk of blood clot formation**

g. **Neurologic signs:** Transient blurred vision, reversible paralysis, headaches, focal seizures, myoclonic jerking

h. **Motor abnormalities:** Flaccidity, depressed reflexes, tremors or fasciculations

i. Nausea, vomiting, and abdominal pain and Kussmaul respirations characteristic of DKA are not present in HHS.

j. **The physical examination**: Hypotension, tachycardia.

7. **Investigations:**

Investigations	Findings in Hyperglycemic hyperosmolar state.
Plasma glucose	(> 600 mg/dL)
Serum osmolarity	> 320 mOsm/kg
Serum bicarbonates	> 15 meq/l
Arterial pH	>7.30
Urine or serum ketone	(~+ on dipstick) and absent-to-low ketonemia
Blood urea/creatinine	May be high
Serum sodium	135-145
Anion gap	A small anion gap (metabolic acidosis may be present secondary to increased lactic acid.)

8. **Diagnosis:**

Diagnostic features include above lab findings plus

a. Profound dehydration, up to an average of 9L

b. Some alteration in mental status

c. Prerenal azotemia.

9. **Management:**

a. General measures

1. Nasogastric tube is inserted in patients with shock, coma.
2. Insert Foley's catheter
3. Monitor glucose (Hourly), serum ketones, electrolyte, arterial blood gas analysis, urine ketones and glucose
4. Monitor BP, pulse, neurological status, fluid intake & output charting

b. Intravenous fluids:

1. Correct fluid deficit by intravenous fluids administration
2. People with HHS have 8 to 12 liters of fluid deficit
   a. Fluid replacement: 2-3 L of 0.9% saline over (10-20 ml/kg/hour) for first 1 to 3 hours
   b. In later stage, when serum sodium > 155 meq/l then 1/2 NS (0.45%) used
3. 5% dextrose given if blood glucose reaches normal level.
4. Serum osmolarity and central venous pressure should be monitored to avoid unnecessary fluid overload, especially in cardiac renal impaired patients.

c. Electrolyte replacement:

1. In initial insulin therapy and fluid resuscitation K^+ concentration decreases.
2. K replacement is necessary in early treatment:

Serum K^+	Management
< 3.3 meq/l	Hold insulin Give 40 meq/l (⅔ as KCl and ⅓ KPO^4) until $K^+ \geq 3.3$ meq/l
$\geq$ 5 meq/l	Do not give k^+ but check potassium every 2 hr.
$\geq$ 3.3 meq/l and < 5 meq/l	Give 10 meq/l K^+ in each litre of fluid (⅔ as KCl and ⅓ as KPO^4) to keep serum K^+ at 4-5 meq/l.

d. Insulin therapy:

1. Start continuous infusion of regular insulin
2. HHS insulin therapy begins with an IV insulin bolus of 0.1 unit/kg followed by IV insulin at a constant infusion rate of 0.1 unit/kg per hour.
3. If the serum glucose level does not fall, increase the insulin infusion rate by two folds.
5. If blood glucose < 250 mg/dl then add dextrose 5% to prevent hypoglycemia
4. The insulin infusion should be continued until the patient has resumed oral diet and able to take food by mouth then can be transferred to SC insulin regimen.

e. Identify & treat the precipitating factor

f. Prevention of complications

1. Hypoglycemia
2. Hypokalemia
3. Hyperglycemia
4. Cerebral edema

DIABETIC KETOACIDOSIS

1. **Definition:** Characterized by a plasma glucose 250 mg/dl-600mg/dl, arterial pH 6.8-7.30 or serum bicarbonate level < 15 meq/l and moderate ketonemia with ketonuria.

   a. This is most frequent encountered endocrine emergency

   b. It is more common in type I diabetes but can occur in Type II DM.

   c. Develops over a period of several hours or days

   d. It occurs due to inadequate administration of exogenous insulin or due to stressful conditions

   e. Insulin deficiency leads to hyperglycemia, osmotic diuresis resulting in dehydration and electrolyte abnormality.

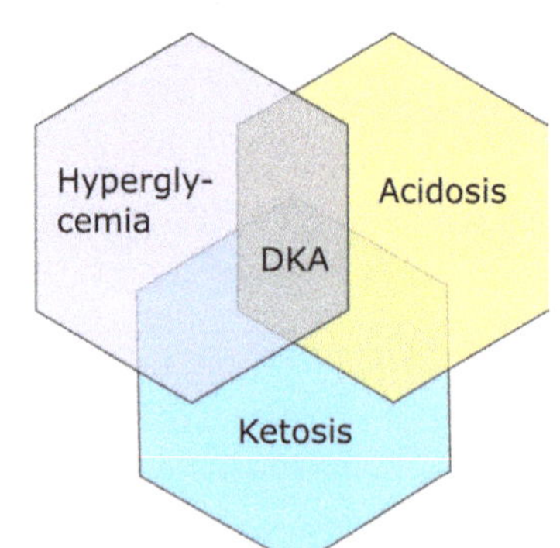

2. **Stressful condition:**

Infection (Pneumonia, gastroenteritis, URI, meningitis, cholecystitis or pancreatitis)	Pregnancy
Myocardial infarction, stroke	Emotional stress (adolescence)
Endocrine disorder (Hyperthyroidism, Cushing's syndrome, acromegaly, pheochromocytoma)	Trauma, Interruption in insulin therapy, high dose steroids or thiazides Drugs -cocaine

3. In this situation, there is an increase in production of counter regulatory hormones namely Epinephrine, glucagon, corticosteroids and growth hormones and hence the dose of insulin needs to be increased.

4. **Clinical features:**

   a. Altered consciousness, stupor or coma

   b. Weakness

   c. Anorexia

   d. Nausea

   e. Vomiting

   f. Abdominal pain

   g. Polydipsia

   h. Polyuria

   i. Breathlessness

5. **Clinical finding:**

   a. Fruity or musty odor (acetone)

   b. Loss of skin turgor, dry tongue, dehydration/hypotension

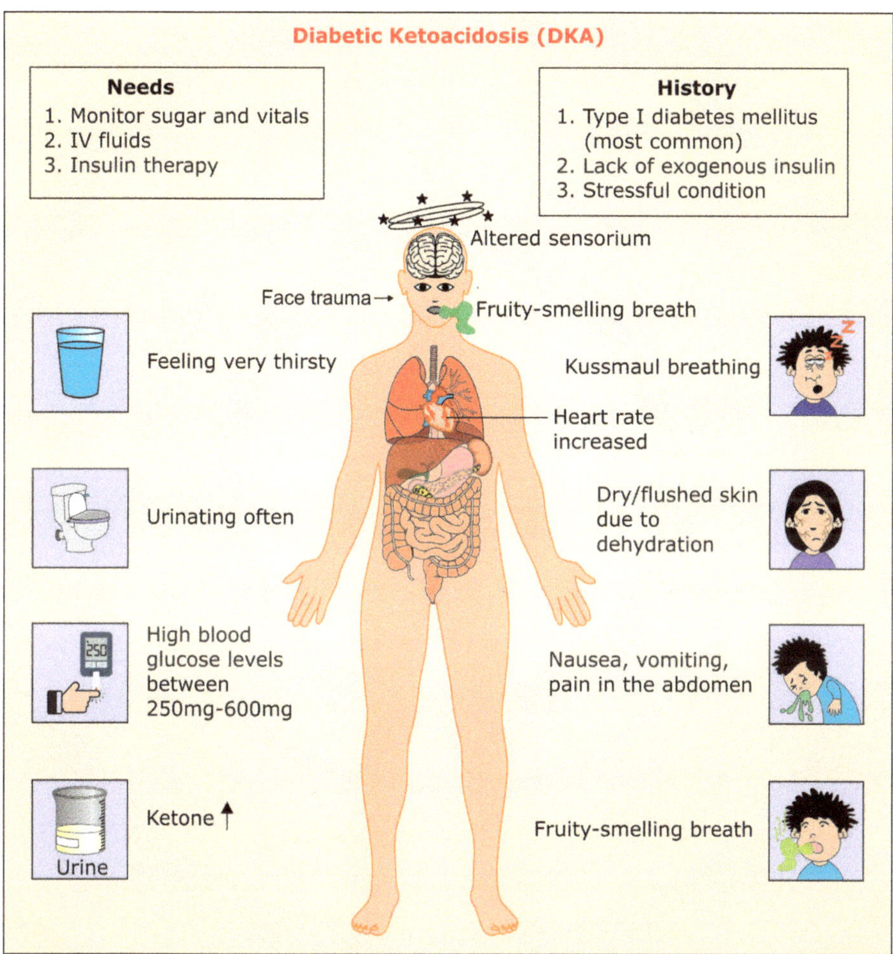

c. Sunken eyes (Decreased IOP)
d. Hypothermia
e. Tachycardia
f. Hyporeflexia (Decreased K)
g. Hypotonia
h. Stupor or coma
i. Kussmaul's breathing depending on metabolic acidosis
j. Abdominal distension

6. **Investigation:**
   a. **Serum glucose:** > 300 mg/dl
   b. **Arterial blood gas analysis:** Metabolic acidosis pH < 7.3, serum bicarbonate < 15 meq/l (due to accumulation of beta hydroxybutyrate and acetoacetic acid)

c. **Ketonemia: (**Beta HBA/AAA ratio if 3:1 mild, if 15:1 severe)

d. **Serum electrolyte:** (Sodium - low, high or normal; Potassium - low, high or normal; Phosfate - may be normal)

e. **Complete blood count:** (WBC count may be increased in infection)

f. **Serum creatinine:** (BUN increased due to depletion of volume)

g. **Urine ketones positive**

h. **ECG:** Monitoring done to understand potassium disturbance during insulin infusion

7. **Management:**

   a. **General measures:**

      1. NG tube inserted in patients with shock, coma to prevent aspiration of gastric content.
      2. Foley's catheterization
      3. Monitor glucose (hourly), serum ketones, electrolyte, ABG, urine ketones and glucose
      4. Oxygen therapy, monitor BP, pulse, Neurological status

   b. **Intravenous Fluids and insulin therapy:**

      1. Fluid used: 0.9% saline/RL or 0.45% saline
      2. In DKA total volume deficit of 6 lit (3 lit intracellular and 3 lit extracellular)
      3. **In normal cardiac function patients:**
         a. Initially normal saline is administered 0.9%
         b. Fluid replacement: 2-3 L of 0.9% saline over (10-20 ml/kg/hour) for first 1 to 3 hours
         c. In later stage when Na > 155 meq/l then 1/2 NS (0.45%) used
         d. If blood glucose < 250 mg/dl then add dextrose 5% to prevent hypoglycemia
      4. **Insulin therapy:**
         a. Do not start until K > 3.5 meq/l (If K < 3 meq/l give K correction and then start insulin infusion) in normal saline
         b. Bolus: 0.1 unit/kg or 10 -15 units IV stat
         c. Infusion rate: 0.1 unit/kg/hour and observe for response
         d. If no response by 2-4 h with initial insulin infusion rate then increase infusion by 2-3 folds

e. Rapid correction of hyperglycemia (Correction > 100 mg/dl/hr) can cause osmotic encephalopathy so, 50 to 75 mg/dl/hr correction is sufficient.

f. Once oral intake resumes then discontinue parenteral IV infusion and start subcutaneous insulin.

g. Give subcutaneous injection of insulin 30-60 min before stopping IV insulin.

5. **Potassium:**

> 5.5 meq/l	No KCl
3.5-5.5 meq/l	20 meq KCl
<3.5 meq/l	40 meq/l
<2.5 meq/l	80 meq/L

a. **Signs of hypokalemia:** Hyporeflexia, gastroparesis, abnormal ECG (Q-T prolongation, U wave and ST depression)

6. **Bicarbonates**

a. Use is controversial

b. **Indications.:**

1. Life threatening hyperkalemia
2. Lactic acidosis
3. Severe acidosis
4. Acidosis induced respiratory or cardiac dysfunction
5. Bicarbonate < 5 meq/l

7. **If intravenous line is not accessible:**

Regular insulin given in the deltoid as loading dose

HYPOGLYCEMIA

1. **Hypoglycemia:** Blood sugar decreases to below normal levels
2. The lower limit of the fasting plasma glucose concentration is normally 70 mg/dL
3. It is the major complication of insulin treatment and is also common with oral hypoglycemic agents (OHA) especially in old age patients.
4. It should be suspected in any patient with an altered level of consciousness, or a seizure
5. It is a medical emergency that requires urgent treatment.
6. **Etiology:**
   a. **Medication:**
      1. Oral hypoglycemic agents
      2. Insulin
      3. Thiazides diuretics
      4. Quinine
      5. Alcohol
      6. Others

   b. **Critical illness**
      1. Hepatic diseases
      2. Renal or cardiac failure
      3. Sepsis
      4. Exhaustion caused by lack of nourishment.

   c. **Hormone deficiency**
      1. Cortisol (Addison's disease)
      2. Glucagon and epinephrine (in insulin-deficient diabetes)
      3. Hypopituitarism

   d. **Personal cultural and social factors**
      1. Fasting during shravan, ramzan
      2. Strenuous activity

   e. **Non–islet cell tumor**

f. **Endogenous hyperinsulinism**

1. **Insulinoma:** Excessive insulin secretion
2. **Insulin secretagogue:** Increase in production and secretion of insulin
3. **Idiopathic**

7. **Clinical features:**

a. **Symptoms and signs of hypoglycemia:**

Sympathetic over-activity	Neuroglycopenia
1. Palpitation	1. Coma
2. Sweating	2. Focal neurological deficit, hemiplegia and amnesia
3. Anxiety	3. Headache
4. Tremors	4. Fatigue
5. Shivering	5. Impaired consciousness
6. Vomiting	6. Dizziness
7. Irritable	7. Inappropriate behavior
8. Cool, clammy skin	8. Difficulty in speech/slurred speech
	9. Confusion, drowsiness
	10. Generalised or focal seizures

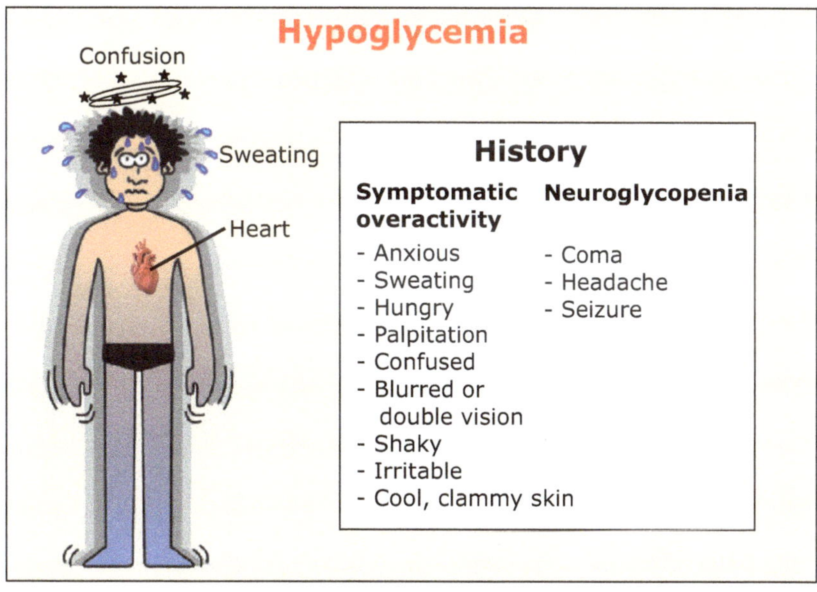

8. **Diagnosis:**

a. The documentation of hypoglycemia is done by the **Whipple triad:**

1. Clinical features of hypoglycemia

2. Documentation of low plasma glucose level < 55
3. Relief of symptoms/Glucose return normal after intake of glucose

b. **When the cause of the hypoglycemic episode is uncertain, following investigation should be performed before initiating treatment:**
   1. Plasma insulin
   2. C-peptide
   3. Proinsulin
   4. β-hydroxybutyrate levels

9. **Test for insulinoma:**
   a. An insulinoma is a tumor of the pancreas that is derived from beta cells and secretes insulin.
   b. Insulin level of 20 U/ml or more even blood glucose level below 40 mg/dl.
   c. **Following blood tests are used to diagnose insulinoma:**
      1. **Blood glucose level : Low**
      2. **Insulin level : High**
      3. **C-peptide suppression test**
   d. Diagnosis is confirmed by localizing the tumor with CT Scan or MRI scan
   e. The definitive treatment is surgery.

10. **Management**
   a. **If the person is conscious and able to swallow:**
      1. Give orange, apple or grape juice
      2. Fruit juices contain a higher proportion of fructose
      3. Glucose tablets or candy is appropriate
   b. **If patient is unconscious should not be given orally:**
      1. Secure intravenous line and give intravenous 25% of dextrose followed by glucose infusion with glucose monitoring.
      2. If IV access cannot be established (in fatty patients, collapsed veins), then in this patient administer 1 to 2 milligrams of glucagon by an intramuscular injection/subcutaneous route.
   c. **Treat the underlying cause:**
      1. **Stop the drug or doses are reduced if it is the cause:** Most of the cases are due to OHA or insulin induced hypoglycemia

2. **Stop alcohol consumption**
3. Anticholinergic may be useful in delaying gastric emptying
4. Treatment of underlying critical or other illness
5. Treatment of insulinoma
6. Treatment of autoimmune hypoglycemia by steroid or immunosuppressive drugs

HYPOCALCEMIC TETANY

1. Hypocalcemia is defined as a state in which total calcium concentration in serum falls below the lower limit of normal i.e. 8.5 mg/dl.
2. Normal calcium homeostasis is maintained by parathyroid hormone, vit D and calcitonin.
3. Normal range of serum calcium (8.5 to 10.5 mg/dl or 2.1 to 2.6 mmol/dl)
4. **Causes:**

   Hypocalcemia may occur in acute, subacute and chronic forms

   1. **Reduced intake or absorption**

      Malabsorption, Vit D deficiency, Vit D resistance
   2. **Endocrine diseases:** Hypothyroidism (Post surgery, due to autoimmune disease), Hypoparathyroidism .
   3. **Critical illness:** Acute pancreatitis, end stage sepsis, AKI or CKD, liver disease, burns, malignancy
   4. **Drugs:** Diuretic therapy, glucagon, heparin, protamine
   5. **Other:** Hypomagnesemia, HyperPhosfatemia, hypoalbuminemia, plasma pheresis, alkalosis, citrated blood transfusion
5. **Clinical features**:

   a. **Mental symptoms:**
      1. Depression
      2. Irritability
      3. Psychosis
      4. Convulsions
      5. Confusion

   b. **Neurological features:**
      1. Numbness
      2. Paraesthesia (Oral, perioral and acral paresthesias, tingling and needles sensation in and around the mouth and lips, and in the extremities of the hands and feet. This is often the earliest symptom of hypocalcemia.)

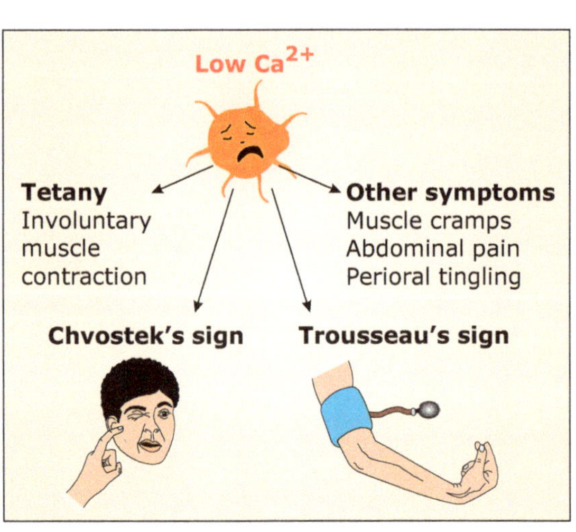

3. Carpopedal and generalized tetany (Unrelieved and strong contractions of the hands, and in the large muscles of the rest of the body) are seen.
4. Seizures
5. **Signs in tetany**
    a. **Trousseau sign:** In Latent tetany within 3 minutes (Eliciting carpal spasm by inflating blood pressure cuff and maintaining the cuff pressure above systolic)
    b. **Chvostek's sign:** (Tapping the inferior portion of the cheekbone will produce facial spasms)
6. Tendon reflexes are diminished or absent in tetany

c. **Cardiac features:**

1. **Effects on cardiac output:**
    a. Decreased heart rate
    b. Decreased heart contractility

Hypocalcemia

Trousseau's Sign

Inflation of BP apparatus cuff and maintaining cuff pressure above systolic for 3 minutes

Response: Carpopedal spasm characterized by

- Adduction of the thumb
- Flexion of the thumb
- Flexion of the metacarpophalangeal joints
- Extension of the interphalangeal joints
- Flexion of the wrist

Chvostek's Sign

Tapping of the inferior part of cheek bone

Response: Twitching of the lip to spasm of all facial muscles

d. **Ophthalmic features:**

1. Cataract
2. Optic neuritis
3. Papilledema

6. **Diagnosis and investigation**

a. **Total & Ionised serum calcium:** Low

b. **Serum Phosfate concentration:** Elevated in hypoparathyroidism or in advanced CKD patients

c. **Serum magnesium level:** May be low

d. **On ECG:** Prolongation of the QTc

7. **Management:**

   a. **Mild hypocalcemia**

      1. In mild cases, doses of both calcium and vitamin-D (often as 1, 25-$(OH)_2$-D_3 i.e. calcitriol) are given orally.

   b. **Severe hypocalcemia**

      1. Intravenous 10% calcium gluconate administered

         Initial 2 ampoules (1 ampoule = 90 mg elemental calcium) infused in normal saline over 10 min followed by infusion of 60 ml (5-6 ampoules) in 500 ml of glucose (1 mg/min) at a rate of 0.5 -2.0 mg/kg/hour.

      2. If tetany is not relieved by the calcium, magnesium administration may be tried

      3. Maintenance doses of both calcium and vitamin-D (often as 1, 25-$(OH)_2$-D_3 i.e. calcitriol) are often necessary to prevent further decline.

   c. **In respiratory alkalosis:** Hypocalcemia due to hyperventilation can be overcomed by the use of 5% CO_2 in oxygen or by rebreathing expired air.

CHAPTER

12 Hematology

THROMBOCYTOPENIA

1. **Thrombocytopenia** is a condition characterized by abnormally low levels of platelets in the blood.
2. A normal platelet count ranges from 150,000 to 450,000 per microliter of blood
3. Platelets are derived from the fragmentation of megakaryocyte
4. One third of platelets after leaving bone marrow are sequestrated in the spleen, while the other two thirds circulate for platelet function and remains for 7-10 days
5. Platelet production is regulated by the hormone thrombopoietin (TPO), which is synthesized in the liver and kidney.
6. Thrombocytopenia with bleeding is a medical emergency that should be managed actively.
7. **Thrombocytopenia results from following processes:**

a. Decreased bone marrow production

b. Increased platelet destruction

8. Most common cause of thrombocytopenia is auto-immunological in young patients
9. Exposure to drugs, infections, toxins, gram negative septicemia and DIC are common causes of thrombocytopenia.

10. **Causes of thrombocytopenia:**

Impaired production	Increased destruction
1. Sepsis, systemic viral or bacterial infection 2. Aplastic anemia, Fanconi anemia 3. Vitamin B_{12} deficiency (Megaloblastic anemia) 4. Leukemia or myelodysplastic syndrome 5. Hepatic failure 6. Hereditary syndromes	1. Autoimmune thrombocytopenic purpura 2. Thrombotic thrombocytopenic purpura (TTP) 3. Disseminated intravascular coagulation 4. Systemic lupus erythematosus 5. Hemolytic-uremic syndrome 6. Antiphospholipid syndrome 7. Post-transfusion purpura: Delayed adverse reaction to blood or platelet transfusion in which platelets are destroyed by alloantibodies 8. Hypersplenism: Portal hypertension 9. Heparin induced

Drug induced (Some drugs are responsible for thrombocytopenia)	Other causes
Abciximab, Tirofiban, Eptifibatide, heparin, Acetaminophen, Amiodarone, Amlodipine, Gold, Haloperidol, Heparin, Ibuprofen, Quinine, Quinidine, Tranilast, Trimethoprim/sulfamethoxazole, Vancomycin.	1. Snakebite 2. Niacin toxicity 3. Lyme disease

11. **Clinical features:** Vary from asymptomatic or mild disease to life threatening complications (visceral bleeding)

    a. **The common sites of bleeding:**

    1. Intracranial bleeding
    2. Mucous membrane and gum bleeding
    3. Nasal bleeding
    4. Genitourinary tract bleeding
    5. Skin: Purpura, Petechiae, Ecchymosis

    b. **The severity of bleeding**

    1. **Mild:** Patient is asymptomatic and bleeding time remains normal
    2. **Moderate:** Bleeding may occur on trauma, administration of drugs, surgery and bleeding time prolongs
    3. **Severe:** May lead to bruising, purpura or bleeding with minimal trauma
    4. **Very severe**: May lead to spontaneous bleeding

12. **Clinical evaluation:**

    a. The history and physical examination, blood investigation are useful in the initial evaluation of thrombocytopenic patients

    b. **History of patient:**

        1. History related to bleeding (Internal or external)
        2. Recent viral infection/bacterial infection
        3. Ask for any recent drug intake or chemotherapy, blood transfusion
        4. Connective tissue disorder: e.g. Systemic lupus erythematosus
        5. Past history of similar episode
        6. Family history
        7. Obstetrics history

    c. **Physical findings on examination:**

        1. Petechiae, purpura, ecchymosis, nasal or gum bleeding
        2. Facial puffiness
        3. Splenomegaly
        4. Lymphadenopathy, joint involvement, rash (Connective tissue disorder)
        5. Hypotension due to hemorrhage

    d. **Investigation:**

        1. **Complete Blood count:** Decreased in number of platelets
        2. **Bleeding time:** Prolonged
        3. **Bone marrow study:** Normal or increased number of megakaryocytes
        4. **Peripheral blood film:** For any abnormality in platelets &

           Reticulocyte count to be done for bone marrow response.
        5. **Renal function test:** Deranged in renal disease (Hemolytic-uremic syndrome)
        6. **Liver function test:** Deranged in liver disease (Liver failure)
        7. **Coagulation profile:** To rule out coagulation disorder
        8. **Serology** for viral and connective tissue disorder
        9. **Detection of platelet antibody**
        10. **Imaging study:** ultrasonography for splenomegaly and CT scan for any intracranial bleed.

13. **Management**

a. **General measures:** It includes precautionary measures to avoid bleeding (Unless indicated).

   1. Avoid trauma
   2. Avoid intramuscular injection
   3. Avoid use of NSAIDs
   4. Avoid urethral catheterization, and enema
   5. Apply firm pressure at venous puncture site after collecting sample or IV administration to avoid bleeding.

b. **Measures for hemostasis:**

   1. **Local measures to stop active bleed**
      i. Compression bandage
      ii. Use local hemostatic agents
      iii. Nasal packing for nasal bleeding
   2. **Systemic measures to stop active bleeding**
      i. Platelet and FFP transfusion: Indicated for patients with active bleeding or at high risk of bleeding in severe thrombocytopenia.
      ii. Investigation to know the cause and complications
   3. **Treatment of underlying cause**
      i. **Withdrawal of offending drug/toxin**
      ii. **Antibiotics for infection**
      iii. **Immune ITP:** IVIG & anti-D, steroids, TPO receptor antagonist, splenectomy
      iv. **Heparin induced TCP:** Prompt discontinuation of heparin and use of alternative anticoagulants, if bleeding risk does not outweigh thrombotic risk.
      v. **Thrombotic thrombocytopenic purpura:**
         - **Plasma exchange:** Mainstay of treatment of TTP
         - **Immunomodulatory therapies:** Rituximab, vincristine, cyclophosphamide, and splenectomy successful in refractory or relapsing TTP, including
      vi. **Treatment of hemolytic-uremic syndrome:**

DISSEMINATED INTRAVASCULAR COAGULATION

1. Clinicopathologic syndrome characterized by excessive, uncontrolled formation of intravascular fibrin in response to excessive blood protease activity that overcomes the natural anticoagulant mechanisms.
2. DIC occurs in acute or chronic form.
3. The most common causes are sepsis or severe infection, malignant conditions and obstetric complications
4. Excessively formed fibrin deposit in blood vessels can reduce blood flow to many vital organs which finally results into multiorgan failure.
5. As in widespread thrombosis clotting factors and platelets are used up, bleeding may occur.
6. **Causes:**
   a. **Sepsis or severe infection:** Bacterial (Gram-negative and Gram-positive sepsis), viral, fungal, or protozoan infections
   b. **Massive tissue injury:** Massive trauma, severe burn injury, Malignant hyperthermia, rhabdomyolysis, extensive surgery
   c. **Obstetric complications:** abruptio placentae, pre-eclampsia or eclampsia, septic abortion, post partum hemorrhage, retained products of dead fetus
   d. **Malignant disease e.g. leukemia**
   e. **Hemolytic transfusion reactions:** (i.e., ABO incompatibility, haemolytic reactions)
   f. **Toxins:** i.e. snake venom, insect venom
   g. **Others:** Heat stroke, shock, liver diseases
7. **Clinical features: Signs and symptoms of widespread and excessive thrombosis as per organ involved:**
   1. **Heart:** Chest pain, if clot in cardiac vessels (Myocardial infarction)
   2. **Lungs:** Dyspnea and chest pain occur when clot formation in the pulmonary blood vessel (Pulmonary embolism).
   3. **Brain:** Slurred speech, facial deviation, limb weakness (Ischemic stroke)
   4. **Lower limb:** Swelling, redness, pain in lower leg (Deep vein thrombosis)
      a. **Signs and symptoms related to bleeding**
         1. **Internal bleeding**
            i. Hematuria
            ii. Melena

iii. Hematemesis

iv. Severe headache, altered mental status, vomiting, blurred vision, diplopia, due to intracranial bleed

2. **External bleeding**

i. Bleeding from gum mucosa

ii. Nasal bleeding

iii. Skin: Petechiae, purpura

iv. Bleeding from venepuncture site

3. **Signs and symptoms of hemorrhagic shock**

i. Altered mental status

ii. Hypotension

iii. Tachycardia

iv. Pallor

v. Cold extremities

8. **Investigations:** The diagnosis is based on the presence of clinical and/or laboratory abnormalities of coagulation profile or thrombocytopenia

a. **Peripheral blood smear examination:** presence of schistocytes (fragmented red cells) in the blood smear

b. **Platelet count:** Thrombocytopenia

c. **PT and aPTT and TT:** Prolongation

d. **Fibrinogen level:** Reduced due to depletion of coagulation protein

e. **Fibrin degradation products:** Elevated levels of FDP. The most sensitive test for DIC is the FDP level.

f. **D dimer test: Increased** (This test is very specific for detection of fibrin degradation products)

g. **Clotting time:** Prolonged

9. **Management:**

a. **Supportive measures:**

1. Measures to control active bleeding: Nasal packing, local hemostatic agents application, compression bandage at venepuncture site
2. IV fluid administration to maintain mean arterial pressure
3. Oxygen therapy
4. Correction of electrolyte abnormalities

5. Strictly monitor fluid intake and output
6. Inotropic support if required
7. Intubation and ventilatory support if required.

b. **Treat the underlying or precipitating cause:**

1. Antibiotics for sepsis
2. Termination of pregnancy if obstetrics complication
3. Anti-snake venom in snake bite

c. **Replacement therapy:**

1. **Administration of FFP and/or platelet concentrates:** indicated for patients with active bleeding or at high risk of bleeding in severe thrombocytopenia
2. **Blood transfusion:** Transfusion is needed if severe blood loss is due to surgery, trauma associated with DIC.
3. **Cryoprecipitate (plasma fraction enriched for fibrinogen, FVIII, and VWF): Indicated in** Low levels of fibrinogen or brisk hyperfibrinolysis

d. **Anticoagulant therapy:**

1. Drugs to control coagulation such as heparin, antithrombin III, or antifibrinolytic drugs can be used.
2. In acute DIC, the use of heparin is likely to aggravate bleeding.
3. Use of antithrombin III has shown rapid improvement in coagulation profile and shortened the duration of DIC.

CHAPTER

13

Dog Bite, Snake Bite and Poisoning

DOG BITE

1. Rabies is a viral infection that causes inflammation of the brain.
2. It spreads when an infected animal scratches or bites the another animal
3. It is transmitted through the saliva of an infected animals.
4. Rabies disease have a 100% fatality rate.
5. The incubation period is from days to months to years
6. Bites on the face, head and neck have a shorter incubation period.
7. **Clinical features**
   a. **Prodromal symptoms**
      1. Fever
      2. Malaise
      3. Headache
      4. Nausea, Vomiting
      5. Tingling at the site of exposure
      6. Pain, paraesthesia at site

b. **CNS involvement (In encephalitic rabies)**

1. Hydrophobia
2. Hypersalivation (Autonomic stimulation)
3. Seizures
4. Acute laryngeal spasm
5. Violent movement
6. Uncontrolled excitement
7. Barbinski reflex is positive

c. **CNS involvement (Paralytic rabies)**

1. The stage of excitement is absent
2. Paraplegia or Hemiplegia (acute ascending paralysis)
3. Deep reflexes are absent

8. **Management of dog bite**

a. After confirmed or suspected exposure, vaccination must be started immediately.

b. The treatment is according to the type of wound, exposure and status of the animal.

c. First wash the wound with large quantities of water and soap.

Category	Type of contact with a suspect rabid domestic or wild animals or animal unavailable for observation	Recommended treatment
I	Touching or feeding to animals, licks on intact skin, contact with animal but definitely not with its saliva	None if reliable case history is available In case of doubt vaccinate with on D0, D7, D28 by IM or ID
II	Nibbling of uncovered skin, minor scratches, superficial bites (except on head, neck, shoulder girdle, arms or hands) or abrasions **without bleeding**, licks on broken skin	Administer vaccine immediately by IM or ID as per schedule Stop treatment if the animal remains healthy throughout the period of 10 days.
III	Single or multiple major transdermal bites or scratches especially on head, face, neck, shoulder girdle, arms or hands or contamination of mucous membrane with saliva.	Administer the anti-rabies Immunoglobulin or rabies Immunoserum and vaccinate Immediately as per scheduled by IM or ID

Note: Any wound with bleeding is considered Cat III and requires immunoglobulin.

d. **Route of administration:**

1. **Intramuscular route:** 0.5 ml dose of vaccine is administered intramuscularly in the deltoid in adults and in anterolateral aspect of the thigh in young children.

Do not administer in the gluteal region due to poor absorption.

2. **Intradermal route:** The 0.1 ml dose of vaccine is administered intradermally in each upper arm (over the right and left deltoid)

   If the dose goes intramuscular or subcutaneously instead intradermal then give it intradermally in the nearby site immediately.

e. **Schedule for administration of rabies vaccine:**

Route of administration dose	Intramuscular (IM)	Intradermal (ID)
1st dose	Zero dose	Zero dose
2nd dose	Day 3	Day 3
3rd dose	Day 7	Day 7
4th dose	Day 14	Day 28
5th dose	Day 28	-
6th dose	Day 90 (optional)	-

f. **ID regimen approved in india:**

1. 2 site regimen (Updated thai red-cross intradermal regimen)
2. Uses PVRV, HDCV, PCEC.
3. "2-2-2-0-2" on 0, 3, 7, 14, 28 days, on 14 no dose given
4. A dose of vaccine in volume of 0.1 ml is given intradermally at two different lymphatic drainage sites.

g. **Oxford regimen:** Use only with PCEC or HPCV with dose 0.1 ml

Scheduled: 8-0-4-0-1-1 on 0, 3, 7, 14, 28, 90 days

h. **How to give vaccine:**

1. Using aseptic techniques, reconstitute a vial of freeze - dried vaccine with the diluent.
2. A 1 ml syringe with insulin syringe draws 0.2 ml (upto 20 units if 100 units syringe is used or 8 units if a 40 units syringe is used) 0.1 ml at two sites.

i. **Wound management:**

1. **Do's:** Wash under tap water with soap
2. **Don't:**
   a. Don't apply irritants like soil, oil
   b. Try to avoid the suturing if required then 1-2 loose sutures and only after administration of immunoglobulin

j. **Passive immunisation:**

1. **Indications for passive immunisation**
   a. All category III bite irrespective of status of biting animal
   b. Category II exposure in immunocompromised or immunosuppressed individuals including HIV infected people and AIDS patients.
2. Immunoglobulin is life saving in Cat III bite
3. In re-exposure cases (Previously completed postexposure prophylaxis) RIG is not indicated.
4. RIG is more effective if given immediately within 24 hours of animal bite along with the first dose of vaccine.
5. However RIG can be infiltrated even after a week or later, if the person has not received antirabies vaccine, but it is always good to administer RIG at the earliest.
6. Dose of Human rabies immunoglobulin (HRIG): 20 IU/kg.
7. Dose of equine rabies immunoglobulin (ERIG): 40 IU/kg.
8. Infiltrate ERIG in the depth and all around the wound
9. Infiltrate immunoglobulin as much as possible into and around the wound remaining amount (If any) to be infiltrated intramuscularly at a site away from the site where the vaccine has been administered.
10. **RIG should be given in special situation:**
    a. Such as person who consumed unboiled milk of rabid animal
    b. Cat-III exposure even by vaccinated animals

k. **Pre-exposure prophylaxis:**

1. Important in high risk groups like veterans, medical, paramedical staff treating rabies patients.
2. Dog catchers, forest staff, zoo personnel recommended for the pre-exposure prophylaxis.
3. 3 doses given in series by IM route on 0, 7, 21 or 28 days.
4. 2 doses given in series by ID route on 0, 3 days.
5. Booster dose is advised if antibody titre is less than 0.5 ml/IU.

l. **Re-exposure management:**

1. Re-exposure after a full course: vaccinate with 2 booster doses on day 0 and day 3.
2. Rabies immunoglobulin is not needed
3. All incomplete/partial vaccination cases are treated as fresh cases.

SNAKE BITE

1. Snake bite is an acute life threatening time limiting medical emergency.
2. In india, there are about 250 species, out of which about 50 species are poisonous
3. Most common snake bite being krait.
4. **Common poisonous snakes:**
   a. The cobra (Nag, naja tripudians, naja naja, kala samp)
   b. The king cobra
   c. The common krait
   d. The banded krait
   e. Russell's viper or daboia
   f. Sea snake
5. **For medical purposes, snakes are classified as:**
   1] **Poisonous:**
      A] **Colubridae:**
         a) **Elapidae:** Cobra and krait
         b) **Hydrophidae:** Sea snake
      B] **Viperidae:**
         a) Includes vipers
   2] **Non poisonous**
6. **On the basis of poison, the snakes are classified as:**
   1] **Elapids: Neurotoxic**
   2] **Vipers: Vasculotoxic**
   3] **Sea snake: Myotoxic**
7. The proteins in the snake venom are present in the form of enzymes, peptides and polypeptides and they exert their effect in following ways:
   a. **Elapsid venom:** It is neurotoxic and they block neuromuscular junction and thus decrease output of acetyl choline .

      It affect central nervous system, respiration and heart functions.
   b. **Viperine venom:** It has mainly hemolytic, hemorrhagic, necrotic effect and thus causes intravascular hemolysis.
   c. **Sea snake venom:** It is myotoxic and causes severe muscle pain, myoglobunuria, and hypokalemia in patient.

Signs and Symptoms

	Local manifestation	Systemic manifestation
Elapids (Neurotoxic)	Mild in the form of burning, redness, swelling, and inflammation at the site of bite	Vomiting, lethargy, salivation, extraocular muscle paralysis, ptosis, difficulty in speaking and swallowing, muscle weakness and pain, paralysis, convulsions
Vipers (vasculotoxic)	Intense pain, swelling, irritation, cellulitis, cyanosis, oozing of blood, serum and formation of blisters containing serosanguinous or rarely serous fluid.	Vomiting, unconsciousness, intravascular hemolysis, petechial hemorrhages, bleeding from body orifices and hypotension
Sea snakes (Myotoxic)	Initially painful but soon painless	Vomiting, circulatory collapse, muscular pain, muscle stiffness, myoglobinuria, hyperkalemia, and serum transaminase levels

Investigations

1. **Complete blood count:** Thrombocytopenia, hemoconcentration
2. **Blood film:** Schistocytes seen due to microangiopathic hemolysis.
3. **20 minutes whole blood clotting test:**

   Test: 2 ml of freshly drawn venous blood from patient is kept in plain glass tube for 20 minutes.

   Result: If blood remain unclotted even after 20 min then it means the patient has hypofibrinogenemia as a result of venom-induced consumption coagulopathy..
4. **In vasculotoxic venomation, for coagulopathy:** BT, CT, PT, aPTT, platelets, Serum Fibrinogen, FDP, LDH.
5. **Serum electrolyte:** Hyperkalemia is seen in the sea snake bite due to extensive rhabdomyolysis
6. **Arterial blood gases:** Metabolic acidosis, low bicarbonate may be seen
7. Aminotransferases and muscle enzymes (e.g. Creatine kinase, aldolase etc.) will be elevated if there is severe muscle (Local and generalized).
8. **Renal function test:** Blood urea nitrogen, serum creatinine raised in renal failure
9. **Urine examination:** Tested for presence of myoglobinuria, hemoglobinuria
10. ECG for arrhythmias,myocardial damage, evidence of hyperkalemia.
11. **Chest X-ray:** To detect pulmonary edema, pleural effusion, secondary bronchopneumonia.

Treatment

I] First aid:

1) Assure the patient if the patient is anxious, as 70% of all snakebites are from non-venomous species

2) Clean the wound with soap and water, or iodine and cover with sterile dressing.

3) **Immobilise the limb:** Movement can accelerate the spread of venom and Immobilize the limb in the same way as a fractured limb with the help of splint, bandages and cloths.

4) Remove the bandage or tourniquet in the hospital.

5) Advise a patient to lie on one side in the recovery position so that the airway remains clear, in case of vomiting

6) **Transport the patient immediately to hospital.**

7) **Don'ts in management wound:**

   a. Do not suck the venom

   b. Do not give local incision (Cause damage to nerve and causes local bleeding)

   c. Do not use the hazardous chemicals or medicines on the wound

   d. Do not cauterise the wound which seals the poison within tissue.

II] Use of antisnake venom serum:

A. Polyvalent anti-snake venom is obtained from horses

B. Horses are hyperimmunized against the venom of the common poisonous snakes, i.e., cobra, common krait, Russell's viper and saw scaled viper.

1) ASV is available in the form of lyophilised powder in an ampoule

2) Start administartion of ASV as soon as indicated to reverse effect of systemic venom.

3) **Dose:**

   a. **Dose of neuroparalytic snake bites:** ASV 10 vials diluted in 500 ml of distilled water or normal saline and infused over a period of 30 mins followed by 2nd dose of 10 vials after 1 hour if no improvement within 1 hour is seen.

   b. **Dose for vasculotoxic snake bite:** 10 vials of ASV stat over 30 minutes as infusion, followed by 6 vials 6 hourly as bolus therapy till clotting normalizes and/or local swelling subsides.

4) **If any signs and symptoms of reaction/hypersensitivity after PAV infusion then:**

   a. Stop PAV infusion

   b. Administer 0.5 mg 1:1000 adrenaline i.m for adults (0.01 mg/kg for children)

   c. Give hydrocortisone and antihistamine to provide longer term protection

   d. Still no improvement after 10 to 15 min give a second dose of adrenaline

   e. Once the condition has improved restart antiserum infusion

5) **Supportive measures:**

a. Careful assessment of airway, breathing, circulation and mental status is necessary.

b. Hypoxia: Start oxygen administartion.

c. In respiratory failure, ventilator support is needed.

d. Treatment of hypotension or shock by IV fluids or by inotropic support.

e. **Acute kidney injury:** Conservative or dialysis may be needed.

f. Identify and treat hyperkalemia by calcium gluconate.

g. Management of metabolic acidosis by sodium bicarbonate.

6) **Treatment of bitten part**

a. Inject tetanus toxoid booster or tetanus antitoxin

b. A broad spectrum antibiotic should be given if there is severe tissue damage

c. Use paracetamol as analgesic and avoid aspirin use as it increases a risk of bleeding.

d. Surgical debridement of the blebs, bloody vesicles, and superficial necrosis may be necessary.

7) **Treatment of hematological abnormality**

a. Bleeding and clotting abnormalities can respond well to antisnake venom

b. Keep watch on the prothrombin time while treating a case of viper bite

c. In some cases fresh frozen plasma, cryoprecipitate (fibrinogen, factor VIII), fresh whole blood or platelet concentrates may be required.

8) **Use of anticholinesterase**

a. If neuroparalysis signs are present then atropine sulfate (0.6 mg for adults) or glycopyrronium is given by intravenous injection followed by neostigmine 1.5 mg IV and repeat dose of neostigmine 0.5 mg with atropine every 30 min. for 5 doses.

b. To counteract the muscarinic effects of neostigmine, atropine is given.

c. The patient is observed over the next 30-60 minutes (Neostigmine) for improvement.

d. Ptosis may disappear and respiratory function may improve with its use.

CARBOLIC ACID (PHENOL)

1. It is largely used as an antiseptic as well as disinfectant
2. It is one of the most popular suicidal poison used.
3. Acute poisoning can occur by ingestion, inhalation, accidental exposure
4. **Signs and symptoms:**
   a. **Local:**
      1. **Skin:**
         a. Initially it causes no pain, but by the time pain is felt due to burn injury
         b. It causes burning and numbness due to nerve ending damage.
         c. Local effects of phenol includes erythema, inflammation and necrosis.
      2. **Digestive tract:**
         a. Severe hot burning pain is felt by a patient which extends from a mouth to the stomach, which is followed by tingling sensation & later on anesthesia due to irritation of tract and nerve ending damage.
         b. Deglutition and speech becomes painful and difficult
         c. Patient complains of nausea, vomiting and abdominal pain.
      3. **Respiratory tract:**
         a. Carbolic acid affects the respiratory system by inhalation or aspiration.
         b. Pulmonary and laryngeal edema develops due to irritation of respiratory tract.
   b. **Systemic effects:**
      1. **CNS:**
         a. CNS depressant
         b. Headache, giddiness
         c. Altered mental status
         d. Convulsion
      2. **CVS:**
         a. Pulse is rapid, feeble, and irregular
         b. Sweating
         c. Dusky cyanosis
      3. **RS:**
         a. Breathlessness, Pulmonary edema, bronchitis, bronchopneumonia.
         b. Progressive respiratory failure may occur in patients.

4. **Hepatic:** Liver necrosis

5. **Treatment: Divided into three parts**

a. **Limit absorption**

1. Contaminated clothing should be removed
2. Contaminated skin should be washed with soap and water.
3. Gastric lavage should be done with activated charcoal, olive oil, castor oil, cotton seed oil, magnesium or sodium sulfate or saccharated lime with which phenol combines and form harmless products.
4. The stomach wash should be repeated until no odor of phenol is left & washings are clear.

b. **To provide necessary support to body to withstand the effect of poisoning**

1. Make proper assessment of airway, breathing, circulation and neurological status.
2. Maintain clear airway
3. Assisted ventilation if indicated (Pulmonary edema, pneumonia, respiratory failure)
4. If the patient is unconscious then provide artificial respiration
5. Circulatory support byIV fluid administration
6. Hemodialysis, if renal failure
7. Anticonvulsant therapy, if patients have convulsions.

c. **Assist the body for excretion.**

1. Sodium bicarbonate is given in saline to dilute carbolic acid and to increase excretion by diuresis.

RAT KILL POISON (ZINC PHOSPHIDE)

1. The zinc phosphide is used as a rodenticide
2. It is a 10 gm packet containing black colored powder.
3. It is available by different names in market like ratol, kilrat, rometan etc.
4. Zinc phosphide produces toxic phosphine gas when comes in contact with water or HCl of the stomach, which is responsible for its toxic effects.
5. Zinc phosphide poisoning occurs only by ingestion.
6. It is fat soluble & not water soluble so it remains in the stomach for a longer duration.
7. **Clinical features:**
   a. **GI tract**

      Nausea, vomiting, burning epigastric pain, abdominal pain, diarrhea

   b. **Cardiovascular system**

      Hypotension or shock, cardiac arrhythmias, myocardial ischemia, myocarditis, pericarditis, congestive cardiac failure

   c. **Respiratory system**

      Cough, breathelessness, cyanosis, acute pulmonary edema, type I and type II respiratory failure

   d. **Hepatobiliary system**

      Jaundice, hepatomegaly, liver failure

   e. **Renal system**

      Renal failure

   f. **Central nervous system**

      Restlessness, anxiety, fear, delirium, convulsion and coma.
8. **Investigation**
   a. **Complete blood count**
   b. **Liver function test:** Raised transaminases, prothrombin time
   c. **Blood urea/creatinine:** Normal or raised if acute renal failure develops
   d. **Arterial blood gas:** Hypoxemia, hypocarbia, metabolic acidosis may be seen
   e. **Serum electrolyte:** Hypokalemia and Hypomagnesemia
   f. **Blood phosphine level by Liquid gas chromatography:** High
   g. **Chest X-ray:** Non cardiogenic pulmonary edema.

h. **PT and INR:** May be increased.

i. **ECG:** Changes of myocarditis, arrhythmias (SVT or VT or ST segment changes)

9. **Management**

a. **To delay absorption**

1. Gastric lavage with KMnO4 so as to remove or oxidized unabsorbed poison
2. A slurry of activated charcoal to be given as soon as possible to absorb PH3
3. Liquid paraffin or magnesium sulfate can be given to accelerate its excretion from the gut.

b. **To enhance excretion**

1. Maintain adequate hydration and renal perfusion so as to excrete absorbed phosphine.
2. If renal perfusion is low then low dose dopamine started.

c. **To reduce organ toxicity**

1. Most of the organ toxicity is due to hypoxia and oxidant injury produced by PH3
2. No antidote for PH3
3. N acetyl cysteine, a glutathione precursor, has been commonly used in rat kill poisoning. It is given as loading dose of 150 mg/kg in 200 ml D5W over 1 hour followed by 50 mg/kg in 500 ml D5W over 4 hour then 100 mg/kg in 1000 ml D5W over 16 hours.

d. **Supportive measures**

1. Assessement of airway, breathing, circulation & mental status of patient.
2. Maintain clear airway
3. Oxygen therapy: If patient is having respiratory distress or hypoxemia.
4. Secure IV line & start IV fluids administration for dehydration correction.
5. NPO & insert Ryle's tube
6. Inotropic support with dopamine, dobutamine, noradrenaline.
7. Correct metabolic acidosis with sodium bicarbonate
8. Identify and correct electrolyte imbalance
9. FFP, whole blood transfusion is indicated in severe case of hemolysis or abnormal bleeding parameters.
10. Treatment of arrhythmias with antiarrhythmic drugs: Cardiac arrhythmias occur secondary to electrolyte abnormalities such as hyperkalemia, hypocalcemia & treated with magnesium sulfate, digoxin.

ORGANOPHOSPHORUS POISONS

1. OrganoPhosfates are a group of insecticides which are antiacetyl -cholinesterase.
2. The organoPhosfates are used as insecticides, petroleum additives and as chemical warfare agents.
3. Carbamates are another group of insecticides which act at the same site but have slightly different mechanisms of action.
4. Mode of poisoning is more suicidal than accidental.
5. They are the esters of phosphoric acid and forms two series of compounds
   a. Alkyl Phosfate
   b. Aryl Phosfate
6. **Action:**
   a. Organophosphorus compounds are powerful inhibitors of carboxylic esterase enzymes, including acetylcholinesterase and pseudocholinesterase
   b. Organophosphorus compounds bind firmly to the esterase enzyme, inactivating it by phosphorylation at the myoneural junctions and synapses of the ganglions.

Signs and Symptoms of Acute OP Poisoning

Signs and symptoms appear when cholinesterase level drops significantly of its normal activity.

I] **Muscarinic manifestation:**

These symptoms can be easily remembered by the acronym SLUDGE

S- Salivation

L- Lacrimation

U- Urination

D- Defecation

G- GI distress

E- Emesis

Bronchial tree	Bronchoconstriction, increased bronchial secretion, dyspnea, pulmonary edema
G.I.T	Anorexia, salivation, nausea, vomiting, cramps, diarrhea, fecal incontinence, tenesmus. Pancreatitis may develop.
Sweat gland	Increased sweating
Salivary glands	Increased salivation
Lacrimal glands	Increased lacrimation
C.V.S	Bradycardia or tachycardia, arrhythmias, hypotension
Pupils	Miosis, occasionally unequal or dilated
Ciliary body	Blurred vision
bladder	Urinary incontinence

II] Nicotinic manifestation:

1) **On Striated muscles:** Initial stimulus results in contraction, later there is paralysis due to persistent depolarisation

   a) Muscle weakness occurs due to accumulation of acetylcholine

   b) Muscular fasciculations, cramps, weakness, areflexia

2) **On Sympathetic ganglia:**

   Hypertension, tachycardia, pallor, mydriasis

III] CNS manifestation:

Restlessness, headache, tremor, anxiety, drowsiness, confusion, slurred speech, ataxia, generalised weakness, coma, GTCS convulsions, depression of respiratory and cardiovascular centres.

Mild poisoning	Nausea, malaise, fatigue, minimal muscle weakness, cramping without diarrhea
Moderate poisoning	SLUDGE and/or tremors, weakness, fasciculation, confusion, lethargy, anxiety
Severe poisoning	SLUDGE and respiratory insufficiency, weakness, fasciculation, coma, paralysis, seizure, autonomic dysfunction.

Diagnosis

1. **History of consumption of insecticides poison**
2. **Characteristic clinical feature**
   a. Muscarinic features

   b. Nicotinic features
   c. Central nervous system features
3. **Clinical improvement after atropine:**
   a. In normal person it causes marked atropinization
   b. In case of poisoning, symptoms are not relieved without atropinization
4. **Inhibition of cholinesterase:** Assay to measure a decrease in cholinesterase in plasma (**Definitive and gold standard method)**

Investigations

1. **Complete blood count:** Neutrophilic leukocytosis
2. **ECG:** QTc prolongation due to cholinergic stimulation of heart
3. **Arterial blood gas:** Metabolic acidosis
4. **Serum electrolyte:** Electrolyte imbalance may present
5. **Serum amylase:** Raised due to cholinergic stimulation of pancreas.
6. **Chest X-ray:** Aspiration pneumonitis pulmonary edema may be evident
7. **Liver function test:** Deranged hepatic enzymes
8. **Renal function test:** Serum creatinine, BUN may be raised in acute kidney injury.
9. **Urine examination:** Proteinuria/glycosuria
10. **Plasma SChE:** More useful in diagnosis of acute poisoning.
11. **Cholinesterase level:** Low level

Treatment

1. **Identify the toxin**
2. **Classify the organophosphorus or non organophosphorus poison**
3. **Goal of treatment**
   a. Reduce absorption of the toxin
   b. Enhance elimination
   c. Neutralize toxin
4. **Immediate management includes:**
   a. Check the patency of airway
   b. Assess the blood pressure, pulse rate, breathing, mental status

c. Position to patient: Head low position, left lateral position to avoid aspiration of secretions

d. Oxygen therapy if hypoxemia or severe respiratory distress present

e. Secure IV line & start fluid administration

f. Insert Foley's catheter

g. Start atropine

5. **Decontamination:**

a. The patient is removed from the source of exposure

b. Contaminated cloth to be removed

c. Exposed areas are washed with soap and water

d. Eyes are decontaminated with water only

6. **Reduce absorption of the toxin**

a. Lavage only if patient arrives within 1 hour of consumption

b. Ipecacuanha (Plant derived syrup for induction of vomiting) induced emesis is contraindicated in OP poisoning

c. When the poison is ingested activated charcoal (1gm/kg) used for gastric lavage

7. **Atropine sulfate**

a. Arrest the muscarine effects of postganglionic parasympathetic activity and arrest the CNS effect

b. No effect on nicotinic manifestations

c. Oxygenation should be achieved before atropine to avoid the increased risk of ventricular tachyarrhythmias associated with hypoxia

d. Its use is stopped if B.P. falls and heart rate exceeds 140 beats/min.

e. 2 to 5 mg iv given as a bolus dose

f. If there is no effect then dose can be doubled after every 10 to 15 min, until muscarinic symptoms are relieved

g. Atropine should be continued until the tracheobronchial tree is cleared of the secretion and most secretions are dried (Clear lung field on auscultation).

h. **Atropine toxicity:** Fever + confusion + absent bowel sounds.

i. If toxicity then stop infusion for 1 hour and restart after the patient becomes calm and fever subsides with less dose.

Before atropine	After atropinization
1. Pulmonary secretions	1. Dry lungs filled
2. Sweating	2. Dry axilla
3. Pinpoint pupils	3. No longer pinpoint pupils
4. Hypotension	4. BP more than 80 mm of Hg
5. Bradycardia	5. Heart rate more than 80 beats/min
6. Hyperactive bowel sounds	6. Bowel sounds Only present

8. **Specific cholinesterase reactivators** like Diacetyl monoxime (DAM), or 2-Pyridine aldoxime methiodide, or Pralidoxime chloride:
   a. It is used to regenerate AchE by competing the Phosfate moiety of OP compound and release it from cholinesterase enzyme.
   b. Its action is marked at nicotinic site
   c. It is used to improve muscle strength & respiratory depression
   d. The adult dose of 1 to 2 gm given in 5% dextrose solution given 5 min or in 150 ml of saline and infused over half an hour
   e. This dose should be repeated at 6 to 12 hours interval for 24 to 48 hours
   f. Pralidoxime decrease the amount of atropine required for atropinization and also potentiates the action of atropine
   g. Infusion is stopped when
      1. Muscle fasciculation and weakness are resolved
      2. Reactivation and increased level of SCh E.
   h. Infusion is continued till the patient has no symptoms for 12 hours without atropine use.
9. **Other supportive management**
   a. **To prevent the pulmonary infections:** Broad spectrum antibiotics are used.
   b. **If renal failure:** Conservative or hemodialysis may be needed.

SEDATIVE AND HYPNOTIC POISONING

1. The term Sedative and hypnotic group includes several pharmcological groups
2. A **sedative** or **tranquilliser** is a substance that induces sedation by reducing anxiety and exerting a calming effect.
3. Hypnotics are commonly known as **sleeping pills**, are a class of psychoactive drugs whose main function is to induce sleep.
4. Overdose of this agent causes global central nervous system depression.
5. They are taken in overdose for suicidal purposes.
6. Sedative and hypnotic drugs are classified as follows
   a. **Benzodiazepines** (It includes anti-anxiety, hypnotic and anticonvulsant)
   b. **Barbiturates (It includes sedatives, hypnotics & antiepileptics)**
   c. **Non benzodiazepines** e.g. zolpidem, zaleplon, zopiclone

A) BENZODIAZEPINE POISONING

a. **Mode of action**

Benzodiazepines enhance the effect of the neurotransmitter gamma-aminobutyric acid (GABA) at the $GABA_A$ receptor, resulting in sedative, hypnotic (Sleep-inducing), anxiolytic (Anti-anxiety), anticonvulsant, and muscle relaxant properties.

b. **Classification of benzodiazepines**

Ultrashort acting	Short acting	Long acting
1. Midazolam	1. Alprazolam	1. Diazepam
2. Triazolam	2. Lorazepam	2. Clonazepam
3. Estazolam	3. Oxazepam	3. Flurazepam
4. Temazepam		4. Nitrazepam
		5. Prazepam
		6. Quazepam
		7. Chlordiazepoxide

c. **Effect of benzodiazepines**

1. Sedation can progress to hypnosis and finally stupor with increasing dose
2. In preanesthetic doses patients have amnesia.
3. They are unable to cause true general anesthesia as awareness is present in patient.
4. It increases total sleep time

d. Clinical features

1. Initially patient has paradoxical excitation characterised by over talkativeness, excitement.
2. Weakness and hypotonia
3. Hypotension
4. Constricted pupils
5. Drowsiness, stupor
6. Coma
7. Respiratory depression
8. Ataxia, dysarthria

e. Diagnosis

1. History of consumption of benzodiazepines
2. On the basis of clinical features
3. Identification of metabolites of benzodiazepines in urine
4. Response to antidote i.e. Flumazenil

f. Management

1. **General measures:**
   a. Nasogastric tube insertion and Foley's catheterisation.
   b. Monitor pulse, blood pressure, respiration, mental status.
   c. Serial monitoring of blood investigation
2. **Avoid the absorption of drug:**
   Removal of unabsorbed drug by giving repeated gastric lavage and administration of activated charcoal
3. **Use of antidote:**
   a. Flumazenil is antidote of benzodiazepines
   b. Flumazenil is competitive benzodiazepines receptor antagonist
   c. It can reverse the effect of central nervous system and respiratory depression.
   d. The initial dose is 0.2 mg, given intravenously, and this can be repeated at 1–6 minute intervals, if necessary, to a cumulative dose of 1 mg.
4. **Circulatory support:**
   a. Start intravenous fluid administration
   b. If the hypotension still persists then inotropic support is required.
5. **Respiratory support:**
   a. O_2 therapy
   b. Maintain patent airway
   c. Intubation is done in patients with severe respiratory depression.

B) BARBITURATE POISONING

Barbiturates are used as a sedative, hypnotic and as an antiepileptic

a. **Mode of action**

Barbiturates act as a positive allosteric modulators and, at higher doses, act as agonists of $GABA_A$ receptors.

b. **Classification:**

Ultra short acting	Short acting	Intermediate acting	Long acting
1. Methohexital	1. Hexa barbital	1. Amlo barbital	1. Phenobarbitone
2. Thiopental	2. Secobarbital	2. Butabarbital	2. Barbital
	3. Pentobarbital		3. Pyrimidone

c. **Actions**

1. **CNS depression:** Depending on dose, at low dose causes calming effect and in higher dose may induce coma.
2. **Respiratory depression**
3. **Enzyme induction:** Barbiturates induce P450 microsomal enzymes in the liver.

d. **Clinical features:**

1. **Central nervous system:** Depression stupor, areflexia, or coma.
2. **Respiratory depression:** Shallow breathing
3. **Cardiovascular system:** Hypotension weak & rapid pulse, cold extremities
4. **Renal system:** Acute renal failure, oliguria

e. **Diagnosis and investigations**

1. History of consumption of barbital drugs in large quantities.
2. Signs and symptoms of poisoning
3. Serum barbital level is mandatory to confirm diagnosis and also for treatment.
4. **Investigation:**
   a. **Complete blood examination**
   b. **Blood sugar**
   c. **Renal function**
   d. **Liver function**
   e. **Electrocardiogram**
   f. **Chest X-ray**

f. **Management**

1. **General measures**
   a. Nasogastric tube insertion and Foley's catheterisation.
   b. Monitor pulse, blood pressure, respiration, mental status.
   c. Serial monitoring of blood investigation
2. **To reduce the absorption of drug.**
   Gastric lavage with activated charcoal & emesis is useful in reduction of absorption of drug.
3. **To remove absorbed drug**
   a. **Removal by forced alkaline diuresis**
      1. Useful in long acting barbiturates poisoning
      2. **Complication of diuresis:** Pulmonary edema, circulatory overload, electrolyte disturbance.
   b. **Catharsis:** Excrete the drug through stool
   c. **Removal by peritoneal or hemodialysis**
      1. Useful in short and long acting barbiturates
      2. Indicated in renal failure and pulmonary edema
      3. Deep coma with areflexia, hypotension and respiratory depression.
4. **Respiratory support:** Oxygen supplementation and if required Assisted ventilation.
5. **Circulatory support:** Maintain central venous pressure with intravenous fluids and if required inotropic support.

OPIATE POISONING

a. The opiates are derived from the juice of poppy flower

b. Different types of opiates :-

   1. Natural opiate: Opium, morphine, codeine
   2. Semi-synthetic opiate: Hydrocodone, oxycodone, hydromorphone and oxymorphone
   3. Synthetic opiate: Fentanyl, methadone, tramadol and propoxyphene

c. Opiates are used as narcotic analgesia in medicine.

d. High doses of opiates can result in overdose or poisoning

e. The duration of effect of opiates varies from a few hours (heroin) to days (methadone)

f. **Clinical features**

   1. Euphoria, analgesia, sedation
   2. Respiratory depression slow & shallow breathing
   3. Constriction of pupils
   4. Hypotension, bradycardia
   5. Hypothermia
   6. Stupor or coma
   7. Gastrointestinal symptoms: Nausea, vomiting, constipation
   8. Convulsions can occur in tramadol, meperidine, dextromethorphan
   9. Methadone has been associated with prolonged QT interval and torsades de pointes.

g. **Treatment**

   1. **Supportive measures**

      a. Oxygen inhalation: if needed mechanical ventilation
      b. Start IV fluids for resuscitation
      c. Gastric lavage to remove the unabsorbed poison if oral intake is the cause
      d. Activated charcoal is used to remove unabsorbed drugs
      e. If no response to IV fluids then start inotropic support to raise the blood pressure
      f. Monitor vitals i.e pulse, blood pressure, respiration and temperature.

2. **Specific antidote**

   a. Naloxone: It is an opioid antagonist

      Dose: Initial dose of 0.4–1.2 mg given IV, IM or subcutaneously and if required dose may be repeated after every 5 min.

   b. Repeated dose is needed in long acting opiates.

   c. If there is no response to above treatment then poisoning from multiple drugs may be considered (Benzodiazepines, cocaine, alcohol).

3. **Other measures**

   a. Care of unconscious patients (Intermittent airway suction to avoid aspiration, keep bed & bedding free from moisture, change patients position frequently to avoid bed sores).

   b. Treatment of convulsion and cardiac arrhythmia, if occurs

   c. Prevention and treatment of aspiration pneumonia

Section

7

Skin Emergencies

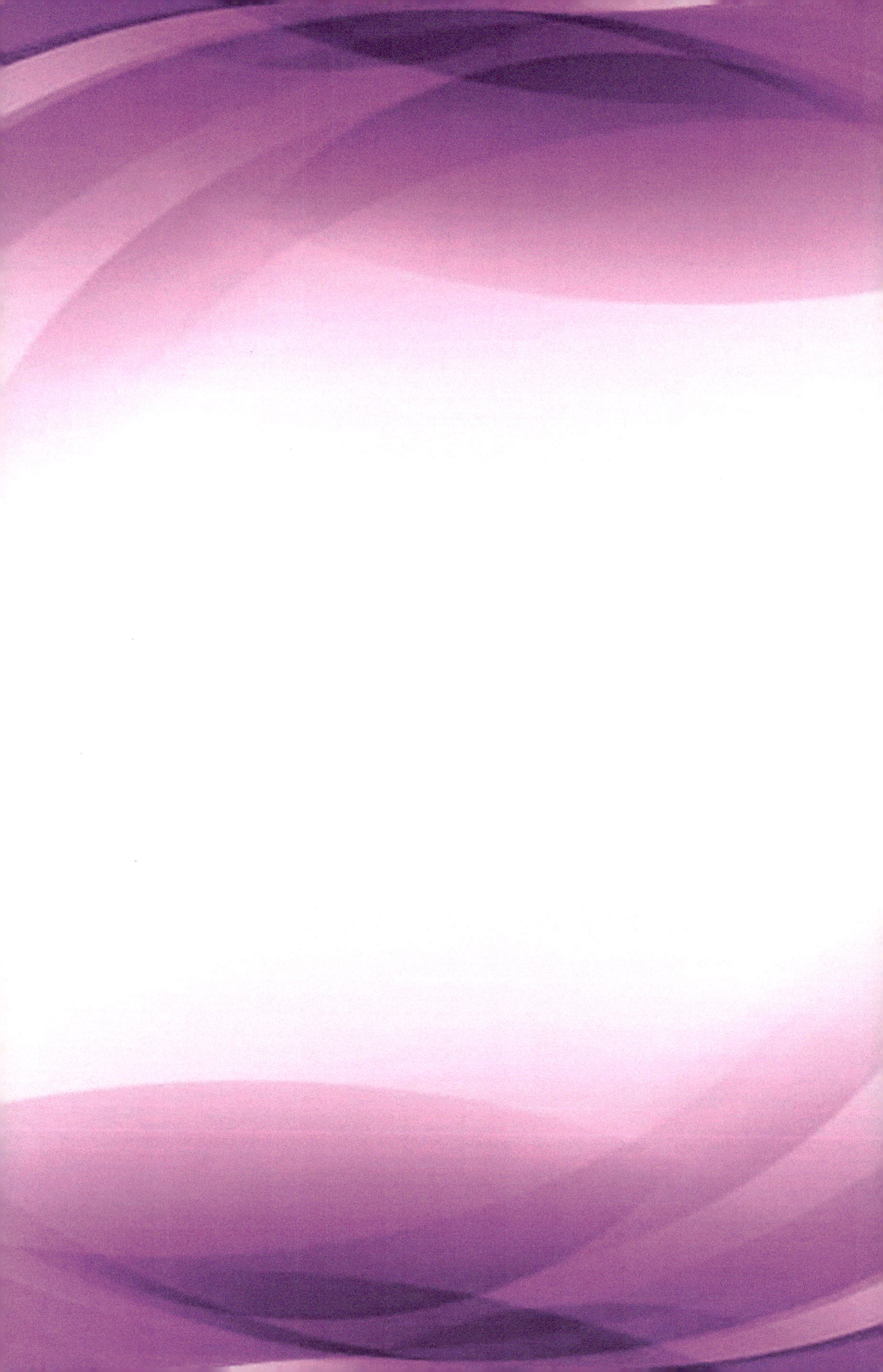

CHAPTER

14 Skin Emergencies

ACUTE URTICARIA AND ANGIOEDEMA

ACUTE URTICARIA

1. **Definition:** Condition characterised by transient, well -demarcated, edematous pruritic plaques which usually fade within hours.
2. Urticaria occurs due to infection or as result of immunological reaction
3. **Classification:**
   a. In acute urticaria the lesions last for less than 6 weeks.
   b. In chronic urticaria the lesion lasts for more than 6 weeks.
4. Urticaria is due to dermal vessel dilation followed by exudation of plasma.
5. **Common causes of acute urticaria and angioedema:**

Exogenous
Inhaled: Pollen grains, plant hairs, feathers
Ingestant: Drugs like sulfonamides, chloroquine, NSAIDs and Food like seafood, milk, tomatoes, eggs, food additives and preservatives e.g. azo dyes & benzoates
Injectants: Drugs like insulin, penicillins, radioactive contrast media
Contactants: Bee stings, bug bites, animal excreta and plants
Blood transfusion reaction
Serum sickness
Vaccine
Endogenous
Infections: URTI, biliary pancreatitis and cholecystitis
Parasitic infestations: Helminthiasis, amebiasis and giardiasis.
Immunological disease: Systemic lupus erythematosus
Physical urticaria: Heat, Pressure, cold, aquagenic

6. **Clinical features:**

   1. **Appearance of wheals**

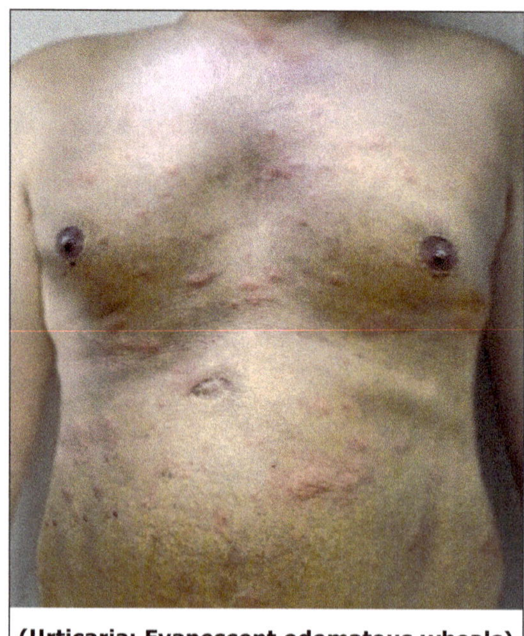

(Urticaria: Evanescent edematous wheals)

A Wheal consists of three typical features:

a. A central swelling of variable size, almost invariably surrounded by a reflex erythema

b. Wheals are associated with itching or sometimes burning/stinging sensations

c. Its fleeting nature, usually patients skin returns to its normal appearance within 1–24 h, but may remain for indefinite period.

2. **Distribution:**

   a. Any part of the body can be affected (eyelids, lips, tongue, genitalia, palms, soles, GI tract)

   b. Trunk is more commonly involved than extremities or face

   c. Mucosal surfaces may involve and may become swollen, lips being the commonest region affected.

3. **Systemic symptoms:**

   a. Rhinitis, difficulty in breathing, sensation of heaviness in chest, wheezing, vomiting, and abdominal pain may be present along with skin lesions.

b. Require urgent treatment to avoid the complication of bronchospasm laryngeal edema.

c. Hypotension, shock

7. **Investigations:**

1. **Laboratory investigations (for infections):**

a. Complete blood count

b. Differential leukocyte count

c. Urine and stool examination

2. **Allergy test (Not done routinely):** Intradermal scratch test or an estimation of serum IGE levels directed specifically at each allergen.

8. **Treatment:** Urticaria needs to be treated immediately to avoid serious complications laryngeal edema and bronchospasm.

a. **Antihistamines:** In widespread urticaria, accompanied by bronchospasm, initially intramuscular antihistamines e.g injection chlorpheniramine (avil) 2CC stat (in adults) should be given.

In milder cases oral antihistamines is given

Sedatives	Non sedatives
Pheniramine 25 mg TDS	Levocetirizine 5-10 mg/day
Hydroxyzine 10 mg TDS	Desloratadine 10-20 mg/day
Cetirizine 10 mg OD or BD	Fexofenadine 180 mg ODor BD
Loratidine 10 mg OD or BD	Mizolastine 10 mg OD
	Bilastine 20 mg OD

b. **Corticosteroids:** IM or IV intravenous hydrocortisone

E.g Injection hydrocortisone 200 mg stat (For adults)

c. **Adrenaline:** If there is no response, with above treatment intramuscular or subcutaneous adrenaline 0.5 ml of 1:1000 solution brings about prompt relief.

d. **Cyclosporine:** Given in severe cases of autoimmune urticaria.

ANGIOEDEMA

1. Angioedema is an acute circumbcribed edema that remains for a short period of time.
2. It results due to dermal edema as well as subcutaneous edema
3. It usually affects the most distensible tissues such as lips, eyebrows, eyelids, earlobes, external genitalia and mucous membrane of mouth, tongue, larynx.
4. Angioedema may occur with or without urticaria
5. Pathogenesis of this condition is also similar to urticaria
6. It may be histamine/bradykinin induced.
7. **Angioedema lesions:**

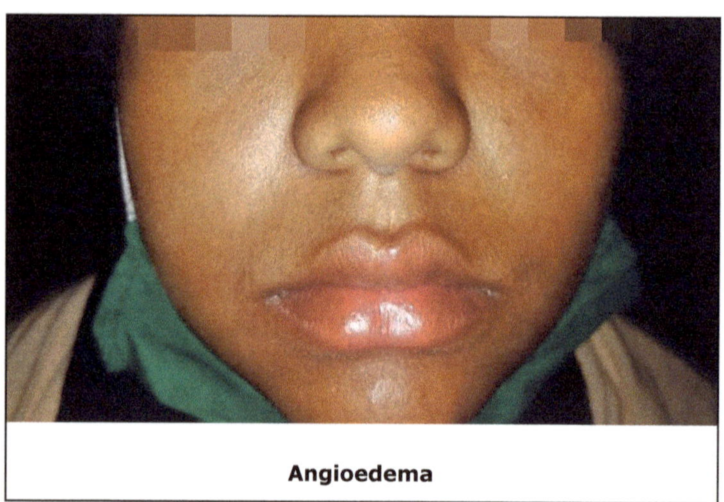

Angioedema

   a. Sudden, marked & non tender swelling of the lower dermis and subcutaneous space.
   b. Pain
   c. Frequent involvement of mucous membranes
   d. Angioedema needs upto 72 hours for resolution.
8. **Distribution:**
   a. Eyelids and lips are the commonest sites
   b. Hands, forearms, scrotum, vulva and penis may be affected
9. **Treatment: As like urticaria**

   Most dangerous manifestation of angioedema is the involvement of laryngeal mucosa which causes obstruction of airways and should be treated immediately by the subcutaneous adrenaline or sometimes tracheostomy may be required

STEVENS-JOHNSON SYNDROME AND TOXIC EPIDERMAL NECROLYSIS

Stevens-Johnson syndrome and toxic epidermal necrolysis

1. Steven Johnson syndrome (SJS) and toxic epidermal necrolysis (TEN) are life-threatening dermatological emergencies and are considered as part of the disease spectrum (SJS, SJS/TEN, TEN) with SJS being less severe and TEN causing a severe form of disease.
2. Stevens-Johnson/toxic epidermal necrolysis (SJS/TEN) have clinicopathological and etiological similarities and hence are better explained together.
3. Adolescents & young adults are commonly affected as compared to children & elderly.
4. Most of the cases requires immediate hospitalization and intensive care to avoid complications.
5. Possible complications of SJS/TEN include dehydration, sepsis, pneumonia and multiple organ failure.
6. **Causes of Stevens-Johnson/toxic epidermal necrolysis (SJS/TEN):**
   a. **Disorder of the immune system:** SJS is thought to arise from a disorder of the immune system.

      The immune reaction can be triggered by drugs or infections.

   b. Most of the cases are drug induced.
   c. Specific drug classes show higher risk for development of SJS/TEN in people of specific ethnic groups with certain HLA phenotypes.

Drug class	Associated drugs
Sulfonamides	Cotrimoxazole, sulfasalazine, sulfadiazine
Antiepileptics	Phenytoin, carbamazepine, barbiturates, lamotrigine
Antiviral	Nevirapine, abacavir
Antitubercular	Rifampicin, ethambutol, INH
Antibiotics	Cephalosporins, fluoroquinolones, penicillin group, vancomycin
Non-steroidal anti inflammatory drugs (NSAIDs)	Diclofenac, ibuprofen, piroxicam

   d. **Infections:** Second most common trigger particularly in children

      E.g. Mycoplasma pneumoniae, cytomegalovirus etc.

   e. **Genetic factors:** Associated with a predisposition to SJS.
   f. The exact cause of SJS is unknown in 25 to 50% of cases.

7. Morphology and distribution:

	Stevens Johnson syndrome	Toxic epidermal necrolysis
Morphology	**M**ost lesions begins as tender dusky red patches of erythema **M**ost part of lesion turn dark red to brown-black except rim that remains erythematous **A**ppearance of flaccid blisters followed by a sheet like detachment leaving behind erosions**.** **S**evere erosions of oropharynx may be painful enough to prevent eating or talking **T**ypical **target lesions/Bull's eye lesion or iris lesions** are **absent.**	**O**n whole body large patches of tender darkish erythema develops **F**luid begins to collect under epidermis forming vesicles that collapse to form bullae within 24-48 hours. **L**arge flaccid bullae collapse, their roof shed off leaving behind large erosions which ooze serosanguinous fluid. **A**pplications of a rotational shearing force with thumb over erythematous skin or even on apparently normal skin leading to peeling of skin preferably on bony prominence. **(Pseudo Nikolsky's sign)**
Distribution	**M**ucocutaneous junctions, mucosae and periorificial regions are preferentially or exclusively involved. **S**evere ocular involvement leads to keratitis, corneal ulceration and resultant complication.	**I**nvolvement of mucous membranes of oro-pharyngeal, conjunctival, anogenital and nasal. **S**evere ocular involvement leads to keratitis, corneal ulceration and resultant complication.

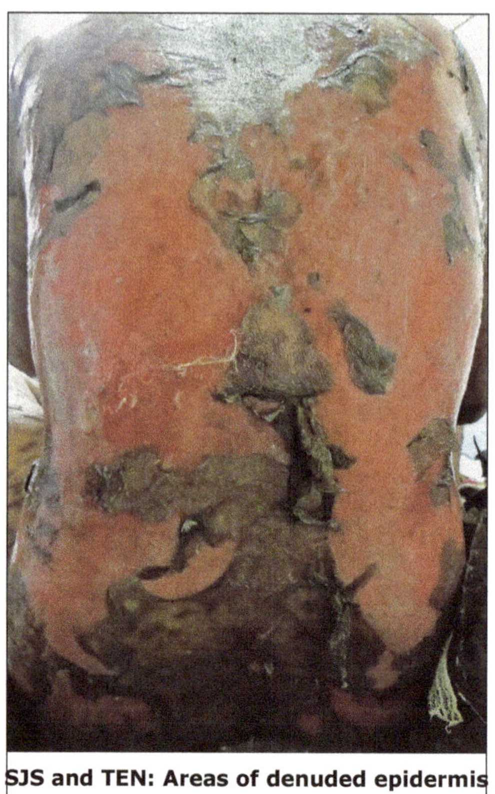

SJS and TEN: Areas of denuded epidermis

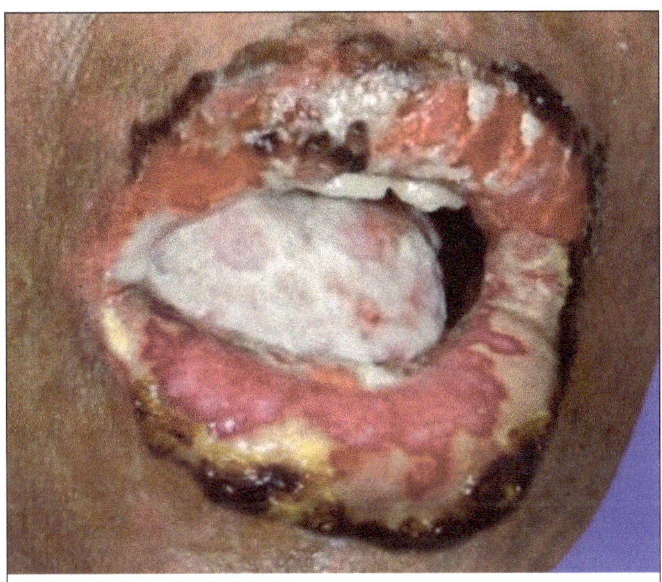

Multiple erosions and crusts are present on the lips of this patient with Stevens-Johnson syndrome

8. **Treatment**

   a. Admission to ICU

   b. Remove the cause (prompt removal of all suspected drugs)

   c. Supportive therapy (skin care, correction of electrolyte imbalance, maintain temperature, fluid management (Input/output charting to guide fluid administration), parenteral nutrition, oral and eye care)

   d. Specific therapy includes administration of systemic steroids or oral cyclosporine 3-5 mg/kg/day or IVIG (Intravenous immunoglobulin 2 gm/kg in divided doses).

PEMPHIGUS

1. It is an autoimmune disorder characterized by the formation of recurrent vesicles or bullae on apparently normal skin with or without involvement of mucosa.
2. Young, middle aged population is commonly affected (20-40 years)
3. In pemphigus, autoantibodies form against desmoglein.
4. Desmoglein is a cell surface molecule typically found in desmosomes which forms the "glue" that attaches adjacent epidermal cells via attachment points called desmosomes.
5. When autoantibodies attack desmogleins, the cells become separated from each other and the epidermis becomes "unglued", a phenomenon called acantholysis.
6. This phenomenon causes blisters that ruptures to form skin erosions.
7. **Types of pemphigus**
   a. **Pemphigus vulgaris**

      Variant pemphigus vegetans

   b. **Pemphigus foliaceus**

      Variant endemic pemphigus foliaceus and pemphigus erythematosus

   c. **Pemphigus herpetiformis**
   d. **IgA pemphigus**

      Variant intradermal neutrophilic and subcorneal pustular type

   e. **Paraneoplastic pemphigus**
   f. **Drug induced pemphigus**
8. **Clinical features:**

	Pemphigus vulgaris	Pemphigus foliaceus
Skin lesion	1. Persistent painful oral erosions & they are large and deep. 2. Followed by multiple vesicles over trunk and extremities. 3. Lesions grow into flaccid and fragile blisters. 4. Blisters may get infected.	1. Differs from vulgaris by the superficial & small nature of the erosion. 2. The vesicles are thin roofed, rupture easily 3. If left untreated becomes extensive leading to erythroderma and may be fatal. 4. Spares the mucosae
Skin sites	Face, scalp, upper trunk, flexures and periungual	Face, scalp, exposed and seborrhoeic

(Continued)

	Pemphigus vulgaris	Pemphigus foliaceus
Skin around the bullae	Normal	Normal
Bullae	Large, flaccid	Small, flaccid
Erosions	Superficial and large	Superficial and small
Antibody attacks on	Desmoglein 3 (a protein in the epidermal layer) and Desmoglein 1	Desmoglein 1

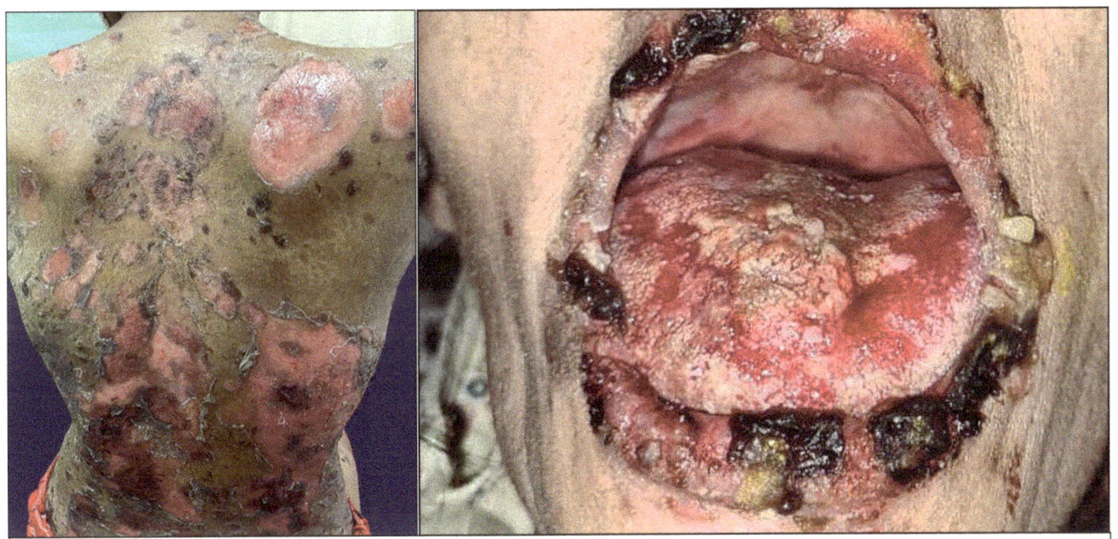

Pemphigus vulgaris

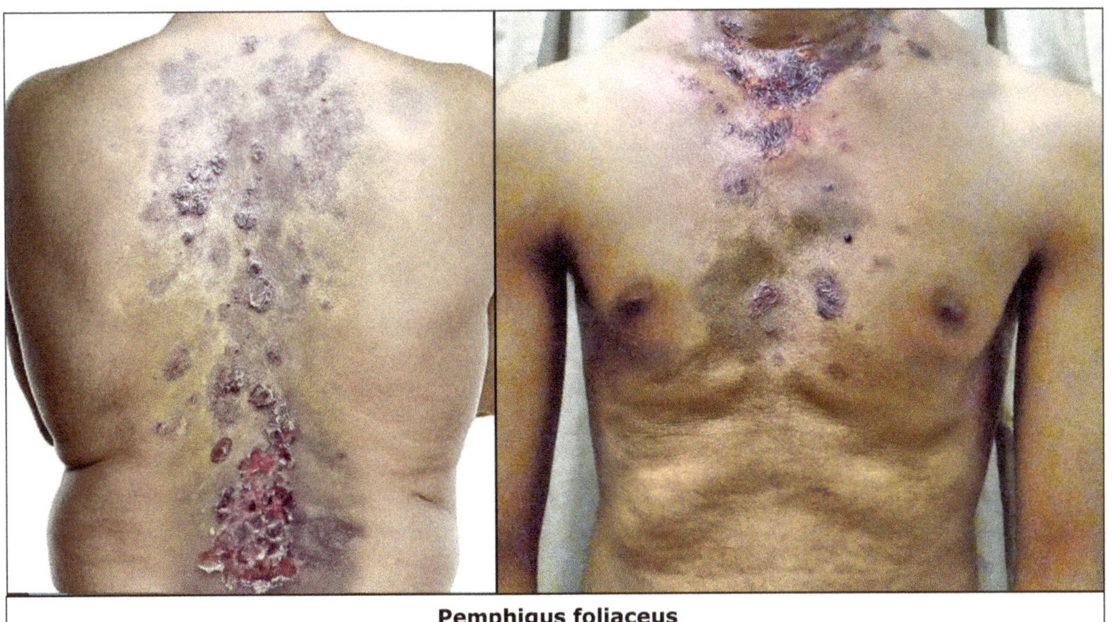

Pemphigus foliaceus

Nikolsky's sign positive: The sign is elicited by applying lateral pressure with thumb on the skin over a bony prominences leading to formation of an erosion.

9. The least common and most severe type of pemphigus is **paraneoplastic pemphigus** (PNP) (This disorder is a complication of cancer).

10. **Diagnosis and investigation:**

    1. **Tzanck smear:** Smear is taken after rupturing an intact blister and scrapping is taken from the base with scalpel on glass slide and stained with giemsa

       It reveals acantholytic cells with large dense nuclei and a rim of cytoplasm.

    2. **Skin biopsy and histopathological examination:**

       a. Biopsy taken from the fresh blister.

       b. On histopathological examination reveals the intraepidermal cleft

       c. The cleft is subcorneal in pemphigus foliaceous and its variants and suprabasal in pemphigus vulgaris and its variants

       d. Direct suprabasal acantholytic cells are seen in the cleft

    3. **Immunofluorescence:** Antibodies appear as IgG deposits along the desmosomes between epidermal cells, & fishnet pattern appears

    4. **ELISA:** Anti-desmoglein (I & III) antibodies can also be detected in a blood sample using the ELISA technique.

11. **Management:**

    a. Hospitalization

    b. Maintain fluid and electrolyte balance

    c. Treatment of Infection by the use of antibiotics

    d. Local anesthetic agent before taking a meal to avoid pain due to oral lesions while eating.

    e. General supportive measures include $KMNO_4$ compresses & application of topical antibiotics.

    f. Immunosuppression:

       1. Systemic steroid: Prednisolone 1-2 mg/kg/day orally

       2. Cytotoxic agents: Cyclophosphamide or azathioprine (1 mg/kg/day) Cytotoxic agents along with corticosteroids reduces the amount of dose of steroids needed.

       3. Intravenous gamma globulin: Intravenous gamma globulin (IVIG) may be useful in severe cases, especially paraneoplastic pemphigus

       4. Rituximab: An anti-CD20 antibody, which can be used

STAPHYLOCOCCAL SCALDED SKIN SYNDROME

1. **Definition:** It is a generalised superficial exfoliative disease caused by the group 2 staphylococcal strain (Staphylococcal aureus in most cases) that elaborates staphylococcal exfoliative toxin resulting in superficial blisters.
2. It is also called as Ritter's disease
3. Both children and adults can be affected
4. Children are more commonly affected than adults.
5. Adults are affected due to associated significant comorbidities such as renal failure, immunosuppressant therapy, hepatic failure, alcoholism, malignancy, or human immunodeficiency virus infection when they are affected.
6. **Clinical features:**
   a. The primary infection begins focally in the conjunctiva, ear, urinary tract or skin.
   b. Initially patients present with systemic symptoms like irritability, malaise and fever, then within 24-48 hours, a very tender rash develops.
   c. The rash typically starts on the face, flexures (groin, axilla, neck, trunk & spares acral and periorificial area)with erythema and fissures, soon after this large thin blisters are formed.
   d. Patient progress to develop diffuse markedly erythematous rash with significant tenderness and then desquamation.
   e. If untreated, extensive loss of surface layer of the skin and which results into fluid loss, electrolyte imbalance & hypothermia.
   f. Finally patient may lead to death due to hypovolemia & severe sepsis.
7. **Diagnosis:**
   a. The diagnosis of SSSS is made **clinically.**
   b. Isolation of S. aureus: from blood, mucous membranes, or skin biopsy
   c. **Skin biopsy:** Reveals separation of the superficial layer of the epidermis **(intraepidermal separation)**
   d. Nikolsky sign: Positive

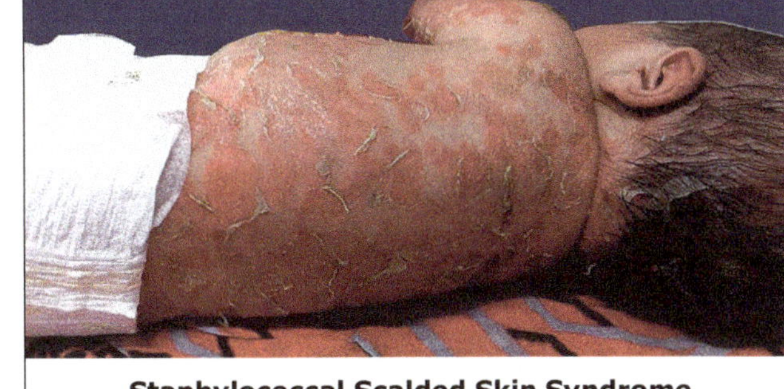

Staphylococcal Scalded Skin Syndrome

8. **Treatment:**
   a. Supportive care
      1. Maintain and electrolyte balance
      2. Antipyretics
      3. Local skin care
   b. Antibiotics
      1. Parenteral antibiotics: Most of the strains have penicillinases

      In penicillin resistant patients: Nafcillin, oxacillin, or vancomycin are used.

HERPES ZOSTER

1. Viral disease characterized by a painful skin rash with blisters in a dermatomal distribution.
2. It occurs due to reactivation of dormant varicella -zoster virus under conditions of stress.
3. It commonly affects elderly persons
4. **Precipitating factors:** Physical or mental stress, or an immunocompromised state like HIV disease or lymphoma or steroids, ultraviolet rays, systemic administration of immunosuppressant.
5. **Clinical features:**
   a. Early symptoms may include fever, malaise, headache
   b. Pain and hyperaesthesia occurs first before development of skin lesions in affected segments.
   c. Pain can be mild to severe in the affected dermatome, with stinging, tingling, aching, numbing or throbbing, and sensations.
   d. Skin lesions appear in one to three groups over 3-5 days.
   e. Grouped vesicles on an erythematous, edematous base in unilateral segmental pattern are typical.
   f. Skin changes limited to a dermatome, normally resulting in a stripe or belt-like pattern that is restricted to one side of the body and does not cross the midline
   g. In an immunocompromised patient more than one dermatome is involved.
   h. In severe cases, such groups of vesicles are very closely placed forming coalescing vesicles with erythematous background.

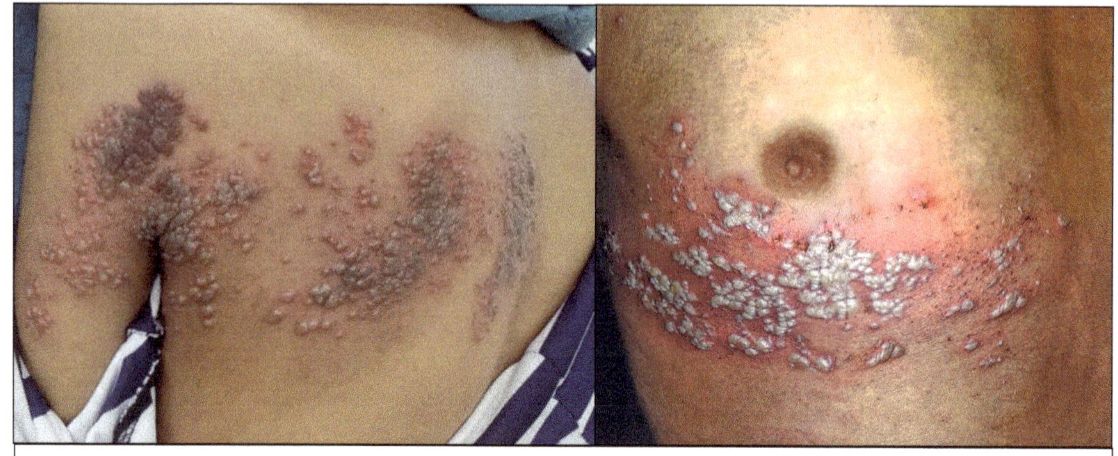

Herpes zoster

i. After a week the tops of vesicles become dry depressed leading to crust formation.

j. Crusts falls off within 10-15 days leaving behind dyspigmentation.

6. **Treatment**

   a. **Antiviral therapy**

      1. Early treatment reduces the postherpetic neuralgia

      2. Dose: oral acyclovir 800 mg 5 times a day for 5 to 7 days with plenty of oral fluids to facilitate renal excretion of drug.

      3. Administered early in the course of disease (within 2-3 days)

   b. **Analgesics**

   c. **Antiepileptics:** Pregabalin, if postherpetic neuralgia disturbing sleep.

   d. **Antibiotics:** for secondary infection with lesions.

7. **Complications**

   a. **Secondary bacterial infections**

   b. **Postherpetic neuralgia**

   c. **Related to nerve segment affected**

      1. **Ophthalmic:** keratoconjunctivitis, extraocular muscle palsy

      2. **Facial:** Facial palsy, deafness, vertigo

      3. **Upper cervical:** Unilateral paralysis of diaphragm

   d. **Systemic complications:** Meningoencephalitis, myelitis and radiculitis

   e. **Ulcerative or gangrenous lesions in severe cases in immunocompromised patients.**

Section 8

Psychiatry Emergencies

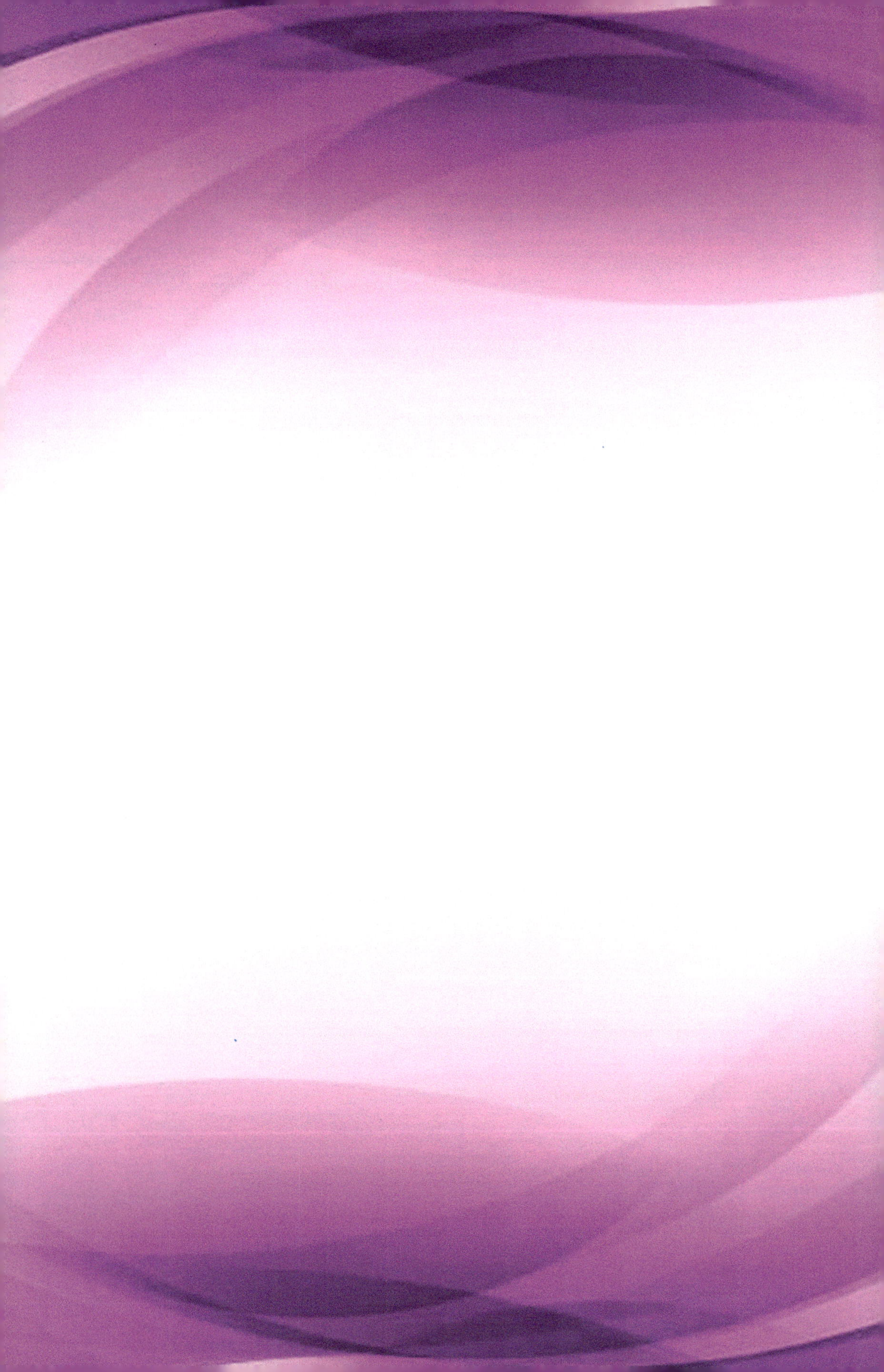

CHAPTER

15 Introduction of Psychiatric Emergencies

SCHEME FOR TAKING PSYCHIATRIC HISTORY

1. **Sociodemographic data (**Name, age, sex, marital status, mother tongue, other languages known, education, occupation, address, income, religion)
2. **Informant (**name, relationship, adequacy of information, reliability of information)
3. **Presenting chief complaints in chronological order**
4. **History of present illness** (Detailed and coherent information of symptoms i.e onset, precipitating factors, course and associated disturbances)
5. **Past psychiatric and medical history**
   a. **Symptoms of each episode, interval period, precipitating factors**
   b. **Treatment history (Drugs, dosage & duration, compliance, resistance to treatment)**
6. **Family history of psychiatric illness/medical illness**
7. **Personal history (birth and early development, behavior during childhood, childhood illness, school, occupational, sexual or marital history, substance use, appetite, bowel, bladder, diet)**

8. **Premorbid personality (Personality prior to beginning of mental illness)**

   It includes social relationship, intellectual activities, mood, character, attitude work and responsibilities, interpersonal relationship, energy, fantasy life and habits)

9. **General and systemic examination**

10. **Mental state examination**

    a. Level of consciousness

    b. Appearance and general behavior

    c. Speech and motor activity

    d. Affect and mood

    e. Thought and perception

    f. Attitude and insight

    g. Cognitive ability (attention, language, memory, constructional ability and praxis, abstract reasoning)

11. **Differential diagnosis**

12. **Diagnosis**

INTRODUCTION OF PSYCHIATRIC EMERGENCIES

1. **Definition:**A psychiatric emergency is any disturbance in thoughts, feelings, or actions for which immediate therapeutic intervention is necessary.
2. Emergency physicians are usually focused on evaluating and treating non-psychiatric patients in the ED.
3. Lack of experience is a problem in management of psychiatric emergencies.
4. Negative attitude towards the psychiatric patient may lead to poor patient outcomes.
5. The most important question for the emergency doctor to know is whether the problem is medical, psychiatric or both.
6. We can differentiate medical condition from psychiatric illness with help of detailed history, physical examination, mental status examination & investigations of patient.
7. Features that points the medical cause rather than psychiatric cause
   a. **Acute onset**
   b. **Geriatric age**
   c. **First episode**
   d. **Medical illness history**
   e. **Neurological symptoms** like LOC, head injury, vomiting, change in vision
   f. **Classic neurological signs** include diminished alertness, disorientation, impairment of concentration, memory impairment, impairment in attention, concentration.
   g. **Other neurological signs** include disturbances in speech, movement, gait
   h. **Constructional apraxia:** inability to draw the clock or cube.
8. Medical conditions such as diabetes mellitus, thyroid disease, acute intoxications, withdrawal states, head injury can present with significant altered mental status which mimic psychiatric illness.
9. Such medical conditions may be life-threatening if not treated promptly.
10. After medical clearance, if we understand that the cause of illness is psychiatric then go for proper psychiatric evaluation
11. The other part of the psychiatric evaluation is to place patient into one of three risk categories: low (can be discharged home); moderate/(needs further psychiatric assessment); and high (inpatient psychiatric admission indicated)
12. The physician must make an initial diagnosis, identify the precipitating factors and immediate needs and treatment.
13. Suicidal behavior and severe behavioral disturbances are two commonly faced conditions in the emergency department.

SUICIDAL PATIENTS

1. According to WHO definition, suicide is a deliberate act to end ones life.
2. The highest rate of suicide is seen in younger age groups i.e. < 30 years of age.
3. The suicide risk is highest for primary psychiatric disorder, substance use disorder and least for organic disorders
4. Depression accounts for nearly half the number of patients committing suicide followed by alcohol abuse and schizophrenia.
5. **Presentation to emergency department**

Attempted suicide	Self harm under influence of substance	Self harm in response to an inner cry for help
Impulsive in response to trigger (inner or external) Secondary to underlying depressive or mood disorder Secondary to underlying psychiatric process in response to commanding hallucinations E.g Patients with schizophrenia	Intoxication or withdrawal from substance e.g alcohol intoxication presenting with suicidal burn	An attempt to draw attention towards inner psychological distress (Parasuicidal behavior) Intent of die may be low e.g in certain personality disorders like borderline personality disorder

6. **Assessment of suicidal behavior includes**
   a. A thorough psychiatric examination with special focus on identifying risk and protective factors along with identifying modifiable risk factors

   Risk factors for suicides (As per national strategy for suicide prevention: goals and objectives for action 2001)

Biopsychosocial risk factors	Environmental risk factors	Sociocultural risk factors
1. Presence of psychiatric disorder, alcohol or substance abuse disorders 2. Hopelessness 3. High risk behavior e.g. rage, anger 4. A history of psychological trauma or abuse 5. Major physical illness malignancy 6. A family history of suicide 7. History of previous suicide attempts	1. Job and financial losses 2. Relational or social losses	1. Lack of social support and sense of isolation 2. Stigma associated with help seeking behavior 3. Barrier to accessing healthcare, especially treatment for mental health and substance abuse 4. Socio-cultural beliefs

   b. Specific enquiry about suicidal thoughts, plans and behaviors

Warning signs	**a. Thoughts:** Hopelessness, feeling trapped in problems, no reason for living, having no sense of purpose in life **b. Behavior:** Rage, anger, revenge seeking behavior, engaging in dangerous tasks without thinking, as if there is no way out, increase in consumption or drug abuse, anxiety, inability of sleep or sleeping all the time, withdrawing from friends, family, or society.
History	Past history of psychiatric illness, family history of mental illness or suicidal behavior, past medical or surgical history, past history of suicidal behavior

c. Determine the degree of suicidal risk i.e. low, moderate and high

7. **Management:**

a. Most suicides among psychiatric patients are preventable, if properly assessed or treated.

b. **The main goals in management with suicidal behaviors are–**

1. To diagnose and treat the underlying medical complication which may predispose patient to suicidal attempt or suicidal behavior.
2. To protect patient from self harm till the suicide crisis is over.
3. To diagnose and treat the underlying psychiatric illness predisposing the patient to suicidal behavior.
4. To resolve the acute problem that precipitated the present suicidal crisis

c. **The decision to hospitalize a patient depends on**

1. Risk of self harm which may take place soon
2. Severity of underlying psychiatric illness
3. Presence of active suicidal ideation
4. Patient's living status
5. Patient's and the family's ability to deal with crisis & social support
6. Risk factors for suicide.

d. Not all such patients require hospitalization; some can be treated on an outpatient basis.

e. In a hospital, patients can receive antidepressant or antipsychotic medications as indicated, individual therapy, group therapy, family therapy, social support and sense of security.

f. Antidepressants are necessary for treatment of depressive patients.

g. Mood stabilizers and antipsychotic medications are useful in the treatment of bipolar patients and those with psychotic depression.

h. ECT may be needed for some severely depressed patients, or in those with strong suicidal ideation.

AGITATED AND VIOLENT PATIENTS

1. Aggression, violence, psychomotor excitement, and agitation can be clinical presentations of many underlying conditions ranging from medical disorder to a variety of mental illnesses.
2. The risk of violence is especially high in those communities where there is easy availability to alcohol/substance abuse such as cocaine, amphetamine.
3. **Common causes of aggression and violence**
    a. Schizophrenia
    b. Mania, hypomania, depression
    c. Personality disorder especially antisocial type/Borderline personality disorder
    d. Alcohol intoxication or withdrawal
    e. Substance intoxication with cocaine, amphetamines
    f. Substance withdrawal
    g. Organic mental disorder and brain damage, epilepsy and dementia
    h. Post traumatic stress disorder (Less common)
    i. Child and adolescent behavior disorders
4. Persons who are paranoid or in a state of catatonic excitement require tranquilization.
5. Agitated patients are managed based on
    a. Control aggression
    b. Underlying psychiatric diagnosis
6. **Management:**
    a. Prevention of assault on health workers:
    1. Adequate security staff to control the patient, if needed.
    2. Access to examination rooms and treatment areas should be limited
    3. Preventive measures to prevent an assault on our health care workers includes give respect and always be polite with patient, keep safe distance and remove nearby dangerous objects.
    4. Restraints are used as a last option when patients are less likely to control themselves and do not respond to other measures of behavioral control.
    5. Patients may be restrained temporarily for a small time period.

    b. Drugs used for controlling aggression
    1. If the patient is willing to take drugs then give orally, however, usually the

parenteral route is necessary.

2. **Lorazepam 2 mg** given intramuscularly is effective dosage up to a maximum of 10 mg & it is equally effective as haloperidol.
3. The most commonly used drug is **haloperidol 5-10 mg** which is given as a single dose in combination with **promethazine 25-50 mg** intramuscularly has a tranquilising as well as sedative effect.
4. Give intravenous medication with great care to avoid respiratory arrest.

c. Once the patient comes under control, then carry out a careful physical examination, detailed history from relatives, laboratory investigations to know the cause of violent behavior.

d. Once the diagnosis is made from history the specific treatment is initiated based on underlying psychiatric diagnosis.

MANIC EPISODE

1. **Manic episode:** An elevated, expansive, or irritable mood is the hallmark of a manic episode.
2. This period of abnormal mood must last at least 1 week
3. Hypomania is an episode of manic symptoms that does not meet the criteria of mania.
4. Onset may be acute or insidious
5. **Etiology:**
   a. Manic disorders can arise spontaneously or follow depressive illness, surgery, infection, substance intoxication or withdrawal
   b. Disturbed sleep, childbirth, unfavorable/difficult life condition
   c. Antidepressant medication, amphetamines can precipitate manic episodes.
   d. Family history of bipolar mood disorder
   e. Seasonal changes: Some patients experience hypomania and mania in spring season.
6. **Clinical features:**
   a. Heightened, grandiose or agitated mood
   b. Over Cheerfulness
   c. Over-talkative
   d. Hyperactive
   e. Sleeplessness/decreased need of sleep
   f. Flight of ideas
   g. Easily distracted
   h. Exaggerated self esteem
   i. High risk activity, impaired judgment
7. **Mental state examination:**
   a. **Appearance and general behavior:**
      1. Patient's appearance is flamboyant and tends to attract attention
      2. Excited, over talkative and frequently hyperactive
      3. Some are grossly psychotic and have severe behavioral disturbance so require physical restraints and sedatives.

b. **Mood, Affect and Feelings:**
   1. Mood is usually described as great or happy
   2. Affect is usually elevated, expansive or euphoric

c. **Speech and thought:**
   1. Their speech is often disturbed
   2. More intense, speech becomes louder, more rapid, and difficult to interpret.
   3. Speech is filled with puns, jokes, rhymes, plays on words, and irrelevancies.
   4. Delusion of grandeur is commonly associate.

d. **Cognition:** Cognitive functioning in the manic state is impaired.

e. **Perceptual Disturbances:**
   1. May have hallucination

f. **Impulse control: Impaired**

g. **Judgment and Insight:**
   1. Impaired judgment is a hallmark of manic patients.
   2. Manic patients also have little insight.

8. **Treatment: (Psychotherapy and Pharmacotherapy)**
   1. Hospitalizations
   2. Restraints, if necessary
   3. **Acute mania: Benzodiazepines/antipsychotics (Olanzapine) for behavioral control**
   4. **Prophylaxis of mania: Lithium/Mood stabilizer**

PANIC ATTACK

1. **An acute intense attack of anxiety accompanied by feelings of impending doom is known as panic attack**
2. Panic disorder is an anxiety disorder characterized by recurrent unexpected panic attacks
3. It lasts from minutes to hours.
4. It can occur in other psychiatric illnesses such as phobias, post traumatic stress disorder (PTSD).
5. Panic attack can occurs due physiological effect of substance (e.g. a drug of abuse, a medication) or in medical disorders such as endocrine disorder (e.g. Hypo- and hyperthyroidism, hyperparathyroidism, hypoglycemia associated with insulinomas), Cardiopulmonary disorders (e.g. acute myocardial infarction, arrhythmias, chronic obstructive pulmonary disease, and asthma)
6. **Clinical features:**
   a. The first panic attack is often completely spontaneous.
   b. After the first attack patient constantly worries about repeated attacks and tries to avoid situations that can cause an attack.

Psychological symptoms	Physical symptoms
1. Extreme fear 2. Sense of impending doom/fear of dying 3. Derealization (feelings of unreality) or depersonalization (being detached from one-self/going crazy)	1. Palpitations, pounding heart, or accelerated heart rate 2. Sweating 3. Shaking 4. Sensations of shortness of breath or unable to inhale 5. Feeling of choking 6. Chest pain or discomfort 7. Abdominal discomfort 8. Feelings dizzy, unsteady, light headed or faint 9. Paresthesias (numbness or tingling sensations)

   c. A formal mental status examination during a panic attack may reveal that the patient has continuous repetitive thoughts (rumination), difficulty speaking (e.g., stammering), and impaired memory.
   d. Patient may have fear of death due to cardiac or respiratory problems during panic attack.
   e. Hyperventilation can produce respiratory alkalosis due to more CO_2 wash out during rapid and deep breathing.

f. Breathing into a paper bag or using that mask allows you to rebreathe CO_2 will helps to reduce respiratory alkalosis.

g. Depressive symptoms are commonly associated with the panic disorder.

7. **Treatment:**

   a. The two most effective treatments are Pharmacotherapy and cognitive-behavioral therapy.

   b. Family and group therapy

   c. In acute attack: Benzodiazepines give quick relief.

      e.g. Alprazolam, clonazepam

   d. All SSRIs are effective for panic disorder.

   e. Paroxetine and paroxetine CR (SSRI) are often preferred.

8. When pharmacotherapy becomes effective, then treatment should generally continue for 8 to 12 months.

SCHIZOPHRENIA

1. Schizophrenia is one of the most common serious mental disorders
2. The disorder usually begins before the age of 25 years, persists throughout life, and affects persons of all social classes.
3. A combination of genetic and environmental factors play a role in the development of schizophrenia.
4. Environmental factors associated with the development of schizophrenia include the living environment, drug use, and prenatal stressors.
5. **Five subtypes of schizophrenia have been described, predominantly based on clinical presentation (Listed in ICD 10):**
   a. **Paranoid**
   b. **Disorganized**
   c. **Catatonic**
   d. **Undifferentiated**
   e. **Residual**
6. **Diagnosis of schizophrenia is based entirely on the psychiatric history and mental status examination.**
7. **Signs and symptoms**

Positive symptoms	Negative symptoms	Cognitive deficits
1. Delusions 2. Hallucinations 3. Disorganised speech and thinking 4. Purposeless abnormal motor activity or aggressive behavior	1. Reduced expression of emotions via facial expression or by voice 2. Reduced speech 3. Inability to experience pleasure 4. Withdrawal from society 5. Inability to begin and sustain activity 6. Unwillingness in performing daytoday tasks	1. Poor executive functioning 2. Poor working memory 3. Poor attention

8. **Treatment:**
   a. **Antipsychotic medications:** It includes typical (D2 blocker) e.g. Trifluperazine, flupenthixol, haloperidol and atypical antipsychotics (Act via other mechanisms) e.g. clozapine, quetiapine, olanzapine, risperidone.
   b. **Psychosocial interventions:** Including psychotherapy, can increase the clinical improvement.

c. **Hospitalization is indicated for**

    1. Diagnostic purposes
    2. For stabilization of psychiatric drug dosage
    3. To ensure safety of patient and people around them
    4. For grossly impaired or inappropriate behavior, & unble to take care of basic needs.

9. **Treatment of Acute Psychosis phase of schizophrenia:**

    a. Acute psychotic symptoms require immediate attention.

    b. Acute agitation treated with antipsychotics.

    c. Benzodiazepines are used for behavioral management

    d. Hospitalisation, if necessary.

    e. Few important precautions during hospitalisation

        1. Keep away from sharp objects
        2. Close watch on patients
        3. Supervised medications

ACUTE AND TRANSIENT PSYCHOTIC DISORDER

1. These syndromes are to be considered as psychiatric emergencies.
2. The heterogeneous group of acute and transient psychotic disorders are characterized by three typical features, listed below in descending order of priority
   a. **Suddenness of onset (within 2 weeks or less)**
   b. **Presence of typical syndromes with polymorphic (changing and variable) symptoms or typical schizophrenic symptoms**
   c. **Presence of associated acute stress**
3. If abrupt in onset (occurs < 48 hours) then outcome is better.
4. Complete recovery occurs within 3 months of onset or less (i.e. within few days or weeks) & some patients may have persistent & disabling symptoms.
5. **Treatment**
   a. **Short-term treatment:**
      1. **Acute psychotic syndromes needs early hospitalization**
         - To make a careful physical, mental examination and clinical evaluation
         - To isolate the patient from stressful enviroment
         - To reduce the acute psychotic symptoms
      2. **Antipsychotic drugs**
         - Antipsychotic treatment started after physical, mental, clinical evaluation & laboratory findings.
         - Most commonly atypical antipsychotics are used but typical antipsychotics can also be used.
      3. **Benzodiazepines:** Given for behavioral control for short term.
      4. **Frequent monitoring to assess drug response**
      5. **Look for adverse effects of drugs**
      6. **Sociotherapy (occupational or intensive) and psychotherapy (reality–adaptive–supportive).**

ALCOHOL INTOXICATION

1. Acute alcohol intoxication is a condition associated with drinking a large amount of alcohol in a short time.
2. It is a serious medical condition and requires immediate attention.
3. Alcohol depresses the nervous system but initially patient has euphoric effects which is due to suppression of inhibition of cerebral cortex
4. Alcohol intoxication leads to harmful or fatal events i.e. road traffic accidents, machinery accidents and assaults
5. **Signs and symptoms of alcohol intoxication**
   a. Slurred speech
   b. Dizziness
   c. Incoordination
   d. Unsteady gait
   e. Nystagmus
   f. Impairment in attention or memory
   g. Stupor or coma
   h. Double vision
6. **Differential diagnosis:**
   a. Head injury
   b. Hypoglycemia
   c. Postictal phase
   d. Hepatic encephalopathy
   e. Encephalitis
   f. Meningitis
   g. Intoxication of other drugs
7. **Treatment:**
   a. Maintain a patent airway and adequate ventilation
   b. Monitor blood pressure, pulse, respiratory rate, temperature
   c. Check blood sugar for hypoglycemia
   d. Check for head injury
   e. Intravenous fluid with multivitamins and glucose

ALCOHOL WITHDRAWAL

1. Alcohol withdrawal state is a group of symptoms of variable clustering and severity occurring on absolute or relative withdrawal of substance after repeated and usually prolonged and high dose of alcohol.
2. Alcohol withdrawal leads to seizures, delirium and autonomic hyperactivity.
3. Any of three following symptoms:
   a. Tremors of outstretched hand, tongue or eyelids
   b. Sweating
   c. Nausea, vomiting
   d. Tachycardia, hypertension
   e. Psychomotor agitation
   f. Headache
   g. Insomnia
   h. Weakness/malaise
   i. Transient visual, tactile, auditory hallucination or illusions.
   j. Generalised tonic clonic seizure
4. The classic sign of alcohol withdrawal is tremulousness, although the following spectrum of symptoms can be seen.

Alcohol spectrum symptoms	Tremulousness	Psychotic and perceptual symptoms	Seizures	Alcohol delirium
Time since cessation of alcohol drink	6 to 8 hours	8 to 12 hours	12 to 24 hours	First 24 hours

   - Watch for the development of DTs for the first week of withdrawal
5. **Treatment of alcohol withdrawal: Benzodiazepines**

   Choice of benzodiazepines also depends on liver function test
   1. **If deranged: Lorazepam (Preferred)**
   2. **If normal: Chlordiazepoxide, Lorazepam.**

Clinical problems	Drugs
Mild to moderate agitation and tremulousness	Chlordiazepoxide Diazepam
Hallucinations	Lorazepam
Extreme agitation	Chlordiazepoxide
Withdrawal seizures	Diazepam
Delirium tremens	Lorazepam

ALCOHOL WITHDRAWAL SEIZURES

1. Seizures associated with alcohol withdrawal are typically, generalized and tonic-clonic in character.
2. It is difficult to establish an underlying cause of seizures in primary assessment of alcoholic patients in emergency department and hence it needs further evaluation.
3. Role of anticonvulsant medications in the management of alcohol withdrawal seizures is limited.
4. Seizure activity in chronic alcoholic patients should be promptly evaluated for other causative factors, such as head injuries, meningitis, encephalitis, brain tumors cerebrovascular accidents
5. **Treatment:**
   a. The primary medications to control alcohol withdrawal symptoms are the benzodiazepines
   b. Benzodiazepines can be given either orally or parenterally
   c. Carbamazepine can be used in alcohol withdrawal seizure as they have dual action (Anticraving & anticonvulsant).
   d. Multivitamin therapy specially thiamine deficiency is common in patients with chronic alcohol use.
   e. Parenteral thiamine administration is given for a minimum of 5 days in the treatment of patients with alcohol dependence followed by oral thiamine supplementation for 3-6 months.

ALCOHOL DELIRIUM

1. Patients with alcohol withdrawal symptoms should be carefully monitored to prevent progression to withdrawal delirium.
2. This is the most severe form of withdrawal syndrome that occurs within the first week.
3. Alcohol withdrawal delirium is a medical emergency that can be life threatening if not treated properly.
4. Physical illness (e.g., hepatitis or pancreatitis) predisposes to this syndrome more than the person with good physical health
5. **Symptoms:**
   a. Violent or suicidal behavior
   b. Fluctuating orientation and disturbance in attention (Hallmark of delirium)
   c. Hallucinations (Most frequently visual or tactile)
   d. Global confusion
   e. Sleep disturbance
   f. Autonomic hyperactivity clinically manifests as tachycardia, diaphoresis, fever, anxiety, insomnia and hypertension
6. **Treatment:**
   a. The best treatment for DTs is **prevention.**
   b. Benzodiazepine:
      1. Orally 50 to 100 mg of chlordiazepoxide (librium) is given every 4 hourly and if administration of oral medication is not possible then give intravenous benzodiazepines such as lorazepam.

   c. Diet plan: A high-calorie, high-carbohydrate diet, with multivitamins supplementation.
   d. Dehydration correction: Vomiting & dehydration often occurs in alcohol withdrawal which leads to dehydration & it is corrected with oral or intravenous fluids.
   e. Supportive psychotherapy of relatives of patient is an essential part in the treatment of DTs

DELIRIUM (OTHER THAN ALCOHOL)

Definition: It is the most common acute organic mental disorder characterized by an acute decline in the level of consciousness and disorientation as well as disturbance in the perception and restlessness.

1. Sudden in onset (Hours or days)
2. **Clinical features:**
   a. **Emotional instability:** Fear, anger, depression, anxiety, irritability, euphoria or apathy.
   b. **Impairment of consciousness:** Clouding of consciousness ranging from drowsiness to stupor and coma.
   c. **Impairment of attention:** Difficulty in shifting, focusing and sustaining attention.
   d. **Perceptual disturbances:** Illusion, hallucination, most often visual.
   e. **Disturbance of cognition:** Impairment of memory (recent and immediate), abstract thinking and comprehension
   f. **Disturbance in the sleep wake cycle**
3. Rapid improvement occurs in patients when the causative factor is identified and treated.
4. **Etiological factors:**

Central nervous system	Seizures, migraine, head trauma, sub arachnoid hemorrhage, non hemorrhagic stroke, brain tumor, brain abscess, transient ischemic attack, metabolic encephalopathy
Metabolic disorder	Electrolyte abnormalities, diabetes mellitus, hypoglycemia, hyperglycemia or insulin resistance
Systemic illness	a. Infection (e.g. sepsis, malaria, viral, pneumonia, urinary tract infection, syphilis or abscess.) b. Post trauma (e.g. fractures) c. Severe dehydration d. Severe burn e. Heat stroke
Medications	a. Narcotic analgesics b. Antibiotics, antiviral and antifungal c. High dose steroids d. General anesthetic agents e. Antiarrhythmic drugs: e.g. digoxin, disopyramide f. Antihypertensives: Diuretics, beta-blocker g. Central nervous system drugs: Benzodiazepines, tricyclic antidepressants

(Continued)

Cardiac	Heart failure, cardiac arrhythmias, shock, myocardial infarction
Pulmonary	Chronic obstructive pulmonary disorder, hypoxia, hypercapnia
Hematological	Anemia, leukemia, blood dyscrasia.
Renal	Renal failure, SIADH, uremia
Hepatic	Hepatic failure, hepatitis, cirrhosis
Drugs of abuse	Intoxication and withdrawal
Toxins	Intoxication and withdrawal of heavy metals and aluminium

5. **Treatment:**
   a. In treating delirium, the primary goal is to treat the underlying cause
   b. **Pharmacotherapy:**
      1. Pharmacological treatment is used for behavioral management depending on cause and insomnia.
         - **Behavioral management**
           i. **Low dose antipsychotic drugs:** e.g. Haloperidol, Quetiapine
           ii. **Benzodiazepines:** e.g. Lorazepam (especially if there is a history of alcohol dependence and withdrawal)

           Use benzodiazepines with caution in patients with a history of head injury.
         - **Insomnia:** Benzodiazepines with short or intermediate half-lives (e.g., Lorazepam 1 to 2 mg at bedtime) are best used.

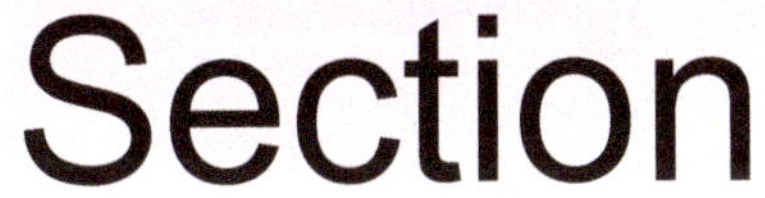

9

Pediatric Emergencies

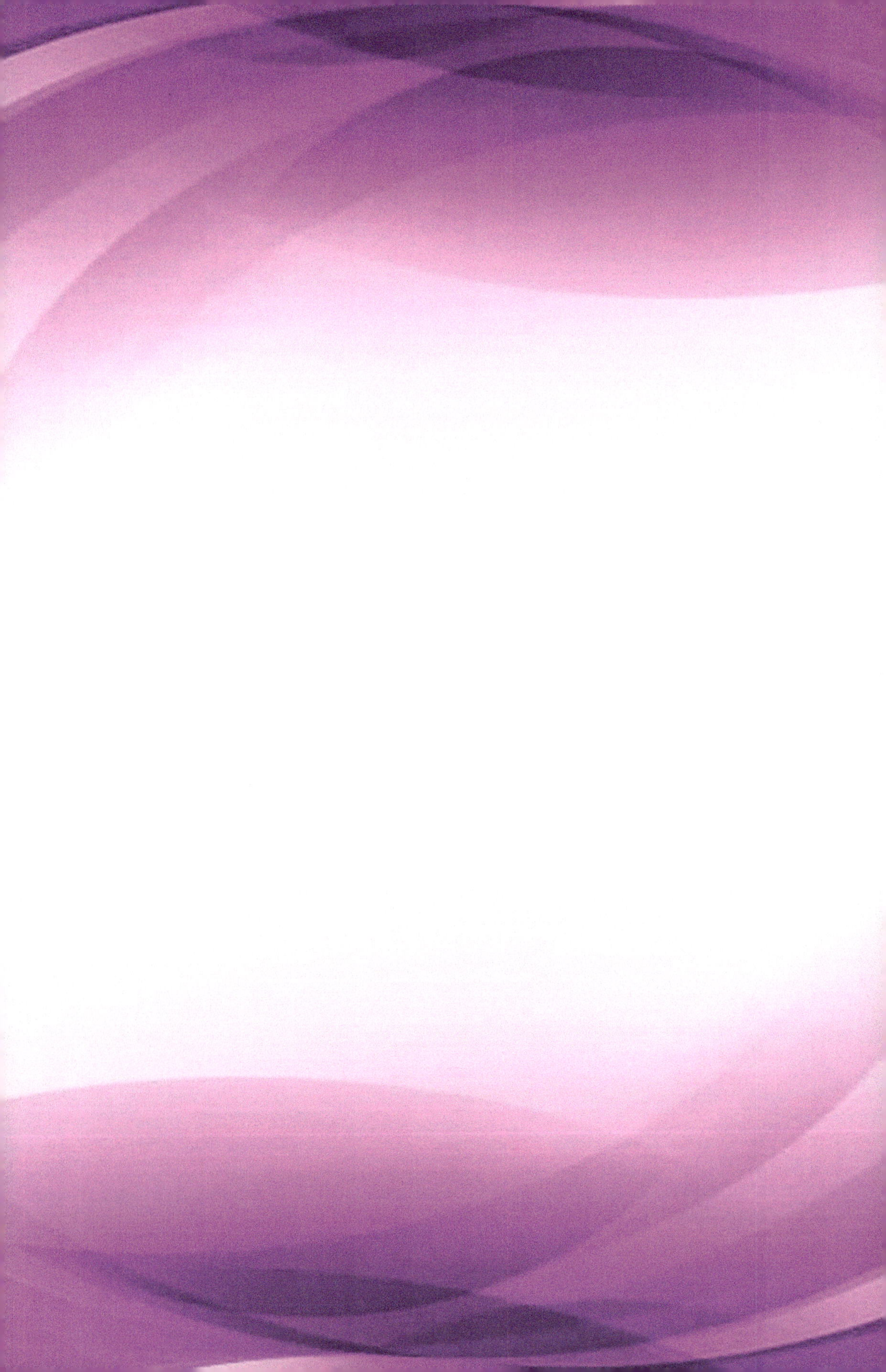

CHAPTER

16 Pediatric Emergencies

ASSESSMENT OF A SICK CHILD

1. Assessment of a sick child is important to recognise the management of a seriously ill child as early as possible.
2. **Assessment of sick child includes**
    a. Pediatric assessment triangle: Appearance, breathing and circulation
    b. Primary survey based on basic life support (ABCDE)
    c. Secondary survey (Detailed physical examination, vital signs, focused examination)
    d. Ongoing assessment
3. **Pediatric assessment triangle/first impression**

Appearance	Assessment is done under TICLS mnemonic	
	Tone	**I**s the child active, moving around lethargic?
	Interaction (Mental status)	**H**ow alert is the child? **I**s the child interested in interacting with the surrounding or the caretaker (mother)?
	Consolability	**C**an the child be comforted by the caretaker?
	Look	**D**oes the child have a fixed gaze or glassy-eyed stare? (Dull, dazed, or uncomprehending expression)

(Continued)

	Speech/cry	Strong and vigorous or weak or hoarse?
	Tone	Is child active, moving around
Breathing	Check adequacy of airway, oxygenation and ventilation. Chest movement and breathing pattern Listen for abnormal air sounds Look for signs of increased work of breathing	
Circulation to skin	Look at the skin and mucous membrane for abnormal color	

4. Primary survey (Assessment and management done simultaneously)

It is helpful to detect immediate life threatening problems that can compromise basic life functions

Airway	Check the patency of airway Look for signs of obstruction (e.g. stridor, dyspnea, hoarseness of voice) If the child is unresponsive and cannot talk, cry or cough, evaluate for possible airway obstruction. Look inside the mouth for any foreign body and if present remove it under direct vision. If a foreign body is suspected but not visualised, a combination of back blows and chest thrusts is recommended in infants and In older children back blows in a forward leaning position is recommended Use airway adjuvants to maintain patency of airway Intubation to provide optimum condition and to minimise the potential for aspiration.
Breathing	Position of child (Flat, tripod, sniffing) Is nasal flaring present? Uses accessory muscles of breathing or minimal movement of chest wall Is there sternal, supraclavicular, substernal, or intercostal retraction present? Cyanosis present or not Respiratory rate Auscultation of chest for abnormal sounds
Circulation	To assess cardiovascular function and tissue perfusion. Pulse rate, volume of pulse (weak or strong), Capillary refilling time Extremities cool or warm Is skin color normal, pale, mottled?

(Continued)

Mental status	Level of consciousness seen by AVPU mnemonic.	
	Alert	Not necessarily oriented to time and place or neurologically normal.
	Verbal	Not fully awake only responsive to verbal stimuli
	Pain	Only responds to painful stimuli and is difficult to wake up.
	Unresponsive	Unresponsive to any stimuli, completely unconscious.
Exposure	**P**roper exposure of the child is necessary for completing the initial physical assessment. **I**t is necessary to see any type of rash, fever, injury and swelling. **I**t is helpful for completion of initial physical examination.	

5. **Secondary survey (Focuses on advanced life support interventions and management)**

   Help to detect less immediate threats to life

Complete history	SAMPLE mnemonic.
	Signs/symptoms: Onset and nature of symptoms, signs of Respiratory distress as per age. **A**llergies:Known drug reaction **M**edications: Exact names, doses and frequency of drugs, and timing of last dose **P**ast history:Previous illness and Immunisation **L**ast food and liquid intake

6. **Ongoing assessment:** To assess the effectiveness of the emergency interventions provided and identify any missed injuries or conditions.

CROUP

1. Croup is a viral infection of the upper respiratory tract
2. It is the most common cause of upper airway obstruction.
3. The viral infection leads to swelling inside the trachea which interferes with normal breathing.
4. The most severe form develops with bacterial superinfection which may extend from the larynx & trachea to the bronchus.
5. It occurs most commonly among the ages of 6 months to 3 years.
6. Croup usually worsens at night.
7. **Signs and symptoms:**
   a. **Signs**
      1. Tachypnea
      2. Tachycardia
      3. Cyanosis
      4. Air entry may be normal, decreased, minimal or absent.
      5. **Steeple on X-ray:** Edema develops which narrows the airway lumen.

   b. **Symptoms**
      1. Classic symptoms of croup include barking cough, stridor and a hoarse voice.
      2. Low grade fever
      3. Runny nose
8. These symptoms are mild, moderate or severe.
9. Viral croup score depends on stridor, air entry, retractions (suprasternal, sternal, subcostal), cyanosis and level of consciousness.
10. **Westley croup score:**

Chest wall retraction	None	0
	Mild	+1
	Moderate	+2
	Severe	+3
Stridor	None	0
	With agitation	+1
	At rest	+2

(Continued)

Cyanosis	None	0
	With agitation	+4
	At rest	+5
Level of consciousness	Normal	0
	Disoriented	+5
Air entry	Normal	0
	Decreased	+1
	Markedly decreased	+2

11. If croup score > 7 it indicates ICU admission and nebulization of adrenaline and steroids.
12. The first step is to exclude other obstructive conditions of the upper airway, especially epiglottitis, a foreign body, subglottic stenosis, angioedema, retropharyngeal abscess and bacterial tracheitis.
13. **Management**

Mild croup	Moderate	Severe
Regular observation **M**inimal interference **C**ontinue feed **S**teroids	**F**requent observation **M**inimal interference **N**il by mouth, IV fluids **A**BC assessment **H**umidified oxygen **I**nhalation of nebulized adrenaline	**A**void instrumentation of the throat and excess handling to avoid complete obstruction. **N**il by mouth, IV fluids **A**BC assessment **H**umidified oxygen **I**nhalation of nebulized adrenaline **I**V steroids **I**ntubate if the patient is in impending respiratory arrest.

14. **Dose of steroids:**

    Dexamethasone 0.6 mg/kg stat, repeat 0.2 mg/kg/dose 12 hourly in moderate and 8 hourly in severe cases

    Nebulized budesonide: 2 mg in 4 ml NS used in single dose

    Prednisolone: 1-2 mg/kg/day x 24 hours.

15. **Nebulized adrenaline**
    a. If a patient is having severe symptoms, 3 doses of adrenaline given at 20 min intervals.
    b. Adrenaline is indicated in patients with severe stridor and retractions at rest.
16. If oxygen is needed, avoid agitation by the mask and give oxygen by holding the oxygen source near the child's face.

17. Indication for intubation in croup

a. Need for oxygen/cyanosis despite supportive treatment.
b. Lethargy/drowsiness
c. Marked respiratory distress with severe obstruction
d. Increased work of breathing with decreased intensity of stridor.

EPIGLOTTITIS

1. Inflammation of epiglottitis resulting most commonly from bacterial infections or a non infectious process like inhalation or caustic burn.
2. Acute in onset
3. It is a true medical emergency which may cause complete airway obstruction
4. Occurs most commonly between 3 and 7 years of age & is rare in infancy.
5. Intensity of symptoms are the same throughout the day but in croup the increase in the evening/night hours.
6. **Signs and symptoms**
   a. **Symptoms**
      1. High grade fever
      2. Change in voice
      3. Dysphagia
      4. Toxic appearance
      5. Drooling of saliva
      6. Anxiety
      7. May be sitting in tripod position (Leaning forward with weight on out-stretched hands)

   b. **Signs**
      1. Tachypnea
      2. Tachycardia
      3. Inspiratory Stridor
      4. Pale, mottled, Cyanotic skin
      5. Neck swelling and tenderness may present
7. **Investigation:**

   X-ray lateral view of neck: Shows engorged epiglottitis (a "thumbprint sign")
8. **Diagnosis**
   a. Diagnosis is clinical.
   b. It may be confirmed by direct inspection using a laryngoscope, showing large, cherry red and swollen epiglottitis.
   c. As this may provoke airway spasms, it should be performed in an intensive care unit.

9. **Management**

   a. **Limit agitation**

   b. **Oxygen supplementation:** To avoid agitation by the mask, give oxygen by holding the oxygen source near the child's face

   c. **Dose of steroids:**

      1. **Dexamethasone** 0.6 mg/kg stat, repeat 0.2 mg/kg/dose 12 hourly in moderate and 8 hourly in severe cases

      2. **Nebulized budesonide:** 2 mg in 4 ml NS used in single dose

   d. **Nebulized adrenaline**

      1. If a patient is having severe symptoms, 3 doses of adrenaline are given at 20 min intervals.

      2. Adrenaline is indicated in patients with severe stridor and retractions at rest.

   e. Take assistance from ENT surgeons and anesthetists

   f. If the patient is not improving then consider early intubation by the use of inhalational anesthesia.

   g. Nasotracheal intubation is prefered.

   h. **IV antibiotics:** Such as ceftriaxone and possibly vancomycin or clindamycin can be given. If an allergy to penicillins is present, trimethoprim/sulfamethoxazole or clindamycin can be given as an alternative.

BRONCHIOLITIS

1. It is an acute inflammatory disease of lower respiratory tract which results in the obstruction in small airways in lungs which occur due to viral infection.
2. Seasonal viruses are responsible for bronchiolitis and respiratory syncytial virus (RSV), Rhinovirus, Parainfluenza viruses, Influenza virus, Adenovirus and Coronavirus. RSV is the most common cause.
3. Occurs in early childhood
4. The duration of illness in children with age < 2 years is 5-21 days
5. Two pathological processes result into lower airways obstruction
   a. Inflammatory edema of mucosal lining of bronchus which results in narrowing
   b. Excess mucus production
6. **Signs and symptoms:**
   a. **Symptoms**
      1. Running nose
      2. Low/high grade fever
      3. Dry cough
   b. **Signs**
      1. Agitation
      2. Inspiratory or expiratory wheeze
      3. Cyanosis
      4. Intercoastal or suprasternal retraction
      5. Tachypnea
      6. Tachycardia
      7. Increased work of breathing such as nasal flaring or grunting that develops over one to three days
      8. Signs of dehydration
      9. Low oxygen saturation
7. **Signs and symptoms of severe disease**
   a. Poor feeding
   b. Significant decreased activity in patient
   c. Oxygen saturation < 92% on room air
   d. Tachypnea

   e. Increased work of breathing (accessory muscle use)
   f. Decreased urine output
   g. Cyanosis

8. **Differential diagnosis**
   a. Congestive cardiac failure
   b. Bacterial pneumonia
   c. Foreign body aspiration
   d. Cystic fibrosis
   e. Congenital lung anomaly

9. **Management**
   a. Supportive care is important in bronchiolitis (supplemental oxygen therapy, IV fluids)
   b. Nebulized bronchodilators (epinephrine/salbutamol), Nebulized Hypertonic saline, Dexamethasone + Inhaled epinephrine are effective in management.
   c. ICU admission of patients with signs and symptoms of severe disease monitoring.
   d. Monitor for signs of impending respiratory failure (Increased work of breathing, inability to maintain oxygen saturation or a rising PCO_2)
   e. **Oxygen therapy and mechanical ventilation**
      1. Supplementation of oxygen, if saturation less than 92%
      2. Humidified high flow nasal cannula or nasal CPAP.
      3. Decision to start positive pressure ventilation depends on the clinical condition of the patient.
      4. If required then intubate the patient
   f. **Nebulisation with saline:** To reduce the airway edema.
   g. **Nebulized with ipratropium in patient age < 6 months, salbutamol for patients with age > 6 months:**
      1. Smooth muscles relaxant (more useful in the asthmatic patient to reduce bronchospasm and for patient with age > 6 months since before this age, smooth muscles are not developed).
      2. Single nebulisation is given and observed for improvement in air entry, decreased work of breathing and oxygen saturation
      3. If yes, further doses are administered.

h. **Nebulisation with adrenaline:**

1. Used to reduce the edema of bronchial mucosa by vasoconstriction
2. Given 2-4 hourly with saline, only if there is clinical improvement after first nebulisation (dose 0.5 ml/kg with saline)

i. **Nutrition and fluid therapy**

1. Maintaining the hydration is very important in bronchiolitis
2. Hydration correction is done by using nasogastric tube or IV fluids
3. Monitor continuously the sodium, potassium and hydration.

j. Antibiotics are useful in patients with sepsis and in those whose radiological findings suggest progressive infiltrative changes.

ASTHMA

1. In acute severe asthma patients have progressively worsening bronchospasm and respiratory dysfunction which fails to respond to conventional therapy.
2. Acute asthma exacerbation is a frequent cause of emergency department visits.
3. Airway obstruction occurs in patients due to hyper-responsiveness of the airway to various allergens.
4. The most common triggers for asthma exacerbations in both younger and older children are viral respiratory tract infections.
5. **Signs and symptoms that defines severe asthma attack**
   a. Altered level of consciousness
   b. Inability to speak or feed
   c. Severely diminished or absent breath sounds
   d. Use of accessory muscles while breathing
   e. Tachypnea and tachycardia
   f. Low oxygen saturation on pulse oximetry
6. **Clinical features**
   a. Signs
      1. Tachypnea
      2. Tachycardia
      3. Use of accessory muscles of respiration
      4. Altered mental status due to hypoxemia
      5. Extent and loudness of wheezing (chest becomes silent in severe asthma)

   b. Symptoms: Symptoms are usually worse at night and in the early morning or in response to exercise or cold air.
      1. Difficulty in breathing
      2. Unable to talk and feed
      3. Chest tightness
      4. Coughing
7. **Assessment of severity**
   a. Depends on the neurological status, physical exhaustion, inability to complete a sentence, cyanosis, accessory muscle use, air entry, loudness of wheeze, ABG, heart rate and respiratory rate

b. On that basis patient is classified into mild/moderate, severe and danger signs

c. In mild or moderate asthma patient may need admission

d. In severe asthma, patient may need ICU admission

e. In severe asthma with danger signs patient may need ICU admission with intubation.

8. **Diagnosis:**

Diagnostic steps for asthma:

1. **Patient with respiratory symptoms (Typical of asthma)**

   If no typical symptoms of asthma then take further history and do tests for alternative diagnosis.

2. **Detailed history/examination for asthma (To support diagnosis)**

3. **Perform spirometry (Support diagnosis)**

4. **The diagnosis should be confirmed and evidence documented for further reference, before starting controller therapy.**

9. **Management of asthma (as per GINA 2019 guidelines):**

Steps	**Preferred controller (To prevent exacerbation and control symptoms)**	**Other controller**	**Reliever**
Step 1	—	Low dose ICS taken whenever SABA taken (Indirect incidence) **Or** Daily low dose ICS.	As needed short -acting β2 agonist (SABA)
Step 2	Daily low dose inhaled corticosteroid **(ICS)**	Daily low dose inhaled corticosteroid Leukotriene receptor antagonist (LTRA) or Low dose ICS taken whenever SABA taken	As needed short acting β2 agonist (SABA)
Step 3	Low dose ICS-LABA or medium dose ICS	Low dose ICS +LTRA	As needed short acting β2 agonist (SABA)
Step 4	Medium dose ICS -LTRA Refer for expert advice	High dose ICS-LABA or add on tiotropium, or add on LTRA	As needed short acting β2 agonist (SABA)
Step 5	Refer for phenotypic assessment ± add-on therapy, e.g. anti-IgE	Add-on anti-IL5, or add-on low dose OCS, but consider side-effects	As needed short acting β2 agonist (SABA)

Acute asthma Management includes:

	Acute Severe
Oxygen	**Supply to maintain O_2 > 92%**
Salbutamol	**Nebulisation with salbutamol** (3 doses with 20 min. Interval) **Respule:** (1 respule =0.63 mg) **Solution:** Wt < 20 kg: 0.5 ml with 3 ml NS Wt > 20 kg: 1 ml with 3 ml NS
Ipratropium nebulization	**Given with salbutamol** < 1 year: 0.5 ml > 1 year: 1 ml
Steroids	**IV methylprednisolone** **Dose:** 2 mg/kg stat then 1 mg/kg 6 hourly
Adrenaline	0.1 ml/kg (1:10, 000) SC 20 min interval for maximum 3 doses
Terbutaline	0.005 to 0.01 ml/kg SC 20 min interval for maximum 3 doses
Magnesium sulfate	IV 50 mg/kg in 10 ml nS over 30 minutes
Terbutaline infusion	0.05 -01 ug/kg/min infusion, reduce dose if HR is increased by more than 20/min or ST changes
Aminophylline	Loading dose 5-10 mg/kg/hr followed by 0.5 -1.0 mg/kg/hr
Mechanical intubation	Required in patients with danger signs

DEHYDRATION

1. **Dehydration is defined when the patient having a total body water deficit associated with disruption of metabolic processes.**
2. It occurs when the total body water loss is greater than intake.
3. **Causes of dehydration**
   a. **Related to intake**
      1. Poor feeding
   b. **Related to loss**
      1. Acute gastroenteritis
      2. Vomiting
      3. Burns
      4. Diabetes
4. **Types of dehydration**
   a. **Mild:** Total body water fluid loss reaches 5% or less
   b. **Moderate:** Total body water fluid loss reaches 5-10%
   c. **Severe:** Total body water fluid loss reaches more than 10%
5. **Clinical features**

Clinical features	Mild	Moderate	Severe
Mental status	Consciousness, alert	Normal, drowsiness, irritable, restless	Unconsciousness, lethargic, apathetic
Eyes	Normal	Slightly shrunken	Deeply shrunken
Tears	Present	Decreased	Absent
Mouth and tongue	Moist	Dry	Parched
Thirst	Thirsty, drinks normally	Thirsty, eager to drink	Drink poorly;unable to drink
Skin folds	Instant recoil	Recoil in < 2 sec	Recoil in > 2 sec
Extremities	Warm	Cold	Cold, mottled, cyanotic.
Capillary refill	Normal	Prolonged	Prolonged
Heart rate	Normal	Normal to increased	Tachycardia, bradycardia in most severe cases
Respiration rate	Normal	Normal to fast	Deep

6. **Management**

   a. **Child with no dehydration (< 5%), gets treatment Plan A.**

   b. **Child with mild-moderate dehydration (5-10%), gets treatment Plan B.**

   c. **Child with severe dehydration (> 10%), gets treatment Plan C.**

Therapeutic options	**Mild dehydration (plan A)**	**Moderate dehydration (plan B) (Hospitalisation)**	**Severe dehydration (plan C) (Hospitalisation)**
Oral fluids	More than normal intake	100-200 ml clear fluids within 4-6 hours	Nil
ORS	Optional	75 ml/kg over 3- 4 hours, orally or via nasogastric tube	20 ml/kg/hr for 6 hours (IV fluids preferable as pt.is unable to drink)
Intravenous fluids (RL or NS) can be given after initial bolus after urine is passed	Usually not required	In patients with worsening clinical condition RL or NS 75-100 ml/kg over 3-4 hours	**Infants:** 30 ml/kg in 1st hour 70 ml/kg in next 5 hours **Older children:** 30 ml/kg in 30 min 70 ml/kg in next 2.5 hours Repeat 2nd bolus of 30 ml/kg (If signs of dehydration persist after first bolus)
Maintenance therapy	Usual oral fluids **< 10 kg body weight:** 60–120 ml for each episode of loose motion or vomiting **> 10 kg:** 120–240 ml/episode	Continue ORS for stool replacement and oral feeds **< 10 kg body weight:** 60–120 ml for each episode of loose motion or vomiting **> 10 kg:** 120–240 ml/episode	If child is able to drink, commence clear fluids Maintenance IV fluids may be required along with replacement of stool losses with ORS **< 10 kg body weight:** 60–120 ml for each episode of loose motion or vomiting **> 10 kg:** 120–240 ml/episode
	(Instruction to mother) **B**reast fed babies should be given milk and ORS **G**ive fluids as much as child wants **F**luids like rice water, koko, soup, water, ORS	**C**heck signs of clinical worsening **R**eassess state of dehydration after 4 hours: If improves then Plan A If persistent Plan B If worsening Plan C Give zinc supplement for 10–14 days	**R**eassess the child every 1-2 hours. **If** hydration status is not improving, give the IV fluid more rapidly **St**art ORS as soon as patient is able to drink at 5 ml/kg/hour **C**ontinue to observe child until child has no signs of dehydration, then move to Plan A

ACUTE FEBRILE ILLNESS

1. Fever is the most common symptom due to which many parents bring their children to the emergency department.
2. It can be a result of a simple self limiting infection or a life threatening disorder.
3. It plays an important role in fighting infections and occurs due to release of endogenous pyrogenic mediators called cytokines.
4. Fever can be classified as:
   a. **Mild: 36.8 to 38.3 Degree**
   b. **High: 38.3 to 39.4 Degree**
   c. **Very high: Above 39.4 Degree**
5. **Pattern of fever**

Pattern of fever	Characteristic of fever	Examples
Continuous fever	Fever that does not fluctuate more than 2 degree celsius/F throughout the day	Bacterial pneumonia, infective endocarditis, miliary tuberculosis.
Remittent	Fever that fluctuate more than 2 degree celsius/F, but never comes to normal body temperature throughout the day	Typhoid
Intermittent	Fever that presents only some time of the day with normal temperature in between.	Malaria
Hectic	Fever spike variation between highest and lowest is more than 5 degree celsius/F throughout the day.	Septicemia
Relapsing	Repeated episodes of fever separated by intervals of apparent recovery.	Pel ebstein fever

6. **Causes of fever**
   a. **Viral infection:** Influenza, chicken pox, rubella, measles, infective hepatitis, dengue fever
   b. **Bacterial infection:** Pharyngitis, laryngitis, tonsillitis, typhoid, paratyphoid, urinary tract infection, bacterial endocarditis, tuberculosis, leptospirosis
   c. **Protozoal:** Malaria, Amebic liver abscess
   d. **Post Vaccination fever:** e.g. MMR, measles
   e. **Dehydration:** Excess of fluid loss from body due to AGE

f. **Malignancy:** Hodgkin's lymphoma, leukemia

g. **Iatrogenic:** Injection site abscess, Due to atropinization

h. In neonates until and unless proved otherwise fever is due to septicemia

7. **History:**

a. **History of present illness:** Duration and grade of fever, method of measurement, dose and frequency of antipyretic and associated symptoms to know possible cause.

Possible cause	Associated signs and symptoms
1. Viral infections	Upper respiratory tract infection Non specific viral infection
2. Influenza infection	Cough, arthralgia, headache, anorexia
3. Viral illness with rash	Chicken pox, rubella, measles
4. Otitis media	Earache, hearing loss
5. Tonsillitis	Sore throat, enlarged tonsillar gland
6. Pneumonia	Tachypnea, chest indrawing, crackles on auscultation, cough
7. Septic arthritis	Swelling and painful joints
8. Urinary tract infection	Suprapubic or loin pain, vomiting, dysuria, frequency
9. Blood infection	Toxic shock syndrome, streptococcal or meningococcal septicemia, malaria
10. Kawasaki disease	Vasculitis, large lymph nodes, red eyes, lips, palms and soles

b. **Factors that predispose to infection**

1. **Neonates:** Prematurity, Premature rupture of membranes, positive prenatal test for sexually transmitted diseases, group B streptococcus, cytomegalovirus.

2. **Children:** Recent exposure to infections of caretaker or family members, indwelling catheter, travel history to endemic areas, exposure to animals (mosquitoes, ticks, rats, farm animals, reptiles **).**

c. **Past medical history: Previous history of infections or fever, conditions which predispose to fever** (Congenital heart disease, immunodeficiency, cancers, sickle cell anemia)

d. **Family history:** Autoimmune disorders or hereditary conditions

e. **Drug history:** To rule out drug induced fever

8. **Clinical assessment, investigation and management**

Patients are divided into low, intermediate and high risk depending on signs and symptoms.

	Low risk	Intermediate risk	High risk
Color	Normal color of skin, lip and tongue	Pallor	Pale/mottled/ashen/blue
Activity	**S**tay awake or awaken quickly. **C**hild interested in interacting in surroundings or he/she is playing with a caretaker (mother). **S**ocial smile	**W**akes after prolong stimuli **D**ecreased activity/ Lethargic/Dull **C**hild shows lack of interested in interacting in surroundings or he/she is playing with a caretaker **N**o smile	**W**akes after prolonged stimuli and does not remain awake for a long time/ unresponsive **D**ecreased activity **N**o smile
Hydration	**N**ormal skin and eyes **M**oist mucous membrane	**D**ry skin and mucous membranes **P**oor feeding in infants **R**educed urine output **C**RT more than equal to 3	**D**ry skin and mucous membranes **U**nable to take feed **R**educed skin turgor and urine output
Respiratory	**N**o nasal flaring, grunting **N**o tachypnea **N**o adventitious sounds heard **N**ormal oxygen saturation (97 to 99%)	**N**asal flaring present **T**achypnea (RR > 50 Bpm age 6-12 months, RR > 40 Bpm age > 12 months) **C**repts **O**xygen saturation less than or equal to 95%	**G**runting **T**achypnea (RR > 60 Bpm) **M**oderate to severe chest indrawing **C**yanosis **C**repts **O**xygen saturation less than 90%
Other	**N**o associated signs and symptoms	**H**igh grade fever **F**ever > 5 days **L**ymphadenopathy of sizes more than 2 cm. **S**welling of joint or limbs	**V**ery high grade fever **N**on blanching rash **C**linical bleeding **E**vidence of shock **B**leeding from orifices **N**eck stiffness **S**tatus epilepticus **F**ocal neurological signs **F**ocal seizures

(Continued)

	Low risk	Intermediate risk	High risk
Investigations	Assess for pneumonia Perform a test for urine tract infection. Do not perform routine tests and chest X-rays.	Urine test Complete blood count Blood culture C reactive protein Chest X-ray if respiratory signs and symptoms Lumbar puncture if a child younger than 1 year.	Urine test Complete blood count Blood culture C reactive protein Chest X-ray if respiratory signs and symptoms (Portable) Lumbar puncture Serum electrolyte Blood gas analysis
Management	Outpatient management Oral antipyretics if fever Tepid sponge bath Observe baby for 3 days Explain all dangerous signs and symptoms to the caretaker or relatives.	Admit in ward Oral (If able to take orally)/Parenteral antibiotics Antipyretics Hydration correction Treatment of cause of fever Tepid sponge bath	Admit in ICU Oxygen therapy Parenteral antibiotics **IV** Antipyretics Hydration correction Find and Treatment of cause of fever

Some important points to be remembered:

1. Avoid rational use of antibiotics
2. Lumbar puncture is to be done before first antibiotic dose
3. Use antibiotics depending on pathogenic species responsible in that age group and also based on culture & sensitivity.
4. Age appropriate antibiotics dosing and toxicities must also be considered.
5. Consider optimal duration of antibiotic therapy needed in specific infection to treat.
6. **Some common antibiotics and dosage:**
   a. **Amoxicillin: Milder infection** 25 to 50 mg/kg/day q 8-12 hourly oral **severe infections** 80-100 mg/kg/day orally. (C/I Jaundice, hepatic dysfunction, penicillin allergy)
   b. **Amoxicillin with clavulanic acid:** 25 to 50 mg/kg/day q 8-12 hourly oral and 50–100 mg/kg/day q 6–8 hours IV.

c. **Azithromycin:** 10 mg/kg/day single dose empty stomach oral on day 1 and then 5 mg/kg/day during next 4 days (avoid administration in infants below 6 months)

d. **Cefixime:** 8 mg/kg/day once or twice a day orally for enteric fever 20 mg/kg/day (hypersensitivity to cephalosporin)

e. **Ceftriaxone sodium:** 50–75 mg/kg/day IV q 12–24 hour, for meningitis use 100 mg/kg/day q 12 hourly (C/I penicillin or cephalosporin hypersensitivity and also ceftriaxone is contraindicated before 1 year of age to avoid Hyperbilirubinemia).

f. **Meropenem:** 60 mg/kg/day q 8 hour IV, for neonatal sepsis 20 mg/kg/dose q 12 hours, meningitis 40 mg/kg/dose q 8 hours.

7. **Paracetamol dose:** 10–15 mg/kg/dose oral q 4–6 hours maximum upto 60 mg/kg/dose (C/I hepatic damage and nephropathy).

SEIZURES

1. **Definition:**

   Paroxysmal, sudden, involuntary disturbance in neurological function caused by abnormal or excessive neuronal discharge.

2. **Convulsions:** Visible manifestation of seizures (If seizures manifest as motor Act)

3. **Epilepsy:** Chronic disease diagnosed by more than or equal to 2 unprovoked seizures in a time frame of more than 24 hours.

4. **Types of seizures (Two broad types)**

   a. **Focal seizures:** Abnormal electrical discharge in one or more area of one side of the brain.

   1. **Simple:** Consciousness is not impaired

   2. **Complex:** Consciousness is impaired

   b. **Generalized seizures:** Involves both sides of the brain.

   Patient has loss of consciousness, postictal state.

5. **Causes of seizures**

   a. **Epilepetic seizures**

      1. **Idiopathic** (in most of the patients) unknown cause but presumed genetic.

      2. **Secondary:**

         a. Cerebral vascular occlusion

         b. Cerebral malformation

         c. Cerebral damage (hypoxic, ischemic, congenital infections)

         d. Cerebral tumors

         e. Neurodegenerative disorder

         f. Neurocutaneous syndromes: tuberous sclerosis, neurofibromatosis.

   b. **Non epileptic seizures**

      1. **Febrile seizures**

      2. **Meningitis, encephalitis**

      3. **Metabolic**

         a. Hypoglycemia

         b. Hypocalcemia

         c. Hypomagnesemia

         d. Hypo or hypernatremia

4. **Head injury**
5. **Toxins or poisoning**

6. **Clinical features**

Symptoms (Depend on types of seizure)

a. **Subtle seizures:**
   1. Random or roving eye movement, eye blinking, eyes rolling up, staring look
   2. Sucking, smacking, chewing or protruding tongue
   3. Bicycling or pedalling movement of the leg
   4. Long pause in breathing
   5. Struggling movement

b. **Absence seizures:**
   1. A brief altered state of consciousness and staring episodes.
   2. During seizures the mouth or face may move or the eyes may blink.
   3. Abrupt onset and termination
   4. **Types: Typical and Atypical**

c. **Tonic:**
   1. Stiffening or tightening of the muscles
   2. Increased tone of muscles

d. **Clonic:**

   Rhythmic jerking movements that may involve the muscles of the face, tongue, arms, legs or other regions of the body.

e. **Myoclonic:**

   Sudden jerking in a group of muscles, may occur several times a day.

f. **Generalized tonic clonic:**
   1. Stiffening or tightening of muscles (tonic), rhythmic jerking movements (clonic) of arms & legs, followed by the postical phase.

g. **Infantile spasm:**
   1. Occurs in infants before six months of age.
   2. Mostly observed when the child is waking up, or when they are trying to go to sleep.
   3. The infant usually has brief periods of movement of the neck, trunk, or legs that last for a few seconds.

h. **Febrile seizures:**
   1. Associated with fever
   2. More commonly seen in children between the age of 6 months and 5 years

7. **Diagnosis:**
   a. Detailed history
   b. Eye witness
   c. Video if available

8. **Investigation:** First seizure episode should be evaluated for potentially life-threatening causes of seizures, such as meningitis, systemic sepsis, head injury, substance abuse or accidental ingestion of drugs or other toxins.
   a. **Evaluation for infection:**
      1. **Complete blood count**
      2. **CRP**
      3. **Lumbar puncture for CSF examination**
      4. **Culture:** Blood, urine, CSF.
   b. **Evaluation for metabolic cause:**
      Serum electrolyte and blood sugar
   c. **Skin markers:** For neurocutaneous syndromes or neurological abnormality
   d. **Brain imaging:** Cerebral infarction, bleeding, space occupying lesion
   e. **EEG:** Measurement of electrical activity in the brain
      Important for diagnosis and monitoring of the patient

9. **Steps in diagnosis and management of the patient with a history of seizures**
   a. **Did the child have a seizure?**
      1. **No seizure then consider following differential**
         - Benign paroxysmal vertigo
         - Breath holding spells
         - Cough syncope
         - Pseudoseizures
         - Rage attack
         - Benign myoclonus of infancy
         - Tics
         - Narcolepsy
         - Night terror

2. **If seizure is present then**
   - **First seizure**
     i. Investigate for metabolic cause
     ii. CT and MRI
     iii. EEG
     iv. CSF examination

If above investigations are:

Abnormal	Normal	Normal other investigations except EEG
Control Seizures **T**reat underlying cause (Hypoglycemia, metabolic abnormalities, meningitis, temporal lobe tumor, etc.) **A**ntiepileptic drugs, if necessary	**N**o continuous drug treatment required. **C**lose observation **P**rescribe rescue medications (rectal diazepam) for seizures longer than 5 min	**C**onsider drug therapy then look for **a. Good control then** 1. Antiepileptic drug level and toxicity monitoring a. Complete Blood Count (CBC) b. Liver function test c. Behavior d. Learning ability 2. Regular follow-up **b. Poor control** 1. Antiepileptic drug dose adjustment 2. Prolonged EEG recording and video monitoring for possible epilepsy 3. Do CT and MRI again for underlying cause 4. Frequent follow up

   - **Recurrent seizures**
     i. Improper dose
     ii. Incorrect drug
     iii. Drug interaction
     iv. Drug compliance
     v. Metabolic cause
     vi. Underlying space occupying lesion

10. **Management of seizure:**
    a. **General measures**
       1. **Maintain airway patency by chin lift or oral airway**

2. **NG tube insertion:** To avoid aspiration
3. Secure the IV line as early as possible.
4. **Breathing:** Correct hypoxia with oxygen therapy.
5. **Circulation:** Assess the pulse rate, blood pressure and CRT/perfusion

b. **During convulsion**

1. Move patient away from the dangers
2. Give left lateral decubitus position
3. Do not put anything in mouth
4. Clean the secretions from mouth

c. **Febrile seizures management**

1. **Fever:** Find the cause
2. In febrile seizures, always rule out meningitis
3. **Physical methods**
    - Tepid sponging
    - Fanning
    - Light clothing
4. **Drugs:** Paracetamol

d. **Treatment of specific cause**

1. **Provoked seizures:** Due to underlying specific medical condition and these seizures respond well to treatment.
2. **An unprovoked seizure:** One that has no apparent cause.
3. **Febrile seizures:** Treat hyperthermia aggressively.
4. **Treat Metabolic causes:** Treat hypoglycemia, hypocalcemia, hyponatremia
5. **Bacterial meningitis:** Broad spectrum antibiotics
6. **Viral encephalitis:** Acyclovir
7. **Cerebral malaria:** Antimalarial

e. **Pharmacological therapy**

1. **Control seizures**
2. **Deciding the long term therapy after a first seizure:**
    - Need of long term therapy depends on neurodevelopment of patient, family history, EEG and MRI reports .

3. **Selection of antiepileptics drugs in long term therapy**
   - **Focal seizures and epilepsies:** Oxcarbazepine (DOC) and levetiracetam
   - **Absence seizures:** Ethosuximide, valproate (DOC)
   - **Primary generalized tonic-clonic seizures:** Levetiracetam, lamotrigine, Topiramate.
   - **Juvenile myoclonic epilepsy:** Levetiracetam, lamotrigine
   - **Infantile spasms:** (ACTH) hormone (DOC), vigabatrin
4. **Counselling to family members and patient**

STATUS EPILEPTICUS

1. **Definition:** Continuous seizures which last more than 5 minutes or two or more discrete seizures between which there is incomplete recovery of consciousness.
2. **Management:**
   a. Admit in ICU
   b. Support airway, breathing, circulation
   c. Sequence of drug therapy
      1. **To control the seizures immediately** (while administrating be ready to deal with respiratory and hemodynamic complications)
      a. **Benzodiazepines**

         Lorazepam (0.05 to 0.1 mg/kg, max 4 mg), repeated every 10-15 minutes for 3 doses

         Midazolam (0.05 to 0.1 mg/kg, max 5 mg), repeated 10 minutes for 3 doses

         Diazepam: used less frequently
      2. **To control recurrence**
         - **Phenytoin** (Loading dose 15-20 mg/kg, max 1 gm and repeat dose of 10 mg/kg Or fosphenytoin (drug of choice) 30 mg/kg, max 1 gm)
         - **Levetiracetam** (Loading dose 20-30 mg/kg, maintenance dose 10-20 mg, max 80 mg/kg/day, not exceeding 3 gm/day)
         - **Sodium Valproate (Loading dose 20-30 mg/kg)**
         - **Phenobarbitone (standard dose = 20 mg/kg)**

           Max loading dose 1 gm
      3. **Drugs in refractory cases**
         - **Midazolam infusion**

           Loading dose: 0.15 mg/kg followed by infusion of 1-10 mcg/kg/min
         - **High dose phenobarbitone:**

           10 mg/kg repeated boluses until seizure control is achieved.
         - **Thiopentone infusion**

           Loading dose: 3-5 mg/kg slowly

Section

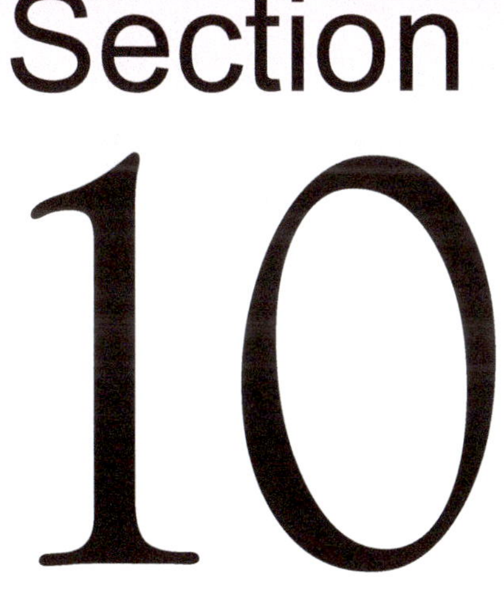

Reference Range of Different Investigation

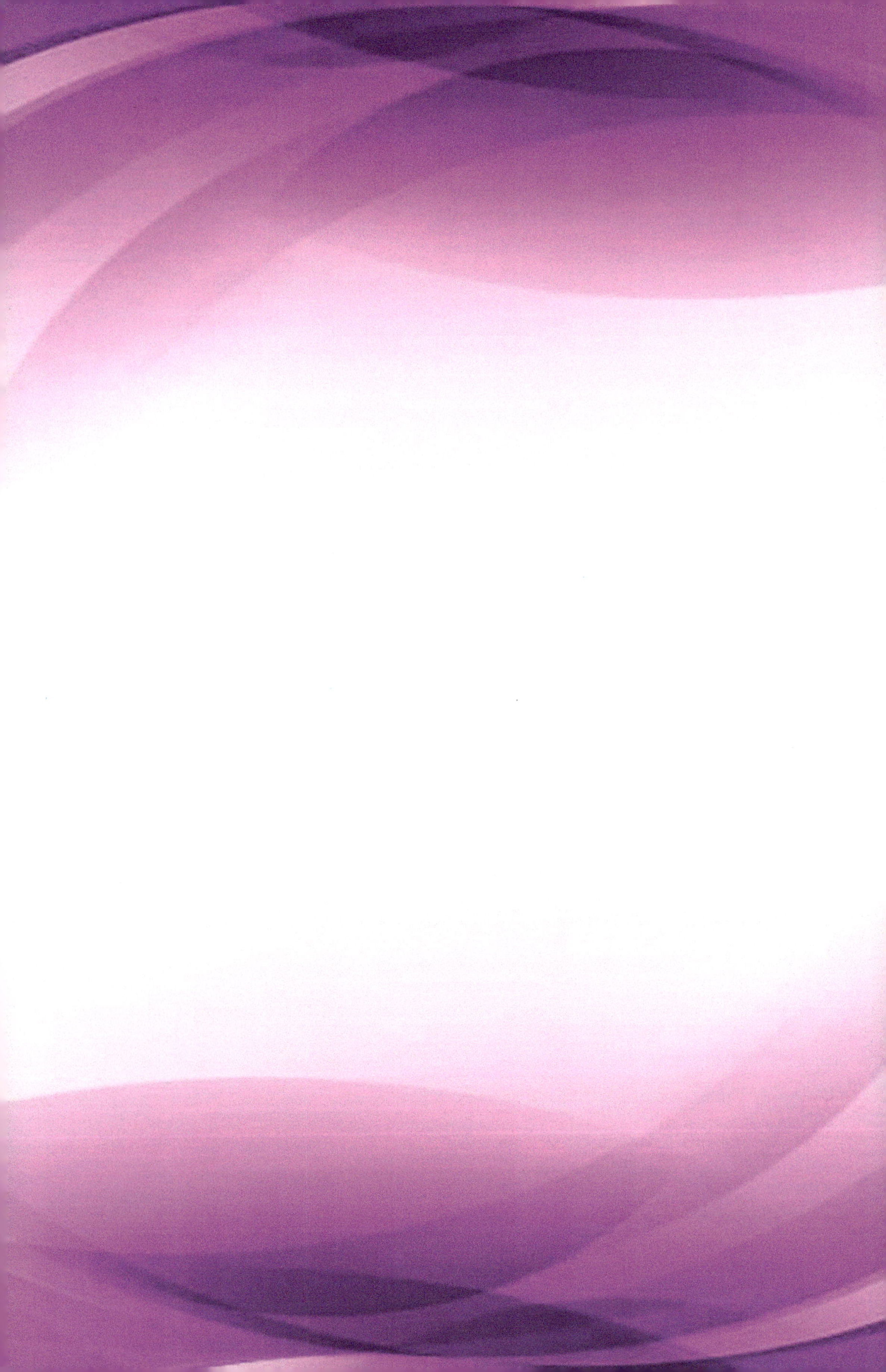

CHAPTER

17

Reference Range of Different Investigation

Complete blood count	**Hb**	M: 13 to17 F : 12 to15
	Erythrocyte count	M: 4.5 to 5.5 million per cu.mm F: 3.8 to 4.8 million per cu.mm
	Leukocyte count	4000-11000
	RBC indices P.C.V M.C.V M.C.H M.C.H.C R.D.W S.D	 M: 40 to 50%, F: 36 to 46% 83 to 99 femtoliters 27 to 32 pico-grams 31.5 to 34.5% 39 to 46 fl
	W.B.C differential count Neutrophils Eosinophils Lymphocytes Basophils Monocytes	 40 to 70% 00 to 06% 20 to 40% 00 to 02% 02 to 10%
	Platelets	1, 50, 000 to 4, 00, 000 per cu.mm
ESR	0 to 15 mm/hr	
CRP	0.0 to 0.6 mg/l	
Liver function test	Total bilirubin	0.2 to 1 mg%
	Direct	Upto 0.2%
	Indirect	
	SGPT	8 to 30 U/l
	SGOT	7 to 27 U/l
	Total proteins	6 to 8 gm%
	Serum albumin	3 to 5 gm%
	Serum globulin	2 to 3.5 gm%

Renal function test	Blood urea	15 to 40 mg%
	Serum creatinine	0.5 to 1.5 gm%
	Serum uric acid	2.5 to 7.2 mg%
	Serum amylase	0 to 86 IU/lit
	Serum calcium	7.5 to 10.5 mg%
Lipid profile	Total cholesterol	150 to 250 mg%
	HDL	30 to 65 mg%
	LDL	80 to160 mg%
	VLDL	10 to 30 mg%
	Serum triglycerides	10 to190 mg%
	cholesterol:HDL ratio	< 3: Low risk > 5: High risk
Coagulation profile	Platelets	
	PT (prothrombin time)	12 to 14 sec
	APTT (activated partial thromboplastin time)	25 to 40 sec
	INR	< or = 1.1
	BT (bleeding time)	1 to 3 minutes
	CT (clotting time)	2 to 7 minutes
Serum electrolyte	Sodium	136-146 meq/l
	Potassium	3.5 to 4.5 meq/l
	Chloride	96-106 mmol/L
Blood sugar	Fasting blood sugar	Normal: < 100 Impaired: 100 to 125 Diabetes mellitus > or = 126
	Two hours after meal (post meal)	Normal: < 140 Impaired: 140 to 199 Diabetes mellitus > or = 200
HBA1C	Normal	4.0 to 5.9%
	Prediabetes	6 to 6.4%
	Diabetic	> 6.5%

Urine routine	**Color**	Pale yellow
	Appearance	Clear
	Chemical examination Protein Sugar Bile salts Bile pigments Blood	 Absent Absent Absent Absent Absent
	Microscopic examination Epithelial cells Pus cells Red blood cells Yeast cells Amorphous material Trichomonas vaginalis Calcium oxalate (crystals)	 Absent 0 to 1/hpf Absent Absent Absent Absent Absent
D dimer	< 1 ug/mL	
Thyroid profile	T3	0.79 to 1.58 ng/ml
	T4	4.0 to 11.0 ug/dl
	TSH	0.39-4.31 uIU/ml
Iron profile	Serum iron	50 to 150 ug/dl
	Total iron binding capacity	350 to 450 cug/dl
	% transferrin saturation	30 to 40%
	Serum ferritin	15 to 300 ug/L
CPK -MB	Upto 25 U/lit	
Serum lipase	0 to 60 U/lit	
Serum amylase	20 to 90 IU/lit	
RA factor	0 to 20 IU/ml	
ASO	0 to 200 IU/ml	
Vitamin D	8.4 to 10.4 mg/dl	
Peripheral smear	RBCs	Normal in number, morphology and distribution
	Parasites	Not seen
	WBCs	Normal in number, morphology and distribution
	Platelets	Adequate in number
	Immature cells	Np immature cells are seen

Widal test	S. Typhi H antigen titre	> 1:200 (Positive)
	S.Typhi O antigen titre	> 1:100 (Positive)
	S. Typhi H antigen & O antigen rising titre	A rising titre (Positive)
ABG analysis	pH	7.35 to 7.45
	$PaCO_2$	35-45 mmHg
	PaO_2	80-100 mmHg
	SaO_2	93-100%
	HCO_3^-	22-26 meq/l
	%metHb	< 2.0%
	%CoHb	< 3.0%
Follicle stimulating hormone test	M: 4-25 U/L F: 4-30 U/L	
ACTH Catecholamines	Morning < 80 pg/mL or < 18 pmol/L Evening < 50 pg/mL or < 11 pmol/L	
	50 micrograms in 24 hours of urine sample	
Vanillyl mandelic acid	Daily excretion 2-6 mg/day	
Lactate dehydrogenase	45-90 U/L	
Schilling test	250-835 pgs/mL	
Troponin	I: 0 to 0.4 Ng/L T: 0 to 0.01 Ng/L	
BNP	< 100 PG/ml	Likely not in exacerbation of HF
	100 to 400 PG/ml	May be or may be not
	> 400 PG/ml	Most likely
NT -BNP	< 300 PG/ml (all ages)	

INDEX

www.ingramcontent.com/pod-product-compliance
Ingram Content Group UK Ltd.
Pitfield, Milton Keynes, MK11 3LW, UK
UKHW061133310726
14090UKWH00037B/1220